国际经典内科学教科书

第10版

Cecil Essentials of Medicine

希氏内科学精要

中英双语版

原　著　Edward J. Wing, MD, FACP, FIDSA
Former Dean of Medicine and Biological Sciences
Professor of Medicine
Warren Alpert Medical School of Brown University, Providence, Rhode Island

Fred J. Schiffman, MD, MACP
Sigal Family Professor of Humanistic Medicine
Vice Chair, Department of Medicine
Warren Alpert Medical School of Brown University, Providence, Rhode Island

中英双语版　编辑委员会　主任委员　王　辰

U0196945

第7分册

内分泌疾病与代谢疾病·女性健康·男性健康·骨与骨矿物质代谢疾病

主　译　宁　光　朱　兰　姜　辉　夏维波　潘　慧

北京大学医学出版社

XISHI NEIKEXUE JINGYAO（DI 10 BAN） DI 7 FENCE NEIFENMI JIBING YU DAIXIE JIBING·NÜXING JIANKANG·NANXING JIANKANG·GU YU GU KUANGWUZHI DAIXIE JIBING（ZHONGYING SHUANGYU BAN）

图书在版编目（CIP）数据

希氏内科学精要 ：第 10 版 . 第 7 分册，内分泌疾病与代谢疾病·女性健康·男性健康·骨与骨矿物质代谢疾病 ：汉、英 /（美）爱德华·温（Edward J. Wing），（美）弗雷德·谢夫曼（Fred J. Schiffman）原著；宁光等主译 . -- 北京 ：北京大学医学出版社，2024. 11. -- ISBN 978-7-5659-3267-0

Ⅰ. R5

中国国家版本馆 CIP 数据核字第 2024ZX1544 号

北京市版权局著作权合同登记号：图字：01-2024-4518

Elsevier (Singapore) Pte Ltd.
3 Killiney Road, #08-01 Winsland House I, Singapore 239519
Tel: (65) 6349-0200; Fax: (65) 6733-1817

Cecil Essentials of Medicine, Tenth Edition
Copyright © 2022 by Elsevier, Inc. All rights are reserved, including those for text and data mining, AI training, and similar technologies.
Publisher's note: Elsevier takes a neutral position with respect to territorial disputes or jurisdictional claims in its published content, including in maps and institutional affiliations.
Previous editions copyrighted 2016, 2010, 2007, 2004, 2001, 1997, 1993, 1990, and 1986.
ISBN-13: 978-0-323-72271-1

This translation of Cecil Essentials of Medicine, Tenth Edition by Edward J. Wing and Fred J. Schiffman was undertaken by Peking University Medical Press and is published by arrangement with Elsevier (Singapore) Pte Ltd.
Cecil Essentials of Medicine, Tenth Edition by Edward J. Wing and Fred J. Schiffman 由北京大学医学出版社进行翻译，并根据北京大学医学出版社与爱思唯尔（新加坡）私人有限公司的协议约定出版。
《希氏内科学精要（第 10 版） 第 7 分册 内分泌疾病与代谢疾病·女性健康·男性健康·骨与骨矿物质代谢疾病（中英双语版）》（宁光 朱兰 姜辉 夏维波 潘慧 主译）
ISBN: 978-7-5659-3267-0
Copyright © 2024 by Elsevier (Singapore) Pte Ltd. and Peking University Medical Press.
All rights reserved. No part of this publication may be reproduced or transmitted in any form or by any means, electronic or mechanical, including photocopying, recording, or any information storage and retrieval system, without permission in writing from Elsevier (Singapore) Pte Ltd. and Peking University Medical Press.

注　意

本译本由北京大学医学出版社独立完成。相关从业及研究人员必须凭借其自身经验和知识对文中描述的信息数据、方法策略、搭配组合、实验操作进行评估和使用。由于医学科学发展迅速，临床诊断和给药剂量尤其需要经过独立验证。在法律允许的最大范围内，爱思唯尔、译文的原文作者、原文编辑及原文内容提供者均不对译文或因产品责任、疏忽或其他操作造成的人身及（或）财产伤害及（或）损失承担责任，亦不对由于使用文中提到的方法、产品、说明或思想而导致的人身及（或）财产伤害及（或）损失承担责任。

Published in China by Peking University Medical Press under special arrangement with Elsevier (Singapore) Pte Ltd. This edition is authorized for sale in the People's Republic of China only, excluding Hong Kong SAR, Macau SAR and Taiwan. Unauthorized export of this edition is a violation of the contract.

希氏内科学精要（第 10 版） 第 7 分册 内分泌疾病与代谢疾病·女性健康·男性健康·骨与骨矿物质代谢疾病（中英双语版）

主　　译：宁　光　朱　兰　姜　辉　夏维波　潘　慧
出版发行：北京大学医学出版社
地　　址：（100191）北京市海淀区学院路 38 号 北京大学医学部院内
电　　话：发行部 010-82802230；图书邮购 010-82802495
网　　址：http://www.pumpress.com.cn
E-mail：booksale@bjmu.edu.cn
印　　刷：北京信彩瑞禾印刷厂
经　　销：新华书店
策划编辑：高　瑾
责任编辑：梁　洁　　责任校对：靳新强　　责任印制：李　啸
开　　本：889 mm×1194 mm　1/16　印张：20.5　字数：768 千字
版　　次：2024 年 11 月第 1 版　2024 年 11 月第 1 次印刷
书　　号：ISBN 978-7-5659-3267-0
定　　价：138.00 元

版权所有，违者必究

（凡属质量问题请与本社发行部联系退换）

中英双语版 编辑委员会

主任委员

王 辰

委 员（按姓氏笔画排序）

王 洁	王伊龙	王建祥	巴 一	代华平	宁 光	宁晓红	朱 兰
任景怡	刘海鹰	李小鹰	李梦涛	李雪梅	杨爱明	张福杰	郑金刚
房静远	赵 晶	赵明辉	郝 伟	姜 辉	栗占国	贾继东	夏维波
黄 慧	黄晓军	曹 彬	彭 斌	潘 慧			

第 1 分册　内科学概论 · 呼吸与危重症医学 · 术前和术后照护

　　　　　主译　王 辰　代华平　赵 晶　黄 慧

第 2 分册　心血管疾病

　　　　　主译　郑金刚　任景怡

第 3 分册　肾脏疾病

　　　　　主译　李雪梅　赵明辉

第 4 分册　胃肠疾病 · 肝脏与胆道系统疾病

　　　　　主译　房静远　杨爱明　贾继东

第 5 分册　血液疾病

　　　　　主译　黄晓军　王建祥

第 6 分册　肿瘤疾病

　　　　　主译　王 洁　巴 一

第 7 分册　内分泌疾病与代谢疾病 · 女性健康 · 男性健康 · 骨与骨矿物质代谢疾病

　　　　　主译　宁 光　朱 兰　姜 辉　夏维波　潘 慧

第 8 分册　肌肉骨骼与结缔组织疾病

　　　　　主译　栗占国　李梦涛

第 9 分册　感染性疾病

　　　　　主译　刘海鹰　张福杰　曹 彬

第 10 分册　神经疾病 · 老年医学 · 缓和医疗 · 酒精和物质使用

　　　　　主译　彭 斌　王伊龙　李小鹰　宁晓红　郝 伟

医学名词审定指导

任慧玲　李晓瑛　冀玉静　张燕舞　李军莲

　　让我国医学生与国际医学生站在同一起跑线上的首要之事，是为其提供具有世界先进水平的标准教材。我们应争取使每一位医学生都能接触到内容经典、充分代表现代医学水平的国际权威原文教材并力求准确翻译，提供原文与中文双语对照版本，使医学生和医生在学习中形成双语医学词语、概念、概念间逻辑及由此构成的医学知识体系。在这样的思想驱动下，国际经典内科学教科书《希氏内科学精要（第10版）》中英双语版应运而生。

　　《希氏内科学》原著以其论述严谨准确、系统全面，被誉为"标准的内科学参考书"。自 1927 年首次出版以来，在内科学领域渐享世界级声誉，成为全球众多优秀医学院校，包括哈佛医学院、斯坦福大学医学院、约翰斯·霍普金斯大学医学院、牛津大学医学部、剑桥大学医学院、墨尔本大学医学院、新加坡国立大学医学院及多伦多大学医学院等普遍采用的内科学参考书。首版《希氏内科学精要》则诞生于 1986 年，旨在凝炼其全本的精华和要点，以最为简洁明确的方式向以医学生为主体的医学界精辟传达《希氏内科学》的核心信息，包括书中所体现出的人文精神。此后，每版精要本都力求凝炼地反映当时最新医学成果和医疗实践指南，愈来愈成为各国医学生、住院医师、专培医师及教师学习和传授内科学的主要教本，在世界医学教材体系中居引领地位。《希氏内科学》和《希氏内科学精要》两个版本不仅在英语国家被广泛使用，更被翻译为葡萄牙语、西班牙语、希腊语、意大利语、日语、简体中文版，为全球医学界广泛采用。

　　中国的医学生、住院医师、专培医师需要培养国际专业信息获取能力。将精要本原文引进并准确翻译，以中英文对照的形式呈现，便于读者进行双语对照阅读和学习，使之在学习理解国际标准医学内容的同时，学习好中英文医学词语，为国际医学交流打好基础。相信此举对于提高我国的医学教育水平，培养国际型医学人才至为有益。

　　《希氏内科学精要》精练地涵盖了内科学的所有主要领域，包括心血管疾病、呼吸疾病与危重症、消化疾病、肾脏疾病、内分泌和代谢疾病、风湿疾病、血液疾病、肿瘤、感染性疾病、神经与老年疾病等，构建了较为系统的知识体系。在翻译引进过程中，我们遵循将相关内容集中的原则，将原书按系统器官拆分为十个分册，使其更具有专科阅读的对应性，以更加灵活轻便的形式为读者提供多样化的阅读选择。

为确保译文质量，我们在译者遴选上采取了严谨的标准。从《希氏内科学（第26版）》翻译团队中择优选取责任心强、译文优质的译者，同时吸纳了临床医学专业"101"计划核心教材的编者团队。每个分册均由主译专家带领各自译者团队完成翻译、审校、交叉互审、通审四级审校工作。这些译者具备扎实的英语与专业能力，他们在翻译过程中，深入理解原文，准确阐述作者思想，并多角度审视译文的准确性、流畅性与风格一致性，确保译文的忠实性、规范性与可读性，在不同的语言和文化间架起坚实的桥梁。尤其值得称赞的是，对原著中疏漏或不够完善之处，译文中以"译者注"的形式加以适当解释和说明，使译文内容在忠实于原著的基础上更为准确。

本书读者定位于具有一定学习能力和基础的高等医学院校医学专业 8 年制、5 年制学生以及相关医学专业人员，可作为医务人员的内科学参考书、住院医师规范化培训和专科医师规范化培训辅导教材、研究生入学考试辅导教材、内科学教师参考书、内科学各专科医师复习回顾其他专科知识的重要读本。

呼吸与危重症医学教授

中国医学科学院院长

北京协和医学院校长

2024 年 11 月

对学习者教科书重要。

对学医者内科学重要。

世界上的内科学教科书，

首推《希氏内科学精要》。

中文是中国医生主要执业用语。

英文是国际医学交流的主要文字。

学习医学，当以双语对应阅读为好。

如此，可获纵横国际之效。

本书力求有助于此。

In Memoriam

Thomas E. Andreoli, MD

Dr. Thomas Andreoli, along with Drs. Lloyd Hollingsworth (Holly) Smith, Jr., Fred Plum, and Charles C.J. Carpenter, was one of the four founding editors of *Cecil Essentials of Medicine.* He served as editor for editions one through eight before he passed away on April 14, 2009. Dr. Andreoli was born in the Bronx, New York, in 1935, attended Catholic primary and high schools, and graduated from St. Vincent College and the Georgetown School of Medicine. He trained as a resident at Duke University under legendary Chair of Medicine Dr. Eugene Stead, who recognized him as a brilliant physician and scientist and encouraged his research career. Dr. Andreoli received his research training at the NIH and then in the laboratory of Dr. Tosteson at Duke. His research focused on the biochemical and biophysical properties of renal tubular cell membranes and their role in water and electrolyte transport. He made fundamental discoveries on the normal renal physiology, illuminating the way to subsequent work by many others on renal health and disease. His research was recognized with numerous awards and election to honorific societies both in the United States and in Europe. Dr. Andreoli also served as editor of *The American Journal of Physiology: Renal Physiology* and Editor in Chief of *Kidney International.*

Tom's national prominence and leadership qualities were recognized early in his career when he became head of Nephrology at the University of Alabama in Birmingham. There he helped faculty and trainees develop outstanding research, organized clinical services, and created a hemodialysis program to build one of the outstanding Divisions of Nephrology in the country. In 1979, Dr. Andreoli was appointed Chair of the Department of Internal Medicine at the University of Texas, Houston, where he assembled an outstanding faculty focused on research, clinical care, and teaching. In 1988, he accepted the position as Chairman of Internal Medicine at the University of Arkansas School of Medicine, a position he held until his death. There he again assembled a distinguished faculty who were outstanding researchers but also dedicated to outstanding clinical care and teaching. Morning report and clinical rounds with Dr. Andreoli were rigorous and riveting, focusing on the individual patient, not only their diagnoses and treatment but also on each patient's personal concerns and well-being. Dr. Andreoli was revered by medical students, his house staff, faculty, and colleagues, and I (EJW) personally can attest to what he regarded as his most cherished role—the mentorship and education of the next generation of physicians.

One of Dr. Andreoli's great interests was *Cecil Essentials of Medicine,* for which he was the editor/chief editor for eight of its ten editions, an interest that reflected his commitment to the education of students, house staff, and other physicians in the "essentials" of Internal Medicine.

Dr. Andreoli was devoted to his family. He was married to Elizabeth Berglund Andreoli from 1987 until his death. He was previously married to Dr. Kathleen Gainor Andreoli, mother of his three children and their ten grandchildren. Being of Italian ancestry and from Bronx, New York, it is not surprising that Dr. Andreoli was a passionate fan of the New York Yankees, Italian opera, which he could sing in Italian, and Frank Sinatra.

Dr. Andreoli's legacy lives on in his numerous previous students, house staff, colleagues, and in this book.

托马斯·安德里奥利博士

托马斯·安德里奥利（Thomas E. Andreoli）博士携手李奥德·霍灵斯沃斯·史密斯［Lloyd Hollingsworth（Holly）Smith］博士、弗雷德·普拉姆（Fred Plum）博士和查尔斯·卡彭特（Charles C.J. Carpenter）博士同为《希氏内科学精要》的创始编者。他在 2009 年 4 月 14 日去世前，曾担任该书第 1 至第 8 版的编者。安德里奥利博士于 1935 年出生于美国纽约布朗克斯区，就读于天主教小学和中学，后毕业于圣文森特学院和乔治城大学医学院。他在杜克大学医学院接受住院医师培训期间师从著名内科主任尤金·斯特德（Eugene Stead）博士，后者将其视为杰出的医生和科学家，并鼓励他投身科研事业。安德里奥利博士在美国国立卫生研究院接受科研训练后，前往杜克大学托斯特森（Tosteson）博士的实验室继续深造。他重点研究肾小管细胞膜的生化和生物物理特性及其在水和电解质转运中所发挥的作用。他在正常肾脏生理学方面的重要发现为后续关于肾脏健康和疾病的研究铺平了道路。安德里奥利博士的研究工作荣获多个学术奖项，并入选美国和欧洲的多个荣誉学会。他还担任《美国生理学杂志：肾脏生理学篇》（The American Journal of Physiology：Renal Physiology）的编辑以及《国际肾脏杂志》（Kidney International）的主编。

安德里奥利博士担任阿拉巴马大学伯明翰分校肾脏病学系主任后不久，即因其杰出领导力而赢得全美业内声誉。他帮助本校师生们取得科研突破，负责临床业务的组织实施，并因开创血液透析业务而使该科跻身全美顶级肾脏内科之列。1979 年，安德里奥利博士被任命为得克萨斯大学休斯敦分校内科学系主任，他在该系组建了一支科研、临床诊疗和教学并重的优秀教职团队。自 1988 年起，他担任阿肯色大学医学院内科学系主任，直至辞世。在这里他再次组建了一支卓越的教职团队，他们不仅科研工作出色，临床诊疗和教学工作也出类拔萃。安德里奥利博士带领的晨会报告和查房非常严谨而引人入胜，不仅尽心竭力于每位患者的诊断和治疗，还关注到他们每个人的个体情况和福祉。安德里奥利博士深受医学生、住院医师、教职人员和同事的崇敬，我（EJW）可以证明，他最珍视的角色当属培养和教育下一代医生。

安德里奥利博士对《希氏内科学精要》倾注了满腔热忱，先后担任了该书 10 版中 8 版的编者 / 主编，践行他为医学生、住院医师和其他各科医生们传授内科学"精要"的承诺。

安德里奥利博士高度重视家庭。他与第二任妻子伊丽莎白·伯格兰德·安德里奥利（Elizabeth Berglund Andreoli）的婚姻从 1987 年延续到辞世。他与第一任妻子凯瑟琳·盖娜·安德里奥利（Kathleen Gainor Andreoli）博士育有三个子女和十个孙辈。作为意大利裔和纽约布朗克斯人，安德里奥利博士是纽约洋基队、意大利歌剧（他能用意大利语演唱）和美国著名歌手、演员、主持人弗兰克·辛纳屈（Frank Sinatra）的忠实拥趸。安德里奥利博士将永远被他的众多学生、住院医师和同事怀念，并因本书而流芳百世。

Charles C.J. Carpenter, MD

Dr. Charles C.J. Carpenter joined Drs. Thomas Andreoli, Lloyd Hollingsworth Smith, Jr., and Fred Plum as a founder of *Cecil Essentials of Medicine*. He served as editor for seven editions and was followed in that role by Dr. Ivor Benjamin and then Dr. Edward Wing. Sadly, Chuck passed away on March 19, 2020, surrounded by his wife and children. He was Professor Emeritus of Medicine at The Warren Alpert Medical School of Brown University and Physician-in-Chief Emeritus at The Miriam Hospital.

Chuck was born in Savannah, Georgia, on January 5, 1931. He attended college at Princeton and medical school at Johns Hopkins where he also did his house staff training, including chief residency, and then joined the Johns Hopkins faculty. With his young family, he travelled to Calcutta, India, where he carried out landmark studies for the treatment of cholera.

Before coming to Brown in 1986, he was Chair of Medicine at Baltimore City Hospital and Case Western Reserve University.

His contributions to medical science and clinical care were many. While in Calcutta, using basic scientific evidence coupled with practical approaches, Dr. Carpenter developed "oral rehydration therapy" to address the cholera epidemic there. This treatment has saved millions of lives. While at Case, one of his innovations was to develop the nation's first Division of Geographic Medicine because of his strong belief that all physicians should be medical citizens of the world. In 1987, as he became deeply involved in the clinical management of persons living with HIV, he initiated a unique program in which Brown University faculty and trainees assumed responsibility for all HIV care in the Rhode Island State prison system.

Dr. Carpenter served as Chairman of the American Board of Internal Medicine and President of the Association of American Physicians. He has been a member of the NIH AIDS Executive Committee, the National Advisory Allergy and Infectious Diseases Council, and the USPHS AIDS Task Force. He was Chair of the Antiretroviral Treatment Panel of the International AIDS Society-USA and authored their recommendations on antiretroviral treatment. He also served as Chair of the Treatment Committee to evaluate the President's Emergency Plan for HIV/AIDS Relief. He became the director of the Brown University International Health Institute and the director of the Lifespan/Brown Center for AIDS Research with several Boston hospitals.

Throughout his career, Dr. Carpenter was the recipient of many international, national, and regional awards, accepting each with characteristic humility. With both small and large groups of learners, Chuck made certain that every member of his team was well educated, and each felt that they contributed to the well-being of their patients. His ability to sit calmly at the bedside, hold the patient's hand, comfort them, and listen in a genuinely focused way, influenced so many physicians. He was truly grateful for the opportunity to care for those less fortunate than he, and the feeling of being privileged to do so was clearly transmitted to all. Dr. Carpenter was a wonderful blend of profound compassion combined with the adherence to scholarship and teaching. Sir William Osler wrote that physicians should "Do the kind thing and do it first." Chuck lived by this precept. Vigor and insight characterized his approach to clinical and ethical challenges, always with younger colleagues at his side. In a recent tribute to him, many emphasized that Dr. Carpenter dedicated his life to his patients, many of whom were the most vulnerable members of society. We hope that we will have some of his strength and use his example as our compass as we are challenged to reduce suffering and improve the health of all for whom we are responsible.

He is survived by his wife of 61 years, Sally; three sons, Charles, Murray, and Andrew; and seven grandchildren.

查尔斯·卡彭特博士

查尔斯·卡彭特（Charles C.J. Carpenter）博士与 托马斯·安德里奥利（Thomas E. Andreoli）博士、李奥德·霍灵斯沃斯·史密斯（Lloyd Hollingsworth Smith）博士和弗雷德·普拉姆（Fred Plum）博士共同开创了《希氏内科学精要》。他共担任了 7 版的编者，嗣后由艾弗·本杰明（Ivor Benjamin）博士和爱德华·温（Edward Wing）博士接任。查尔斯·卡彭特博士于 2020 年 3 月 19 日在妻子和子女们的陪伴下辞世。他曾担任布朗大学沃伦·阿尔珀特医学院的内科学系名誉教授和米里亚姆医院的名誉主任医师。

查尔斯·卡彭特博士于 1931 年 1 月 5 日出生于美国佐治亚州萨凡纳市。他在普林斯顿大学获得学士学位后进入约翰斯·霍普金斯大学医学院，并完成了包括住院总医师在内的住院医师培训，随后加入了约翰斯·霍普金斯大学的教职团队。他曾携妻子和年幼的孩子前往印度加尔各答，在当地对霍乱的治疗进行了具有里程碑意义的研究工作。

在 1986 年入职布朗大学之前，他曾担任巴尔的摩市医院和凯斯西储大学医学院的内科学主任。

他在医学科学研究和临床诊疗领域建树颇多。在加尔各答期间，基于基础科学证据及临床实践，查尔斯·卡彭特博士开创了"口服补液疗法"以遏制当地的霍乱疫情。这一疗法拯救了数百万人的生命。秉承医生无国界的世界公民理念，他在凯斯西储大学做了一项开创性工作，建立了美国首个地缘医学部（研究地理环境因素对人体健康和疾病影响的学科）。1987 年，他深度参与人类免疫缺陷病毒（HIV）携带者的临床管理，并发起了一个独特的项目——由布朗大学教职团队和医学生们承担罗德岛州监狱系统内所有艾滋病相关诊疗工作。

查尔斯·卡彭特博士曾担任美国内科医师委员会主席和美国医师协会主席。他曾是美国国立卫生研究院艾滋病行政委员会、美国国家过敏与传染病咨询委员会以及公共卫生服务部艾滋病工作组的成员。他还曾担任国际艾滋病学会–美国分会抗逆转录病毒治疗组主席，并撰写了抗逆转录病毒治疗建议。他还担任过艾滋病治疗委员会主席，该委员会负责评估美国总统防治艾滋病紧急救援计划；曾担任布朗大学国际健康研究所所长，以及大学与多家波士顿当地医院合办的生命周期 / 布朗大学艾滋病研究中心主任。

查尔斯·卡彭特博士在职业生涯中获得过诸多国际性、全美和地区性奖项，同时展现其谦逊品格。无论学员人数多寡，查尔斯·卡彭特博士都会确保人人都能受到良好教育，并让他们感到自己也对患者的健康做出了贡献。他能够安静地坐在病床边，握住患者的手，安慰他们，并全神贯注地听取患者倾诉，这一举动深深地感染了许多医生。他十分珍视诊治不幸染病者的机会，并且能够将这种殊荣感传递给所有人。查尔斯·卡彭特博士完美地融汇了对患者的宅心仁厚与对学术和教学的坚守。威廉·奥斯勒（William Osler）爵士曾写道，医生应该"行善事，为人先"，而这正是查尔斯·卡彭特博士一生奉行的信条。他在面对临床和伦理挑战时充满活力和洞察力，始终重视提携年轻同事。许多人的悼词中都重点指出，查尔斯·卡彭特博士将毕生致力于患者福祉，其中许多人属于社会上最弱势群体。我们希望，在我们面临减少患者痛苦及改善其健康状况的挑战时，能够拥有他的力量，并以他为榜样获得指引。

查尔斯·卡彭特博士与妻子萨丽（Sally）共度了 61 年的婚姻时光，育有查尔斯（Charles）、穆雷（Murray）和安德鲁（Andrew）三子以及七个孙辈。

ABOUT THE EDITORS

Dr. Edward J. Wing was an editor of *Cecil Essentials of Medicine*, editions 8 and 9, and is the lead editor of edition 10. He graduated from Williams College in 1967 and from the Harvard Medical School in 1971. He was a resident in Internal Medicine at the Peter Bent Brigham and completed an Infectious Diseases Fellowship at Stanford University. Joining the faculty at the University of Pittsburgh in 1975, he focused his NIH-funded research on mechanisms of cell-mediated immunity as well as various clinical aspects of Infectious Diseases. From 1990 to 1998, the University and UPMC appointed him as Physician-in-Chief at Montefiore Hospital, then Chief of Infectious Diseases, and finally Interim Chair of Medicine.

In 1998, Dr. Wing became Chair of Medicine at Brown University (1998–2008) where he consolidated the department across hospitals, practice plans, and training programs. As Dean of Medicine and Biological Sciences at Brown University (2008–2013) he strengthened ties with affiliated hospitals (Lifespan and Care New England), increased research, and oversaw the construction of a new medical school building. International exchange programs with medical schools in Kenya, the Dominican Republic, and Haiti were established during his years as chairman and dean. Dr. Wing has cared for patients with HIV since the beginning of the epidemic in outpatient clinics. He continues to be active in research, clinical care, and teaching.

Dr. Fred J. Schiffman, who along with Dr. Edward Wing is editor of *Cecil Essentials of Medicine*, 10th edition, attended Wagner College and then the New York University School of Medicine, from which he graduated in 1973. He performed his early house staff training at Yale-New Haven Hospital and then spent two years at the National Cancer Institute. He returned to Yale as Chief Medical Resident followed by a hematology fellowship. He became Medical Director of Yale's Primary Care Center before coming to Brown University in 1983, where he has been a leader in the medical residency program as well as Associate Physician-in-Chief at The Miriam Hospital.

Dr. Schiffman holds The Sigal Family Professorship in Humanistic Medicine at The Warren Alpert Medical School of Brown University. His scholarly interests include the structure and function of the human spleen and the intersection of the arts and medical care. He has directed or championed many projects and programs, including those that encourage and reinforce wellness and resilience in patients, families, and caregivers. He began a novel program that places medical students and physicians with other nonmedical professionals as they share in the viewing of works of art in the Museum of the Rhode Island School of Design. Dr. Schiffman recently led a Brown University edX course entitled, "Artful Medicine: Art's Power to Enrich Patient Care," with worldwide participation. Dr. Schiffman has also edited texts on hematologic pathophysiology, consultative hematology, and the anemias.

爱德华·温（Edward J. Wing）博士是《希氏内科学精要》第 8 版和第 9 版的编者，以及第 10 版的主编。他先后于 1967 年和 1971 年毕业于威廉姆斯学院和哈佛医学院。他曾在彼得·本特·布里格姆医院任内科住院医师，后在斯坦福大学完成了传染病学的专科医师（Fellowship）课程。自 1975 年加入匹兹堡大学医学院以来，他通过美国国立卫生研究院资助的研究项目，探索细胞介导免疫的机制以及传染病学各领域的临床诊疗工作。1990—1998 年期间，他先后被匹兹堡大学及其医学中心任命为蒙特菲奥里医院的主任医师、传染病科主任，后担任内科临聘主任。

1998 年起，温博士担任布朗大学医学院的内科主任（1998—2008 年）。在此期间，他在不同医院、实践计划和培训项目间对内科进行整合。在担任布朗大学医学与生物科学院院长（2008—2013 年）期间，他加强了与各附属医院（Lifespan 医院和 Care New England 医院）间的联系，提升了科研工作的水准，并为医学院建成了一座新楼。在担任主任和院长期间，他还建立了与肯尼亚、多米尼加共和国和海地的医学院的国际交流项目。温博士自艾滋病流行初期便在门诊诊治艾滋病患者，并始终工作在科研、临床和教学一线。

弗雷德·谢夫曼（Fred J. Schiffman）博士与爱德华·温（Edward Wing）博士共同担任《希氏内科学精要》第 10 版的主编。他就读于瓦格纳学院，随后进入纽约大学医学院，并于 1973 年毕业。他在耶鲁大学附属纽黑文医院接受早期住院医师培训，随后在美国国家癌症研究所工作了两年。回到耶鲁大学后，他担任住院总医师，然后完成了血液学专科医师课程，随后成为耶鲁初级保健中心医学主任。他于 1983 年入职布朗大学，领导医学住院医师项目并担任米里亚姆医院的副主任医师。

谢夫曼博士担任布朗大学沃伦·阿尔珀特医学院人文医学系的西格尔家庭医学教授。他的学术兴趣涵盖人体脾脏的结构和功能，以及艺术与医疗的交叉融合。他主持或参与了许多项目和计划，其中包括许多旨在鼓励和加强患者、家人和医护人员的福祉与康复能力的项目。他所创办的一个新项目可以让医学生和医生与其他非医学专业人士一起，共同欣赏罗德岛设计学院博物馆的艺术作品。谢夫曼博士近期还主持了布朗大学名为"艺术与医学：艺术赋能患者照护"的 edX 课程，此课程的参与者来自全球多个国家。谢夫曼博士还出版了有关血液病理生理学、血液科会诊和贫血的著作。

原著者名单

Jinnette Dawn Abbott, MD

Rajiv Agarwal, MD

Marwa Al-Badri, MD

Hyeon-Ju Ryoo Ali, MD

Jason M. Aliotta, MD

Khaldoun Almhanna, MD, MPH

Mohanad T. Al-Qaisi, MD

Zuhal Arzomand, MD

Akwi W. Asombang, MD, MPH

Su N. Aung, MD, MPH

Christopher G. Azzoli, MD

Christina Bandera, MD

Debasree Banerjee, MD

Mashal Batheja, MD

Jeffrey J. Bazarian, MD, MPH

Selim R. Benbadis, MD

Ivor J. Benjamin, MD, FAHA, FACC

Eric Benoit, MD

Marcie G. Berger, MD

Clemens Bergwitz, MD

Nancy Berliner, MD

Jeffrey S. Berns, MD

Pooja Bhadbhade, DO

Ratna Bhavaraju-Sanka, MD

Tanmayee Bichile, MD

Ariel E. Birnbaum, MD

Charles M. Bliss, Jr., MD

Andrew S. Blum, MD, PhD

Bryan J. Bonder, MD

Russell Bratman, MD

Glenn D. Braunstein, MD

Alma M. Guerrero Bready, MD

Richard Bungiro, PhD

Anna Marie Burgner, MD, MEHP

Jonathan Cahill, MD

Andrew Canakis, DO

Benedito A. Carneiro, MD, MS

Brian Casserly, MD

Abdullah Chahin, MD, MA, MSc

Philip A. Chan, MD

Kimberle Chapin, MD

William P. Cheshire, Jr., MD

Waihong Chung, MD, PhD

Emma Ciafaloni, MD

Joaquin E. Cigarroa, MD

Michael P. Cinquegrani, MD

Andreea Coca, MD, MPH

Harvey Jay Cohen, MD

Scott Cohen, MD, MPH

Beatrice P. Concepcion, MD, MS

Nathan T. Connell, MD, MPH

Maria Constantinou, MD

Roberto Cortez, MD

Timothy J. Counihan, MD, FRCPI

Anne Haney Cross, MD

Cheston B. Cunha, MD, FACP

Joanne S. Cunha, MD

Susan Cu-Uvin, MD

Noura M. Dabbouseh, MD

Kwame Dapaah-Afriyie, MD, MBA

Erin M. Denney-Koelsch, MD

Andre De Souza, MD

An S. De Vriese, MD, PhD

Neal D. Dharmadhikari, MD

Leah Dickstein, MD

Don Dizon, MD, FACP, FASCO

Robyn T. Domsic, MD, MPH

Kim A. Eagle, MD

Michael G. Earing, MD

Pamela Egan, MD

Wafik S. El-Deiry, MD, PhD, FACP

Mitchell S. V. Elkind, MD, MS

Tarra B. Evans, MD

Michael B. Fallon, MD

Dimitrios Farmakiotis, MD

Francis A. Farraye, MD

Ronan Farrell, MD

Panayotis Fasseas, MD, FACC

Mary Anne Fenton, MD

Fernando C. Fervenza, MD, PhD

Sean Fine, MD

Arkadiy Finn, MD

Timothy Flanigan, MD

Brisas M. Flores, MD

Andrew E. Foderaro, MD

Theodore C. Friedman, MD, PhD

Joseph Metmowlee Garland, MD, AAHIVM

Eric J. Gartman, MD

Abdallah Geara, MD

Raul Macias Gil, MD

Timothy Gilligan, MD, FASCO

Michael Raymond Goggins, MB BCh BAO, MRCPI

Geetha Gopalakrishnan, MD

Vidya Gopinath, MD

Susan L. Greenspan, MD, FACP

Osama Hamdy, MD, PhD

Johanna Hamel, MD

Sajeev Handa, MD, SFHM

Mitchell T. Heflin, MD, MHS

Robert G. Holloway, MD, MPH

Christopher S. Huang, MD

Zilla Hussain, MD

T. Alp Ikizler, MD

Iris Isufi, MD

Carlayne E. Jackson, MD

Paul G. Jacob, MD, MPH

Matthew D. Jankowich, MD

Niels V. Johnsen, MD, MPH

Jessica E. Johnson, MD

Rayford R. June, MD

Tareq Kheirbek, MD, ScM, FACS

Alok A. Khorana, MD, FACP, FASCO

Sena Kilic, MD

David Kim, MD

James Kleczka, MD

James R. Klinger, MD

Patrick Koo, MD, ScM

Pooja Koolwal, MD

Mary P. Kotlarczyk, PhD

Nicole M. Kuderer, MD

Awewura Kwara, MD

Jennifer M. Kwon, MD, MPH

Richard A. Lange, MD, MBA

Jerome Larkin, MD

Alfred I. Lee, MD, PhD

Daniel J. Levine, MD

David E. Lewandowski, MD

Kelly V. Liang, MD, MS

Kimberly P. Liang, MD, MS

David R. Lichtenstein, MD

扫描二维码了解更多信息

Douglas W. Lienesch, MD

Geoffrey S.F. Ling, MD, PhD

Ester Little, MD, FACP

Yi Liu, MD

Nicole L. Lohr, MD, PhD

John R. Lonks, MD, FACP, FIDSA, FSHEA

Gary H. Lyman, MD, MPH

Jeffrey M. Lyness, MD

Shane Lyons, MD, MRCPI, MRCP(UK)

Diana Maas, MD

Talha A. Malik, MD, MSPH

Sonia Manocha, MD

Susan Manzi, MD, MPH

Frederick J. Marshall, MD

F. Dennis McCool, MD

Russell J. McCulloh, MD

Kelly McGarry, MD, FACP

Eavan Mc Govern, MD, PhD

Robin L. McKinney, MD

Anthony Mega, MD

Shivang Mehta, MD

Douglas F. Milam, MD

Maria D. Mileno, MD

Abhinav Kumar Misra, MBBS, MD

Orson W. Moe, MD

Niveditha Mohan, MBBS

Larry W. Moreland, MD

Alan R. Morrison, MD, PhD

Steven F. Moss, MD

Christopher J. Mullin, MD, MHS

Sinéad M. Murphy, MB, BCh, MD, FRCPI

Sagarika Nallu, MD, FAAP, FAAN, FAASM

Javier A. Neyra, MD, MSCS

Ghaith Noaiseh, MD

Thomas A. Ollila, MD

Steven M. Opal, MD

Biff F. Palmer, MD

Jen Jung Pan, MD, PhD

Anna Papazoglou, MD

Aric Parnes, MD

Nayan M. Patel, DO, MPH

Ari Pelcovits, MD

Mark A. Perazella, MD

Michael F. Picco, MD, PhD

Kate E. Powers, DO

Laura A. Previll, MD, MPH

Nilum Rajora, MD

Adolfo Ramirez-Zamora, MD

John Reagan, MD

Rebecca Reece, MD

Harlan Rich, MD, AGAF, FACP

Jennifer H. Richman, MD

Lisa R. Rogers, DO

Ralph Rogers, MD

Michal G. Rose, MD

James A. Roth, MD

Sharon Rounds, MD

Jason C. Rubenstein, MD

Abbas Rupawala, MD

Jenna Sarvaideo, DO

Ramesh Saxena, MD, PhD

Fred J. Schiffman, MD, MACP

Ruth B. Schneider, MD

Kristin A. Seaborg, MD

Anil Seetharam, MD

Stuart Seropian, MD

Jigme Michael Sethi, MD

Sanjeev Sethi, MD, PhD

Elizabeth Shane, MD

Esseim Sharma, MD

Shani Shastri, MD, MPH

Barry S. Shea, MD

Lauren Shevell, MD, MPH

Joseph A. Smith, Jr., MD

Robert J. Smith, MD

Davendra P.S. Sohal, MD, MPH

Christopher Song, MD, FACC

Thomas Sperry, MD

Jeffrey M. Statland, MD

Emily M. Stein, MD

Jennifer L. Strande, MD, PhD

Rochelle Strenger, MD

Thomas R. Talbot, MD, MPH

Christopher G. Tarolli, MD, MSEd

Yael Tarshish, MD

Pushpak Taunk, MD

Philip Tsoukas, MD

Allan R. Tunkel, MD, PhD

Jeffrey M. Turner, MD

Zoe G.S. Vazquez, MD

Stacie A. F. Vela, MD

Paul M. Vespa, MD, FCCM, FAAN, FANA, FNCS

Wanpen Vongpatanasin, MD

Marcella D. Walker, MD

Eunice S. Wang, MD

Sharmeel K. Wasan, MD

Thomas J. Weber, MD

Brandon J. Wilcoxson, MD

Edward J. Wing, MD, FACP, FIDSA

Ellice Wong, MD

John J. Wysolmerski, MD

Rayan Yousefzai, MD

Thomas R. Ziegler, MD

Rebecca Zon, MD

ACKNOWLEDGMENTS

Dr. Schiffman and I wish to thank first of all, the authors of the 128 chapters that make up the tenth edition of *Cecil Essentials of Medicine.* They have worked diligently to compose the material for each chapter and apply their mastery as they added the newest information, in clear language, to the text. Their efforts are apparent in the excellence of the book, and we are immensely grateful for their work. We wish to also thank Marybeth Thiel, Jennifer Ehlers, and Dan Fitzgerald from Elsevier who guided and supported our work as editors and whose expertise has made this volume possible. Finally, we are always thankful to our wives, Dr. Rena Wing and Ms. Gerri Schiffman, without whose love, support, and especially humor, this book would not have happened.

致　谢

　　谢夫曼博士和我首先要致谢《希氏内科学精要》第 10 版全书 128 章的各位作者。感谢他们精益求精地撰写每一章节，并运用其专业知识，以简明的语言将前沿资讯呈现在书中。正是他们的辛勤努力确保了本书的卓越地位，对他们唯有由衷的感激。我们还要感谢爱思唯尔出版集团的玛丽贝丝·蒂尔（Marybeth Thiel）、詹妮弗·埃勒斯（Jennifer Ehlers）和丹·菲茨杰拉德（Dan Fitzgerald），他们对本书的编辑工作给予了指导和支持，其专业水准保障了本书的完稿。最后，要特别感谢我们的妻子——蕾娜·温（Rena Wing）博士和盖瑞·谢夫曼（Gerri Schiffman）女士，对她们的爱和支持，特别是积极乐观的心态始终心存感激，她们为本书的圆满完成发挥了不可或缺的作用。

总目录

第7分册

内分泌疾病与代谢疾病·女性健康·
男性健康·骨与骨矿物质代谢疾病

第7分册译者名单

主 译

宁 光 朱 兰 姜 辉 夏维波 潘 慧

译 者（按姓氏笔画排序）

王 鸥	中国医学科学院北京协和医院	陈 蓉	中国医学科学院北京协和医院
王林杰	中国医学科学院北京协和医院	林浩成	北京大学第三医院
卢 琳	中国医学科学院北京协和医院	周 翔	中国医学科学院北京协和医院
宁 光	上海交通大学医学院附属瑞金医院	郑清月	中国医学科学院北京协和医院
朱 兰	中国医学科学院北京协和医院	赵宇星	中国医学科学院北京协和医院
朱 军	北京大学第一医院	赵维纲	中国医学科学院北京协和医院
朱惠娟	中国医学科学院北京协和医院	段 炼	中国医学科学院北京协和医院
阳洪波	中国医学科学院北京协和医院	段佳丽	中国医学科学院北京协和医院
苏 婉	中国医学科学院北京协和医院	姜 艳	中国医学科学院北京协和医院
杜函泽	中国医学科学院北京协和医院	姜 辉	北京大学第一医院
李 梅	中国医学科学院北京协和医院	袁 涛	中国医学科学院北京协和医院
李乃适	中国医学科学院北京协和医院	夏维波	中国医学科学院北京协和医院
吴 寒	山东大学附属生殖医院	梁思宇	中国医学科学院北京协和医院
陈 伟	中国医学科学院北京协和医院	童安莉	中国医学科学院北京协和医院
陈 适	中国医学科学院北京协和医院	潘 慧	中国医学科学院北京协和医院

第 1 篇　内分泌疾病与代谢疾病　Endocrine Disease and Metabolic Disease

第 2 篇　女性健康　Women's Health

第 3 篇　男性健康　Men's Health

第4篇 骨与骨矿物质代谢疾病 Diseases of Bone and Bone Mineral Metabolism

CECIL ESSENTIALS OF
MEDICINE

Endocrine Disease and Metabolic Disease

Women's Health

Men's Health

Diseases of Bone and Bone Mineral Metabolism

Endocrine Disease and Metabolic Disease

内分泌疾病与代谢疾病

Hypothalamic-Pituitary Axis

Diana Maas, Jenna Sarvaideo

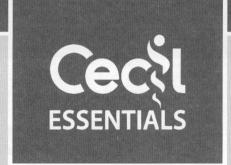

ANATOMY AND PHYSIOLOGY

The pituitary gland sits in the skull base in a bony structure called the sella turcica. It weighs approximately 600 mg and is composed of three lobes, the adenohypophysis (anterior lobe), the neurohypophysis (posterior lobe), and the intermediate lobe. The intermediate lobe regresses in humans at about 15 weeks' gestation and is absent in the adult normal pituitary gland. The infundibular stalk, which contains the portal plexus circulation, connects the hypothalamus to the pituitary gland. The pituitary gland is surrounded by important structures that can be compromised by its enlargement, including the optic chiasm, located superior to the gland, and the cavernous sinuses, located on both sides of the gland. The cavernous sinuses each contain the internal carotid artery and cranial nerves III, IV, V1, V2, and VI (Fig. 1.1).

The anterior pituitary gland produces six hormones that are produced by specific cell types within the gland: adrenocorticotropic hormone (ACTH), follicle-stimulating hormone (FSH), luteinizing hormone (LH), growth hormone (GH), prolactin (PRL), and thyroid-stimulating hormone (TSH or thyrotropin). These hormones are regulated by stimulatory and inhibitory peptides produced within the hypothalamus and are transported to the anterior pituitary gland by the infundibular portal system. The posterior pituitary gland makes up about 20% of the total pituitary mass and stores and secretes two major peptide hormones: vasopressin (AVP or antidiuretic hormone) and oxytocin. These neurohypophyseal hormones are synthesized by the supraoptic and paraventricular nuclei of the hypothalamus and transported to the posterior lobe in neurosecretory granules along the supraopticohypophyseal tract (Table 1.1).

On imaging studies, the normal adult pituitary gland has a flat superior border and a vertical height of approximately 8 to 10 mm. The anterior pituitary is homogeneous in signal on magnetic resonance imaging (MRI), the preferred imaging method, and enhances homogeneously after intravenous administration of a contrast agent (see Fig. 1.1). The posterior pituitary lobe is distinguished from the anterior lobe on T1-weighted MRI as a bright spot in the posterior aspect of the gland, best seen on a sagittal view. The bright appearance is thought to result from the presence of AVP and/or phospholipid vesicles within the normal neurohypophysis.

PITUITARY TUMORS

Pituitary tumors account for approximately 10% to 15% of intracranial tumors. They are the most common tumors in the sella, accounting for more than 90% of masses that develop in that area, and they are usually benign. Their true incidence is difficult to determine because they are often asymptomatic, but the prevalence is about 10% to 20% in radiologic studies. Most pituitary tumors are slow growing, but some have higher growth rates and can be invasive. Pituitary carcinomas are very

rare and are defined by the presence of a metastasis that is noncontiguous with the original tumor, or cerebrospinal fluid dissemination.

Pituitary tumors are classified by size and secretory capacity. Tumors that are smaller than 10 mm in diameter are called *microadenomas*, whereas lesions 10 mm or larger are called *macroadenomas*. Hormone-producing tumors are called *secretory adenomas,* and those that do not secrete a hormone are known as *nonsecretory adenomas.* Pituitary tumors may be composed of any of the anterior pituitary cell types, with multiple cell types forming plurihormonal tumors. Prolactin-secreting pituitary tumors are the most common type. Table 1.2 reviews the prevalence of the various pituitary tumors, and Table 1.3 describes the screening tests used to determine the secretory status of a new pituitary tumor.

The clinical manifestations of pituitary tumors are usually signs and symptoms caused by hormone overproduction or underproduction or mass effect. Common clinical features of pituitary mass effect include headaches, visual field defects, and cranial nerve palsies. Superior extension of a tumor compresses the optic chiasm, causing bitemporal hemianopsia; lateral extension into the cavernous sinuses results in ophthalmoplegia, diplopia, or ptosis due to compression of cranial nerves III, IV, or VI or facial pain due to compression of V1 or V2. Compromise of normal pituitary tissue by a tumor can cause hormone loss or hypopituitarism. Screening tests for and causes of pituitary hormone deficiency are shown in Tables 1.3 and 1.4 , respectively.

DISORDERS OF ANTERIOR PITUITARY HORMONES

Prolactin

Definition and Epidemiology

The mature prolactin polypeptide contains 199 amino acids and is formed after a 28-amino-acid signal peptide is proteolytically cleaved from the prolactin prohormone (pre-prolactin). Prolactin synthesis and secretion by pituitary lactotrophs is under tonic inhibitory control by hypothalamic-derived dopamine, which keeps prolactin at its basal levels. Factors stimulating prolactin synthesis and secretion, in addition to reduced dopamine availability to the lactotrophs, include thyrotropin-releasing hormone (TRH), estrogen, vasoactive intestinal polypeptide (VIP), AVP, oxytocin, and epidermal growth factor.

Prolactin levels physiologically increase during pregnancy. After delivery, prolactin induces and maintains lactation of the breast. Hyperprolactinemia, regardless of the etiology, can cause hypogonadism through its inhibitory effect on gonadotropin release, infertility, galactorrhea, and/or bone loss from the hypogonadism.

Prolactinomas and hyperprolactinemia are more common in women, with a peak prevalence between 25 and 35 years of age. The mean prevalence of patients medically treated for hyperprolactinemia is approximately 20 per 100,000 in men and approximately 90 per 100,000 in women. Prolactinomas are rare in childhood or adolescence.

下丘脑－垂体轴

段炼 译 朱惠娟 潘慧 审校 宁光 通审

解剖学和生理学

垂体位于颅底一个被称作蝶鞍的骨质结构中。它的重量约 600 mg，由 3 个叶组成，腺垂体（前叶）、神经垂体（后叶）和中间叶。人类的中间叶在妊娠约 15 周时退化，在成人正常垂体中已不存在。漏斗柄包含门静脉丛循环，连接下丘脑和垂体。垂体周围的重要结构包括位于垂体上方的视交叉和位于垂体两侧的海绵窦，这些结构可能因垂体增大而受损。双侧海绵窦包含颈内动脉和颅神经Ⅲ、Ⅳ、V1、V2、Ⅵ（图 1.1）。

垂体前叶可合成 6 种激素，由腺体内的特定细胞产生：促肾上腺皮质激素（ACTH）、卵泡刺激素（FSH）、黄体生成素（LH）、生长激素（GH）、催乳素（PRL）和促甲状腺激素（TSH）。这些激素受下丘脑产生的刺激和抑制肽类的调节，并通过漏斗门静脉系统传输至垂体前叶。垂体后叶约占垂体总重量的 20%，储存和释放两种主要的肽类激素：血管升压素［又称精氨酸血管升压素（AVP）或抗利尿激素］和催产素。这些神经垂体激素由下丘脑的视上核和室旁核合成，并以神经分泌颗粒的形式沿着视上垂体束运送至后叶（表 1.1）。

在影像学检查中，正常成人的垂体上缘平坦，垂直高度为 8～10 mm。磁共振成像（MRI）是首选的影像学方法，MRI 可显示垂体前叶信号均匀，静脉注射造影剂后呈均匀强化（图 1.1）。与垂体前叶信号不同，垂体后叶在 MRI T1 加权像中表现为腺体后部的亮点，在矢状位上显示最为清楚。高信号被认为是由于正常神经垂体内含有 AVP 和（或）磷脂囊泡。

垂体瘤

垂体瘤占颅内肿瘤的 10%～15%。垂体瘤是鞍区最常见的肿瘤，占鞍区肿物的 90% 以上，且常为良性病变。由于通常无症状，垂体瘤的真实发病率很难确定，但在影像学研究中的患病率为 10%～20%。大多数垂体瘤生长缓慢，但有些肿瘤生长速度较快，并具有侵袭性。垂体癌非常罕见，其定义为存在与原发肿瘤非毗邻部位的转移或脑脊液播散。

垂体瘤可依据大小和分泌功能进行分类。直径 < 10 mm 的肿瘤被称为微腺瘤，而直径 ≥ 10 mm 的肿瘤被称为大腺瘤。产生激素的肿瘤被称为分泌性腺瘤，不分泌激素的肿瘤被称为非分泌性腺瘤。垂体瘤可由任何一种类型的垂体前叶细胞组成，由多种细胞类型形成的肿瘤被称为多激素腺瘤。垂体催乳素瘤是最常见的肿瘤类型。表 1.2 总结了各种垂体瘤的患病率，表 1.3 介绍了用于确诊新发垂体瘤分泌状态的筛查试验。

垂体瘤的临床表现通常是由激素分泌过多、分泌不足或肿物占位效应所致的体征和症状。垂体肿物占位效应的常见临床特征包括头痛、视野缺损和颅神经麻痹。肿物向上延伸可压迫视交叉，引起双眼颞侧偏盲；肿物向侧方延伸侵入海绵窦，由于颅神经Ⅲ、Ⅳ或Ⅵ受压，可导致眼肌麻痹、复视或上睑下垂，或由于颅神经V1 或 V2 受压引起面部疼痛。肿瘤累及正常垂体组织可导致激素缺乏或垂体功能减退。垂体激素缺乏的筛查试验和病因分别见表 1.3 和表 1.4。

垂体前叶激素异常

催乳素

定义和流行病学

成熟的 PRL 多肽含有 199 个氨基酸，由催乳素前体激素（前催乳素）通过蛋白水解剪切掉一个含有 28 个氨基酸的信号肽而形成。垂体催乳激素细胞合成和分泌 PRL 受下丘脑源性多巴胺的张力性抑制作用的调节，从而使 PRL 维持在基础水平。除了降低多巴胺对催乳激素细胞的作用活性外，刺激 PRL 合成和分泌的因素还包括促甲状腺激素释放激素（TRH）、雌激素、血管活性肠肽（VIP）、AVP、催产素和表皮生长因子。

在妊娠期，PRL 水平会生理性升高。分娩后，PRL 诱导并维持乳房泌乳。无论病因如何，高催乳素血症可通过抑制促性腺激素的释放而导致性腺功能减退症，继而引起不孕症、溢乳和（或）骨量丢失。

催乳素瘤和高催乳素血症在女性中更常见，发病高峰年龄为 25～35 岁。接受药物治疗的高催乳素血症在男性中的平均患病率约为 20/100 000，在女性中约为 90/100 000。催乳素瘤在儿童或青少年中较为罕见。

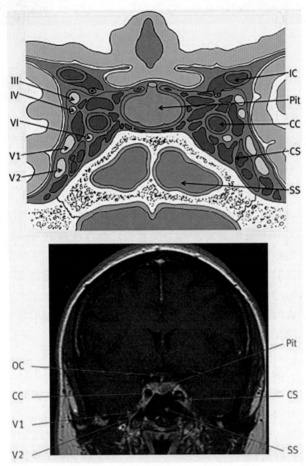

Fig. 1.1 Coronal section and corresponding magnetic resonance imaging scan of the pituitary gland and surrounding structures, including cranial nerves III (oculomotor), IV (trochlear), V1 (trigeminal, ophthalmic branch), V2 (trigeminal, maxillary branch), and VI (abducens). *CC,* Carotid artery (intracavernous); *CS,* cavernous sinus (left); *IC,* internal carotid artery; *OC,* optic chiasm; *Pit,* pituitary gland; *SS,* sphenoid sinus. (From Jesurasa A, Kailaya-Vasan A, Sinha S: Surgery for pituitary tumors, Surgery 29:428-433, 2011, Figure 1.)

Clinical Presentation

The clinical presentation of a prolactinoma varies with the age and gender of the patient. Typically, the patient is a young woman with menstrual irregularities, galactorrhea, and infertility. Galactorrhea occurs in 50% to 80% of affected women. Men may report a decrease in libido and erectile dysfunction as a result of hypogonadism caused by reduced secretion of LH and FSH. Typically, however, their tumors are diagnosed after symptoms of tumor compression appear, including headache, neurologic deficits, and vision changes. Galactorrhea and gynecomastia are rare in men. Because of the early presentation of menstrual irregularities in women, microprolactinomas are more common in women; macroprolactinomas are more frequent in men and in postmenopausal women.

Diagnosis and Differential Diagnosis

Hyperprolactinemia is diagnosed by a serum prolactin above the upper limit of normal. This can be drawn at any time of day. For prolactinomas, serum prolactin levels typically parallel tumor size. A prolactin level greater than 250 ng/mL is usually diagnostic of a prolactinoma, but smaller prolactinomas may have lower levels. Dynamic testing is not needed to diagnose hyperprolactinemia.

Two types of artifacts can occur during the standard measurement of prolactin: the presence of macroprolactin and the hook effect. When a patient with mild hyperprolactinemia does not have the expected clinical features of hyperprolactinemia (e.g., galactorrhea, menstrual disturbance, infertility), one should consider the presence of macroprolactin. Macroprolactin is a polymeric form of prolactin that is biologically inactive. Most commercially available prolactin assays do not detect macroprolactin, but it can be detected inexpensively in the serum by polyethylene glycol precipitation. The estimated incidence of macroprolactin accounting for a significant proportion of hyperprolactinemia is 10% to 20%. The hook effect should be considered in a patient who has a very large pituitary mass and only a mild elevation in prolactin. The hook effect is an assay artifact that occurs when very high serum prolactin concentrations saturate antibodies in the standard two-site immunoradiometric assay, resulting in falsely low levels. This artifact can be overcome by repeating the prolactin measurement on a 1:100 serum sample dilution.

Physiologic increases in prolactin occur with pregnancy, physical or emotional stress, exercise, and chest wall stimulation. Mild to moderate hyperprolactinemia (25 to 200 ng/mL) in the presence of a larger pituitary mass is more likely to be caused by a non–prolactin-secreting tumor with infundibular stalk compression and inhibition of dopamine transport to the lactotroph. Other common causes for hyperprolactinemia are shown in Table 1.5. Some drugs such as metoclopramide and risperidone can increase prolactin to greater than 200 ng/mL.

Treatment and Prognosis

Medical management with a dopamine agonist—bromocriptine or cabergoline—is the recommended treatment. The dopamine agonists normalize prolactin, decrease tumor size, and restore gonadal function in more than 80% of patients with prolactinomas. Because of the rapidity and efficacy of the dopamine agonists in treating these tumors, they are also the initial treatment for macroprolactinomas that have caused compromise in vision, neurologic deficits, or pituitary dysfunction.

Cabergoline, the newer agent, is preferred to other dopamine agonists because it has higher efficacy in normalizing prolactin levels and shrinking tumor size and has fewer side effects. The most common side effects seen with dopamine agonists are nausea, vomiting, orthostatic lightheadedness, dizziness, and nasal congestion. Because of the concern for cabergoline-related cardiac valvulopathy that was reported in patients who had Parkinson's disease treated with higher doses of cabergoline than used in prolactinomas, baseline echocardiogram and regular cardiac auscultation is recommended in patients taking greater than 2 mg weekly. Transsphenoidal resection of the tumor is indicated for patients who cannot tolerate the dopamine agonists or who do not respond to medical treatment. No treatment is required for patients who have microprolactinomas that are asymptomatic.

Studies have shown that dopamine agonists may be safely withdrawn in patients who have maintained normal prolactin levels for 2 years and who have no visible tumor on low doses of dopamine agonist. Once the dopamine agonist is discontinued, prolactin levels should be checked every 3 months for 1 year and then annually. An MRI should be obtained only if the prolactin level becomes elevated again. Recurrence risk after drug withdrawal ranges from 26% to 69% and is predicted by the initial prolactin level and tumor size.

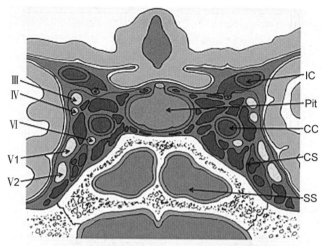

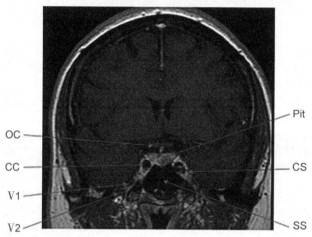

图 1.1　垂体及其周围结构的冠状面和 MRI 图像，包括颅神经Ⅲ（动眼神经）、Ⅳ（滑车神经）、V1（三叉神经，眼支）、V2（三叉神经，上颌支）和Ⅵ（外展神经）。CC，颈动脉（海绵窦内）；CS，海绵窦（左）；IC，颈内动脉；OC，视交叉；Pit，垂体；SS，蝶窦（引自 Jesurasa A，Kailaya-Vasan A，Sinha S：Surgery for pituitary tumors，Surgery 29：428-433，2011，Figure 1.）

临床表现

催乳素瘤的临床表现因患者的年龄和性别不同而异。年轻女性的典型表现为月经不规律、溢乳和不孕症。50%～80% 的女性患者会发生溢乳。男性患者可能会主诉性欲减退和勃起功能障碍，这是由于 LH 和 FSH 分泌减少导致患者性腺功能减退症。然而，这些患者通常是在表现出肿瘤压迫症状之后才被诊断出来，包括头痛、神经功能损伤和视力改变。溢乳和男性乳房发育在男性患者中很少见。由于月经不规律是女性患者的早期表现，催乳素微腺瘤在女性中更为常见，而催乳素大腺瘤在男性和绝经后女性中更为常见。

诊断和鉴别诊断

血清 PRL 水平高于正常值上限即可诊断高催乳素血症，可在一天中的任何时间检测 PRL。在催乳素瘤患者中，血清 PRL 水平通常与肿瘤大小相平行。当 PRL > 250 ng/ml 时，通常可诊断催乳素瘤，但体积较

小的催乳素瘤患者的 PRL 水平可能较低。诊断高催乳素血症不需要动态检测。

在标准测定 PRL 的过程中会出现两种类型的假象：巨催乳素和钩状效应。当患者仅有轻度高催乳素血症但无预期的相关临床特征（如溢乳、月经紊乱、不孕症）时，应考虑存在巨催乳素。巨催乳素是催乳素的一种多聚体形式，但缺乏生物活性。大多数可用的 PRL 测定方法不能检测巨催乳素，但可采用廉价的聚乙二醇沉淀法进行检测。巨催乳素在高催乳素血症中的估计发生率为 10%～20%。当患者有巨大垂体占位但 PRL 水平仅轻度升高时，应考虑钩状效应。钩状效应是一种假性检测结果，当血清 PRL 水平过高时，可使标准的双位点免疫放射分析法中的抗体饱和，导致检测结果呈假性降低。这一假象可通过 1∶100 稀释血清后重复测定 PRL 来避免。

生理性 PRL 水平升高可见于妊娠、躯体或情绪应激、运动、胸壁刺激。当较大的垂体占位合并轻中度高催乳素血症（25～200 ng/ml）时，很可能是由于非 PRL 分泌瘤所致，伴漏斗柄受压且阻断了多巴胺对催乳激素细胞的抑制作用，其他引起高催乳素血症的常见病因见表 1.5。部分药物（如甲氧氯普胺和利培酮）也可使 PRL > 200 ng/ml。

治疗和预后

催乳素瘤的药物治疗推荐使用多巴胺受体激动剂——溴隐亭或卡麦角林。多巴胺受体激动剂能够使 80% 以上的催乳素瘤患者的 PRL 水平恢复正常，缩小肿瘤体积，并恢复性腺功能。由于多巴胺受体激动剂在治疗这些肿瘤方面具有快速性和有效性，因此也可作为引起视力损害、神经功能损伤或垂体功能障碍的催乳素大腺瘤的初始治疗方案。

卡麦角林是一种疗效优于其他多巴胺受体激动剂的药物，这是因为它在促使 PRL 水平正常化和缩小肿瘤体积方面具有更好的效果，且副作用更少。多巴胺受体激动剂最常见的副作用包括恶心、呕吐、直立性头晕、眩晕和鼻塞。由于在帕金森病患者（剂量大于催乳素瘤的治疗剂量）中报道了卡麦角林相关的心脏瓣膜病变，因此推荐每周服用超过 2 mg 卡麦角林的催乳素瘤患者应在基线接受超声心动图和常规心脏听诊。经蝶窦肿瘤切除术适用于不能耐受多巴胺受体激动剂或药物治疗无效的患者。无症状的催乳素微腺瘤患者无须治疗。

研究表明，对于 PRL 水平正常持续 2 年或服用低剂量多巴胺受体激动剂时影像学检查未见肿瘤的患者，可以安全停药。一旦停用多巴胺受体激动剂，应在停药后的第 1 年内每 3 个月检测 1 次 PRL 水平，此后每年检测 1 次。只有当 PRL 水平再次升高时，再行 MRI 检查。停药后的复发风险为 26%～69%，可通过初始 PRL 水平和肿瘤体积来预测。

TABLE 1.1   Pituitary–Target Organ Hormone Axis

Hypothalamic Hormone	Pituitary Target Cell	Pituitary Hormone Affected	Peripheral Target Gland	Peripheral Hormone Affected
Stimulatory				
Anterior Lobe of Pituitary Gland				
Thyrotropin-releasing hormone (TRH)	Thyrotroph	Thyroid-stimulating hormone (TSH)	Thyroid gland	Thyroxine (T_4) Triiodothyronine (T_3)
Growth hormone-releasing hormone (GHRH)	Somatotroph	Growth hormone (GH)	Liver	Insulin-like growth factor-I (IGF-I)
Gonadotropin-releasing hormone (GnRH)	Gonadotroph	Luteinizing hormone (LH)	Ovary Testis	Progesterone Testosterone
		Follicle-stimulating hormone (FSH)	Ovary Testis	Estradiol Inhibin
Corticotropin-releasing hormone	Corticotroph	Adrenocorticotrophic hormone (ACTH)	Adrenal gland	Cortisol
Posterior Lobe of Pituitary Gland				
Vasopressin (AVP)			Kidney	
Oxytocin			Uterus	
			Breast	
Inhibitory				
Somatostatin	Somatotroph	Growth hormone (GH)	Liver	IGF-I
	Thyrotroph	Thyroid stimulating hormone (TSH)	Thyroid	T_4 and T_3
Dopamine	Lactotroph	Prolactin (PRL)	Breast	

TABLE 1.2   Prevalence of Pituitary Tumors

Tumor	Prevalence (%)
Prolactin-secreting adenomas	40-45
Gonadotropin-secreting adenomas	20
Growth hormone–secreting adenomas	10-15
Adrenocorticotrophic hormone–secreting adenomas	10-15
Null cell adenomas	5-10
Thyroid-stimulating hormone–secreting adenomas	1-2

TABLE 1.3   Biochemical Tests for Pituitary Disorders

Disorder	Tests
Pituitary Tumor	
GH-secreting adenomas	IGF-I
	OGTT: measure blood sugar and GH (0, 60, 120 min)
PRL-secreting adenomas	Basal serum prolactin
ACTH-secreting adenomas	24-hr urine-free cortisol and creatinine level
	1-mg overnight dexamethasone suppression test
	11 PM salivary cortisol
	Serum ACTH
TSH-secreting adenomas	Serum TSH, Free T_4, Free T_3, alpha subunit
Gonadotropin-secreting adenomas	FSH, LH, alpha subunit estradiol (women), testosterone (men)
Hypopituitarism	
GH deficiency	IGF-I
	Glucagon stimulation test
	Arginine-GHRH (GHRH not available in the United States)
	Arginine-L-DOPA
	ITT
Gonadotropin deficiency	Women: basal estradiol, LH, FSH
	Men: 8 AM fasting testosterone (total; free), LH, FSH
TSH deficiency	Serum TSH, free T_4
ACTH deficiency	8 AM fasting ACTH and cortisol
	Cosyntropin-stimulation test (1 µg and 250 µg)

ACTH, Adrenocorticotropic hormone; *CRH,* corticotropin-releasing hormone; *FSH,* follicle-stimulating hormone; *GH,* growth hormone; *GHRH,* growth hormone-releasing hormone; *IGF-I,* insulin-like growth factor-I; *ITT,* insulin tolerance test; *LH,* luteinizing hormone; *OGTT,* oral glucose tolerance test; *PRL,* prolactin; *T₄,* thyroxine; *TFT,* thyroid function test; *TSH,* thyroid-stimulating hormone.

Growth Hormone

Definition

GH is a single-chain polypeptide hormone consisting of 191 amino acids that is synthesized, stored, and secreted by the anterior pituitary somatotrophs. GH secretion is regulated by two factors derived from the hypothalamus: growth hormone–releasing hormone (GHRH) and somatostatin. GHRH stimulates somatotroph GH release, and somatostatin inhibits it. GH stimulates secretion of insulin-like growth factor-I (IGF-I) by the liver. IGF-I circulates in the blood attached to binding proteins; although there are six binding proteins in serum, more than 80% of IGF-I is bound to a protein called IGFBP3. Postnatally and through puberty, GH and IGF-I are critical in determining longitudinal skeletal growth, skeletal maturation, and bone mass. In adulthood, they are instrumental in the maintenance of skeletal architecture and bone mass. GH also has effects on the metabolism of carbohydrates, lipids, and proteins by antagonizing insulin action, increasing lipolysis and free fatty acid production, and increasing protein synthesis.

Growth Hormone Deficiency

Epidemiology. Childhood-onset GH deficiency is most commonly idiopathic, but it may be genetic or associated with congenital anatomic malformations in the brain or sellar region. The most common cause of GH deficiency in adults is a pituitary macroadenoma and its treatment;

表 1.1　垂体靶腺激素轴

下丘脑激素	垂体靶细胞	受调节的垂体激素	外周靶腺	受调节的外周激素
刺激作用				
垂体前叶				
促甲状腺激素释放激素（TRH）	促甲状腺激素细胞	促甲状腺激素（TSH）	甲状腺	甲状腺素（T_4）
				三碘甲状腺原氨酸（T_3）
生长激素释放激素（GHRH）	生长激素细胞	生长激素（GH）	肝	胰岛素样生长因子 - I
				（IGF- I ）
促性腺激素释放激素（GnRH）	促性腺激素细胞	黄体生成素（LH）	卵巢	孕酮
			睾丸	睾酮
		卵泡刺激素（FSH）	卵巢	雌二醇
			睾丸	抑制素
促肾上腺皮质激素释放激素（CRH）	促肾上腺皮质激素细胞	促肾上腺皮质激素（ACTH）	肾上腺	皮质醇
垂体后叶				
血管升压素（AVP）			肾	
催产素			子宫	
			乳腺	
抑制作用				
生长抑素	生长激素细胞	生长激素（GH）	肝	IGF- I
	促甲状腺激素细胞	促甲状腺激素（TSH）	甲状腺	T_4 和 T_3
多巴胺	催乳激素细胞	催乳素（PRL）	乳腺	

表 1.2　垂体瘤的患病率

肿瘤类型	患病率（%）
催乳素分泌腺瘤	40 ～ 45
促性腺激素分泌腺瘤	20
生长激素分泌腺瘤	10 ～ 15
促肾上腺皮质激素分泌腺瘤	10 ～ 15
零细胞腺瘤	5 ～ 10
促甲状腺激素分泌腺瘤	1 ～ 2

生长激素

定义

　　GH 是一种含 191 个氨基酸的单链多肽激素，由垂体前叶生长激素细胞合成、储存和分泌。GH 的分泌受来源于下丘脑的两个因素的调节：生长激素释放激素（GHRH）和生长抑素。GHRH 刺激生长激素细胞释放 GH，而生长抑素则抑制 GH 释放。GH 可促进肝脏分泌胰岛素样生长因子 - I（IGF- I ）。血循环中的 IGF- I 附着于结合蛋白上；血清中含有 6 种结合蛋白，但超过 80% 的 IGF- I 与 IGFBP3 结合。在出生后及整个青春期，GH 和 IGF- I 在决定骨骼纵向生长、骨骼成熟和骨量方面至关重要。在成年期，它们在维持骨骼结构和骨量方面发挥重要作用。GH 对碳水化合物、脂肪和蛋白质的代谢也有影响，可通过拮抗胰岛素的作用，增加脂肪分解和游离脂肪酸的产生，并增加蛋白质合成。

生长激素缺乏症

　　流行病学　儿童期起病的 GH 缺乏症多为特发性，但也可能是遗传性，或与大脑或鞍区先天性解剖畸形有关。成人 GH 缺乏症最常见的原因是垂体大腺瘤及

表 1.3　垂体疾病的生化检测

疾病	检测
垂体瘤	
GH 分泌腺瘤	IGF- I
	OGTT：检测血糖和 GH（0、60 min、120 min）[译者注：原文不准确，应为 GH（0、30 min、60 min、90 min、120 min）]
PRL 分泌腺瘤	基线血清 PRL
ACTH 分泌腺瘤	24 h 尿游离皮质醇和肌酐水平
	1 mg 过夜地塞米松抑制试验
	23：00 唾液皮质醇
	血清 ACTH
TSH 分泌腺瘤	血清 TSH、游离 T_4、游离 T_3、α 亚基
促性腺激素分泌腺瘤	FSH、LH、α 亚基、雌二醇（女性）、睾酮（男性）
垂体功能减退症	
GH 缺乏	IGF- I
	胰高血糖素兴奋试验
	精氨酸 -GHRH 兴奋试验（GHRH 在美国未上市）
	精氨酸-左旋多巴
	ITT
促性腺激素缺乏	女性：基线雌二醇、LH、FSH
	男性：08：00 空腹睾酮（总睾酮；游离睾酮）、LH、FSH
TSH 缺乏	血清 TSH、游离 T_4
ACTH 缺乏	08：00 空腹 ACTH 和皮质醇
	促皮质素兴奋试验（1 μg 和 250 μg）

ACTH，促肾上腺皮质激素；FSH，卵泡刺激素；GH，生长激素；GHRH，生长激素释放激素；IGF- I，胰岛素样生长因子 - I ；ITT，胰岛素耐量试验；LH，黄体生成素；OGTT，口服葡萄糖耐量试验；PRL，催乳素；T_4，甲状腺素；TSH，促甲状腺激素。

TABLE 1.4   Causes of Pituitary Hormone Deficiency

Causes	Examples
Sellar masses	Pituitary macroadenomas, craniopharyngiomas
Treatment of sellar, parasellar, and hypothalamic tumors	Pituitary/hypothalamic surgery, radiotherapy, radiosurgery (gamma knife)
Infiltrative diseases	Lymphocytic hypophysitis, hemochromatosis, sarcoidosis
Trauma	Head injury, perinatal trauma
Vascular	Sheehan syndrome, pituitary apoplexy
Medications	Opiates, glucocorticoids
Infections	Fungal, tuberculosis
Genetic	Combined or isolated pituitary hormone deficiencies
Developmental	Pituitary hypoplasia or aplasia, midline cerebral and cranial malformations
Empty sella	

TABLE 1.5   Causes of Hyperprolactinemia

Causes	Examples
Medications	Methyldopa, estrogens, metoclopramide, domperidone, neuroleptics and antipsychotics
Hypothalamic-infundibular stalk damage	Infiltrative disorders (sarcoidosis), brain irradiation, trauma, surgery, tumors
Pituitary	Prolactinomas, non-PRL-secreting pituitary macroadenomas with stalk compression
Medical	Renal failure, primary hypothyroidism

deficiency of one or more pituitary hormones occurs in 30% to 60% of such cases. The incidence of hypopituitarism 10 years after irradiation of the sellar region is approximately 50%.

Clinical presentation. Children with GH deficiency exhibit growth retardation, short stature, and fasting hypoglycemia. Manifestations of adult GH deficiency include reduced bone density, decreased muscle strength and exercise performance, decreased lean body mass with increase in fat mass and abdominal adiposity, glucose intolerance and insulin resistance, abnormal lipid profile including elevated low-density lipoprotein (LDL) and triglyceride levels with decreased high-density lipoprotein (HDL), depressed mood, and impaired psychosocial well-being.

Diagnosis and differential diagnosis. Because of the pulsatile nature of pituitary GH secretion, a single random measurement of serum GH is not helpful to diagnose GH deficiency. In adults with GH deficiency due to a pituitary tumor and concomitant hypopituitarism involving any three other pituitary hormones, a low IGF-I level is sufficient to diagnose GH deficiency, and provocative testing is not warranted. Falsely low IGF-I levels are seen in malnutrition, acute illness, celiac disease, poorly controlled diabetes mellitus, and liver disease. In children, there tends to be greater variation in IGF-I levels that do not correspond to the true GH status, so provocative testing is required.

The historical "gold standard" stimulatory test is insulin-induced hypoglycemia (insulin tolerance test or ITT). Symptomatic hypoglycemia with a serum glucose level lower than 45 mg/dL is a potent stimulus for GH secretion; the normal GH response is greater than 10 ng/mL in children and greater than 5 ng/mL in adults. Because of the unavailability in the United States of GHRH, which is as sensitive and specific as the ITT in stimulating GH secretion, glucagon stimulation is being used, especially in adults with ischemic heart disease or seizures. A normal adult response with the glucagon stimulation test is defined as a GH peak greater than 3 ng/mL for those with normal weight, but in obese patients, a cutoff of 1 ng/mL is used.

Treatment and prognosis. The US Food and Drug Administration (FDA) has approved recombinant human growth hormone (hGH) in both the adult and pediatric populations. It is used in conditions involving complete absence of GH associated with severe growth retardation or partial GH deficiency resulting in short stature. Short stature is defined as height more than 2.5 standard deviations below the mean for age-matched normal children, growth velocity less than the 25th percentile, delayed bone age, and predicted adult height less than the mean parental height. Other conditions approved by the FDA to use hGH include Turner syndrome, Prader-Willi syndrome, chronic kidney disease, AIDS-associated muscle wasting, *SHOX* gene deficiency, Noonan syndrome, and children born small for gestational age. Combined clinical evaluations, along with an inadequate pituitary GH response to provocative testing, are used in the assessment of childhood GH deficiency. Higher doses of GH are recommended for children without GH deficiency disorders or with partial GH deficiency.

In adults, hGH is administered as a daily subcutaneous injection starting at 0.1 to 0.3 mg, with dose increases at 6-week intervals based on clinical response, side effects, and IGF-I levels. Absolute contraindications to hGH therapy in adults include active neoplasm, intracranial hypertension, and proliferative diabetic retinopathy; uncontrolled diabetes and untreated thyroid disease are relative contraindications. Side effects of hGH therapy are usually transient and include arthralgias, fluid retention, carpal tunnel syndrome, and glucose intolerance. Additional side effects in children include slipped capital femoral epiphysis and hydrocephalus.

Acromegaly or Growth Hormone Hypersecretion

Definition and epidemiology. Acromegaly is literally translated as abnormal enlargement of the extremities of the skeleton. It is caused by hypersecretion of GH in adulthood. In children, excessive GH secretion before closure of the epiphyseal growth plate leads to gigantism. In both cases, the cause is almost always a GH-secreting pituitary tumor. Approximately 30% of GH-secreting pituitary adenomas are bihormonal and also secrete prolactin. The incidence of acromegaly is about 2 to 4 per million population, and the mean age at diagnosis is 40 to 50 years. GH-secreting tumors are caused by a clonal expansion of pure somatotrophs or mixed somatomammotrophs. A variety of genetic abnormalities can be found in GH-secreting pituitary adenomas including McCune-Albright syndrome, multiple endocrine neoplasia type 1 and 4, Carney complex, and familial isolated pituitary adenoma.

表1.4	垂体激素缺乏的病因
病因	**举例**
鞍区占位	垂体大腺瘤、颅咽管瘤
蝶鞍肿瘤、鞍旁肿瘤和下丘脑肿瘤的治疗	垂体 / 下丘脑手术、放疗、放射外科治疗（伽马刀）
浸润性疾病	淋巴细胞性垂体炎、血色病、结节病
创伤	头部外伤、围产期创伤
血管因素	希恩综合征、垂体卒中
药物	阿片类药物、糖皮质激素
感染	真菌、结核
遗传	联合性或孤立性垂体激素缺乏
发育因素	垂体发育不良或未发育、脑中线或头颅畸形
空泡蝶鞍	

表1.5	高催乳素血症的病因
病因	**举例**
药物	甲基多巴、雌激素、甲氧氯普胺、多潘立酮、镇静剂和抗精神病药
下丘脑-漏斗柄损伤	浸润性疾病（结节病）、颅脑照射、创伤、手术、肿瘤
垂体	催乳素瘤、非催乳素分泌垂体大腺瘤伴垂体柄受压
内科	肾衰竭、原发性甲状腺功能减退症

其治疗；30% ～ 60% 的患者缺乏 1 种或多种垂体激素。鞍区放疗后 10 年垂体功能减退的发生率约为 50%。

临床表现　儿童 GH 缺乏症表现为生长迟缓、身材矮小和空腹低血糖。成人 GH 缺乏症的表现包括骨密度降低、肌力和运动表现下降、瘦体重减少伴脂肪含量增加和腹型肥胖、糖耐量异常和胰岛素抵抗、血脂异常 [包括低密度脂蛋白（LDL）和甘油三酯水平升高，高密度脂蛋白（HDL）水平下降]，以及心境低落和社会心理健康受损。

诊断和鉴别诊断　由于垂体呈脉冲性分泌 GH，单次随机测定血清 GH 不能帮助诊断 GH 缺乏症。在因垂体瘤导致 GH 缺乏并伴有垂体功能减退（影响任意 3 种其他垂体激素）的成人患者中，IGF-Ⅰ 水平降低即可诊断 GH 缺乏症，无须进行激发试验。IGF-Ⅰ 水平假性降低可见于营养不良、急性疾病、乳糜泻、糖尿病控制不佳和肝脏疾病。在儿童中，IGF-Ⅰ 水平的变化更大，与真实的 GH 分泌状态不相符，因此需要进行激发试验。

既往被作为"金标准"的激发试验是胰岛素诱发的低血糖试验 [胰岛素耐量试验（ITT）]。血糖＜ 45 mg/dl 的症状性低血糖是对 GH 分泌的强刺激；正常 GH 反应为儿童＞ 10 ng/ml，成人＞ 5 ng/ml。在美国，由于无法使用 GHRH（与 ITT 刺激 GH 分泌的敏感性和特异性相似），可采用胰高血糖素刺激试验，尤其是患有缺血性心脏病或癫痫发作的成人患者。体重正常的成人对胰高血糖素刺激试验的正常反应是 GH 峰值＞ 3 ng/ml，但在肥胖症患者中，其诊断阈值为 1 ng/ml。

治疗和预后　美国食品药品监督管理局（FDA）已批准重组人生长激素（hGH）用于治疗成人和儿童患者。hGH 适用于 GH 完全缺乏引起的严重生长迟缓或 GH 部分缺乏导致的身材矮小。身材矮小的定义是身高低于年龄匹配的正常儿童身高均值 2.5 个标准差以上、生长速度低于第 25 百分位数、骨龄落后，且预测成年身高低于父母的平均身高。hGH 的其他获批适应证包括特纳综合征（Turner 综合征）、普拉德-威利综合征（Prader-Willi 综合征）、慢性肾脏病、艾滋病相关性肌肉萎缩、*SHOX* 基因缺失、努南综合征（Noonan 综合征），以及出生时小于胎龄儿的儿童。儿童 GH 缺乏症的评估包括临床评估和激发试验（垂体不能适当分泌 GH）。对于未患 GH 缺乏性疾病或患有 GH 部分缺乏症的儿童，建议使用更大剂量的 hGH。

在成人患者中，每日皮下注射 hGH 的起始剂量为 0.1 ～ 0.3 mg，基于临床反应、副作用和 IGF-Ⅰ 水平，每间隔 6 周可增加 1 次剂量。成人患者接受 hGH 治疗的绝对禁忌证包括活动性肿瘤、颅内高压、增殖性糖尿病视网膜病变；相对禁忌证包括未控制的糖尿病和未经治疗的甲状腺疾病。hGH 治疗的副作用通常较为短暂，包括关节痛、体液潴留、腕管综合征和糖耐量异常。儿童的其他副作用包括股骨头骨骺滑脱和脑积水。

肢端肥大症或生长激素过量分泌

定义和流行病学　肢端肥大症是指肢端骨骼的异常增大。它是由成年期 GH 分泌过多所致。在儿童中，GH 过量分泌发生在骨骺生长板闭合前，可导致巨人症。在这两种情况下，其病因几乎都是垂体 GH 分泌腺瘤。约 30% 的垂体 GH 分泌腺瘤可分泌 GH 和 PRL。肢端肥大症的发病率为（2 ～ 4）/1 000 000，平均诊断年龄为 40 ～ 50 岁。GH 分泌腺瘤是由单纯生长激素细胞或混合性生长激素催乳素细胞的克隆扩增引起的。垂体 GH 分泌腺瘤可能存在多种遗传异常，包括 McCune-Albright 综合征、多发性内分泌腺瘤病 1 型和 4 型、卡尼综合征（Carney 综合征）和家族性孤立性垂体腺瘤。

TABLE 1.6	Clinical Features of Acromegaly
Change	**Manifestations**
Somatic Changes	
Acral changes	Enlarged hands and feet
Musculoskeletal changes	Arthralgias
	Prognathism
	Malocclusion
	Carpal tunnel syndrome
Skin changes	Sweating
	Skin tags
	Nevi
Colon changes	Polyps
	Carcinoma
Cardiovascular symptoms	Cardiomegaly
	Hypertension
Visceromegaly	Tongue
	Thyroid
	Liver
Endocrine-Metabolic Changes	
Reproduction	Menstrual abnormalities
	Galactorrhea
	Decreased libido
Carbohydrate metabolism	Impaired glucose tolerance
	Diabetes mellitus
	Insulin resistance
Lipids	Hypertriglyceridemia

Clinical presentation. Acromegaly is a rare disease, and the rate of change of symptoms and signs is slow and insidious. The usual period from earliest onset of symptoms and signs to diagnosis is 8 to 10 years, during which time many patients undergo medical and surgical treatments for many of the metabolic abnormalities and morbidities caused by GH excess. Characteristic clinical findings of this disease include physical changes of the bone and soft tissue and multiple endocrine and metabolic abnormalities (Table 1.6).

Diagnosis and differential diagnosis. Measurement of serum IGF-I can be used to diagnose excess GH in most patients with acromegaly. An alternative is an oral glucose tolerance test using a 75 g glucose load. Normally, glucose suppresses GH levels to less than 1 ng/mL after 2 hours; in patients with acromegaly, GH levels may paradoxically increase, remain unchanged, or decrease but not below 1 ng/mL. Most acromegalic patients have GH-secreting pituitary tumors, and approximately 70% of cases of acromegaly present with pituitary macroadenomas. Rarely, GH hypersecretion is caused by ectopic GHRH-secreting tumors, including hypothalamic hamartomas and gangliocytomas, pancreatic islet cell tumors, small cell carcinoma of the lung, carcinoid, adrenal adenomas, and pheochromocytomas. Ectopic GH secretion has also been reported in pancreatic, lung, and breast cancers.

Treatment and prognosis. Treatment of acromegaly requires both treatment of the tumor and normalization of GH and IGF-I levels, along with management of the comorbidities and metabolic abnormalities caused by the excess GH. Treatment often requires the use of multiple modalities to achieve adequate control of the disease. Primary therapy is almost always transsphenoidal surgery, with the cure rate being directly proportional to tumor size. Patients with intrasellar microadenomas have a 75% to 95% cure rate with surgery.

In patients with noninvasive macroadenomas, surgical removal results in normalization of GH and IGF-I in 40% to 68% of patients.

Approximately 40% to 60% of tumors are not controlled with surgery alone because of cavernous sinus invasion or intracapsular intra-arachnoid invasion. Additional treatment options include primary medical therapy or primary surgical debulking of the tumor followed by medical therapy for hormonal control and/or radiation therapy for treatment of residual tumor. Conventional radiotherapy can normalize GH and IGF-I levels in more than 60% of patients, but the maximum response takes 10 to 15 years to achieve. Focused single-dose gamma knife radiotherapy has a 5-year remission rate of 29% to 60%. Hypopituitarism is seen in more than 50% of patients within 5 to 10 years after radiotherapy.

Currently, three drug classes are used to treat acromegaly: dopamine agonists, somatostatin receptor ligands (SRLs) such as octreotide, lanreotide, and pasireotide, and GH receptor antagonists. SRLs work mainly through the somatostatin receptor subtypes 2 and 5 (except pasireotide works through receptor subtypes 1, 2, 3, and 5), causing a decrease in tumor GH secretion. In acromegaly, SRLs are indicated for first-line treatment when there is low probability of surgical cure, after a failed surgical cure of GH hypersecretion, and to provide GH and IGF-I control while waiting for radiotherapy to achieve its maximum effect. SRLs reduce GH and IGF-I levels to normal in 40% to 65% of patients and shrink tumor size in approximately 50% of cases. Side effects of SRLs include diarrhea, abdominal cramping, flatulence, and cholelithiasis (15%).

Pegvisomant is the only GH receptor antagonist available. It works by blocking the peripheral action of GH through blockade of the GH receptors located on the liver. Pegvisomant is indicated for patients who have persistent elevation in IGF-I even with maximum doses of SRLs. This drug is highly effective in the treatment of acromegaly and normalizes IGF-I levels in 97% of patients; transient elevation in liver function enzymes is seen in 25% of those treated and tumor growth in fewer than 2%. After starting pegvisomant, GH levels are often elevated and are no longer helpful in guiding treatment.

Cabergoline is the most efficacious of the dopamine agonists for treatment of acromegaly, but it is effective in fewer than 10% of patients, working best in bihormonal PRL and GH-secreting tumors.

Thyroid-Stimulating Hormone
Definition

TSH is a glycoprotein secreted from the thyrotroph cells of the anterior pituitary. It is composed of alpha and beta subunits with the beta subunit giving its specific biological activity. Its release is regulated by TRH (stimulatory) and somatostatin (inhibitory). In addition, it is subject to the negative feedback of thyroid hormones released from the thyroid gland. Assessment of the pituitary-thyroid axis requires checking levels of TSH as well as thyroid hormones released by the thyroid gland (i.e., thyroxine [T_4] and triiodothyronine [T_3]).

Deficiency of TSH

Definition and epidemiology. Deficiency of TSH leads to secondary hypothyroidism. The diminished secretion of TSH from the pituitary provides inadequate stimulation to the thyroid gland for thyroid hormone release. The estimated prevalence of TSH deficiency is about 1 in 80,000 to 120,000 individuals. The more common causes of TSH deficiency are found in Table 1.4 , listing causes of hypopituitarism.

Clinical presentation. The usual signs and symptoms of hypothyroidism are weight gain, fatigue, cold intolerance, and constipation. If the condition is caused by an underlying sellar tumor, symptoms of mass effect may also be present, depending on the size of the tumor.

表 1.6　肢端肥大症的临床特征	
改变	**临床表现**
躯体改变	
肢端改变	手和足增大
肌肉骨骼变化	关节痛
	下颌前突
	咬合不正
	腕管综合征
皮肤改变	多汗
	皮赘
	色素痣
结肠改变	息肉
	结肠癌
心血管症状	心脏肥大
	高血压
内脏肥大	舌体
	甲状腺
	肝
内分泌 - 代谢性改变	
生殖	月经紊乱
	溢乳
	性欲减退
碳水化合物代谢	糖耐量减低
	糖尿病
	胰岛素抵抗
脂肪代谢	高甘油三酯血症

临床表现　肢端肥大症是一种罕见病，症状和体征的变化速度缓慢且隐匿。从最早出现症状和体征到诊断，通常需要 8 ～ 10 年，在此期间，许多患者因 GH 过量引起的多种代谢异常和并发症而接受药物和手术治疗。该病的特征性临床表现包括骨骼和软组织改变，以及多种内分泌和代谢异常（表 1.6）。

诊断和鉴别诊断　检测血清 IGF- I 可用于诊断大多数肢端肥大症患者存在的 GH 过量分泌。另一种方法是采用 75 g 葡萄糖负荷进行口服葡萄糖耐量试验（OGTT）。正常情况下，在葡萄糖负荷后 2 h，GH 水平可被抑制至＜ 1 ng/ml；在肢端肥大症患者中，GH 水平可能反常性升高、保持不变或降低，但不会＜ 1 ng/ml。大多数患者存在分泌 GH 的垂体瘤，且约 70% 的肢端肥大症患者为垂体大腺瘤。罕见情况下，GH 过量分泌是由分泌 GHRH 的异位肿瘤所致，包括下丘脑错构瘤和神经节细胞瘤、胰岛细胞瘤、小细胞肺癌、类癌、肾上腺腺瘤和嗜铬细胞瘤。已报道的异位分泌 GH 的肿瘤包括胰腺癌、肺癌和乳腺癌。

治疗和预后　肢端肥大症的治疗既需要治疗肿瘤，也需要使 GH 和 IGF- I 水平正常化，同时还要管理由过量 GH 引起的并发症和代谢异常。治疗通常需要联合多种措施来实现对疾病的适当控制。首选治疗几乎均为经蝶窦手术，治愈率与肿瘤大小成正比。鞍内微腺瘤患者的手术治愈率为 75% ～ 95%。对于非侵袭性大腺瘤患者，手术切除可使 40% ～ 68% 患者的 GH 和 IGF- I 水平恢复正常。

40% ～ 60% 的肿瘤因侵犯海绵窦或囊内蛛网膜而无法仅通过手术来控制病情。其他治疗选择包括首选药物治疗或首选减瘤手术后采用药物控制激素水平和（或）放疗控制残余肿瘤。传统的放疗可使超过 60% 患者的 GH 和 IGF- I 水平恢复正常，但需要 10 ～ 15 年才能实现其最大效应。聚焦单次剂量的伽玛刀放疗的 5 年缓解率为 29% ～ 60%。超过 50% 的患者会在放疗后 5 ～ 10 年发生垂体功能减退。

目前有 3 类药物可用于治疗肢端肥大症：多巴胺受体激动剂、生长抑素受体配体（SRL；如奥曲肽、兰瑞肽、帕瑞肽）和 GH 受体拮抗剂。SRL 主要通过生长抑素受体亚型 2 和 5（除帕瑞肽是通过受体亚型 1、2、3 和 5 发挥作用）来抑制肿瘤分泌 GH。在治疗肢端肥大症时，SRL 适用于手术治愈率较低时的一线治疗、手术后 GH 过量分泌未能控制，以及在放疗发挥最大效应前控制 GH 和 IGF- I 水平。SRL 可将 40% ～ 65% 患者的 GH 和 IGF- I 控制在正常范围内，约 50% 患者的肿瘤体积缩小。SRL 的副作用包括腹泻、腹部痉挛、胃肠胀气和胆石症（15%）。

培维索孟是唯一可用的 GH 受体拮抗剂。它通过阻断位于肝脏的 GH 受体而阻止 GH 的外周作用。培维索孟适用于接受最大剂量 SRL 治疗后 IGF- I 水平仍持续升高的患者。该药在肢端肥大症患者中具有很好的疗效，能使 97% 患者的 IGF- I 水平正常化；25% 的患者用药后出现一过性肝酶水平升高，肿瘤体积增大的发生率不足 2%。在启动培维索孟治疗后，GH 水平通常会升高，且对指导治疗不再有帮助。

卡麦角林是治疗肢端肥大症最有效的多巴胺受体激动剂，但仅对不足 10% 的患者有效，治疗同时分泌 PRL 和 GH 的肿瘤的效果最好。

促甲状腺激素
定义

TSH 是由垂体前叶促甲状腺激素细胞分泌的一种糖蛋白。它由 α 亚基和 β 亚基组成，β 亚基赋予其特定的生物学活性。TSH 的释放受 TRH（刺激）和生长抑素（抑制）的调节。此外，TSH 受甲状腺释放的甲状腺激素的负反馈调节。评估垂体 - 甲状腺轴需要检测 TSH 水平和由甲状腺释放的甲状腺激素［即甲状腺素（T_4）和三碘甲状腺原氨酸（T_3）］。

TSH 缺乏

定义和流行病学　TSH 缺乏会导致继发性甲状腺功能减退症。垂体分泌 TSH 减少，从而不能有效刺激甲状腺释放甲状腺激素。TSH 缺乏的估计患病率为 1/（80 000 ～ 120 000）。TSH 缺乏的常见病因见表 1.4。

临床表现　甲状腺功能减退症的常见症状和体征包括体重增加、疲劳、畏寒和便秘。若 TSH 缺乏是由鞍区肿瘤引起，可能还会出现肿瘤占位症状，这取决于肿瘤大小。

Diagnosis and differential diagnosis. Secondary hypothyroidism is characterized by low levels of free T_4 along with low or inappropriately normal TSH. The differential diagnosis includes euthyroid sick syndrome, which is often seen in the setting of an acute illness. This syndrome does not require any intervention, and the laboratory results normalize on repeat testing after resolution of the acute illness.

Treatment and prognosis. Management focuses on replacement of the thyroid hormones, as in primary hypothyroidism. However, measurement of free T_4, rather than TSH, is used as a guide to adjust therapy. Underlying adrenal insufficiency should always be excluded and treated before treatment of secondary hypothyroidism to avoid precipitating an adrenal crisis.

TSH-Secreting Pituitary Tumors

Definition and epidemiology. TSH-secreting pituitary tumors are rare and are characterized by inappropriate release of TSH that is refractory to the negative feedback mechanism of the thyroid hormones released by the thyroid gland. The prevalence of TSH-secreting pituitary adenomas is 1 to 2 cases per million in the general population. The pathogenesis of TSH-secreting pituitary tumors is unknown.

Clinical presentation. The most common age of presentation is in the early fifth decade, and there is no gender predilection. Presenting symptoms can be the result of a mass effect of the tumor or, most commonly, there are symptoms and signs of hyperthyroidism, including weight loss, tremors, heat intolerance, and diarrhea. Diffuse goiter is observed in up to 80% of patients. Many times, these tumors are initially misdiagnosed as primary hyperthyroidism and patients are mistakenly treated with radioactive iodine. Sometimes, the TSH produced by these tumors is biologically inactive and the tumors are diagnosed as an incidental finding on imaging studies.

Diagnosis and differential diagnosis. The diagnosis is made in the setting of elevated or inappropriately normal TSH and alpha subunit along with elevated levels of thyroid hormones (free and total T_4 and T_3). The differential diagnosis includes genetic resistance to thyroid hormone and euthyroid hyperthyroxinemia, which is characterized by normal TSH, high total T_4, normal free T_4, and elevated thyroxine-binding globulin levels. Imaging studies (MRI) should be done only after biochemical confirmation because of the high incidence of incidental pituitary tumors.

Treatment and prognosis. Surgery (transsphenoidal resection) is the first-line treatment. Radiotherapy can be used if surgery is declined or contraindicated, but normalization of thyroid hormones can take years. Medical therapy with somatostatin analogues (e.g., octreotide, lanreotide) is used for first-line drug treatment for persistent hyperthyroidism after surgery. Most patients on SRLs achieve control of symptoms of thyrotoxicosis through normalization of thyroid function as well as reduction in tumor burden.

Adrenocorticotropic Hormone

ACTH is a 39-amino-acid peptide hormone that is formed from a precursor molecule, pro-opiomelanocortin (POMC) and is synthesized and secreted by corticotrophs in the anterior pituitary. It is stimulated by hypothalamic corticotropin-releasing hormone (CRH). ACTH, in turn, stimulates release of glucocorticoids and androgens from the adrenal cortex.

ACTH Deficiency

Definition. ACTH deficiency causes secondary adrenal insufficiency leading to decreased cortisol and adrenal androgens. Aldosterone secretion from the adrenal glands is not impaired because it is maintained via the renin-angiotensin axis. Causes of ACTH deficiency can be found in Table 1.4. Central (secondary and tertiary) adrenal insufficiency is most commonly iatrogenic, caused by the use of steroids for other disease processes.

Clinical presentation. Both primary and central adrenal insufficiency are characterized by weight loss, fatigue, muscle weakness, orthostatic symptoms, nausea, vomiting, diarrhea, and abdominal pain. Biochemical abnormalities include hyponatremia, hypoglycemia, eosinophilia, and anemia. Importantly, hyperpigmentation of the skin and hyperkalemia are seen only with primary adrenal insufficiency, not with ACTH deficiency.

Diagnosis and differential diagnosis. Typically, an 8 AM fasting serum cortisol greater than 10 mcg/dL suggests against adrenal insufficiency whereas a value less than 3 mcg/dL is strongly suggestive of adrenal insufficiency. An inappropriately low morning cortisol and ACTH likely suggests secondary adrenal insufficiency. Many times, it is appropriate to perform an ACTH stimulation test. This test measures the cortisol response to synthetic ACTH or cosyntropin. ACTH and cortisol levels are measured at baseline, followed by cortisol levels at 30 and 60 minutes. A peak plasma cortisol level higher than 14 mcg/dL by liquid chromatography tandem mass spectrometry (LC-MS/MS) is considered a normal response. It is important to keep in mind that if secondary adrenal insufficiency is recent, the adrenal glands may initially respond appropriately to cosyntropin because they have not had time to atrophy.

Treatment. Glucocorticoid therapy in the form of hydrocortisone (10 mg in AM and 5 mg in PM) or prednisone (5 to 7.5 mg/day) should be initiated for replacement. Patient education regarding stress dosing of steroids is important. Mineralocorticoids are usually not needed in patients with central secondary adrenal insufficiency.

ACTH-Secreting Pituitary Tumors (Cushing's Disease)

Definition and epidemiology. ACTH-secreting pituitary tumors (by definition, Cushing's disease) account for about 80% of the cases of Cushing's syndrome; they are usually microadenomas. Cushing's syndrome includes any condition of hypercortisolism regardless of the cause. There is a female preponderance (female-to-male ratio, about 3:1). The chronic stimulation by excessive ACTH causes simple diffuse hyperplasia of the bilateral adrenal glands or sometimes multinodular hyperplasia, both leading to excessive cortisol production.

Clinical presentation. Signs and symptoms of Cushing's disease are related to the hypercortisolism and include central obesity, hirsutism, facial plethora, violaceous striae, supraclavicular and dorsocervical fat pads, and proximal muscle weakness (Fig. 1.2). Additional manifestations of Cushing's disease are type 2 diabetes mellitus, hypertension, dyslipidemia, premature coronary artery disease, osteoporosis, and hypogonadism.

Diagnosis and differential diagnosis. Three different tests are performed in combination to assess for endogenous hypercortisolism. A 24-hour urine collection may show an elevated cortisol level, but this test is not reliable in patients with renal dysfunction. A second test, the 1-mg dexamethasone suppression test, measures an 8 AM fasting cortisol level after a dose of 1 mg dexamethasone given at 11 PM the night before. Cortisol suppression to less than 1.8 µg/dL is considered a normal response. Another diagnostic test is the late-night salivary cortisol measurement, using saliva collected at 11 PM on two consecutive nights. The test relies on a normal sleep cycle. Individuals who are using inhaled or topical steroids are not good candidates because of a high rate of false-positive results. A single positive finding is not sufficient to make this diagnosis and must be repeated and confirmed by doing additional tests. Because of the potential of cyclic ACTH overproduction by these tumors, repeat testing is recommended for individuals with high clinical suspicion but negative initial testing.

诊断和鉴别诊断　继发性甲状腺功能减退症的特征是游离 T_4 水平降低，伴有 TSH 水平降低或在不适当的正常范围内。鉴别诊断包括功能正常甲状腺病综合征，常见于急性疾病状态。该综合征不需要任何干预，在急性疾病缓解后复查实验室检查指标可恢复正常。

治疗和预后　治疗重点是甲状腺激素的替代，如同原发性甲状腺功能减退症的治疗。检测游离 T_4（而非 TSH）可指导治疗方案的调整。在治疗继发性甲状腺功能减退症之前，应先排除潜在的肾上腺皮质功能减退症，避免诱发肾上腺危象。

垂体 TSH 分泌瘤

定义和流行病学　分泌 TSH 的垂体瘤较为罕见，其特征是 TSH 不适当释放，不能被甲状腺释放的甲状腺激素的负反馈调节所抑制。在普通人群中，垂体 TSH 分泌瘤的患病率为（1 ~ 2）/1 000 000。垂体 TSH 分泌瘤的发病机制尚不明确。

临床表现　最常见的发病年龄约为 40 岁，无性别差异。肿瘤占位效应可引起临床症状，甲状腺功能亢进症的症状和体征最为常见，包括体重减轻、震颤、畏热和腹泻。高达 80% 的患者可见弥漫性甲状腺肿。这些肿瘤最初经常被误诊为原发性甲状腺功能亢进症，导致患者错误地接受放射性碘治疗。这些肿瘤产生的 TSH 有时无生物活性，通常是在接受影像学检查时被偶然发现。

诊断和鉴别诊断　诊断基于 TSH 和 α 亚基水平升高或在不适当的正常范围内，同时伴有甲状腺激素（游离 T_4 和 T_3，以及总 T_4 和 T_3）水平升高。鉴别诊断包括遗传性甲状腺激素抵抗和甲状腺功能正常性高甲状腺素血症，其特征是 TSH 水平正常，总 T_4 水平升高，游离 T_4 水平正常，甲状腺素结合球蛋白水平升高。由于偶发垂体瘤的发生率较高，应仅在生化确认后再进行影像学检查（MRI）。

治疗和预后　手术（经蝶窦切除术）是一线治疗。如果患者拒绝手术或有手术禁忌证，可采用放疗，但甲状腺激素恢复正常水平可能需要数年时间。生长抑素类似物（如奥曲肽、兰瑞肽）是手术后持续甲状腺功能亢进症患者的一线治疗药物。大多数患者接受 SRL 治疗后甲状腺功能可恢复正常，且肿瘤负荷减小，进而使甲状腺毒症的症状得到控制。

促肾上腺皮质激素

ACTH 是一种含有 39 个氨基酸的肽类激素，由其前体分子阿黑皮素原（POMC）形成，并由垂体前叶促肾上腺皮质激素细胞合成和分泌。它受到下丘脑促肾上腺皮质激素释放激素（CRH）的刺激。ACTH 可刺激肾上腺皮质释放糖皮质激素和雄激素。

ACTH 缺乏

定义　ACTH 缺乏可引起继发性肾上腺皮质功能不全，导致皮质醇和肾上腺雄激素水平降低。由于醛固酮水平是通过肾素－血管紧张素轴来维持，因此肾上腺分泌醛固酮不受影响。ACTH 缺乏的原因见表 1.4。中枢性（继发性和三发性）肾上腺皮质功能不全最常由医源性病因（治疗其他疾病使用类固醇激素）所致。

临床表现　原发性和中枢性肾上腺皮质功能不全的特征是体重减轻、疲劳、肌无力、直立性症状、恶心、呕吐、腹泻和腹痛。生化检查异常包括低钠血症、低血糖、嗜酸性粒细胞增多症和贫血。重要的是，皮肤色素沉着和高钾血症仅见于原发性肾上腺皮质功能不全，而不是 ACTH 缺乏的表现。

诊断和鉴别诊断　一般情况下，08:00 空腹血清皮质醇 > 10 μg/dl 通常不支持诊断肾上腺皮质功能不全，< 3 μg/dl 则强烈提示肾上腺皮质功能不全。晨起皮质醇和 ACTH 降低可能提示继发性肾上腺皮质功能不全。大多数患者应采用 ACTH 刺激试验。该试验旨在检测皮质醇对合成的 ACTH 或促皮质素的反应。具体方法是测定基线 ACTH 和皮质醇水平，随后在 30 min 和 60 min 检测皮质醇水平。采用液相色谱串联质谱法（LC-MS/MS）测定的血浆皮质醇峰值 > 14 μg/dl 被认为是正常反应。需谨记，如果继发性肾上腺皮质功能不全是近期发生的，肾上腺对促皮质素的最初反应可以是正常的，因为肾上腺还没开始萎缩。

治疗　糖皮质激素治疗的起始方案可选择氢化可的松（上午 10 mg，下午 5 mg）或泼尼松（5 ~ 7.5 mg/d）。有关应激剂量糖皮质激素治疗的患者教育非常重要。继发性肾上腺皮质功能不全患者通常不需要服用盐皮质激素。

垂体 ACTH 分泌瘤（库欣病）

定义和流行病学　垂体 ACTH 分泌瘤（被定义为库欣病）约占库欣综合征病例的 80%；它们通常为微腺瘤。库欣综合征包括各种原因导致的皮质醇增多症。该病多见于女性（女性：男性约为 3：1）。过量 ACTH 的长期刺激可引起双侧肾上腺单纯弥漫性增生或多结节样增生，两者均会导致皮质醇分泌过多。

临床表现　库欣病的症状和体征与皮质醇增多症有关，包括向心性肥胖、多毛、面部多血质、皮肤紫纹、锁骨上和颈背脂肪垫，以及近端肌无力（图 1.2）。库欣病的其他表现包括 2 型糖尿病、高血压、血脂异常、早发冠状动脉疾病、骨质疏松症和性腺功能减退症。

诊断和鉴别诊断　应联合 3 种检测来评估内源性皮质醇增多症。24 h 尿液检测可能显示皮质醇水平升高，但该试验对于肾功能不全的患者并不可靠。第二项检测是 1 mg 地塞米松抑制试验，于前 1 日 23:00 给予 1 mg 地塞米松，08:00 检测空腹血皮质醇水平。皮质醇被抑制至 < 1.8 μg/dl 被认为是正常反应。另一项诊断性检查是午夜唾液皮质醇测定，连续两天 23:00 采集唾液进行检测。这项检查依赖于正常的睡眠周期。吸入或局部使用类固醇的患者不适用该检测，因其假阳性率很高。单项检查的阳性结果不足以做出诊断，必须重复检测并通过额外的检查来确认。由于这些肿瘤过量分泌 ACTH 具有潜在的周期性，推荐对临床上高度怀疑但初始检测结果阴性的患者进行重复检测。

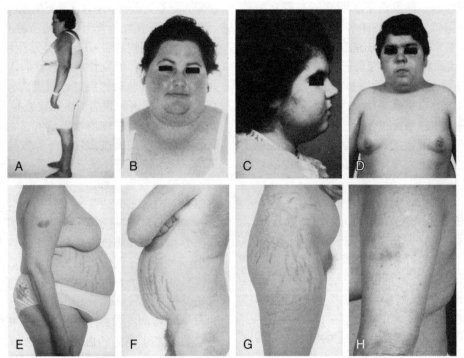

Fig. 1.2 Clinical features of Cushing's syndrome. (A) Centripetal and some generalized obesity and dorsal kyphosis in a 30-year-old woman with Cushing's disease. (B) Moon facies, plethora, hirsutism, and enlarged supraclavicular fat pads in the same woman as in A. (C) Facial rounding, hirsutism, and acne in a 14-year-old girl with Cushing's disease. (D) Central and generalized obesity and moon facies in a 14-year-old boy with Cushing's disease. Typical centripetal obesity with livid abdominal striae in a 41-year-old woman (E) and a 40-year-old man (F) with Cushing's disease. (G) Striae in a 24-year-old patient with congenital adrenal hyperplasia treated with excessive doses of dexamethasone as replacement therapy. (H) Typical bruising and thin skin of a patient with Cushing's disease. In this case, the bruising has occurred without obvious injury. (From Larsen PR, Kronenberg H, Melmed S, et al: Williams Textbook of Endocrinology, ed 10, Philadelphia, 2003, Saunders.)

Pathologic hypercortisolism should be differentiated from physiologic activation of the hypothalamic-pituitary-adrenal axis or pseudo-Cushing's syndrome, which can be observed in conditions such as critical illness, eating disorders, alcoholism, pregnancy, severe neuropsychiatric illness, and poorly controlled diabetes. The desmopressin (DDAVP) stimulation test may be useful to distinguish patients with Cushing's disease from those with pseudo-Cushing's syndrome. Further, pathologic hypercortisolism can be ACTH dependent or independent. Once the diagnosis of ACTH-dependent hypercortisolism is established, a pituitary MRI should be performed looking for a corticotroph adenoma; however, 40% to 45% of ACTH-secreting pituitary tumors are not seen on MRI. In those cases with no or small pituitary tumors and ACTH-dependent Cushing's syndrome, inferior petrosal sinus sampling (IPSS) for ACTH with CRH stimulation differentiates between pituitary and ectopic ACTH overproduction by demonstrating a pituitary-to-peripheral ACTH gradient.

Treatment and prognosis. The treatment involves removal of the pituitary tumor by an experienced neurosurgeon. Options after a failed resection include reoperation, bilateral adrenalectomy, radiotherapy, or pharmacotherapy. Pharmacotherapeutic agents include ketoconazole, metyrapone, mitotane, cabergoline, pasireotide, and mifepristone. In severe cases, intravenous etomidate may be used to stabilize patients for surgery. Long-term remission after resection of a pituitary microadenoma ranges from 69% to 98%, with a recurrence rate of 3% to 19%.

Gonadotropins
Definition

The two gonadotropins, LH and FSH, are glycoprotein hormones that are synthesized and secreted by gonadotrophs in the anterior pituitary. They are both composed of an alpha and a beta subunit, the latter of which gives each its specific biologic function. These hormones bind to the receptors in the gonads (ovaries and testes) and modulate gonadal function. Secretion is regulated both by gonadotropin-releasing hormone (GnRH) from the hypothalamus and by feedback from circulating sex steroids (estrogen and testosterone).

Gonadotropin Deficiency (Hypogonadotropic Hypogonadism)

Definition. Hypogonadotropic hypogonadism is characterized by low levels of sex steroids (estrogen or testosterone) along with low or inappropriately normal FSH and LH.

Clinical presentation. Signs and symptoms depend on the time of onset and the extent of gonadotropin deficiency. If deficiency occurs during fetal life, it can cause ambiguous genitalia. If deficiency occurs after birth but before puberty, it can cause delayed or absent sexual development. Onset after puberty causes menstrual disturbances in women and sexual dysfunction and gynecomastia in men. Osteoporosis and infertility can be present in both sexes.

Diagnosis and differential diagnosis. The diagnosis is made by the presence of low or inappropriately normal FSH and LH levels along with low sex steroids (estrogen or testosterone). Causes of gonadotropin deficiency can be congenital (Kallman syndrome,

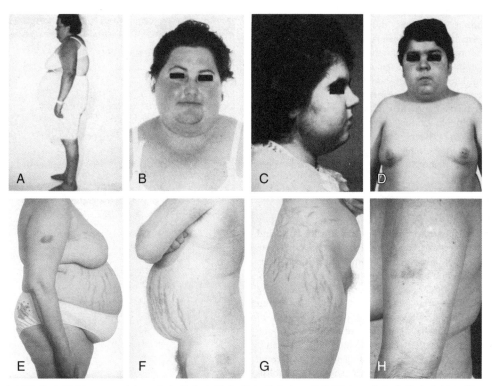

图 1.2　库欣综合征的临床特征。**A**. 一例 30 岁库欣病女性患者表现为向心性肥胖和一些部位的全身性肥胖，以及背侧后凸。**B**. 图 A 同一患者表现为满月脸、多血质、多毛和锁骨上脂肪垫增厚。**C**. 一例 14 岁库欣病女性患者表现为面部圆润、多毛和痤疮。**D**. 一例 14 岁库欣病男性患者表现为向心性肥胖和全身性肥胖、满月脸。**E**. 一例 41 岁女性患者表现为典型向心性肥胖和腹部紫纹。**F**. 一例 40 岁库欣病男性患者表现为典型向心性肥胖和腹部紫纹。**G**. 一例 24 岁先天性肾上腺皮质增生症患者服用过量地塞米松进行替代治疗后出现的紫纹。**H**. 库欣病患者典型的瘀斑和皮肤菲薄，在这种情况下，可在没有明显受伤时发生瘀斑（引自 Larsen PR，Kronenberg H，Melmed S，et al：Williams Textbook of Endocrinology，ed 10，Philadelphia，2003，Saunders.）

　　病理性皮质醇增多症应与下丘脑 – 垂体 – 肾上腺轴的生理性激活或假性库欣综合征区分开来，后者可见于危重疾病、进食障碍、酗酒、妊娠、严重神经精神疾病和控制不佳的糖尿病。去氨加压素（DDAVP）刺激试验可用于鉴别库欣病与假性库欣综合征。此外，病理性皮质醇增多症可为 ACTH 依赖性或非 ACTH 依赖性。一旦确诊为 ACTH 依赖性皮质醇增多症，应进行垂体 MRI 检查寻找垂体 ACTH 分泌瘤；然而，40% ～ 45% 的垂体 ACTH 分泌瘤在 MRI 上不可见。在未发现或垂体瘤较小的 ACTH 依赖性库欣综合征患者中，可采用岩下窦取血（IPSS）检测 ACTH 对 CRH 刺激的反应，并通过垂体 – 外周 ACTH 梯度来区分垂体和异位过量分泌 ACTH。

　　治疗和预后　治疗包括由经验丰富的神经外科医生切除垂体瘤。手术切除失败后的选择包括再次手术、双侧肾上腺切除术、放疗或药物治疗。药物治疗包括酮康唑、美替拉酮、米托坦、卡麦角林、帕瑞肽和米非司酮。在严重病例中，静脉注射依托咪酯可用于稳定病情，以利于后续手术。垂体微腺瘤切除术后的长期缓解率为 69% ～ 98%，复发率为3% ～ 19%。

促性腺激素
定义
　　两种促性腺激素——LH 和 FSH，是由垂体前叶促性腺激素细胞合成和分泌的糖蛋白激素。它们均由 α 亚基和 β 亚基组成，后者赋予其各自特定的生物学功能。这些激素与性腺（卵巢和睾丸）中的受体结合，调节性腺功能。LH 和 FSH 的分泌受下丘脑促性腺激素释放激素（GnRH）和循环中类固醇性激素（雌激素和睾酮）的反馈调节。

促性腺激素缺乏（低促性腺激素性性腺功能减退症）
　　定义　低促性腺激素性性腺功能减退症的特征是类固醇性激素（雌激素或睾酮）水平降低，伴随 FSH 和 LH 降低或在不适当的正常范围内。

　　临床表现　体征和症状取决于起病时间和促性腺激素缺乏的程度。如果促性腺激素缺乏发生在胎儿期，可能导致外生殖器模糊；如果发生在出生后至青春期前，可导致性征发育延迟或不发育。青春期后起病可导致女性月经紊乱，男性出现性功能障碍和男性乳房发育。骨质疏松症和不孕症可见于男性和女性患者。

　　诊断和鉴别诊断　诊断基于 FSH 和 LH 水平降低或在不适当的正常范围，并伴有类固醇性激素（雌激素或睾酮）水平降低。促性腺激素缺乏的病因包括先天性疾

Prader-Willi syndrome, septo-optic dysplasia) or acquired, as in hemochromatosis, hyperprolactinemia, sellar tumors, cranial irradiation, and inflammatory and infiltrative disorders.

Treatment and prognosis. For women, replacement therapy in the form of oral or transdermal estrogen should be continued until the age of natural menopause. Progesterone is essential in women with an intact uterus to prevent endometrial hyperplasia. For men, testosterone replacement is available in multiple forms, including injections, implantable pellets, several gels, and a patch. Exogenous testosterone does not restore fertility and in fact inhibits spermatogenesis. For both men and women, fertility treatment requires the use of gonadotropin therapy.

Gonadotropin-Secreting Pituitary Tumors

Definition and epidemiology. Gonadotropin-secreting pituitary tumors are considered nonfunctional. They are usually large and known as the most common macroadenoma. These tumors can secrete FSH, LH, and/or alpha subunit. Nonfunctioning pituitary adenomas are the second most common pituitary adenoma after prolactinomas. They have a prevalence of 7 to 22 per 100,000 population.

Diagnosis and differential diagnosis. Gonadotropin-secreting pituitary tumors typically manifest with signs and symptoms of mass effect. Patients can also have symptoms of pituitary hormone deficiencies. Hormonal evaluation reveals elevated FSH, LH, and/or alpha subunit in the absence of low estrogen or testosterone. Immunoperoxidase staining on tumor tissue is also needed to establish the diagnosis, especially as seen in postmenopausal women when gonadotropins are appropriately elevated.

Treatment and prognosis. Primary treatment is transsphenoidal surgical removal, which is generally successful. Radiation therapy may be used as an adjunct treatment because of the larger size of these tumors at diagnosis. Medical therapy is not used because no effective therapy exists.

DISORDERS OF POSTERIOR PITUITARY HORMONES

AVP and oxytocin are the two hormones that are produced in the hypothalamus and stored in and released from the posterior pituitary.

Diabetes Insipidus
Definition
Diabetes insipidus (DI) is characterized by AVP deficiency and excretion of large volumes of dilute urine. Central DI (posterior pituitary in origin) can be familial due to an autosomal dominant mutation in the vasopressin gene that affects the functioning of the AVP-producing neurons. It can also be acquired secondary to intrasellar and suprasellar tumors, infiltration of the hypothalamus and posterior pituitary, infection, trauma or surgery, or as part of an autoimmune condition. Table 1.7 gives a more extensive list of causes of diabetes insipidus.

Clinical Presentation
Polyuria (defined as excretion of more than 3 L of urine per day) and polydipsia are the clinical hallmarks of DI.

Diagnosis and Differential Diagnosis
DI can be central, caused by AVP deficiency, or nephrogenic, caused by resistance to AVP. As long as access to free water is maintained and the thirst mechanism is intact, patients with DI are usually able to maintain normal serum sodium levels and osmolality. The water deprivation test is the primary test used to make the

TABLE 1.7	Causes of Diabetes Insipidus
Central Diabetes Insipidus	
Idiopathic	
Familial	
Hypophysectomy	
Infiltration of hypothalamus and posterior pituitary	
Langerhans cell histiocytosis	
Granulomas	
Infection	
Tumors (intrasellar and suprasellar)	
Autoimmune	
Nephrogenic Diabetes Insipidus	
Idiopathic	
Familial	
V_2 receptor gene mutation	
Aquaporin-2 gene mutation	
Chronic renal disease (e.g., chronic pyelonephritis, polycystic kidney disease, or medullary cystic disease)	
Hypokalemia	
Hypercalcemia	
Sickle cell anemia	
Drugs	
Lithium	
Fluoride	
Demeclocycline	
Colchicine	

diagnosis and to differentiate the cause of DI. In patients with DI, the serum sodium level and osmolality increase in response to water deprivation. The response to a synthetic analogue of vasopressin is analyzed if the normal rise in urine osmolality and decrease in urine volume are not seen. Patients with central DI respond to the synthetic analogue by increasing urine osmolality and decreasing urine volume. In contrast, patients with nephrogenic DI do not respond to the synthetic vasopressin. Patients with partial central DI may have a limited response. Primary polydipsia is characterized by increased water intake without a deficiency or resistance to AVP. Patients with primary polydipsia concentrate their urine without the need for synthetic vasopressin. Copeptin, also derived from arginine vasopressin prohormone, is recently being studied as an arginine vasopressin surrogate to differentiate central and nephrogenic DI and primary polydipsia, using a direct measurement of hypertonic saline-stimulated plasma copeptin rather than the indirect water deprivation test.

Treatment
Replacement therapy with DDAVP, an analogue of AVP, is available in oral (desmopressin), parenteral, and intranasal forms. Aqueous vasopressin is a shorter-acting analogue of AVP that can be given subcutaneously in the immediate postoperative period. Because of the transient nature of DI and a possible shift to a transient syndrome of inappropriate secretion of antidiuretic hormone (SIADH) phase in the patient who has undergone pituitary surgery, AVP is given cautiously and not as a scheduled medication in order to avoid hyponatremia.

Syndrome of Inappropriate Secretion of Antidiuretic Hormone

SIADH is covered in the discussion of hyponatremia in "Renal Disease" Chapter 3.

病［卡尔曼综合征（Kallman 综合征）、Prader-Willi 综合征、视隔发育不良］和获得性疾病（如血色病、高催乳素血症、鞍区肿瘤、颅脑照射、炎症性和浸润性疾病）。

治疗和预后　对于女性患者，口服或透皮雌激素替代治疗应持续至自然绝经。对于子宫完整的女性，黄体酮是防止子宫内膜增生所必需的治疗。对于男性患者，睾酮替代治疗有多种形式，包括注射、可植入颗粒、多种凝胶和贴片。外源性睾酮不能恢复生育能力，实际上会抑制精子生成。对于男性和女性患者，生育治疗都需要采用促性腺激素治疗。

垂体促性腺激素分泌瘤

定义和流行病学　垂体促性腺激素分泌瘤被认为是无功能的。它们通常体积很大，是最常见的大腺瘤。这些肿瘤可分泌 FSH、LH 和（或）α 亚基。无功能垂体瘤是第二大垂体瘤，仅次于催乳素瘤。无功能垂体瘤的患病率为（7 ～ 22）/100 000。

诊断和鉴别诊断　垂体促性腺激素分泌瘤的典型表现为肿物占位效应引起的体征和症状。患者还可出现垂体激素缺乏的症状。激素评估可显示在雌激素或睾酮水平并未降低的情况下，FSH、LH 和（或）α 亚基水平升高。需要对肿瘤组织采用免疫过氧化物酶染色以确定诊断，特别是在促性腺激素水平升高的绝经后女性中。

治疗和预后　首选治疗是经蝶窦手术切除，手术成功率高。由于肿瘤在诊断时体积较大，可选择放疗作为辅助治疗。该病缺乏有效药物，故不采用药物治疗。

垂体后叶激素异常

AVP 和催产素是下丘脑产生的两种激素，储存在垂体后叶并从垂体后叶释放。

尿崩症
定义

尿崩症（DI）以 AVP 缺乏和排出大量稀释性尿液为特征。中枢性 DI（起源于垂体后叶）可为家族性，由抗利尿激素基因的常染色体显性突变所致，可影响合成 AVP 的神经元功能。中枢性 DI 也可继发于鞍内和鞍上肿瘤、下丘脑和垂体后叶浸润性疾病、感染、创伤或手术，或作为自身免疫病的一部分。DI 的病因总结于表 1.7。

临床表现

多尿（定义为每天排尿量＞ 3 L）和烦渴是 DI 的临床标志。

诊断和鉴别诊断

DI 包括由 AVP 缺乏导致的中枢性 DI 和由 AVP 抵抗

表 1.7　尿崩症的病因
中枢性尿崩症
特发性
家族性
垂体切除术
下丘脑和垂体后叶浸润性疾病
朗格汉斯细胞组织细胞增生症
肉芽肿
感染
肿瘤（鞍内和鞍上）
自身免疫
肾性尿崩症
特发性
家族性
V_2 受体基因突变
水通道蛋白 -2 基因突变
慢性肾脏病（如慢性肾盂肾炎、多囊肾病或肾髓质囊性病）
低钾血症
高钙血症
镰状细胞贫血
药物
锂剂
氟化物
地美环素
秋水仙碱

引起的肾性 DI。只要能获取自由水且口渴机制保持完好，DI 患者通常能维持正常的血钠水平和血浆渗透压。禁水试验是诊断和鉴别 DI 的首选试验。在禁水后，DI 患者的血钠水平和血浆渗透压会升高。如果未出现尿渗透压升高和尿量减少，需要分析患者对合成血管升压素类似物的反应。中枢性 DI 患者对合成血管升压素类似物的反应是尿渗透压升高且尿量减少。相比之下，肾性 DI 患者对合成血管升压素不会产生反应。部分性中枢性 DI 患者可能会有轻度反应。原发性烦渴的特征是水摄入增加但无 AVP 缺乏或抵抗。原发性烦渴患者不需要合成血管升压素也可浓缩尿液。和肽素也来源于精氨酸加压素激素原，近期被研究作为精氨酸加压素的替代物用于鉴别中枢性和肾性 DI 及原发性烦渴，可在使用高渗盐水刺激后直接测量血浆和肽素而不再采用间接禁水试验。

治疗

DDAVP（AVP 类似物）替代治疗包括口服、肠外给药和鼻内给药。水溶性血管升压素是一种短效 AVP 类似物，可在术后即刻进行皮下注射。在接受过垂体手术的患者中，由于 DI 的一过性特征，以及可能转变为一过性抗利尿激素分泌失调综合征（SIADH），AVP 需谨慎给予且不能作为常规用药，以避免发生低钠血症。

抗利尿激素分泌失调综合征

SIADH 在《肾脏疾病分册》第 3 章 "低钠血症" 中进行讨论。

SUGGESTED READINGS

Biller BM, Grossman AB, Stewart PM, et al: Treatment of adrenocorticotropin-dependent Cushing's syndrome: a consensus statement, J Clin Endocrinol Metab 93:2454–2462, 2008.

Dichtel LE, Yuen KCJ, Bredella MA, et al: Overweight/obese adults with pituitary disorders require lower peak growth hormone cutoff values on glucagon stimulation testing to avoid overdiagnosis of growth hormone deficiency, J Clin Endocrinol Metab 99(12):4712–4719, 2014.

Fenske W, Refardt J, Chifu I, et al: A copeptin-based approach in the diagnosis of diabetes insipidus, N Engl J Med 379(5):428–439, 2018.

Fleseriu M, Petersenn S: Medical management of Cushing's disease: what is the future? Pituitary 15:330–341, 2012.

Freda P, Beckers A, Katznelson L, et al: Pituitary incidentaloma: an Endocrine Society clinical practice guideline, J Clin Endocrinol Metab 96:894–904, 2011.

Melmed S, Casanueva F, Hoffman A, et al: Diagnosis and treatment of hyperprolactinemia: an Endocrine Society clinical practice guideline, J Clin Endocrinol Metab 96:273–288, 2011.

Melmed S, Colao A, Barkan A, et al: Guidelines for acromegaly management: an update, J Clin Endocrinol Metab 94:1509–1517, 2009.

Melmed S: Medical progress: acromegaly, N Engl J Med 355:2558–2573, 2006.

Melmed S: The pituitary, ed 4, 2017, Elsevier.

Nieman L, Biller B, Findling J, et al: The diagnosis of Cushing's syndrome: an Endocrine Society clinical practice guideline, J Clin Endocrinol Metab 93:1526–1540, 2008.

Swearingen B, Biller B: Diagnosis and management of pituitary disorders, New York, 2008, Humana Press.

Ueland GÅ, Methlie P, Øksnes M, et al: The short cosyntropin test revisited: new normal reference range using LC-MS/MS, J Clin Endocrinol Metab 103(4):1696–1703, 2018.

推荐阅读

Biller BM, Grossman AB, Stewart PM, et al: Treatment of adrenocorticotropin-dependent Cushing's syndrome: a consensus statement, J Clin Endocrinol Metab 93:2454–2462, 2008.

Dichtel LE, Yuen KCJ, Bredella MA, et al: Overweight/obese adults with pituitary disorders require lower peak growth hormone cutoff values on glucagon stimulation testing to avoid overdiagnosis of growth hormone deficiency, J Clin Endocrinol Metab 99(12):4712–4719, 2014.

Fenske W, Refardt J, Chifu I, et al: A copeptin-based approach in the diagnosis of diabetes insipidus, N Engl J Med 379(5):428–439, 2018.

Fleseriu M, Petersenn S: Medical management of Cushing's disease: what is the future? Pituitary 15:330–341, 2012.

Freda P, Beckers A, Katznelson L, et al: Pituitary incidentaloma: an Endocrine Society clinical practice guideline, J Clin Endocrinol Metab 96:894–904, 2011.

Melmed S, Casanueva F, Hoffman A, et al: Diagnosis and treatment of hyperprolactinemia: an Endocrine Society clinical practice guideline, J Clin Endocrinol Metab 96:273–288, 2011.

Melmed S, Colao A, Barkan A, et al: Guidelines for acromegaly management: an update, J Clin Endocrinol Metab 94:1509–1517, 2009.

Melmed S: Medical progress: acromegaly, N Engl J Med 355:2558–2573, 2006.

Melmed S: The pituitary, ed 4, 2017, Elsevier.

Nieman L, Biller B, Findling J, et al: The diagnosis of Cushing's syndrome: an Endocrine Society clinical practice guideline, J Clin Endocrinol Metab 93:1526–1540, 2008.

Swearingen B, Biller B: Diagnosis and management of pituitary disorders, New York, 2008, Humana Press.

Ueland GÅ, Methlie P, Øksnes M, et al: The short cosyntropin test revisited: new normal reference range using LC-MS/MS, J Clin Endocrinol Metab 103(4):1696–1703, 2018.

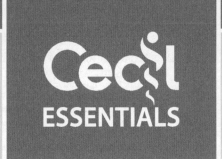

2

Thyroid Gland

Theodore C. Friedman

INTRODUCTION

The thyroid gland secretes thyroxine (T_4) and triiodothyronine (T_3), both of which modulate energy utilization and heat production and facilitate growth. The gland consists of two lateral lobes joined by an isthmus. The weight of the adult gland is 10 to 20 g. Microscopically, the thyroid is composed of several follicles that contain colloid surrounded by a single layer of thyroid epithelium. The follicular cells synthesize thyroglobulin, which is stored as colloid. Biosynthesis of T_4 and T_3 occurs by iodination of tyrosine molecules in thyroglobulin.

THYROID HORMONE PHYSIOLOGY

Thyroid Hormone Synthesis

Dietary iodine is essential for the synthesis of thyroid hormones. Iodine, after conversion to iodide in the stomach, is rapidly absorbed from the gastrointestinal tract. After active transport from the bloodstream across the follicular cell basement membrane, iodide is enzymatically oxidized by thyroid peroxidase, which also mediates the iodination of the tyrosine residues in thyroglobulin, to form monoiodotyrosine and diiodotyrosine. The iodotyrosine molecules couple to form T_4 (3,5,3′,5′-tetraiodothyronine) or T_3 (3,5,3′-triiodothyronine). Once iodinated, thyroglobulin containing newly formed T_4 and T_3 is stored in the follicles. Secretion of free T_4 and T_3 into the circulation occurs after proteolytic digestion of thyroglobulin, which is stimulated by thyroid-stimulating hormone (TSH). Deiodination of monoiodotyrosine and diiodotyrosine by iodotyrosine deiodinase releases iodine, which then reenters the thyroid iodine pool.

Thyroid Hormone Transport

T_4 and T_3 are tightly bound to the serum carrier proteins thyroxine-binding globulin (TBG), thyroxine-binding prealbumin, and albumin. The unbound or free fractions are the biologically active fractions; they represent only 0.04% of the total T_4 and 0.4% of the total T_3.

Peripheral Metabolism of Thyroid Hormones

The normal thyroid gland secretes T_4, T_3, and reverse T_3, a biologically inactive form of T_3. Most of the circulating T_3 is derived from deiodination of circulating T_4 in the peripheral tissues. Deiodination of T_4 can occur at the outer ring (5′-deiodination), producing T_3 (3,5,3′-triiodothyronine), or at the inner ring (5-deiodination), producing reverse T_3 (3,3,5′-triiodothyronine).

Control of Thyroid Function

Hypothalamic thyrotropin-releasing hormone (TRH) is transported through the hypothalamic-hypophyseal portal system to the thyrotrophs of the anterior pituitary gland, stimulating synthesis and release of TSH (Fig. 2.1). TSH, in turn, increases thyroidal iodide uptake and iodination of thyroglobulin, releases T_3 and T_4 from the thyroid gland by increasing hydrolysis of thyroglobulin, and stimulates thyroid cell growth. Hypersecretion of TSH results in thyroid enlargement (goiter). Circulating T_3 exerts negative feedback inhibition of TRH and TSH release.

Physiologic Effects of Thyroid Hormones

Thyroid hormones increase the basal metabolic rate by increasing oxygen consumption and heat production in several body tissues. Thyroid hormones also have specific effects on several organ systems (Table 2.1). These effects are exaggerated in hyperthyroidism and reduced in hypothyroidism, accounting for the well-recognized signs and symptoms of these two disorders.

THYROID EVALUATION

A careful thyroid examination is essential in evaluating a patient with thyroid disease. Thyroid gland function and structure can be evaluated by (1) determining serum thyroid hormone levels, (2) imaging thyroid gland size and architecture, (3) measuring thyroid autoantibodies, and (4) performing a thyroid gland biopsy by fine-needle aspiration (FNA).

Tests of Serum Thyroid Hormone Levels

Measurements of total serum T_4 and total T_3 indicate the total amount of hormone bound to thyroid-binding proteins by radioimmunoassay. Total T_4 and T_3 levels are elevated in hyperthyroidism and low in hypothyroidism. Increased production of TBG (as with pregnancy or estrogen

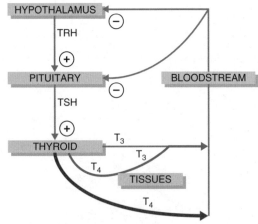

Fig. 2.1 Hypothalamic-pituitary-thyroid axis. T_4 is converted to T_3 in peripheral tissues. *T_3,* Triiodothyronine; *T_4,* thyroxine; *TRH,* thyrotropin-releasing hormone; *TSH,* thyroid-stimulating hormone.

甲状腺

李乃适　译　陈适　潘慧　审校　宁光　通审

引言

甲状腺分泌甲状腺素（T_4）和三碘甲状腺原氨酸（T_3），两者均可调节能量利用和产热，并促进生长。甲状腺由两个经峡部相连的侧叶组成。成人甲状腺的重量为 10～20 g。在显微镜下，甲状腺由含有胶质的多个滤泡组成，胶质被单层甲状腺上皮包围。滤泡细胞合成甲状腺球蛋白，并将其以胶质的形式储存。T_4 和 T_3 的生物合成通过甲状腺球蛋白中酪氨酸分子的碘化来实现。

甲状腺激素生理学

甲状腺激素的合成

膳食碘对甲状腺激素的合成至关重要。碘在胃中转化为碘化物后迅速经胃肠道吸收。从血液中通过滤泡细胞基底膜主动转运后，碘化物被甲状腺过氧化物酶氧化，后者还介导甲状腺球蛋白中酪氨酸残基的碘化，形成单碘酪氨酸和二碘酪氨酸。碘化的酪氨酸分子耦联形成 T_4（3,5,3',5'-四碘甲状腺原氨酸）或 T_3（3,5,3'-三碘甲状腺原氨酸）。一旦碘化，含有新合成的 T_4 和 T_3 的甲状腺球蛋白便会被储存在滤泡中。在促甲状腺激素（TSH）的刺激下，甲状腺球蛋白经蛋白水解消化后分泌游离 T_4 和 T_3 进入循环。单碘酪氨酸和二碘酪氨酸的脱碘由碘酪氨酸脱碘酶介导，释放出的碘会重新进入甲状腺碘池。

甲状腺激素的转运

T_4 和 T_3 紧密结合在血清载体蛋白甲状腺素结合球蛋白（TBG）、甲状腺素结合前白蛋白和白蛋白上。未结合（即游离）的部分为生物活性部分，仅占总 T_4 的 0.04% 和总 T_3 的 0.4%。

甲状腺激素的外周代谢

正常甲状腺分泌 T_4、T_3 和反 T_3（即 T_3 的一种非生物活性形式）。大多数循环 T_3 来自于外周组织中循环 T_4 的脱碘作用。T_4 的脱碘作用可发生在外环（5'-脱碘）或内环（5-脱碘），前者生成 T_3（3,5,3'-三碘甲状腺原氨酸），后者生成反 T_3（3,3,5'-三碘甲状腺原氨酸）。

甲状腺功能的调控

下丘脑的促甲状腺激素释放激素（TRH）通过下丘脑-垂体门静脉系统被输送至垂体前叶的促甲状腺激素细胞，从而刺激 TSH 的合成和释放（图 2.1）。随后，TSH 增加甲状腺对碘的摄取和甲状腺球蛋白的碘化，通过增加甲状腺球蛋白的水解促进甲状腺释放 T_3 和 T_4，并刺激甲状腺细胞的生长。TSH 的过量分泌可导致甲状腺增大（甲状腺肿）。循环中的 T_3 可通过负反馈抑制 TRH 和 TSH 的释放。

甲状腺激素的生理学效应

甲状腺激素可在机体的多个组织中通过增加耗氧量和产热来提高基础代谢率。甲状腺激素对多个器官系统有特定的影响（表 2.1）。这些影响会在甲状腺功能亢进症时增强，在甲状腺功能减退症时减弱，从而能够解释这两种疾病的典型体征和症状。

甲状腺评估

仔细的甲状腺检查对于评估甲状腺疾病患者至关重要。甲状腺功能和结构可通过以下方式评估：①检测血清甲状腺激素水平；②影像学检查评估甲状腺大小和结构；③检测甲状腺自身抗体；④通过细针穿刺抽吸（FNA）进行甲状腺活检。

血清甲状腺激素水平的检测

可通过放射免疫分析法检测血清总 T_4 和总 T_3（反映结合在甲状腺结合蛋白上的激素总量）。总 T_4 和总 T_3 水平在甲状腺功能亢进症时升高，在甲状腺功能减退症时降低。即便没有甲状腺功能亢进症，若 TBG 生成增加（如妊娠或雌激素治疗），总 T_4 和总 T_3 水平也会升高。

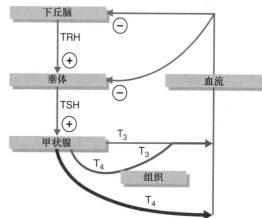

图 2.1　下丘脑-垂体-甲状腺轴。T_4 在外周组织中转化为 T_3。T_3，三碘甲状腺原氨酸；T_4，甲状腺素；TRH，促甲状腺激素释放激素；TSH，促甲状腺激素

therapy) increases the total T_4 and T_3 levels without actual hyperthyroidism. Similarly, total T_4 and T_3 are low despite euthyroidism in conditions associated with low levels of thyroid-binding proteins (e.g., congenital decrease, protein-losing enteropathy, cirrhosis, nephrotic syndrome). Therefore, further tests to assess the free hormone levels, which reflect biologic activity, must be performed. Free T_4 and free T_3 levels can be measured directly or by dialysis or ultrafiltration and have, at most institutions, replaced measuring total T_4 and T_3 levels.

Serum TSH is measured by a third-generation immunometric assay that accurately discriminates between normal TSH levels and levels below the normal range. Thus, the TSH assay can diagnose clinical hyperthyroidism (elevated free T_4 and free T_3 and suppressed TSH) and subclinical hyperthyroidism (normal free T_4 and free T_3 and suppressed TSH). In hyperthyroidism, the free T_3 may be elevated in the presence of a normal free T_4. In primary (thyroidal) hypothyroidism, serum TSH is supranormal because of diminished feedback inhibition. The TSH is usually low but may be normal in secondary (pituitary) or tertiary (hypothalamic) hypothyroidism.

Serum thyroglobulin measurements are useful in the follow-up of patients with papillary or follicular carcinoma. After thyroidectomy and iodine-131 (^{131}I) ablation therapy, thyroglobulin levels should be less than 0.5 ng/mL while the patient is on suppressive levothyroxine treatment. Levels in excess of this value indicate the possibility of persistent or metastatic disease.

Calcitonin is produced by the C cells of the thyroid and has a minor role in calcium homeostasis. Calcitonin measurements are invaluable in the diagnosis of medullary carcinoma of the thyroid and for monitoring the effects of therapy for this entity.

Thyroid Imaging

Technetium-99m (^{99m}Tc) pertechnetate is concentrated in the thyroid gland and can be scanned with a gamma camera, yielding information about the size and shape of the gland and the location of the functional activity in the gland (thyroid scan). The thyroid scan is often performed in conjunction with a quantitative assessment of radioactive iodine (^{123}I) uptake by the thyroid. Functioning thyroid nodules are called *warm* or *hot* nodules; *cold* nodules are nonfunctioning.

Malignancy is usually associated with a cold nodule; 16% of surgically removed cold nodules are malignant.

Thyroid ultrasound evaluation is useful in the differentiation of solid nodules from cystic nodules and to determine which patients should undergo an FNA. The use of thyroid ultrasounds in patients with thyroid nodules is discussed later.

Thyroid Antibodies

Autoantibodies to several different antigenic components in the thyroid gland, including thyroglobulin (TgAb), thyroid peroxidase (TPO Ab, formerly called *antimicrosomal antibodies*), and the TSH receptor, can be measured in the serum. A strongly positive test for TPO Ab indicates autoimmune thyroid disease. Elevated TSH receptor antibody occurs in Graves' disease (see later discussion).

Thyroid Biopsy

FNA of a nodule to obtain thyroid cells for cytologic evaluation is the best way to differentiate benign from malignant disease. FNA requires adequate tissue samples and interpretation by an experienced cytologist.

HYPERTHYROIDISM

Thyrotoxicosis is the clinical syndrome that results from elevated levels of circulating thyroid hormones. Clinical manifestations of thyrotoxicosis result from the direct physiologic effects of the thyroid hormones as well as the increased sensitivity to catecholamines. Tachycardia, tremor, stare, sweating, and lid lag are all caused by catecholamine hypersensitivity.

Signs and Symptoms

Table 2.2 lists the signs and symptoms of hyperthyroidism. Thyrotoxic crisis, or *thyroid storm*, is a life-threatening complication of hyperthyroidism that can be precipitated by surgery, radioactive iodine therapy, or severe stress (e.g., uncontrolled diabetes mellitus, myocardial infarction, acute infection). Patients develop fever, flushing, sweating, significant tachycardia, atrial fibrillation, and cardiac failure. Significant agitation, restlessness, delirium, and coma frequently

TABLE 2.1	Physiologic Effects of Thyroid Hormone
System	**Effects**
Cardiovascular	Increased heart rate and cardiac output
Gastrointestinal	Increased gut motility
Skeletal	Increased bone turnover and resorption
Pulmonary	Maintenance of normal hypoxic and hypercapnic drive in the respiratory center
Neuromuscular	Increased muscle protein turnover and increased speed of muscle contraction and relaxation
Metabolism of lipids and carbohydrates	Increased hepatic gluconeogenesis and glycogenolysis, as well as intestinal glucose absorption
	Increased cholesterol synthesis and degradation
	Increased lipolysis
Sympathetic nervous system	Increased numbers of β-adrenergic receptors in the heart, skeletal muscle, lymphocytes, and adipose cells
	Decreased cardiac α-adrenergic receptors
	Increased catecholamine sensitivity
Hematopoietic	Increased red blood cell 2,3-diphosphoglycerate, facilitating oxygen dissociation from hemoglobin with increased oxygen available to tissues

TABLE 2.2	Signs and Symptoms of Hyperthyroidism
Symptoms	
Palpitations	
Nervousness	
Shortness of breath	
Heat intolerance	
Fatigue and weakness	
Increased appetite	
Weight loss	
Oligomenorrhea	
Signs	
Tachycardia	
Atrial fibrillation	
Wide pulse pressure	
Brisk reflexes	
Fine tremor	
Proximal limb-girdle myopathy	
Chemosis (swelling of conjunctiva)	
Thyroid bruit (Graves' disease)	

同样，尽管甲状腺功能正常，但在甲状腺结合蛋白水平降低（如先天性减少、蛋白丢失性肠病、肝硬化、肾病综合征）的情况下，总 T_4 和总 T_3 水平也会降低。因此，必须进一步检测，以评估反映生物活性的游离甲状腺激素水平。可直接检测或通过透析或超滤检测游离 T_4 和游离 T_3 水平，这在大多数机构已取代了总 T_4 和总 T_3 水平的检测。

通过第三代免疫测定法测定血清 TSH 可以准确区分正常 TSH 水平和低于正常范围的 TSH 水平。因此，TSH 检测可诊断临床甲状腺功能亢进症（游离 T_4 和游离 T_3 水平升高，TSH 被抑制）和亚临床甲状腺功能亢进症（游离 T_4 和游离 T_3 水平正常，TSH 被抑制）。在甲状腺功能亢进症中，游离 T_3 水平可能在游离 T_4 水平正常的情况下升高。在原发性（甲状腺性）甲状腺功能减退症中，由于反馈抑制减弱，血清 TSH 水平升高。在继发性（垂体性）或三发性（下丘脑性）甲状腺功能减退症中，TSH 水平通常低于正常范围，但也可能在正常范围内。

血清甲状腺球蛋白检测可用于甲状腺乳头状癌或滤泡癌患者的随访。在甲状腺切除术和 ^{131}I 消融治疗后，患者在左甲状腺素抑制治疗期间的甲状腺球蛋白水平应 < 0.5 ng/ml，超过此水平提示肿瘤持续存在或肿瘤转移的可能。

降钙素由甲状腺 C 细胞产生，在钙稳态中发挥一定作用。降钙素检测在甲状腺髓样癌的诊断和治疗效果监测中非常有价值。

甲状腺成像

锝 -99m（^{99m}Tc）高锝酸盐可在甲状腺中富集，经伽马照相扫描可获得关于甲状腺大小、形态及甲状腺功能活性区域的定位信息（甲状腺扫描）。甲状腺扫描常与甲状腺放射性碘（^{123}I）摄取的定量评估同时进行。功能性甲状腺结节又称温结节或热结节；冷结节为非功能性。恶性肿瘤通常伴有冷结节；手术切除的冷结节中 16% 为恶性。

甲状腺超声可用于鉴别实性结节和囊性结节，并有助于确定哪些患者应进行 FNA。关于甲状腺超声在甲状腺结节患者中应用的内容详见下文。

甲状腺抗体

血清中可检测到针对甲状腺腺体中不同抗原成分的自身抗体，包括甲状腺球蛋白抗体（TgAb）、甲状腺过氧化物酶抗体（TPOAb；既往被称为抗微粒体抗体）和 TSH 受体。TPOAb 强阳性提示存在自身免疫性甲状腺疾病。TSH 受体抗体水平升高见于格雷夫斯病（Graves 病）（见下文）。

甲状腺活检

对甲状腺结节行 FNA 以获取甲状腺细胞进行细胞学检查是鉴别良恶性疾病的最佳方式。成功的 FNA 需要足够的组织样本并由经验丰富的细胞学专家进行解释。

甲状腺功能亢进症

甲状腺毒症是由于循环中的甲状腺激素水平升高而引起的临床综合征。甲状腺毒症的临床表现源于甲状腺激素的直接生理作用和对儿茶酚胺的敏感性增加。心动过速、震颤、凝视、出汗和眼睑下落迟滞均由对儿茶酚胺过度敏感所致。

体征和症状

表2.2 列出了甲状腺功能亢进症的体征和症状。甲状腺危象是甲状腺功能亢进症危及生命的并发症，其可能由手术，放射性碘治疗或严重应激（如未控制的糖尿病、心肌梗死、急性感染）诱发。患者可出现发热、面部潮红、出汗、明显心动过速、心房颤动和心

表 2.1　甲状腺激素的生理作用	
系统	作用
心血管	加快心率、增加心输出量
胃肠道	增加肠蠕动
骨骼	增加骨转换和吸收
肺	维持呼吸中枢的正常低氧和高二氧化碳驱动
神经肌肉	增加肌蛋白转换，加快肌肉收缩和松弛的速度
脂质和碳水化合物代谢	增加肝脏糖异生和糖原分解，增加肠道的葡萄糖吸收 增加胆固醇合成和降解 增加脂肪分解
交感神经系统	增加心脏、骨骼肌、淋巴细胞和脂肪细胞中 β 受体的数量 减少心脏中 α 受体的数量 增加对儿茶酚胺的敏感性
造血系统	增加红细胞 2,3- 二磷酸甘油酸，促进氧气与血红蛋白的解离 增加组织供氧

表 2.2　甲状腺功能亢进症的体征和症状
症状
心悸
紧张
气短
畏热
疲劳和乏力
食欲增加
体重下降
月经稀发
体征
心动过速
心房颤动
脉压差增大
反射亢进
细颤
近端肢带肌病
结膜水肿（结膜肿胀）
甲状腺杂音（Graves 病）

occur. Gastrointestinal manifestations may include nausea, vomiting, and diarrhea. Hyperpyrexia out of proportion to other clinical findings is the hallmark of thyroid storm.

Differential Diagnosis

Thyrotoxicosis usually reflects excess secretion of thyroid hormones resulting from Graves' disease, toxic adenoma, multinodular goiter, or thyroiditis (Table 2.3 and Fig. 2.2). However, it may be the result of excessive ingestion of thyroid hormone or, rarely, thyroid hormone production from an ectopic site (as in struma ovarii).

Graves' Disease

Graves' disease, the most common cause of thyrotoxicosis, is an auto-immune disease that is more common in women, with a peak incidence between 20 and 50 years of age. One or more of the following features are present: (1) goiter; (2) thyrotoxicosis; (3) eye disease ranging from tearing to proptosis, extraocular muscle paralysis, and loss of sight as a result of optic nerve involvement; and (4) thyroid dermopathy, usually observed as significant skin thickening without pitting in a pretibial distribution (*pretibial myxedema*). (Do not confuse this use of myxedema with that described below under the discussion of the clinical features of *hypothyroidism*.)

Pathogenesis. Thyrotoxicosis in Graves' disease is caused by overproduction of an antibody that binds to the TSH receptor. These thyroid-stimulating immunoglobulins increase thyroid cell growth and thyroid hormone secretion. Ophthalmopathy results from inflammatory infiltration of the extraocular eye muscles by lymphocytes with mucopolysaccharide deposition. The inflammatory reaction that contributes to the eye signs in Graves' disease may be caused by sensitization of lymphocytes to antigens that are common to the orbital muscles and the thyroid.

Clinical presentation. The common manifestations of thyrotoxicosis (see Table 2.2) are characteristic features of younger patients with Graves' disease. In addition, patients may exhibit a diffuse goiter or the eye signs characteristic of Graves' disease. Older patients often do not have the florid clinical features of thyrotoxicosis, and the condition termed *apathetic hyperthyroidism* is exhibited as flat affect, emotional lability, weight loss, muscle weakness, congestive heart failure, and atrial fibrillation resistant to standard therapy.

Eye signs associated with Graves' disease may also occur as a non-specific manifestation of hyperthyroidism from any cause (e.g., thyroid stare). In Graves' disease, a specific inflammatory infiltrate of the orbital tissues leads to periorbital edema, conjunctival congestion and swelling, proptosis, extraocular muscle weakness, or optic nerve damage with visual impairment.

Pretibial myxedema (thyroid dermopathy) occurs in 2% to 3% of patients with Graves' disease and results in a thickening of the skin over the lower tibia without pitting. Onycholysis, characterized by separation of the fingernails from their beds, often occurs in patients with Graves' disease. Thyroid acropachy, or clubbing, may also occur.

Diagnosis. Elevated total or free T_4 or T_3 (or both) and a suppressed TSH confirm the clinical diagnosis of thyrotoxicosis. TSH receptor antibody is usually elevated, and its measurement may be useful in patients with eye signs who do not have other characteristic clinical features. Increased uptake of ^{123}I differentiates Graves' disease from early subacute or Hashimoto thyroiditis, in which uptake is low in the presence of hyperthyroidism. Magnetic resonance imaging or ultrasonography of the orbit usually shows orbital muscle enlargement, whether or not clinical signs of ophthalmopathy are observed.

Treatment. Three treatment modalities are used to control the hyperthyroidism of Graves' disease: antithyroid drugs, radioactive iodine therapy, and surgery. In Europe, Latin America, and Japan, antithyroid drugs are the favored therapy while in the United States, radioactive iodine is the main therapy. However, more recently antithyroid drugs are becoming the mainstay of treatment for Graves' disease worldwide.

Antithyroid drugs. The thiocarbamide drugs propylthiouracil, methimazole, and carbimazole block thyroid hormone synthesis

TABLE 2.3	Causes of Thyrotoxicosis
Common Causes	
Graves' disease	
Toxic adenoma (solitary)	
Toxic multinodular goiter	
Less Common Causes	
Subacute thyroiditis (de Quervain or granulomatous thyroiditis)	
Hashimoto thyroiditis with transient hyperthyroid phase	
Thyrotoxicosis factitia	
Postpartum thyroiditis (probably variant of silent thyroiditis)	
Rare Causes	
Struma ovarii	
Metastatic thyroid carcinoma	
Hydatidiform mole	
TSH-secreting pituitary tumor	

TSH, Thyroid-stimulating hormone.

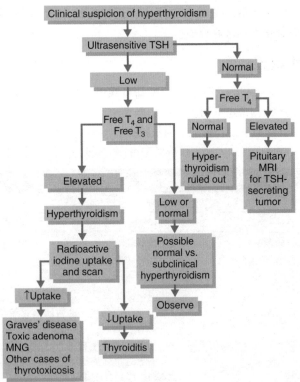

Fig. 2.2 Algorithm for differential diagnosis of hyperthyroidism. *MNG,* Multinodular goiter; *MRI,* magnetic resonance imaging; *RIA,* radioimmunoassay; T_3, triiodothyronine; T_4, thyroxine; *TSH,* thyroid-stimulating hormone.

力衰竭。常见症状还包括激越、躁动不安、谵妄和昏迷。胃肠道表现可能包括恶心、呕吐和腹泻。与其他临床表现不成比例的高热是甲状腺危象的标志。

鉴别诊断

甲状腺毒症反映出甲状腺激素分泌过多，甲状腺激素分泌过多可由 Graves 病、毒性腺瘤、多结节性甲状腺肿或甲状腺炎所致（表 2.3 和图 2.2）。然而，甲状腺毒症也可能由过量摄入甲状腺激素引起，罕见情况下由异位（如卵巢甲状腺肿）产生的甲状腺激素引起。

Graves 病

Graves 病是甲状腺毒症最常见的原因，它是一种自身免疫病，多见于女性，发病高峰年龄为 20 ～ 50 岁。患者可表现出以下 1 种或多种特征：①甲状腺肿；②甲状腺毒症；③眼病，症状范围可从流泪、眼球突出、眼外肌麻痹，到视神经受累导致的失明；④甲状腺皮肤病变，通常表现为胫前皮肤显著增厚且无凹陷（胫前黏液性水肿；勿将此处的黏液性水肿与下文讨论的甲状腺功能减退症中的黏液性水肿混淆）。

发病机制　Graves 病中的甲状腺毒症是由结合 TSH 受体的抗体过量生成所致。这些甲状腺刺激性免疫球蛋白可促进甲状腺细胞的生长和甲状腺激素的分泌。眼病是由淋巴细胞对眼外肌的炎症浸润和黏多糖沉积所致。Graves 病的眼征可能是由眼外肌和甲状腺共有的抗原致敏淋巴细胞引发炎症反应所致。

临床表现　甲状腺毒症的常见表现（表 2.2）是 Graves 病年轻患者的典型特征。此外，患者可能表现出弥漫性甲状腺肿或 Graves 病特有的眼部症状。老年患者甲状腺毒症的临床特征通常不典型，这种情况被称为淡漠型甲状腺功能亢进症，其表现为情感平淡、情绪不稳定、体重减轻、肌无力、充血性心力衰竭和标准治疗难以控制的心房颤动。

表 2.3 甲状腺毒症的病因
常见原因
Graves 病
毒性腺瘤（孤立性）
毒性多结节性甲状腺肿
少见原因
亚急性甲状腺炎（de Quervain 或肉芽肿性甲状腺炎）
桥本甲状腺炎伴一过性甲状腺功能亢进期
人为甲状腺毒症
产后甲状腺炎（可能是无症状性甲状腺炎的变型）
罕见病因
卵巢甲状腺肿
甲状腺癌转移
葡萄胎
垂体 TSH 分泌瘤

TSH，促甲状腺激素。

与 Graves 病相关的眼征也可见于其他原因引起的甲状腺功能亢进症的非特异性表现（如甲状腺凝视）。Graves 病的特异性表现是眼眶组织的炎症浸润，可导致眶周水肿、结膜充血肿胀、眼球突出、眼外肌无力或视神经损伤导致的视力损害。

胫前黏液性水肿（甲状腺皮肤病变）可发生于 2% ～ 3% 的 Graves 病患者，导致胫骨下段皮肤非凹陷性增厚。甲剥离症表现为指甲从甲床上分离，常见于 Graves 病患者，患者也可出现甲状腺杵状指。

诊断　总 T4、总 T3 或游离 T4、游离 T3 水平升高（或均升高）且 TSH 被抑制可证实甲状腺毒症的临床诊断。TSH 受体抗体水平通常升高。检测 TSH 受体抗体在有眼征但无其他特征性临床表现的患者中可能有诊断价值。[123]I 摄取增加可鉴别 Graves 病与早期亚急性或桥本甲状腺炎，后者在甲状腺功能亢进的情况下 [123]I 摄取较低。无论是否出现眼病或眼征，眼眶 MRI 或超声通常显示眼眶肌肉增大。

治疗　控制 Graves 病甲状腺功能亢进症的治疗方法包括 3 种：抗甲状腺药物、放射性碘治疗和手术。在欧洲、拉丁美洲和日本，抗甲状腺药物是首选的治疗方法，在美国，放射性碘是主要的治疗方法。然而，抗甲状腺药物已逐渐成为全球治疗 Graves 病的主要方式。

抗甲状腺药物　丙硫氧嘧啶、甲巯咪唑和卡比马唑等硫脲类药物可通过抑制甲状腺过氧化物酶而阻断

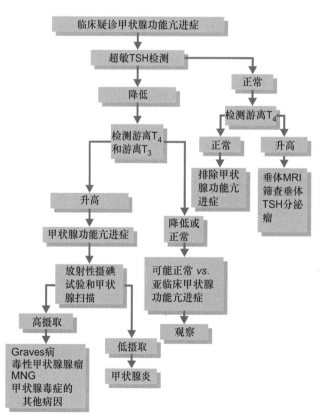

图 2.2　甲状腺功能亢进症的鉴别诊断流程。MNG，多结节性甲状腺肿；MRI，磁共振成像；T3，三碘甲状腺原氨酸；T4，甲状腺素；TSH，促甲状腺激素

by inhibiting thyroid peroxidase. Propylthiouracil also partially inhibits peripheral conversion of T_4 to T_3. Medical therapy is usually administered for a prolonged period (1 to 3 years), with the dose gradually reduced until spontaneous remission occurs. Many patients can remain on low doses of thiocarbamide drugs for long periods of time without significant side effects. One approach is to gradually decrease the dose while maintaining T_4 and T_3 in the normal range, leaving patients on low doses of thiocarbamide drugs if T_4 and T_3 remain high after a gradual taper. After cessation of medication, 40% to 60% of patients remain in remission. Those who experience relapse can either resume therapy with thiocarbamide drugs or undergo definitive surgery or radioactive iodine treatment. Side effects of the thiocarbamide regimen include pruritus and rash (in about 5% of patients), elevated liver function enzymes, cholestatic jaundice, acute arthralgias, and, rarely, agranulocytosis (<0.5% of patients).

Methimazole was found to be more effective at normalizing thyroid hormone levels and led to a lower rate of transaminase elevation and leukopenia than propylthiouracil; it has now become the preferred medical treatment for hyperthyroidism. Methimazole can be given once a day as long as the total dose is 30 mg or less, leading to better compliance, whereas PTU is usually given two to three times a day. At the onset of treatment during the acute phase of thyrotoxicosis, β-adrenergic receptor blockers can be used to help alleviate tachycardia, hypertension, and atrial fibrillation in symptomatic patients. As the thyroid hormone levels return to normal, the treatment with β-blockers is tapered off.

Radioactive iodine. Radioactive iodine (^{131}I) can be used for treating adults with Graves' disease. However, 80% to 90% of patients become hypothyroid after radiotherapy and require lifelong thyroid hormone replacement. As discussed later, a percentage of patients treated with levothyroxine for hypothyroidism continue to have hypothyroid symptoms despite normalization of TSH; this has caused a shift in the paradigm that radioactive iodine is the preferred treatment of hyperthyroidism, with a greater emphasis on using thiocarbamide drugs. ^{131}I has been found to increase the incidence of cancer mortality. ^{131}I is contraindicated in women who are pregnant, but it does not increase the risk of birth defects in offspring conceived after ^{131}I therapy. Patients with severe thyrotoxicosis, very large glands, or underlying heart disease should be rendered euthyroid with antithyroid medication before receiving radioactive iodine, because ^{131}I treatment can cause a release of preformed thyroid hormone from the thyroid gland that could precipitate cardiac arrhythmias and exacerbate symptoms of thyrotoxicosis.

After administration of radioactive iodine, the thyroid gland shrinks; patients become euthyroid and later hypothyroid over a period of 6 weeks to 3 months. Serum free T_4 and TSH levels should be monitored, and replacement with levothyroxine should be instituted when hypothyroidism occurs. Hypothyroidism always occurs after surgical total thyroidectomy, frequently after subtotal thyroidectomy or administration of radioactive iodine, and in a smaller percentage of patients after antithyroid medication; therefore, lifelong monitoring of all patients with Graves' disease is mandated.

Surgery. Either subtotal or total thyroidectomy is the treatment of choice for patients with very large glands and obstructive symptoms, those with multinodular glands, and sometimes in those who desire pregnancy within the next year. It is essential that the surgeon be experienced in thyroid surgery. Preoperatively, patients receive 6 weeks of treatment with antithyroid drugs to ensure that they are euthyroid at the time of surgery. Two weeks before surgery, oral saturated solution of potassium iodide is administered daily to decrease the vascularity of the gland. Permanent hypoparathyroidism and recurrent laryngeal nerve paralysis occur postoperatively in fewer

than 2% of patients, although the rate of transient postoperative hypocalcemia is higher.

Graves' orbitopathy can be treated with glucocorticoids, orbital radiotherapy, or surgery. It was recently found that selenium is effective for Graves' orbitopathy.

Toxic Adenoma

Solitary toxic nodules, which are usually benign, occur more frequently in older patients. The clinical manifestations are those of thyrotoxicosis. Physical examination shows a distinct solitary nodule. Laboratory investigation shows suppressed TSH and significantly elevated T_3 levels, often with only moderately elevated T_4. Thyroid scan shows a hot nodule in the affected lobe with partial or complete suppression of the unaffected lobe. Solitary toxic nodules are usually treated with radioactive iodine. Euthyroidism results if the unaffected lobe has suppressed uptake on a thyroid scan, and often hypothyroidism occurs if the unaffected lobe does not have suppressed uptake. For large nodules, unilateral lobectomy after the administration of antithyroid drugs to render the patient euthyroid may be required.

Toxic Multinodular Goiter

Toxic multinodular goiter occurs in older patients with long-standing multinodular goiter, especially in patients from iodine-deficient regions when they are exposed to increased dietary iodine or iodine-containing radiocontrast dyes. The presenting clinical features are frequently tachycardia, heart failure, and arrhythmias. Physical examination shows a multinodular goiter. The diagnosis is confirmed by laboratory features of suppressed TSH, elevated T_3 and T_4, and a thyroid scan showing multiple functioning nodules. The treatment of choice is often ^{131}I ablation. It is especially effective in patients with small glands and a high degree of radioactive uptake. Larger glands may require surgery.

Subclinical Hyperthyroidism

In subclinical hyperthyroidism, total or free T_4 and T_3 levels are normal and TSH is suppressed. The causes of this condition include early presentation of any form of hyperthyroidism (e.g., Graves' disease, toxic adenoma, toxic multinodular goiter). Because these patients, especially those who are older, are at an increased risk for cardiac dysrhythmias, many patients with a persistently suppressed TSH should be treated with thiocarbamide drugs, β-blockers or, less commonly, radioactive iodine. A decreased bone mineral density is another indication for treatment.

Thyroiditis

Thyroiditis may be classified as acute, subacute, or chronic. Although thyroiditis may eventually result in clinical hypothyroidism, the initial presentation is often that of hyperthyroidism as a result of acute release of T_4 and T_3. Hyperthyroidism caused by thyroiditis can be readily differentiated from other causes of hyperthyroidism by suppressed uptake of radioactive iodine in the thyroid gland, reflecting decreased hormone production by damaged cells.

A rare disorder, acute suppurative thyroiditis, is caused by an infection, usually bacterial. Patients exhibit high fever, redness of the overlying skin, and thyroid gland tenderness; the condition may be confused with subacute thyroiditis. If blood cultures are negative, FNA should identify the organism. Intensive antibiotic treatment and, occasionally, incision and drainage are required.

Subacute Thyroiditis

Subacute thyroiditis (also known as de Quervain thyroiditis or granulomatous thyroiditis) is an acute inflammatory disorder of the thyroid gland that is probably caused by a viral infection and resolves

甲状腺激素的合成。丙硫氧嘧啶还能部分抑制外周 T_4 到 T_3 的转化。药物治疗时间通常较长（1～3年），应逐渐减量，直至出现自发缓解而停药。许多患者可长期服用低剂量硫脲类药物而没有明显的副作用。可在 T_4 和 T_3 维持正常水平时逐渐减量，如果在逐渐减量后 T_4 和 T_3 水平仍然很高，则继续使用低剂量硫脲类药物。停药后，40%～60% 的患者可维持缓解。复发的患者可恢复硫脲类药物治疗，也可接受根治性手术治疗或放射性碘治疗。硫脲类药物的副作用包括瘙痒和皮疹（约 5%）、肝酶水平升高、胆汁淤积性黄疸、急性关节痛、极少数患者会出现粒细胞缺乏症（< 0.5%）。

甲巯咪唑目前已成为治疗甲状腺功能亢进症的首选药物，研究发现，相比于丙硫氧嘧啶，甲巯咪唑能更有效地使甲状腺激素水平恢复正常，且转氨酶升高和白细胞减少的发生率相对较低。丙硫氧嘧啶通常每日服用 2～3 次，而甲巯咪唑可以每日服用 1 次（总剂量 ≤ 30 mg），因此甲巯咪唑的依从性更好。在甲状腺毒症急性期的初始治疗阶段，对于有症状的患者，β 受体阻滞剂可用于缓解心动过速、高血压和心房颤动。随着甲状腺激素水平恢复正常，β 受体阻滞剂可逐渐减量。

放射性碘治疗 放射性碘（^{131}I）治疗可用于成人 Graves 病。然而，80%～90% 的患者在 ^{131}I 治疗后出现甲状腺功能减退症，需要终身使用甲状腺激素替代治疗。部分接受左甲状腺素治疗甲状腺功能减退症的患者仍存在甲状腺功能减退症的症状，尽管 TSH 水平恢复正常，这也限制了 ^{131}I 治疗成为首选治疗，目前仍推荐首选硫脲类药物。研究显示，^{131}I 治疗可升高癌症相关死亡率。孕妇禁用 ^{131}I 治疗，但 ^{131}I 治疗不会增加其后代患出生缺陷的风险。^{131}I 治疗可导致甲状腺释放预先合成的甲状腺激素，从而导致心律失常，加重甲状腺毒症的症状，因此，患有严重甲状腺毒症、腺体明显增大或潜在心脏病的患者在接受 ^{131}I 治疗前，应先使用抗甲状腺药物使甲状腺功能恢复正常。

^{131}I 治疗后，甲状腺会萎缩，在 6 周到 3 个月内，患者的甲状腺功能先恢复正常，然后出现甲状腺功能减退症。应监测血清游离 T_4 和 TSH 水平，发生甲状腺功能减退症时应使用左甲状腺素替代治疗。甲状腺全切除术后患者几乎均会出现甲状腺功能减退症，甲状腺次全切除术或 ^{131}I 治疗后也常出现甲状腺功能减退症，而在使用抗甲状腺药物治疗后的患者出现甲状腺功能减退症的比例较小，因此，所有 Graves 病患者均需终身监测甲状腺功能。

手术 甲状腺次全切除术或全切除术适用于甲状腺明显肿大且有阻塞性症状的患者、多结节性甲状腺肿的患者，以及计划次年妊娠的患者。甲状腺手术的关键在于外科医生的手术经验。患者需在术前接受 6 周的抗甲状腺药物治疗，以确保在手术时甲状腺功能正常。术前 2 周需每日口服碘化钾饱和溶液，以减少腺体血供。不足 2% 的患者在术后发生永久性甲状旁腺功能减退症和

喉返神经麻痹，但术后一过性低钙血症的发生率较高。

Graves 眼病可选用糖皮质激素、眼眶放疗或手术治疗。研究显示，硒对 Graves 眼病有效。

毒性甲状腺腺瘤

甲状腺孤立性毒性结节通常为良性，多见于老年患者，临床表现为甲状腺毒症的症状。体格检查可触及孤立性结节。实验室检查可显示 TSH 受抑制，T_3 水平显著升高，T_4 水平通常仅轻度升高。在甲状腺扫描中，受累侧叶可见热结节，未受累侧叶部分或完全受抑制。孤立的毒性结节通常可采用 ^{131}I 治疗。如果在甲状腺扫描中未受累侧叶有摄取抑制，则 ^{131}I 治疗后甲状腺功能能恢复正常，如果未受累侧叶没有摄取抑制，则 ^{131}I 治疗后常发生甲状腺功能减退症。对于大结节，一般先给予抗甲状腺药物，待患者甲状腺功能恢复正常后进行单侧腺叶切除术。

毒性多结节性甲状腺肿

毒性多结节性甲状腺肿多发生于长期存在多结节性甲状腺肿的老年患者中，特别是来自缺碘地区的患者，在膳食碘增加或使用含碘的放射性造影剂后可出现，临床表现多为心动过速、心力衰竭和心律失常。体格检查可触及多结节性甲状腺肿。实验室检查可见 TSH 受抑制、T_3 和 T_4 水平升高，甲状腺扫描示多个功能性结节可进一步明确诊断。治疗首选 ^{131}I 消融，对于甲状腺小和放射性摄取水平高的患者尤为有效。若甲状腺较大，可能需要手术。

亚临床甲状腺功能亢进症

亚临床甲状腺功能亢进症患者总 T_4、总 T_3，或游离 T_4、游离 T_3 水平正常，TSH 受抑制。其病因可能是所有甲状腺功能亢进症（包括 Graves 病、毒性腺瘤、毒性多结节性甲状腺肿）的早期阶段。亚临床甲状腺功能亢进症患者（特别是老年患者）心律失常的风险增加。因此，多数 TSH 受抑制的患者应使用硫脲类药物、β 受体阻滞剂，部分需要接受 ^{131}I 治疗。骨密度降低是治疗的另一个指征。

甲状腺炎

甲状腺炎可分为急性、亚急性和慢性。虽然甲状腺炎最终可能导致临床甲状腺功能减退症，但最初通常表现为甲状腺功能亢进症，这是由于炎症导致 T_4 和 T_3 迅速释放。甲状腺炎引起的甲状腺功能亢进症与其他原因导致的甲状腺功能亢进症可通过甲状腺摄碘试验鉴别，由于受损的甲状腺细胞产生的激素减少，甲状腺炎患者的碘摄取受抑制。

急性化脓性甲状腺炎较为罕见，通常由细菌感染引起，临床表现为高热、皮肤发红和甲状腺触痛，易与亚急性甲状腺炎相混淆。如果血培养呈阴性，应通过 FNA 明确病原体。通常需要强效抗感染治疗，有时需要切开引流。

亚急性甲状腺炎

亚急性甲状腺炎（又称 de Quervain 甲状腺炎或肉芽肿性甲状腺炎）是一种甲状腺急性炎症性疾病，可能

completely in 90% of cases. Patients with subacute thyroiditis complain of fever and anterior neck pain. The patient may have symptoms and signs of hyperthyroidism. The classic feature on physical examination is an exquisitely tender thyroid gland. Laboratory findings vary with the course of the disease. Initially, the patient may be symptomatically thyrotoxic with elevated serum T_4, depressed serum TSH and low radioactive iodine uptake on the thyroid scan. Subsequently, the thyroid status fluctuates through euthyroid and hypothyroid phases and may return to euthyroidism. An increase in radioactive iodine uptake on the scan reflects recovery of the gland. Treatment usually includes high-dose aspirin or other nonsteroidal anti-inflammatory drugs, but a short course of prednisone may be required if pain and fever are severe. During the hypothyroid phase, replacement therapy with levothyroxine may be indicated.

Postpartum thyroiditis resembles subacute thyroiditis in its clinical course. It usually occurs within the first 6 months after delivery and goes through the triphasic course of hyperthyroidism, hypothyroidism, and then euthyroidism, though it may develop with only hypothyroidism. Some patients have underlying chronic thyroiditis.

Chronic Thyroiditis

Chronic thyroiditis (Hashimoto or lymphocytic thyroiditis), caused by destruction of the normal thyroidal architecture by lymphocytic infiltration, results in hypothyroidism and goiter. Riedel struma is probably a variant of Hashimoto thyroiditis; it is characterized by extensive thyroid fibrosis resulting in a rock-hard thyroid mass. Hashimoto thyroiditis is more common in women and is the most common cause of goiter and hypothyroidism in the United States. Occasionally, patients with Hashimoto thyroiditis have transient hyperthyroidism with low radioactive iodine uptake owing to the release of T_4 and T_3 into the circulation. Chronic thyroiditis can be differentiated from subacute thyroiditis in that in the former, the gland is nontender to palpation and antithyroid antibodies are present in high titer. TPO Ab is usually present early and typically remains present for years. The presence of TgAb does not reflect Hashimoto thyroiditis and does not provide additional information beyond the TPO Ab finding. Serum T_3 and T_4 levels are either normal or low; when they are low, the TSH is elevated. FNA of the thyroid shows lymphocytes and Hürthle cells (enlarged basophilic follicular cells). Hypothyroidism and significant glandular enlargement (goiter) are indications for levothyroxine therapy. Adequate doses of levothyroxine are administered to normalize TSH levels and shrink the goiter. Recent evidence that symptoms of profound fatigue, poor sleep quality, and muscle joint pain persist despite levothyroxine supplementation leading to euthyroidism suggests that symptoms may be related to the autoimmune disease per se rather than hypothyroidism.

Thyrotoxicosis Factitia

Patients with thyrotoxicosis factitia ingest excessive amounts of thyroxine, often in an attempt to lose weight, and exhibit typical features of thyrotoxicosis. Serum T_3 and T_4 levels are elevated and TSH is suppressed, as is the serum thyroglobulin concentration. Radioactive iodine uptake is absent. Patients may require psychotherapy.

Rare Causes of Thyrotoxicosis

Struma ovarii occurs when an ovarian teratoma contains thyroid tissue that secretes thyroid hormone. A body scan confirms the diagnosis by demonstrating uptake of radioactive iodine in the pelvis.

Hydatidiform mole is caused by proliferation and swelling of the trophoblast during pregnancy, with excess production of chorionic gonadotropin, which has intrinsic TSH-like activity. The hyperthyroidism remits with surgical and medical treatment of the molar pregnancy.

HYPOTHYROIDISM

Hypothyroidism is a clinical syndrome caused by deficiency of thyroid hormones. In infants and children, hypothyroidism causes retardation of growth and development and may result in permanent motor and mental retardation. Congenital causes of hypothyroidism include agenesis (complete absence of thyroid tissue), dysgenesis (ectopic or lingual thyroid gland), hypoplastic thyroid, thyroid dyshormonogenesis, and congenital pituitary diseases. Adult-onset hypothyroidism results in a slowing of metabolic processes and is reversible with treatment. Hypothyroidism is usually primary (thyroid failure), but it may be secondary (hypothalamic or pituitary deficiency) or rarely the result of resistance at the thyroid hormone receptor (Table 2.4).

In adults, autoimmune thyroiditis (Hashimoto thyroiditis) is the most common cause of hypothyroidism. This condition may be

TABLE 2.4   Causes of Hypothyroidism
Primary Hypothyroidism
Autoimmune
Hashimoto thyroiditis
Part of polyglandular failure syndrome, type II
Iatrogenic
^{131}I therapy
Thyroidectomy
Drug-Induced
Iodine deficiency
Iodine excess
Lithium
Amiodarone
Antithyroid drugs
Opioids
Glucocorticoids
CTLA-4 inhibitors
PD-1 inhibitors
Congenital
Thyroid agenesis
Thyroid dysgenesis
Hypoplastic thyroid
Biosynthetic defects
Secondary Hypothyroidism
Hypothalamic Dysfunction
Neoplasms
Tuberculosis
Sarcoidosis
Langerhans cell histiocytosis
Hemochromatosis
Radiation treatment
Pituitary Dysfunction
Neoplasms
Pituitary surgery
Postpartum pituitary necrosis
Idiopathic hypopituitarism
Glucocorticoid excess (Cushing's syndrome)
Radiation treatment to the pituitary

由病毒感染引起，90% 患者可痊愈。亚急性甲状腺炎患者通常表现为发热和颈前疼痛，患者可能有甲状腺功能亢进症的症状和体征，体格检查的典型特征是甲状腺触痛。实验室检查结果因病程而异，患者最初可能表现为甲状腺毒性症状，血清 T_4 水平升高，TSH 水平降低，甲状腺扫描示放射性碘摄取减少，随后，甲状腺功能可从正常进展为甲状腺功能减退症，并可能再次恢复正常，甲状腺扫描中放射性碘摄取增加反映腺体功能恢复。治疗通常包括大剂量阿司匹林或其他非甾体抗炎药，但如果出现明显疼痛和高热，可能需要短期使用泼尼松。在甲状腺功能减退期，可使用左甲状腺素替代治疗。

产后甲状腺炎的临床表现与亚急性甲状腺炎相似，通常发生在分娩后 6 个月内，经历甲状腺功能亢进、甲状腺功能减退和甲状腺功能正常这三个阶段，但也可能只发生甲状腺功能减退症。部分患者有潜在的慢性甲状腺炎。

慢性甲状腺炎

慢性甲状腺炎（桥本甲状腺炎或淋巴细胞性甲状腺炎）由淋巴细胞浸润破坏正常甲状腺结构引起，可导致甲状腺功能减退症和甲状腺肿。木样甲状腺炎可能是桥本甲状腺炎的一种变型，其特征为甲状腺广泛纤维化，可出现质硬如石的甲状腺肿块。桥本甲状腺炎在女性中更为常见，是美国甲状腺肿和甲状腺功能减退症最常见的原因。桥本甲状腺炎患者偶尔会出现一过性甲状腺功能亢进症，而放射性碘摄取减少，这是由 T_4 和 T_3 被释放到循环中所致。慢性甲状腺炎需与亚急性甲状腺炎鉴别，前者甲状腺触诊无触痛，抗甲状腺抗体呈高滴度阳性。TPOAb 通常早期出现并持续数年。TgAb 阳性不能反映桥本甲状腺炎，也不能提供比 TPOAb 更多的信息。患者的血清 T_3 和 T_4 水平可正常或偏低，当血清 T_3 和 T_4 水平较低时，TSH 会升高。甲状腺 FNA 镜下可见淋巴细胞和许特莱细胞（Hürthle 细胞；即增大的嗜碱性滤泡细胞）（译者注：原文有误，此处应为嗜酸性滤泡细胞）。甲状腺功能减退症和甲状腺明显肿大（甲状腺肿）是左甲状腺素治疗的指征。给予足量的左甲状腺素可使 TSH 水平恢复正常并使肿大的甲状腺缩小。研究表明，补充左甲状腺素使甲状腺功能正常后仍有患者存在疲劳、睡眠质量差和肌肉关节疼痛的症状，这些症状可能与自身免疫病本身有关，而与甲状腺功能减退症无关。

人为甲状腺毒症

人为甲状腺毒症患者常因试图减重而摄入过量甲状腺素，并表现出甲状腺毒症的典型特征。患者的血清 T_3 和 T_4 水平升高，TSH 水平下降，血清甲状腺球蛋白浓度下降，放射性碘摄取减少至无法测出。患者可能需要心理治疗。

甲状腺毒症的其他罕见病因

当卵巢畸胎瘤含有分泌甲状腺激素的甲状腺组织时，可出现卵巢甲状腺肿，全身扫描显示盆腔内放射性碘聚集可证实诊断。

葡萄胎由妊娠期间绒毛膜滋养层细胞的增殖和水肿引起，并可产生过量的绒毛膜促性腺激素，后者具有 TSH 样活性。通过手术和药物治疗葡萄胎可缓解甲状腺功能亢进症。

甲状腺功能减退症

甲状腺功能减退症是由甲状腺激素缺乏引起的临床综合征。在婴儿和儿童中，甲状腺功能减退症会导致生长迟缓，并可能导致永久性运动发育迟缓和智力低下。甲状腺功能减退症的先天性病因包括甲状腺缺如（甲状腺组织完全缺失）、甲状腺发育不全（异位或舌状甲状腺）、甲状腺发育不良、甲状腺激素合成障碍和先天性垂体疾病。成年起病的甲状腺功能减退症会导致代谢减慢，经治疗可逆转。甲状腺功能减退症通常为原发性（甲状腺功能衰竭），但也可能为继发性（下丘脑或垂体功能障碍），极少数患者是由甲状腺激素受体抵抗所致（表 2.4）。

自身免疫性甲状腺炎（桥本甲状腺炎）是成人甲状腺功能减退症最常见的原因。该病可单独出现，或作

表 2.4　甲状腺功能减退症的病因
原发性甲状腺功能减退症
自身免疫性
桥本甲状腺炎
作为自身免疫性多内分泌腺综合征 II 型的一部分
医源性
^{131}I 治疗
甲状腺切除术
药物性
碘缺乏
碘过量
锂剂
胺碘酮
抗甲状腺药物
阿片类药物
糖皮质激素
CTLA-4 抑制剂
PD-1 抑制剂
先天性
甲状腺缺如
甲状腺发育不全
甲状腺发育不良
生物合成缺陷
继发性甲状腺功能减退症
下丘脑功能障碍
肿瘤
结核
结节病
朗格汉斯细胞组织细胞增生症
血色病
放疗
垂体功能障碍
肿瘤
垂体手术
产后垂体坏死
特发性垂体功能减退症
糖皮质激素过量分泌（库欣综合征）
垂体放疗

isolated, or it may be part of polyglandular failure syndrome type II (Schmidt syndrome), which also includes insulin-dependent diabetes mellitus, adrenal insufficiency, pernicious anemia, vitiligo, gonadal failure, hypophysitis, celiac disease, myasthenia gravis, and primary biliary cirrhosis. Iatrogenic causes of hypothyroidism include ^{131}I therapy, thyroidectomy, and treatment with lithium, amiodarone, opioids, and glucocorticoids, as well as CTLA-4 and PD-1 inhibitors (cancer immunotherapy agents), with the last two drug classes causing painless thyroiditis and transient hyperthyroidism followed by hypothyroidism. Iodine deficiency or excess can also cause hypothyroidism.

Clinical Presentation

The clinical presentation of hypothyroidism (Table 2.5) depends on the age at onset and the severity of the thyroid deficiency. Infants with congenital hypothyroidism (also called *cretinism*) may exhibit feeding problems, hypotonia, inactivity, an open posterior fontanelle, and edematous face and hands. Mental retardation, short stature, and delayed puberty occur if treatment is delayed.

Hypothyroidism in adults usually develops insidiously. Patients often complain of fatigue, lethargy, and gradual weight gain for years before the diagnosis is established. A delayed relaxation phase of deep tendon reflexes (*hung-up* reflexes) is a valuable clinical sign that is characteristic of severe hypothyroidism. Subcutaneous infiltration by mucopolysaccharides, which bind water, causes the edema; this condition, termed *myxedema*, is responsible for the thickened features and puffy appearance of patients with severe hypothyroidism.

Severe untreated hypothyroidism can result in *myxedema coma*, which is characterized by hypothermia, extreme weakness, stupor, hypoventilation, hypoglycemia, and hyponatremia and is often precipitated by cold exposure, infection, or psychoactive drugs. (Do not confuse the uses of myxedema here with *pretibial myxedema* seen in Graves' disease, where it refers to thyroid dermopathy—skin thickening without pitting.)

Diagnosis

Because the initial manifestations of hypothyroidism are subtle, early diagnosis demands a high index of suspicion in patients with one or more of the signs and symptoms (see Table 2.5), though hypothyroidism is often picked up in patients who have a TSH measured as part of routine laboratories. Early symptoms that are often overlooked include menstrual irregularities (usually menorrhagia), arthralgias, and myalgias.

Laboratory abnormalities in patients with primary hypothyroidism include elevated serum TSH and low total and free T_4. A low or low-normal morning serum TSH level in the setting of hypothalamic or pituitary dysfunction characterizes secondary hypothyroidism. Often, the serum total and free T_4 levels are at the lower limits of normal.

Hypothyroidism is often associated with hypercholesterolemia and elevated creatine phosphokinase skeletal muscle (MM) fraction (the fraction representative of skeletal muscle). Anemia is usually normocytic and normochromic but may be macrocytic (with vitamin B_{12} deficiency resulting from associated pernicious anemia) or microcytic (caused by nutritional deficiencies or menstrual blood loss in women). Because TPO Ab is usually positive in Hashimoto thyroiditis, the major cause of hypothyroidism in adults, its measurement is helpful in deciding whether levothyroxine treatment is appropriate in patients with subclinical hypothyroidism (discussed later).

Treatment

Hypothyroidism should be treated initially with synthetic levothyroxine (T_4). Administration of levothyroxine results in physiologic levels of bioavailable T_3 and T_4. Levothyroxine has a half-life of 8 days; consequently, it needs to be given only once a day. The average replacement dose of levothyroxine for adults is 75 to 150 µg/day. In healthy adults, 1.6 µg/kg/day is an appropriate starting dose. In some older patients and patients with cardiac disease, levothyroxine should be increased gradually, starting at 25 µg/day and increasing the dose by 25 µg every 2 weeks; however, most patients can safely be started on a full replacement dose. The therapeutic response to levothyroxine therapy should be monitored clinically and with measurement of serum TSH levels 6 to 8 weeks after a dose adjustment. TSH levels between 0.5 and 2 mU/L are considered optimal. Because TSH measurements are not a useful guide in patients with secondary hypothyroidism (pituitary or hypothalamic dysfunction), these patients should be given levothyroxine until their free T_4 is in the mid- to upper-normal range.

Recent studies have suggested that a percentage of patients treated with levothyroxine for hypothyroidism continue to have hypothyroid symptoms despite normalization of TSH. Furthermore, a large study found that more than 20% of athyreotic patients (those who have absence or functional deficiency of the thyroid gland) treated with levothyroxine replacement did not maintain free T_3 or free T_4 values in the normal range despite normal TSH levels. This reflects the inadequacy of peripheral deiodination to compensate for the absent T_3 secretion. Because of these studies, there is renewed interest (accompanied by a large amount of controversy) in treating hypothyroid patients who have not had an adequate clinical response to levothyroxine replacement with a combination of levothyroxine and liothyronine (a manufactured form of T_3) or with desiccated thyroid preparations that contain levothyroxine and liothyronine.

In patients with myxedema coma, 500 to 800 µg of levothyroxine is administered intravenously as a loading dose, followed by 100 µg/day of levothyroxine, hydrocortisone (100 mg IV intravenously three times daily), and intravenous fluids. Corticosteroids should be given before thyroxine in autoimmune conditions. The underlying precipitating event should be corrected. Respiratory assistance and treatment of hypothermia with warming blankets may be required. Although myxedema coma carries a high mortality rate despite appropriate treatment, many patients improve in 1 to 3 days.

TABLE 2.5	Clinical Features of Hypothyroidism

Children
Learning disabilities
Mental retardation
Short stature
Delayed bone age
Delayed puberty

Adults
Fatigue
Cold intolerance
Weight gain
Constipation
Menstrual irregularities
Dry, coarse, cold skin
Periorbital and peripheral edema
Delayed reflexes
Bradycardia
Arthralgias, myalgias

为自身免疫性多内分泌腺综合征 II 型［施密特综合征（Schmidt 综合征）］的一部分，该综合征还包括胰岛素依赖性糖尿病、肾上腺皮质功能不全、恶性贫血、白癜风、性腺功能减退症、垂体炎、乳糜泻、重症肌无力和原发性胆汁性肝硬化。甲状腺功能减退症的医源性病因包括 ^{131}I 治疗、甲状腺切除术及药物治疗，如锂剂、胺碘酮、阿片类药物、糖皮质激素、CTLA-4 和 PD-1 抑制剂（肿瘤免疫治疗药物）。CTLA-4 和 PD-1 抑制剂可引起无痛性甲状腺炎和一过性甲状腺功能亢进症后的甲状腺功能减退症。碘缺乏或碘过量也可引起甲状腺功能减退症。

临床表现

甲状腺功能减退症（表 2.5）的临床表现取决于发病年龄和甲状腺激素缺乏的严重程度。先天性甲状腺功能减退症（又称呆小病）的婴儿可能表现出喂养困难、肌张力低下、活动减少、后囟未闭、颜面和双手水肿。如未及时治疗，则会出现智力低下、身材矮小和青春期延迟。

成人甲状腺功能减退症通常起病隐匿。患者可在确诊前数年出现疲劳、嗜睡和体重增加。腱反射松弛期延长（悬空反射）是重度甲状腺功能减退症的重要临床特征。黏多糖结合水分沉积于皮下可导致水肿，即黏液性水肿，是重度甲状腺功能减退症患者颜面粗厚和皮肤肿胀的原因。

若未及时治疗，重度甲状腺功能减退症可导致黏液性水肿昏迷，其特征是体温过低、极度虚弱、木僵、通气不足、低血糖和低钠血症，通常由寒冷、感染或精神活性药物诱发。（勿将此处讨论的黏液性水肿与 Graves 病中的胫前黏液性水肿相混淆，后者是指甲状腺皮肤病——皮肤非凹陷性水肿。）

诊断

甲状腺功能减退症的早期表现隐匿，早期诊断需要高度警惕存在 1 种或多种症状和体征（表 2.5）的患者，但通常是在常规检测 TSH 的患者中发现。常被忽视的早期症状

表 2.5　甲状腺功能减退症的临床特点

儿童
学习障碍
智力低下
身材矮小
骨龄延迟
青春期延迟
成人
疲劳
畏寒
体重增加
便秘
月经不规律
皮肤粗糙、干冷
眼眶和四肢水肿
延迟反射
心动过缓
关节痛和肌痛

包括月经不规律（通常为月经过多）、关节痛和肌痛。

原发性甲状腺功能减退症患者的实验室检查异常结果包括血清 TSH 水平升高、总 T_4 和游离 T_4 水平降低。下丘脑或垂体功能障碍时，晨间血清 TSH 水平降低或为正常低值是继发性甲状腺功能减退症的特征，血清总 T_4 和游离 T_4 水平通常处于正常值下限。

甲状腺功能减退症常伴随高胆固醇血症和肌酸磷酸激酶 MM 亚型（代表骨骼肌来源）水平升高。贫血通常为正细胞正色素性贫血，但也可能出现大细胞性贫血（因伴有恶性贫血导致维生素 B_{12} 缺乏）或小细胞性贫血（由营养不良或女性月经失血引起）。由于 TPOAb 在桥本甲状腺炎（成人甲状腺功能减退症的主要原因）中通常呈阳性，因此检测 TPOAb 有助于决定亚临床甲状腺功能减退症患者是否需要进行左甲状腺素治疗（见下文）。

治疗

甲状腺功能减退症的初始治疗应使用合成左甲状腺素。应用左甲状腺素可使具有生物活性的 T_3 和 T_4 处于生理水平。左甲状腺素的半衰期为 8 天，因此仅需每天给药 1 次。成人左甲状腺素平均替代剂量为 75 ～ 150 μg/d。健康成人合适的起始剂量为 1.6 μg/（kg·d）。部分老年患者和心脏病患者应逐渐增加左甲状腺素剂量，从 25 μg/d 开始，每 2 周增加 25 μg；但是，对于大多数患者，以全剂量开始替代治疗也是安全的。临床应监测患者对左甲状腺素的治疗反应，并在剂量调整后的 6 ～ 8 周内检测血清 TSH 水平。0.5 ～ 2 mU/L 通常被认为是 TSH 的最佳水平。对于继发性甲状腺功能减退症（垂体或下丘脑功能障碍）的患者，检测 TSH 无法指导治疗，因此这些患者应调整左甲状腺素剂量直至其游离 T_4 处于正常范围的中上水平。

近期研究指出，部分接受左甲状腺素治疗的甲状腺功能减退症患者的症状仍持续存在，尽管其 TSH 水平已恢复正常。此外，一项大型研究发现，超过 20% 的甲状腺缺如或功能缺陷的患者在接受左甲状腺素替代治疗后，游离 T_3 或游离 T_4 水平仍未达到正常范围，虽然其 TSH 水平恢复正常。这反映了通过外周脱碘不足以代偿 T_3 分泌缺乏。基于这些研究结果，对于左甲状腺素替代治疗后临床反应不充分的甲状腺功能减退症患者，采用左甲状腺素联合碘塞罗宁（一种人工合成的 T_3）或采用含有左甲状腺素和碘塞罗宁的甲状腺干制剂治疗引起了人们的关注，但仍存有争议。

对于黏液性水肿昏迷的患者，先静脉注射 500 ～ 800 μg 左甲状腺素负荷剂量，随后予 100 μg/d 左甲状腺素维持治疗，同时配合氢化可的松（100 mg，静脉注射，3 次/日）和静脉补液。自身免疫病患者应在使用甲状腺素之前给予皮质类固醇。同时消除或纠正潜在的诱发因素。患者可能还需要呼吸支持和用保暖毯治疗低体温。虽然黏液性水肿昏迷经恰当治疗后的死亡率仍较高，但许多患者的症状可在 1 ～ 3 天有所改善。

Subclinical Hypothyroidism

In subclinical hypothyroidism, free or total T_4 and T_3 levels are normal or low-normal, and TSH is mildly elevated. Some of these patients develop overt hypothyroidism. The decision as to when to treat patients who have a mildly elevated TSH level is controversial. It is frequently recommended that patients should be treated with levothyroxine if they have a TSH level greater than 5 mU/L on two occasions and either positive anti–TPO Ab test results or a goiter. If the patient does not have an appreciable goiter and has negative anti–TPO Ab test results, many experts suggest that levothyroxine should be given only if the TSH level is greater than 10 mU/L on two occasions. Other experts suggest treatment at lower TSH levels depending on the presence of TPO antibody.

GOITER

Enlargement of the thyroid gland is called a *goiter*. Patients with goiters may be euthyroid (simple goiter), hyperthyroid (toxic nodular goiter or Graves' disease), or hypothyroid (nontoxic goiter or Hashimoto thyroiditis). Thyroid enlargement (often focal) may also be the result of a thyroid adenoma or carcinoma. In nontoxic goiter, inadequate thyroid hormone synthesis leads to TSH stimulation with resultant enlargement of the thyroid gland. Iodine deficiency (endemic goiter) was once the most common cause of nontoxic goiter. Since the widespread availability of iodized salt, endemic goiter is less common in North America.

Goitrogens are agents that can cause a goiter, and iodine and lithium are the two chemicals or drugs that frequently cause a goiter. Natural goitrogens include thioglucosides found in vegetables such as cabbage, broccoli, Brussels sprouts, turnips, cauliflower, kale, and other greens. Other foods that are goitrogens include soybeans and soybean products, peanuts, spinach, sweet potatoes, and some fruits (e.g., strawberries, pears, and peaches). Thyroid hormone biosynthetic defects can cause goiter associated with hypothyroidism (or, with adequate compensation, euthyroidism).

A careful thyroid examination coupled with thyroid hormone tests can reveal the cause of the goiter. A smooth, symmetrical gland, often with a bruit, and hyperthyroidism are suggestive of Graves' disease. A nodular thyroid gland with hypothyroidism and positive antithyroid antibodies is consistent with Hashimoto thyroiditis. A diffuse, smooth goiter with hypothyroidism and negative antithyroid antibodies may be indicative of iodine deficiency or a biosynthetic defect. Goiters can become very large, extending substernally and causing dysphagia, respiratory distress, or hoarseness. An ultrasound evaluation or radioactive iodine scan delineates the thyroid gland, and measurement of the TSH level determines the functional activity of the goiter.

Hypothyroid goiters are treated with thyroid hormone at a dose that normalizes TSH. Previously, euthyroid goiters were treated with levothyroxine therapy; however, regression with levothyroxine therapy is unlikely and is no longer recommended. Surgery is indicated for nontoxic goiter only if obstructive symptoms develop or substantial substernal extension is present.

SOLITARY THYROID NODULES

Thyroid nodules are common. They can be detected clinically in about 4% of the population and are found in about 50% of the population at autopsy. Benign thyroid nodules are usually follicular adenomas, colloid nodules, benign cysts, or nodular thyroiditis. Patients may have one prominent nodule on clinical examination, but thyroid ultrasound evaluation may reveal multiple nodules. Although most nodules are benign, a small percentage are malignant. Fortunately, most thyroid cancers are low-grade malignancies.

The major etiologic factor for thyroid cancer is childhood or adolescent exposure to head and neck radiation. Previously, radiation was used to treat an enlarged thymus, tonsillar disease, hemangioma, or acne. Exposure to radiation from nuclear plants (e.g., Chernobyl, Ukraine; Fukushima Daiichi, Japan) contributes to an increased incidence of thyroid cancer. Patients with a history of irradiation should have a baseline thyroid ultrasound study, then a repeat study every 5 years.

All patients with a thyroid nodule noticed by the patient or during physical examination by a clinician should undergo a thyroid ultrasound. Patients who are found to have asymptomatic, incidental, nonsuspicious thyroid nodules on imaging performed for other reasons should be referred for diagnostic thyroid ultrasound only if they meet the following criteria: (1) younger than 35 years of age with normal life expectancy and nodule 1 cm or greater, or (2) 35 years of age or older with normal life expectancy and nodule 1.5 cm or greater. Radiologists have a standard report and score on thyroid ultrasounds called TI-RADS that ranges from 1 (looks very benign) to 5 (looks like it might be malignant) (Fig. 2.3). Thus, the TI-RADS helps to distinguish which patient with a thyroid nodule should get a biopsy. If the TI-RADS score is 3 and the nodule is larger than 2.5 cm, if the score is 4 and the nodule is larger than 1.5 cm, or if the score is 5 and the nodule is larger than 1 cm, then an FNA is recommended. If the TI-RADS score is lower and the nodule is smaller, a repeat ultrasound in 1 year is recommended, and for even smaller, more benign looking nodules, no follow-up is needed. FNA should be done under ultrasound guidance if possible.

The Bethesda system for reporting thyroid cytopathology (Table 2.6) is used to report FNA results. Molecular testing can now be performed on FNA specimens to help determine whether follicular lesions have molecular characteristics of malignancy and should be removed.

Although in the past benign thyroid nodules were treated with levothyroxine suppression, this is no longer recommended because it is uncommon for thyroid nodules to shrink substantially with levothyroxine.

THYROID CARCINOMA

The types and characteristics of thyroid carcinomas are presented in Table 2.7. Papillary carcinoma is associated with local invasion and lymph node spread. Indicators of poor prognosis include thyroid capsule invasion, size greater than 2.5 cm, age at onset older than 45 years, tall cell or Hürthle cell variant, and lymph node involvement. Follicular carcinoma is slightly more aggressive than papillary carcinoma and can spread by local invasion of lymph nodes or hematogenously to bone, brain, or lung. Many tumors show both papillary and follicular cell types. Patients may exhibit metastases before diagnosis of the primary thyroid lesion. Anaplastic carcinoma tends to occur in older individuals, is very aggressive, and rapidly causes pain, dysphagia, and hoarseness.

Medullary thyroid carcinoma is derived from calcitonin-producing parafollicular cells and is more malignant than papillary or follicular carcinoma. It is multifocal and spreads both locally and distally. It may be either sporadic or familial. When familial, it is inherited in an autosomal dominant pattern and is part of multiple endocrine neoplasia type IIA (medullary carcinoma of the thyroid, pheochromocytoma, and hyperparathyroidism) or multiple endocrine neoplasia type IIB (medullary carcinoma of the thyroid, mucosal neuromas, intestinal ganglioneuromas, marfanoid habitus, and pheochromocytoma). Elevated basal serum calcitonin levels confirm the diagnosis. Evaluation for *RET* proto-oncogene mutations should be performed

亚临床甲状腺功能减退症

在亚临床甲状腺功能减退症中，游离或总 T_4 和 T_3 水平正常或为正常低值，而 TSH 水平轻度升高。部分患者可能进展为甲状腺功能减退症。对于何时开始治疗 TSH 水平轻度升高的患者仍存有争议。如果患者 TSH 水平在两次检测中均 > 5 mU/L，且 TPOAb 阳性或存在甲状腺肿，通常建议使用左甲状腺素治疗。如果患者无明显甲状腺肿且 TPOAb 阴性，则多数专家建议仅在两次 TSH 水平检测均 > 10 mU/L 时才给予左甲状腺素。部分专家则建议如果 TPOAb 阳性，可在更低的 TSH 水平下启动治疗。

甲状腺肿

甲状腺肿即甲状腺肿大。甲状腺肿可见于甲状腺功能正常（单纯性甲状腺肿）、甲状腺功能亢进（毒性结节性甲状腺肿或 Graves 病）和甲状腺功能减退（非毒性甲状腺肿和桥本甲状腺炎）。甲状腺肿（通常呈局灶性）也可能由甲状腺腺瘤或甲状腺癌所致。在非毒性甲状腺肿中，甲状腺激素合成不足会刺激 TSH 分泌，导致甲状腺增大。碘缺乏（地方性甲状腺肿）曾经是非毒性甲状腺肿最常见的原因。自广泛使用碘盐后，北美地区的地方性甲状腺肿已不常见。

致甲状腺肿大物质是指可引起甲状腺肿的物质，碘和锂是引起甲状腺肿的常见原因。天然致甲状腺肿大物质包括蔬菜中的硫代葡萄糖苷，可见于卷心菜、花椰菜、抱子甘蓝、萝卜、菜花、羽衣甘蓝和其他绿叶蔬菜。其他食物类致甲状腺肿大物质包括大豆及大豆制品、花生、菠菜、红薯和部分水果（如草莓、梨和桃子）。甲状腺激素生物合成缺陷可导致甲状腺肿伴甲状腺功能减退症（或经充分代偿后的甲状腺功能正常）。

通过仔细的甲状腺体格检查和甲状腺激素检测可明确甲状腺肿的病因。甲状腺光滑对称，通常伴有血管杂音和甲状腺功能亢进症，提示为 Graves 病。结节性甲状腺肿伴甲状腺功能减退症及甲状腺抗体阳性，提示为桥本甲状腺炎。甲状腺弥漫性肿大、光滑、伴有甲状腺功能减退症但甲状腺抗体阴性，可能提示碘缺乏或甲状腺激素生物合成缺陷。巨大甲状腺肿可延伸至胸骨后，并引起吞咽困难、呼吸窘迫或声音嘶哑。超声检查或放射性碘扫描可判断甲状腺的形态结构，而 TSH 水平测定可评估甲状腺的功能状态。

伴有甲状腺功能减退症的甲状腺肿可使用甲状腺激素治疗，剂量调整以 TSH 水平恢复正常为目标。甲状腺功能正常的甲状腺肿患者即往也采用左甲状腺素治疗；然而，左甲状腺素治疗不太可能使甲状腺肿消退，因此目前不再推荐。手术治疗适用于非毒性甲状腺肿伴有压迫症状或显著的胸骨后甲状腺肿。

孤立性甲状腺结节

甲状腺结节是常见疾病。普通人群中约有 4% 在临床检查中可发现甲状腺结节，而尸检研究结果显示，约 50% 的人存在甲状腺结节。良性甲状腺结节通常包括滤泡腺瘤、胶质结节、良性囊肿或结节性甲状腺炎。患者在临床检查中可能仅发现 1 个明显的结节，但进一步通过甲状腺超声检查可能显示存在多个结节。尽管大多数结节为良性，但仍有少数结节为恶性。幸运的是，大多数甲状腺癌的恶性程度较低。

甲状腺癌的主要致病因素包括儿童或青少年时期头颈部辐射暴露。在过去，胸腺肥大、扁桃体疾病、血管瘤或痤疮均采用放疗。此外，核电站事故（如乌克兰切尔诺贝利核电站事故和日本福岛第一核电站事故）导致辐射源暴露也使甲状腺癌的发病率显著升高。有辐射暴露史的患者应进行基线甲状腺超声检查，每 5 年复查 1 次。

所有通过自查或临床检查发现甲状腺结节的患者均应进行甲状腺超声检查。因其他原因进行影像学检查时发现的无症状、偶发、非可疑的甲状腺结节患者，仅当满足以下标准时才需要进行诊断性甲状腺超声检查：①年龄 < 35 岁、预期寿命正常且结节 ≥ 1 cm；②年龄 ≥ 35 岁、预期寿命正常且结节 ≥ 1.5 cm。放射科医生在甲状腺超声检查报告中采用甲状腺影像报告和数据系统（TI-RADS），评分范围从 1 分（良性可能性高）到 5 分（恶性可能性高）（图 2.3）。因此，TI-RADS 有助于区分哪些甲状腺结节患者应接受活检。如果 TI-RADS 评分为 3 分且结节 > 2.5 cm，或评分为 4 分且结节 > 1.5 cm，或评分为 5 分且结节 > 1 cm，则建议进行 FNA。如果 TI-RADS 评分较低且结节较小，则建议 1 年后再次进行超声检查；如果结节极小且呈良性，则无须随访。FNA 应尽可能在超声引导下进行。

报告甲状腺细胞病理学的贝塞斯达系统（Bethesda system）（表 2.6）可用于报告 FNA 结果。目前可对 FNA 标本进行分子检测，以帮助确定滤泡性病变是否具有恶性肿瘤的分子特征，从而决定是否需要切除。

虽然既往曾用左甲状腺素抑制良性甲状腺结节，但目前不再推荐使用，因为使用左甲状腺素后甲状腺结节很少出现显著缩小。

甲状腺癌

甲状腺癌的类型和特征见表 2.7。乳头状癌常伴有局部侵袭和淋巴转移。预后不良的指标包括甲状腺包膜侵犯、肿瘤直径 > 2.5 cm、发病年龄 > 45 岁、高柱状细胞或 Hürthle 细胞亚型和淋巴结受累。滤泡癌比乳头状癌更具侵袭性，可通过局部淋巴转移或血行播散至骨、脑或肺。许多肿瘤同时具有乳头状和滤泡状细胞类型。患者可能在诊断原发性甲状腺病变前就已出现转移。未分化癌多见于老年人，具有极强的侵袭性，可迅速引起疼痛、吞咽困难和声音嘶哑。

甲状腺髓样癌源于分泌降钙素的滤泡旁细胞，恶性程度高于乳头状癌或滤泡癌。病变呈多灶性，可出现局部侵犯和远处扩散。甲状腺髓样癌可分为散发性和家族性。家族性甲状腺髓样癌为常染色体显性遗传

ACR TI-RADS

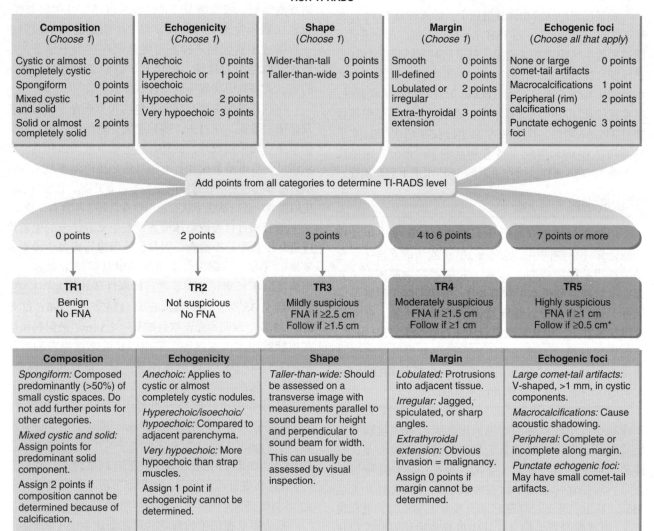

Fig. 2.3   Chart showing five categories on the basis of the ACR Thyroid Imaging, Reporting and Data System (TI-RADS) lexicon, TR levels, and criteria for fine-needle aspiration or follow-up ultrasound. Explanatory notes appear at the bottom.

in patients with medullary carcinoma; if mutations are present, all first-degree relatives should be examined.

Treatment

Lobectomy may be performed for low-risk patients. This includes papillary nodules less than 2.5 cm, TI-RADS score less than 4, absence of neck lymph nodes seen on neck ultrasound, and most follicular tumors. Nodules less than 1 cm with papillary carcinoma can be observed. However, higher risk patients with larger tumors (>3 cm) and/or positive lymph nodes should have a total thyroidectomy. Routine central neck dissection is not needed unless lymph nodes are seen on preoperative imaging or if the surgeon discovers nodes during examination during surgery.

Patients with a lobectomy usually do not need thyroid hormone replacement but should have their TSH monitored. If the TSH goes above range, the patient should be started on levothyroxine. They should have thyroglobulin measured and a thyroid ultrasound every 6 months for the first 2 years and then yearly. A thyroglobulin greater than 30 ng/mL and/or enlarging nodule on the contralateral lobe or lymph nodes draw concern for recurrent disease and should be evaluated for completion of the thyroidectomy.

After total thyroidectomy, patients with low-risk, small carcinomas may be administered doses of levothyroxine sufficient to keep the TSH level in the low-normal or slightly suppressed range and monitored with serum thyroglobulin determinations and yearly neck ultrasound examinations. In the presence of a stable serum TSH level, one should follow the trend in thyroglobulin values with a rising value being concerning. Ideally the thyroglobulin should be less than 0.5 ng/mL, although values less than 2.5 ng/mL may not require an intervention if the thyroid ultrasound does not show detectable thyroid tissue. Patients with large lesions and those at high risk for persistence or metastatic disease should be treated with radioactive iodine with sufficient levothyroxine administration to suppress serum TSH to subnormal levels for about 5 years after thyroidectomy; after that, normal TSH levels can be targeted if no sign of tumor recurrence is seen.

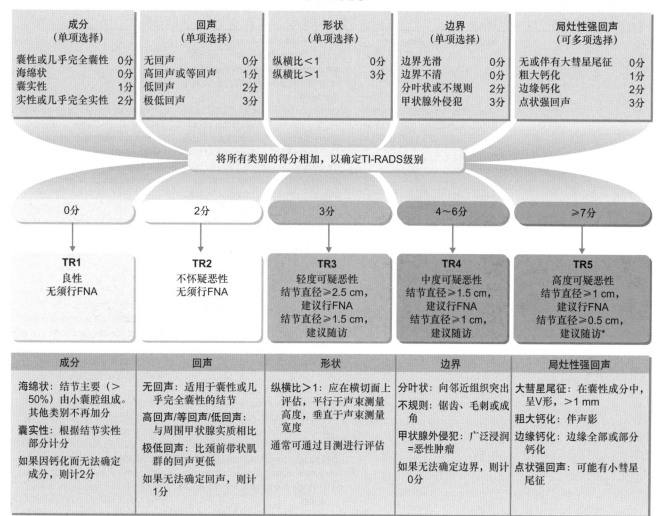

*有关5～9 mm的TR5结节，请参阅乳头状微小癌的讨论

图 2.3　根据 ACR 甲状腺成像、报告和数据系统（TI-RADS）词典、TR 级别、细针穿刺或后续超声检查标准划分的 5 个类别。图片下方为解释性说明

病，并且是多发性内分泌腺瘤病ⅡA 型（包括甲状腺髓样癌、嗜铬细胞瘤和原发性甲状旁腺功能亢进症）或多发性内分泌腺瘤病ⅡB 型（包括甲状腺髓样癌、黏膜神经瘤、肠神经节瘤、马方综合征和嗜铬细胞瘤）的一部分。基础血清降钙素水平升高有助于确诊。甲状腺髓样癌患者应评估 *RET* 原癌基因突变；如果检测到突变，所有一级亲属均应接受检测。

治疗

低风险患者可行甲状腺叶切除术，包括乳头状结节直径＜ 2.5 cm、TI-RADS 评分＜ 4 分、颈部超声检查未显示颈部淋巴结异常，以及大多数滤泡性肿瘤。乳头状癌直径＜ 1 cm 的结节也可随访观察。然而，对于肿瘤较大（直径＞ 3 cm）和（或）淋巴结阳性的高危患者，推荐进行甲状腺全切除术。通常无须常规进行中央区颈淋巴结清扫术，除非术前影像学显示淋巴结异常或外科医生在术中发现淋巴结转移。

对于接受腺叶切除术的患者，甲状腺激素替代治疗通常不是必需的，但应定期监测 TSH 水平。一旦 TSH 超出正常范围，患者应开始使用左甲状腺素治疗。在术后最初两年，患者应每 6 个月进行 1 次甲状腺球蛋白检测和甲状腺超声检查，之后每年进行 1 次。如果甲状腺球蛋白＞ 30 ng/ml 和（或）超声检查发现对侧叶或淋巴结增大的结节，提示可能复发，应评估是否需要进行甲状腺全切除术。

甲状腺全切除术后，对于低风险且肿瘤较小的患者，建议给予足量左甲状腺素治疗，使 TSH 水平维持在正常低值或轻微抑制的范围内，并通过血清甲状腺球蛋白检测和颈部超声检查（每年 1 次）进行监测。在 TSH 水平稳定的情况下，应密切关注甲状腺球蛋白是否有上升趋势。理想情况下，甲状腺球蛋白水平应＜ 0.5 ng/ml，但如果甲状腺超声检查未显示有甲状腺组织，则甲状腺球蛋白＜ 2.5 ng/ml 可能不需要额外干预。对于病灶较大或具有持续性或转移性疾病高风险的患者，术后应给予 [131]I 治疗，并结合足量左甲状腺素，从而使血清 TSH 降低至正常水平以下约 5 年。之后，若未出现肿瘤复发的征象，可调整目标为使 TSH 水平保持在正常范围内。

TABLE 2.6	Bethesda System for Reporting Thyroid Cytopathology		
Bethesda Category	**Diagnosis**	**Disposition**	**Notes**
I	Nondiagnostic/Unsatisfactory	Repeat FNA (under ultrasound guidance)	
II	Benign	Clinical follow-up and a repeat ultrasound and a possible repeat biopsy needed if the patient or provider notices the nodule is growing.	
III	Atypia of Undetermined Significance (AUS) or Follicular Lesion of Undetermined Significance (FLUS)	If pathologist determines a FLUS/AUS reading, one additional biopsy should be performed 3-6 months after the initial biopsy. The repeat FNA should include a sample for molecular testing and if the pathology still shows FLUS/AUS, then the sample should be sent out for molecular testing with the results guiding further treatment. If it is still unclear if surgery is needed, ultrasound should be performed to determine if the nodule grows or changes characteristics (higher TI-RADS score). If it does not grow or change characteristics, the nodule could be watched.	A TPO antibody should also be obtained because FLUS/AUS may occur in the context of a Hashimoto gland and its measurement may assist the pathologist. Molecular testing can be used to determine likelihood of malignancy.
IV	Follicular Neoplasm (FN) or Suspicious for a Follicular Neoplasm (SFN)	If initial biopsy shows FN/SFN, a repeat biopsy should be performed 3-6 months later and include a sample for molecular testing with the results guiding further treatment.	Follicular carcinomas cannot be diagnosed on FNA because definitive diagnosis requires identification of capsular/vascular invasion. Molecular testing can be used to determine likelihood of malignancy.
V	Suspicious for Malignancy	As for malignant	
VI	Malignant	Referral to surgery if nodule is >1 cm. Nodules with papillary carcinoma less than 1 cm may not need to be removed and the option of serial ultrasounds (every 6-12 months) should be discussed with the patient. If the patient feels more comfortable with surgery, that can also be an option.	The most common malignancies of the thyroid are well-differentiated malignancies with a favorable prognosis. Of these, the most common is papillary thyroid carcinoma. Other malignancies include medullary thyroid carcinoma, poorly differentiated thyroid carcinoma, undifferentiated (anaplastic) thyroid carcinoma, squamous cell carcinoma, and malignant lymphoma. Metastases to the thyroid from other malignancies can occur as well

TABLE 2.7	Characteristics of Thyroid Cancers			
Type of Cancer	**Percentage of Thyroid Cancers**	**Age at Onset (Yr)**	**Treatment**	**Prognosis**
Papillary	85	40-80	Lobectomy or thyroidectomy, aggressive cases should receive radioactive iodine ablation	Good
Follicular	10	45-80	Lobectomy or thyroidectomy in aggressive cases	Fair to good
Medullary	3	20-50	Thyroidectomy and central compartment lymph node dissection	Fair
Anaplastic	1	50-80	Isthmusectomy followed by palliative radiograph treatment	Poor
Lymphoma	1	25-70	Radiograph therapy or chemotherapy or both	Fair

表 2.6　用于报告甲状腺细胞病理学的贝塞斯达（Bethesda）系统

贝塞斯达分类	诊断	处理意见	备注
I	无法诊断 / 取材不满意	重复 FNA（超声引导下）	
II	良性	如果患者或医务人员发现结节逐渐增大，则需要临床随访和复查超声检查，并可能进行重复活检	
III	意义不明的非典型增生（AUS）或意义不明的滤泡性病变（FLUS）	如果病理学诊断确定为 FLUS/AUS，应在首次活检后 3～6 个月再进行 1 次活检。若第 2 次活检的病理结果仍为 FLUS/AUS，则应对样本进行分子检测，并根据检测结果指导下一步治疗。如果仍不确定是否需要手术，则应进行超声检查，以评估结节是否增大或有形态学改变（是否导致 TI-RADS 评分升高）。若超声检查显示结节无显著增大或特征性改变，则可进行临床观察和监测	由于 FLUS/AUS 可能在桥本甲状腺炎的背景下出现，检测 TPOAb 可能有助于病理科对病变性质的进一步诊断。分子检测可用于确定恶性肿瘤的可能性
IV	滤泡性肿瘤（FN）或疑似滤泡性肿瘤（SFN）	如果初次活检结果显示为 FN/SFN，应在 3～6 个月后再次进行活检，并采集样本进行分子检测，根据检测结果指导下一步治疗	滤泡癌不能通过 FNA 诊断，因为明确诊断需要识别包膜 / 血管浸润。分子检测可用于确定恶性肿瘤的可能性
V	可疑恶性肿瘤	同恶性肿瘤	
VI	恶性肿瘤	如果结节 > 1 cm，建议转诊至外科进行手术。< 1 cm 的乳头状癌结节可能不需要切除，可与患者讨论进行连续超声随访（每 6～12 个月 1 次）。如果患者更倾向于手术治疗，可切除	甲状腺最常见的恶性肿瘤是预后良好的高分化癌。其中最常见的是甲状腺乳头状癌。其他恶性肿瘤包括甲状腺髓样癌、低分化甲状腺癌、未分化（间变性）甲状腺癌、鳞状细胞癌和恶性淋巴瘤。其他恶性肿瘤也可能发生甲状腺转移

表 2.7　甲状腺癌的特征

癌症类型	占甲状腺癌的比例（%）	发病年龄（岁）	治疗	预后
乳头状癌	85	40～80	甲状腺叶切除术或甲状腺切除术，侵袭性病例应接受放射性碘消融	良好
滤泡癌	10	45～80	侵袭性病例行腺叶切除术或甲状腺切除术	一般至良好
髓样癌	3	20～50	甲状腺切除术和中央区颈淋巴结清扫术	一般
未分化癌	1	50～80	峡部切除术后进行姑息性放疗	差
淋巴瘤	1	25～70	放疗和（或）化疗	一般

A rise in serum thyroglobulin levels suggests recurrence of thyroid cancer and should prompt testing for recurrence and/or metastases. These are evaluated by ^{131}I whole body scans carried out under conditions of TSH stimulation, which increases ^{131}I uptake by the thyroid tissue. Elevated TSH levels can be achieved by withdrawal of thyroxine supplementation for 6 weeks or by treatment with recombinant human TSH administered while the patient maintains therapy with thyroid hormone replacement. The latter avoids symptomatic hypothyroidism. Local or metastatic lesions that take up ^{131}I on whole body scanning can be treated with radioactive iodine after the patient has stopped thyroid hormone replacement, whereas those that do not take up ^{131}I can be treated with surgical excision or local radiograph therapy. Conventional chemotherapy has limited efficacy in the treatment of differentiated thyroid cancer, but newer biologic agents targeting the molecular pathogenesis of these tumors appear promising.

Medullary carcinoma of the thyroid requires total thyroidectomy with removal of the central lymph nodes in the neck. Completeness of the procedure and monitoring for recurrence are determined by measurements of serum calcitonin.

Anaplastic carcinoma is treated with isthmusectomy to confirm the diagnosis and to prevent tracheal compression, followed by palliative radiograph treatment. Thyroid lymphomas are also treated with radiograph therapy, chemotherapy, or both.

The prognosis for well-differentiated thyroid carcinomas is good. The patient's age at the time of diagnosis and sex are the most important prognostic factors. Men older than 40 years of age and women older than 50 years of age have higher recurrence and death rates than do younger patients. The 5-year survival rate for invasive medullary carcinoma is 50%, whereas the mean survival time for anaplastic carcinoma is 6 months.

For a deeper discussion on this topic, please see Chapter 213, ❖ "Thyroid," in *Goldman-Cecil Medicine*, 26th Edition.

SUGGESTED READINGS

Burch HB: Drug effects on the thyroid, N Engl J Med 381(8):749–761, 2019.

Cibas ES, Ali SZ: The 2017 Bethesda system for reporting thyroid cytopathology, Thyroid 27:1341–1346, 2017.

Gullo D, Latina A, Frasca F, et al: Levothyroxine monotherapy cannot guarantee euthyroidism in all athyreotic patients, PloS One 6:e22552, 2011.

Haugen BR, Alexander EK, Bible KC, et al: 2015 American thyroid association management guidelines for adult patients with thyroid nodules and differentiated thyroid cancer: the American Thyroid Association Guidelines Task Force on Thyroid Nodules and Differentiated Thyroid Cancer, Thyroid 26:1–133, 2016.

Ross DS, Burch HB, Cooper DS, et al: 2016 American Thyroid Association Guidelines for Diagnosis and Management of Hyperthyroidism and Other Causes of Thyrotoxicosis, Thyroid 26(10):1343–1421, 2016.

Welch HG, Doherty GM: Saving thyroids—overtreatment of small papillary cancers, N Engl J Med 379:310–312, 2018.

Wiersinga WM: Do we need still more trials on T4 and T3 combination therapy in hypothyroidism? Eur J Endocrinol 161:955–959, 2009.

血清甲状腺球蛋白水平升高通常提示甲状腺癌复发，应立即进行复发和（或）转移的相关检查。TSH 水平升高可增强甲状腺组织对 ^{131}I 的摄取，在 TSH 刺激下进行全身 ^{131}I 扫描可评估复发和（或）转移。提高 TSH 水平可通过停用甲状腺素替代治疗 6 周或在继续使用甲状腺激素替代治疗的同时应用重组人 TSH，后者可避免患者出现甲状腺功能减退症的症状。对于全身扫描识别出的摄取 ^{131}I 的局灶性或转移性病变，可在停用甲状腺激素替代治疗后采用 ^{131}I 治疗；而对于不摄取 ^{131}I 的病变，可通过手术切除或局部放疗。尽管传统化疗对分化型甲状腺癌的疗效有限，但针对肿瘤分子学发病机制的新型生物制剂可能有广阔的治疗前景。

甲状腺髓样癌需要进行甲状腺全切除术和中央区颈淋巴结清扫术。检测血清降钙素水平可评估手术是否完整切除并监测复发。

甲状腺未分化癌可通过切除峡部确诊，并防止气管受压，之后进行姑息性放疗。甲状腺淋巴瘤可采用放疗和（或）化疗。

高分化甲状腺癌的预后较好。诊断时的年龄和性别是最重要的预后因素。40 岁以上男性和 50 岁以上女性的复发率和死亡率均高于年轻患者。侵袭性髓样癌的 5 年生存率为 50%，而未分化癌患者的平均生存期为 6 个月。

有关此专题的深入讨论，请参阅 *Goldman-Cecil Medicine* 第 26 版第 213 章 "甲状腺"。

推荐阅读

Burch HB: Drug effects on the thyroid, N Engl J Med 381(8):749–761, 2019.

Cibas ES, Ali SZ: The 2017 Bethesda system for reporting thyroid cytopathology, Thyroid 27:1341–1346, 2017.

Gullo D, Latina A, Frasca F, et al: Levothyroxine monotherapy cannot guarantee euthyroidism in all athyreotic patients, PloS One 6:e22552, 2011.

Haugen BR, Alexander EK, Bible KC, et al: 2015 American thyroid association management guidelines for adult patients with thyroid nodules and differentiated thyroid cancer: the American Thyroid Association Guidelines Task Force on Thyroid Nodules and Differentiated Thyroid Cancer, Thyroid 26:1–133, 2016.

Ross DS, Burch HB, Cooper DS, et al: 2016 American Thyroid Association Guidelines for Diagnosis and Management of Hyperthyroidism and Other Causes of Thyrotoxicosis, Thyroid 26(10):1343–1421, 2016.

Welch HG, Doherty GM: Saving thyroids—overtreatment of small papillary cancers, N Engl J Med 379:310–312, 2018.

Wiersinga WM: Do we need still more trials on T4 and T3 combination therapy in hypothyroidism? Eur J Endocrinol 161:955–959, 2009.

Adrenal Gland

Theodore C. Friedman

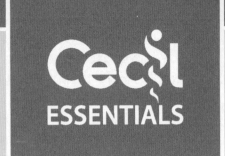

PHYSIOLOGY

The adrenal glands (Fig. 3.1) lie at the superior pole of each kidney and are composed of two distinct regions: the cortex and the medulla. The adrenal cortex comprises three anatomic zones: the outer *zona glomerulosa*, which secretes the mineralocorticoid aldosterone; the intermediate *zona fasciculata*, which secretes cortisol; and the inner *zona reticularis*, which secretes adrenal androgens. The adrenal medulla, lying in the center of the adrenal gland, is functionally related to the sympathetic nervous system and secretes the catecholamines epinephrine and norepinephrine in response to stress.

The synthesis of all steroid hormones begins with cholesterol and is catalyzed by a series of regulated, enzyme-mediated reactions (Fig. 3.2). Glucocorticoids affect metabolism, cardiovascular function, behavior, and the inflammatory and immune responses (Table 3.1). Cortisol, the natural human glucocorticoid, is secreted by the adrenal glands in response to adrenocorticotropic hormone (ACTH), a 39-amino-acid neuropeptide that is regulated by corticotropin-releasing hormone (CRH) and vasopressin (AVP) produced in the hypothalamus (see Chapter 1). Glucocorticoids exert negative feedback on CRH and ACTH secretion. The brain hypothalamic-pituitary-adrenal (HPA) axis (Fig. 3.3) interacts with and influences the functions of the reproductive, growth, and thyroid axes at many levels, with major participation of glucocorticoids at all levels.

The renin-angiotensin-aldosterone system (Fig. 3.4) is the major regulator of aldosterone secretion. Renal juxtaglomerular cells secrete renin in response to a decrease in circulating volume, a reduction in renal perfusion pressure or both. Renin is the rate-limiting enzyme that cleaves the 60-kD angiotensinogen molecule, synthesized by the liver, to produce the bioinactive decapeptide angiotensin I. Angiotensin I is rapidly converted to the octapeptide angiotensin II by angiotensin-converting enzyme in the lungs and other tissues. Angiotensin II is a potent vasopressor; it stimulates aldosterone production but does not stimulate cortisol production. Angiotensin II is the predominant regulator of aldosterone secretion, but plasma potassium concentration, plasma volume, and ACTH level also influence aldosterone secretion. ACTH also mediates the circadian rhythm of aldosterone, and as a result, the plasma concentration of aldosterone is highest in the morning. Aldosterone binds to the type I mineralocorticoid receptor. In contrast, cortisol binds to both the type I mineralocorticoid and type II glucocorticoid receptors. The intracellular enzyme 11β-hydroxysteroid dehydrogenase (11β-HSD) type II, which catabolizes cortisol to inactive cortisone, limits the functional binding to the former receptor. The availability of cortisol to bind to the glucocorticoid receptor is modulated by 11β-HSD type I, which interconverts cortisol and cortisone. Binding of aldosterone to the cytosol mineralocorticoid receptor leads to sodium (Na^+) absorption and potassium (K^+) and hydrogen (H^+) secretion by the renal tubules. The resultant increase in plasma Na^+ and decrease in plasma K^+ provide a feedback mechanism for suppressing renin and, subsequently, aldosterone secretion.

Adrenal androgen precursors include dehydroepiandrosterone (DHEA) and its sulfate and androstenedione. These are synthesized in the zona reticularis under the influence of ACTH and other adrenal androgen-stimulating factors. Although they have minimal intrinsic androgenic activity, they contribute to androgenicity by their peripheral conversion to testosterone and dihydrotestosterone. In adult men, excessive levels of adrenal androgens have negligible clinical consequences, but in women they result in acne, hirsutism, and virilization. Because of gonadal production of androgens and estrogens and the secretion of norepinephrine by sympathetic ganglia, deficiencies of adrenal androgens and catecholamines are not clinically recognized.

SYNDROMES OF ADRENOCORTICAL HYPOFUNCTION

Adrenal Insufficiency

Glucocorticoid insufficiency can be primary, resulting from destruction or dysfunction of the adrenal cortex, or secondary, resulting from ACTH hyposecretion (Table 3.2). Medications and supplements affecting cortisol levels are shown in Table 3.3. Autoimmune destruction of the adrenal glands (Addison's disease) is the most common cause of primary adrenal insufficiency in the industrialized world, accounting for about 65% of cases. Usually, both glucocorticoid and mineralocorticoid secretions are diminished in this condition that, if left untreated, can be fatal. Isolated glucocorticoid or mineralocorticoid deficiency may also occur, and it is becoming apparent that mild adrenal insufficiency (similar to subclinical hypothyroidism, discussed in Chapter 2) should also be diagnosed and, in some cases, treated. Adrenal medulla function is usually spared. About 80% of patients with Addison's disease have antiadrenal antibodies directed at 21α-hydroxylase (CYP21A2), though in clinical practice this may be lower due to poor quality of commercial autoantibody testing.

Tuberculosis used to be the most common cause of adrenal insufficiency. However, its incidence in the industrialized world has decreased since the 1960s, and it now accounts for only 15% to 20% of patients with adrenal insufficiency; calcified adrenal glands can be observed in 50% of these patients. Rare causes of adrenal insufficiency are listed in Table 3.2. Many patients with human immunodeficiency virus (HIV) infection have decreased adrenal reserve without overt adrenal insufficiency.

Addison's disease may be part of two distinct autoimmune polyglandular syndromes. The triad of hypoparathyroidism, adrenal insufficiency, and mucocutaneous candidiasis characterizes *type I polyglandular autoimmune syndrome*, also called autoimmune polyendocrinopathy 1 (APECED), which usually manifests in childhood. Other, less common manifestations include hypothyroidism, gonadal failure,

肾上腺

卢琳　苏婉　译　陈适　童安莉　审校　宁光　通审

生理学

肾上腺（图 3.1）位于每侧肾脏的上极，由 2 个区域组成：皮质和髓质。肾上腺皮质由 3 个解剖区域组成：最外层为球状带，分泌盐皮质激素；中间为束状带，分泌皮质醇；内层为网状带，分泌肾上腺来源的雄激素。肾上腺髓质位于肾上腺的中央，其功能与交感神经系统有关，在应激时可分泌肾上腺素和去甲肾上腺素等儿茶酚胺。

所有类固醇激素的合成均始于胆固醇，并由一系列受调控的、酶介导的反应催化完成（图 3.2）。糖皮质激素可影响代谢、心血管功能、个体行为，以及炎症和免疫反应（表 3.1）。皮质醇是人体天然的糖皮质激素，促肾上腺皮质激素（ACTH）可刺激肾上腺分泌皮质醇，ACTH 是一种含 39 个氨基酸的神经肽，受下丘脑分泌的促肾上腺皮质激素释放激素（CRH）和血管升压素（AVP）的调节（见第 1 章）。糖皮质激素对 CRH 和 ACTH 的分泌起负反馈调节作用。下丘脑-垂体-肾上腺（HPA）轴（图 3.3）与性腺轴、生长激素轴和甲状腺轴的功能在多个层面上相互作用并互影响，糖皮质激素在所有层面均发挥重要作用。

肾素-血管紧张素-醛固酮系统（图 3.4）是醛固酮分泌的主要调节因子。肾球旁细胞在循环容量减少和（或）肾灌注压降低时分泌肾素。肾素是一种限速酶，它能分解由肝脏合成的 60 kD 血管紧张素原，从而产生无生物活性的十肽血管紧张素 I，血管紧张素 I 通过肺和其他组织中的血管紧张素转换酶迅速转化为八肽血管紧张素 II。血管紧张素 II 是一种强效血管收缩剂，它能刺激醛固酮的分泌，但不会刺激皮质醇的分泌。血管紧张素 II 是醛固酮分泌的主要调节剂，但血钾浓度、血容量和 ACTH 水平也会影响醛固酮的分泌。ACTH 参与介导醛固酮的昼夜节律，因此，醛固酮的血浆浓度在早晨最高。醛固酮可结合 I 型盐皮质激素受体。相比之下，皮质醇可同时与 I 型盐皮质激素受体和 II 型糖皮质激素受体结合。细胞内的 II 型 11β-羟基类固醇脱氢酶（11β-HSD）可将皮质醇分解为无活性的皮质素，从而限制了皮质醇与上述受体的功能性结合。皮质醇与糖皮质激素受体结合受 I 型 11β-HSD 的调节，该酶可使皮质醇和皮质素相互转化。醛固酮和盐皮质激素受体结合会导致肾小管重吸收钠离子（Na^+）和分泌钾离子（K^+）、氢离子（H^+）。血浆 Na^+ 增加和血浆 K^+ 减少可反馈性抑制肾素分泌，继而抑制醛固酮的分泌。

肾上腺雄激素前体包括脱氢表雄酮（DHEA）、硫酸脱氢表雄酮和雄烯二酮。它们在 ACTH 和其他肾上腺雄激素刺激因子的影响下在网状带中合成。虽然它们本身的雄激素活性极低，但可通过在外周转化为睾酮和双氢睾酮而发挥雄激素活性。在成年男性中，肾上腺雄激素水平过高的临床表现微乎其微，但在女性中会导致痤疮、多毛和男性化。由于性腺可分泌雄激素和雌激素，交感神经节可分泌去甲肾上腺素，因此肾上腺雄激素和儿茶酚胺缺乏症在临床上并不容易被识别。

肾上腺皮质功能减退
肾上腺皮质功能不全

皮质醇分泌不足可分为原发性（由肾上腺皮质破坏或功能障碍引起）或继发性（由 ACTH 分泌不足引起）（表 3.2）。影响皮质醇水平的药物和补充剂见表 3.3。肾上腺自身免疫病［艾迪生病（Addison 病）］是发达国家人群原发性肾上腺皮质功能不全最常见的原因，约占病例的 65%。在这种情况下，糖皮质激素和盐皮质激素的分泌通常都会减少，如果不及时治疗，可能危及生命。患者也可能出现孤立性糖皮质激素或盐皮质激素缺乏。轻度肾上腺皮质功能不全（类似于第 2 章讨论的亚临床甲状腺功能减退症）也应得到诊断，且在某些情况下需要治疗。约 80% 的 Addison 病患者存在针对 21α-羟化酶（CYP21A2）的抗肾上腺抗体，但在临床实践中，由于可用的自身抗体检测的质量较差，这一比例可能较低。

结核曾是肾上腺皮质功能不全最常见的病因。但是，自 20 世纪 60 年代以来，结核在发达国家的发病率有所下降，目前肾上腺皮质功能不全患者中结核患者仅占 15%～20%；在这些患者中，50% 可观察到钙化的肾上腺。肾上腺皮质功能不全的罕见病因见表 3.2。许多人类免疫缺陷病毒（HIV）感染者的肾上腺储备功能下降，但无明显的肾上腺皮质功能不全表现。

Addison 病可能是两种自身免疫性多内分泌腺综合征的组分。自身免疫性多内分泌腺综合征 I 型［又称自身免疫性多内分泌腺病（APECED）］的特征是甲状旁腺功能减退症、肾上腺皮质功能不全和皮肤黏膜念珠

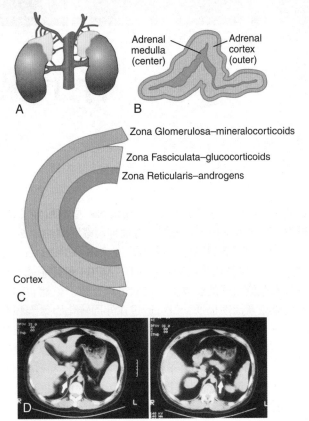

Fig. 3.1 (A) Anatomic location of the adrenal glands. (B) Distribution of adrenal cortex and medulla. (C) Zones of the adrenal cortex. (D) Magnetic resonance images of the abdomen showing the position and relative size of the normal adrenal glands *(arrows)*. (D, From Nieman LK: Adrenal cortex. In Goldman L, Schafer AI, editors: Goldman-Cecil medicine, ed 24, Philadelphia, 2012, Saunders, Figure 234-1.)

gastrointestinal malabsorption, insulin-dependent diabetes mellitus, alopecia areata and totalis, pernicious anemia, vitiligo, chronic active hepatitis, keratopathy, hypoplasia of dental enamel and nails, hypophysitis, asplenism, and cholelithiasis. *Type II polyglandular autoimmune syndrome*, also called *Schmidt syndrome*, is characterized by Addison's disease, autoimmune thyroid disease (Graves' disease or Hashimoto thyroiditis), and insulin-dependent diabetes mellitus. Other associated diseases include pernicious anemia, vitiligo, gonadal failure, hypophysitis, celiac disease, myasthenia gravis, primary biliary cirrhosis, Sjögren's syndrome, lupus erythematosus, and Parkinson's disease. This syndrome usually develops in adults.

Common manifestations of adrenal insufficiency are anorexia, weight loss, increasing fatigue, occasional vomiting, diarrhea, and salt craving. Muscle and joint pain, abdominal pain, and postural dizziness may also occur. Signs of increased pigmentation (initially most significant on the extensor surfaces, palmar creases, and buccal mucosa) often occur secondary to the increased production of ACTH and other related peptides by the pituitary gland. Laboratory abnormalities may include hyponatremia, hyperkalemia, mild metabolic acidosis, azotemia, hypercalcemia, anemia, lymphocytosis, and eosinophilia. Hypoglycemia may also occur, especially in children.

Acute adrenal insufficiency is a medical emergency, and treatment should not be delayed pending laboratory results. In a critically ill patient with hypovolemia, a plasma sample for cortisol, ACTH, aldosterone, and renin should be obtained, and then treatment with

hydrocortisone (100 mg IV bolus) and parenteral saline administration should be initiated. Sepsis-induced adrenal insufficiency is recognized by a basal cortisol level lower than 10 µg/dL or a change in cortisol of less than 9 µg/dL after administration of 0.25 mg ACTH (1-24) (cosyntropin). In severe illness, albumin and cortisol-binding globulin (CBG) are low, resulting in a low level of total cortisol but not free cortisol; therefore, a low total cortisol level may not be diagnostic of adrenal insufficiency in this setting.

In a patient with chronic symptoms suggestive of adrenal insufficiency described previously, a basal early morning plasma cortisol measurement, a 1-hour cosyntropin test, or both, should be performed. These tests are not recommended in patients without symptoms of adrenal insufficiency. In the latter test, 0.25 mg of cosyntropin is given intravenously or intramuscularly, and plasma cortisol is measured after 0, 30, and 60 minutes. A normal response is a plasma cortisol concentration higher than 18 µg/dL at any time during the test. A patient with a basal morning plasma cortisol concentration lower than 5 µg/dL and a stimulated cortisol concentration lower than 18 µg/dL probably has adrenal insufficiency and should receive treatment. A basal plasma morning cortisol concentration between 10 and 18 µg/dL in association with a stimulated cortisol concentration lower than 18 µg/dL probably indicates impaired adrenal reserve and a requirement for receiving cortisol replacement under stress conditions (see later discussion). Birth control pills and oral estrogens increase CBG levels; therefore, a patient on those agents may have a normal basal or cosyntropin-stimulated cortisol level and have a low free cortisol level, making interpretation of the test difficult for these patients.

Once the diagnosis of adrenal insufficiency is made, the distinction between primary and secondary adrenal insufficiency needs to be established. Secondary adrenal insufficiency results from inadequate stimulation of the adrenal cortex by ACTH (see Chapter 1). Hyperpigmentation does not occur. In addition, because mineralocorticoid levels are normal in secondary adrenal insufficiency, symptoms of salt craving, as well as the laboratory abnormalities of hyperkalemia and metabolic acidosis, are not present, although hyponatremia may be observed. Hypothyroidism, hypogonadism, and growth hormone deficiency may also be present. To distinguish primary from secondary adrenal insufficiency, a basal morning plasma ACTH value should be obtained, along with a serum aldosterone level and a measurement of plasma renin activity (PRA). A plasma ACTH value greater than 20 pg/mL (normal, 5 to 30 pg/mL) is consistent with primary adrenal insufficiency, whereas a value lower than 20 pg/mL probably represents secondary adrenal insufficiency. A PRA value greater than 3 ng/mL/hour in the setting of a suppressed aldosterone level is consistent with primary adrenal insufficiency, whereas a value lower than 3 ng/mL/hour probably represents secondary adrenal insufficiency. The 1-hour cosyntropin test is suppressed in both primary and secondary chronic adrenal insufficiency.

Secondary adrenal insufficiency occurs commonly after the discontinuation of exogenous glucocorticoids. Alternate-day glucocorticoid treatment, if feasible, results in less suppression of the HPA axis than does daily glucocorticoid therapy. Complete recovery of the HPA axis can take 1 year or more, and the rate-limiting step appears to be recovery of the CRH-producing neurons.

Under stress, cortisol secretion is increased. Therefore, the concept of adrenal fatigue, proposed by some alternative providers, has no biologic validity.

After stabilization of acute adrenal insufficiency, patients with Addison's disease require lifelong replacement therapy with both glucocorticoids and mineralocorticoids. Many patients are overtreated with glucocorticoids and undertreated with mineralocorticoids. Because overtreatment with glucocorticoids results in insidious weight

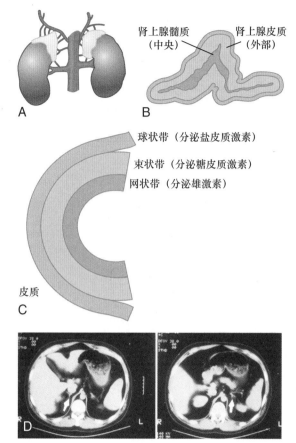

图 3.1　A. 肾上腺的解剖位置。B. 肾上腺皮质和髓质的分布。C. 肾上腺皮质的分区。D. 腹部 MRI 图像，可见正常肾上腺的位置和相对大小（箭头）（D 图引自 Nieman LK：Adrenal cortex. In Goldman L，Schafer AI，editors：Goldman-Cecil medicine，ed 24，Philadelphia，2012，Saunders，Figure 234-1.）

菌病三联征，一般于儿童期起病。其他较少见的表现包括甲状腺功能减退症、性腺功能减退症、胃肠道吸收不良、胰岛素依赖型糖尿病、斑秃和全秃、恶性贫血、白癜风、慢性活动性肝炎、角膜病、牙釉质和指甲发育不全、垂体炎、脾功能不全和胆石症。自身免疫性多内分泌腺综合征Ⅱ型又称施密特综合征（Schmidt 综合征），主要表现为 Addison 病、自身免疫性甲状腺疾病（Graves 病或桥本甲状腺炎）和胰岛素依赖型糖尿病。其他相关疾病包括恶性贫血、白癜风、性腺功能减退症、垂体炎、乳糜泻、重症肌无力、原发性胆汁性肝硬化、干燥综合征、红斑狼疮和帕金森病。该综合征通常于成年期起病。

肾上腺皮质功能不全的常见表现包括厌食、体重减轻、易疲劳、偶尔呕吐、腹泻和嗜盐。患者也可能出现肌肉和关节疼痛、腹痛和体位性头晕。色素沉着（最初位于肢体的伸侧、掌纹和颊黏膜）通常继发于垂体分泌的 ACTH 和其他相关肽增多。实验室检查异常可能包括低钠血症、高钾血症、轻度代谢性酸中毒、氮质血症、高钙血症、贫血、淋巴细胞增多和嗜酸性粒细胞增多。也可能出现低血糖，尤其是儿童患者。

急性肾上腺皮质功能减退是一种内科急症，不应因等待实验室检查结果而延误治疗。对于容量不足的危重患者，应在采集检测皮质醇、ACTH、醛固酮和肾素的血

浆样本后开始氢化可的松（100 mg 静脉推注）和生理盐水治疗。感染中毒症引起的肾上腺皮质功能不全表现为基线皮质醇 < 10 μg/dl 或注射 0.25 mg ACTH（1-24）（促皮质素）后皮质醇增幅 < 9 μg/dl。重症患者的白蛋白和皮质醇结合球蛋白（CBG）水平较低，可导致总皮质醇水平较低，但游离皮质醇水平不受影响；因此，在这种情况下，总皮质醇水平较低不能诊断肾上腺皮质功能不全。

对于有上述提示肾上腺皮质功能不全的慢性症状的患者，应进行清晨基础血浆皮质醇测定和（或）1 h 促皮质素试验。这些检查不建议在无症状的患者中进行。1 h 促皮质素试验是在静脉注射或肌内注射促皮质素 0.25 mg 后，于 0 min、30 min 和 60 min 测量血浆皮质醇。正常反应是试验期间任意时间点的血浆皮质醇浓度 > 18 μg/dl。如果患者清晨基础血浆皮质醇浓度 < 5 μg/dl，而刺激后皮质醇浓度 < 18 μg/dl，则可能为肾上腺皮质功能不全，应接受治疗。清晨基础血浆皮质醇浓度为 10 ~ 18 μg/dl 且刺激后皮质醇浓度 < 18 μg/dl 提示肾上腺储备功能受损，需要在应激条件下补充皮质醇（见下文）。避孕药和口服雌激素可升高 CBG 水平；因此，服用这些药物的患者可能表现为基础或促皮质素刺激后皮质醇水平正常，而游离皮质醇水平较低，导致这些患者的检测结果难以解释。

一旦确诊为肾上腺皮质功能不全，则需要鉴别原发性和继发性肾上腺皮质功能不全。继发性肾上腺皮质功能不全是由 ACTH 对肾上腺皮质的刺激不足所致（见第 1 章），患者不会出现色素沉着。此外，由于继发性肾上腺皮质功能不全患者的盐皮质激素水平正常，因此不会出现嗜盐症状以及高钾血症和代谢性酸中毒等，但可能会出现低钠血症。此外，患者也可能存在甲状腺功能减退症、性腺功能减退症和生长激素缺乏症。测定清晨基础血浆 ACTH、血清醛固酮水平和血浆肾素活性（PRA）有助于鉴别原发性和继发性肾上腺皮质功能不全。血浆 ACTH > 20 pg/ml（正常 5 ~ 30 pg/ml）提示原发性肾上腺皮质功能不全，而血浆 ACTH < 20 pg/ml 提示继发性肾上腺皮质功能不全。在醛固酮水平受抑制的情况下，PRA > 3 ng/（ml·h）提示原发性肾上腺皮质功能不全，而 PRA < 3 ng/（ml·h），则提示继发性肾上腺皮质功能不全。原发性和继发性慢性肾上腺皮质功能不全患者的 1 h 促皮质素试验结果均显示受抑制。

继发性肾上腺皮质功能不全常见于外源性糖皮质激素停药后。如果可行，隔日使用糖皮质激素对 HPA 轴的抑制作用小于每天使用糖皮质激素。HPA 轴完全恢复可能需要 1 年或更长时间，而限速步骤为生成 CRH 的神经元的恢复。

在应激状态下，皮质醇分泌增加。因此，一些学者提出的"肾上腺疲劳"概念尚未得到生物学证实。

急性肾上腺皮质功能不全病情稳定后，Addison 病患者需要终身接受糖皮质激素和盐皮质激素替代治疗。许多患者存在糖皮质激素治疗过度而盐皮质激素

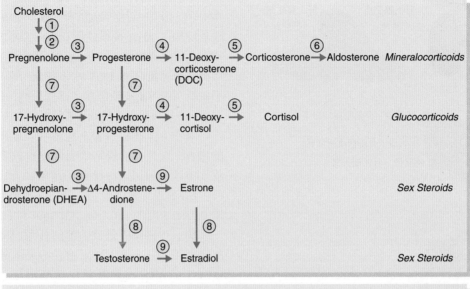

Enzyme Number	Enzyme (Current and Trivial Name)
1	StAR; Steroidogenic acute regulatory protein
2	CYP11A1; Cholesterol side-chain cleavage enzyme/desmolase
3	3β-HSD II; 3β-Hydroxylase dehydrogenase
4	CYP21A2; 21α-Hydroxylase
5	CYP11B1; 11β-Hydroxylase
6	CYP11B2; Corticosterone methyloxidase
7	CYP17; 17α-Hydroxylase/17, 20 lyase
8	17β-HSD; 17β-Hydroxysteroid dehydrogenase
9	CYP19; Aromatase

Fig. 3.2 Pathways of steroid biosynthesis.

TABLE 3.1 Actions of Glucocorticoids

Metabolic Homeostasis
Regulate blood glucose level (permissive effects on gluconeogenesis)
Increase glycogen synthesis
Raise insulin levels (permissive effects on lipolytic hormones)
Increase catabolism, decrease anabolism (except fat), inhibit growth hormone axis
Inhibit reproductive axis
Stimulate mineralocorticoid receptor by cortisol

Connective Tissues
Cause loss of collagen and connective tissue

Calcium Homeostasis
Stimulate osteoclasts, inhibit osteoblasts
Reduce intestinal calcium absorption, stimulate parathyroid hormone release, increase urinary calcium excretion, decrease reabsorption of phosphate

Cardiovascular Function
Increase cardiac output
Increase vascular tone (permissive effects on pressor hormones)
Increase sodium retention

Behavior and Cognitive Function
Daytime fatigue
Nocturnal hyperarousal
Decreased short-term memory
Decreased cognition

Euphoria or Depression
Immune System
Increase intravascular leukocyte concentration
Decrease migration of inflammatory cells to sites of injury
Suppress immune system (thymolysis; suppression of cytokines, prostanoids, kinins, serotonin, histamine, collagenase, and plasminogen activator)

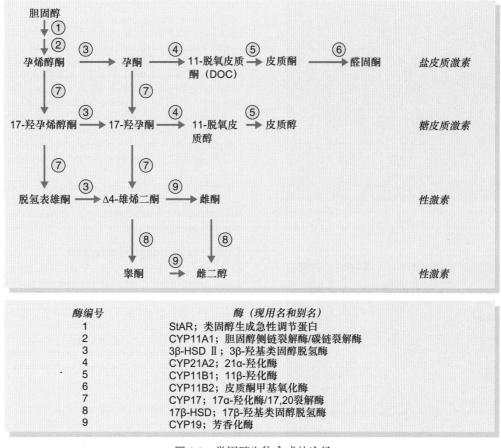

图 3.2　类固醇生物合成的途径

表 3.1　糖皮质激素的作用
代谢平衡
调节血糖水平（糖原合成的允许作用）
增加糖原合成
提高胰岛素水平（对脂肪分解激素产生允许作用）
增加分解代谢，减少合成代谢（脂肪除外），抑制生长激素轴
抑制性腺轴
通过皮质醇刺激盐皮质激素受体
结缔组织
导致胶原蛋白和结缔组织丢失
钙平衡
刺激破骨细胞，抑制成骨细胞
减少肠道对钙的吸收，刺激甲状旁腺激素的释放，增加尿钙排泄，减少对磷酸盐的重吸收
心血管功能
增加心输出量
增强血管张力（对升压激素的允许作用）
增加钠潴留
行为和认知功能
日间疲劳
夜间过度觉醒
短时记忆功能下降
认知功能下降
欣快或抑郁
免疫系统
增加血管内白细胞浓度
减少炎症细胞向受伤部位的迁移
抑制免疫系统（胸腺破坏；抑制细胞因子、前列腺素类激素、激肽、5- 羟色胺、组胺、胶原酶和纤溶酶原激活物）

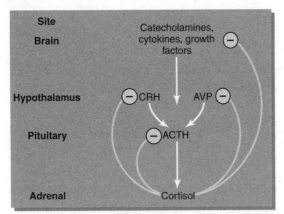

Fig. 3.3 Brain hypothalamic-pituitary-adrenal axis. Minus signs indicate negative feedback. *ACTH,* Adrenocorticotropic hormone; *AVP,* arginine vasopressin; *CRH,* corticotropin-releasing hormone.

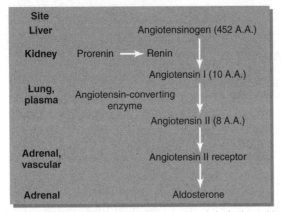

Fig. 3.4 Renin-angiotensin-aldosterone axis. *A.A.,* Amino acids.

gain and osteoporosis, the minimal cortisol dose that can be tolerated without symptoms of glucocorticoid insufficiency (usually joint pain, abdominal pain, or diarrhea) is recommended. An initial regimen of 10 to 15 mg hydrocortisone first thing in the morning plus 5 mg hydrocortisone at about 3:00 PM mimics the physiologic dose and is recommended; a third dose is occasionally needed. Whereas glucocorticoid replacement is fairly uniform in most patients, the requirement for mineralocorticoid replacement varies greatly. The initial dose of the synthetic mineralocorticoid fludrocortisone should be 100 μg/day (often in divided doses), and the dosage should be adjusted to keep the standing PRA value between 1 and 3 ng/mL/hr.

Under the stress of a minor illness (e.g., nausea, vomiting, fever >100.5° F), the hydrocortisone dose should be doubled for as short a period as possible. An inability to ingest hydrocortisone pills may necessitate parenteral hydrocortisone administration. Patients undergoing a major stressful event (e.g., surgery necessitating general anesthesia, major trauma) should receive 150 to 300 mg parenteral hydrocortisone daily (in divided doses) with a rapid taper to normal replacement during recovery. All patients should wear a medical information bracelet and should be instructed in the use of intramuscular emergency hydrocortisone injections or alternatively hydrocortisone suppositories as another option.

Hyporeninemic Hypoaldosteronism

Mineralocorticoid deficiency can result from decreased renin secretion by the kidneys. Resultant hypoangiotensinemia leads to hypoaldosteronism with hyperkalemia and hyperchloremic metabolic acidosis. The plasma sodium concentration is usually normal, but total plasma volume is often deficient. PRA and aldosterone levels are low and unresponsive to stimuli, including hypokalemia. Diabetes mellitus and chronic tubulointerstitial diseases of the kidney are the most common underlying conditions leading to impairment of the juxtaglomerular apparatus. A subset of hyporeninemic hypoaldosteronism is caused by autonomic insufficiency and is a frequent cause of orthostatic hypotension. Stimuli such as upright posture or volume depletion, mediated by baroreceptors, do not cause a normal renin response. Administration of pharmacologic agents such as nonsteroidal anti-inflammatory agents, angiotensin-converting enzyme inhibitors, and β-adrenergic antagonists can also produce conditions of hypoaldosteronism. Salt administration often with fludrocortisone and the α1-receptor agonist midodrine are effective in correcting the orthostatic hypotension and electrolyte abnormalities caused by hypoaldosteronism.

Congenital Adrenal Hyperplasia

Congenital adrenal hyperplasia (CAH) refers to autosomal recessive disorders of adrenal steroid biosynthesis that result in glucocorticoid and mineralocorticoid deficiencies and compensatory increase in ACTH secretion (see Fig. 3.2). Five major types of CAH exist, and the clinical manifestations of each type depend on which steroids are in excess and which are deficient. CYP21A2 deficiency is the most common of these disorders and accounts for about 95% of patients with CAH. In this condition, there is a failure of 21-hydroxylation of 17-hydroxyprogesterone and progesterone to 11-deoxycortisol and 11-deoxycorticosterone, respectively, with deficient cortisol and aldosterone production. Cortisol deficiency leads to increased ACTH release, resulting in adrenal hyperplasia and overproduction of 17-hydroxyprogesterone and progesterone. Increased ACTH production also leads to increased biosynthesis of androstenedione and DHEA, which can be converted to testosterone. Patients with CYP21A2 deficiencies can be divided into two clinical phenotypes: classic 21-hydroxylase deficiency, which usually is diagnosed at birth or during childhood, and late-onset 21-hydroxylase deficiency, which develops during or after puberty. Two thirds of patients with classic CYP21A2 deficiency have various degrees of mineralocorticoid deficiency (salt-losing form); the remaining one third have the non–salt-losing type (simple virilizing form). Both decreased aldosterone production and increased concentrations of precursors that are mineralocorticoid antagonists (progesterone and 17-hydroxyprogesterone) contribute to salt loss.

Late-onset 21-hydroxylase deficiency represents an allelic variant of classic 21-hydroxylase deficiency and is characterized by a mild enzymatic defect. This deficiency is the most common autosomal recessive disorder in humans and is present at high frequency in Ashkenazi Jews. The syndrome usually develops at the time of puberty with signs of virilization (hirsutism and acne) and amenorrhea or oligomenorrhea. This diagnosis should be considered in women who have unexplained hirsutism and menstrual abnormalities or infertility.

The most useful initial measurement for the diagnosis of classic 21-hydroxylase deficiency is that of plasma 17-hydroxyprogesterone. A value greater than 200 ng/dL is consistent with the diagnosis. The diagnosis of late-onset 21-hydroxylase deficiency is based on the finding of an elevated level of plasma 17-hydroxyprogesterone (>1500 ng/dL) 30 minutes after administration of 0.25 mg of synthetic ACTH (1-24).

The aim of treatment for classic 21-hydroxylase deficiency is to replace glucocorticoids and mineralocorticoids, suppress ACTH and androgen overproduction, and allow for normal growth and

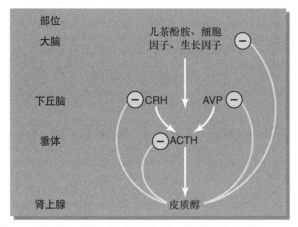

图 3.3　下丘脑 - 垂体 - 肾上腺轴。"－"表示负反馈。ACTH，促肾上腺皮质激素；AVP，精氨酸加压素；CRH，促肾上腺皮质激素释放激素

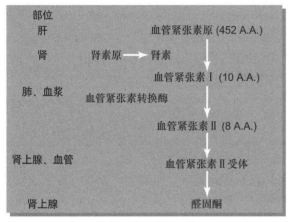

图 3.4　肾素 - 血管紧张素 - 醛固酮轴。A.A.，氨基酸

治疗不足的情况。由于糖皮质激素过度治疗会导致体重增加和骨质疏松症，建议在没有糖皮质激素缺乏症状（通常是关节痛、腹痛或腹泻）的情况下使用可耐受的最小剂量。推荐模拟生理剂量的初始方案，即清晨服用 10 ～ 15 mg 氢化可的松，然后在 15:00 左右服用 5 mg 氢化可的松；偶尔需要服用第三剂。虽然大多数患者的糖皮质激素替代剂量基本一致，但对盐皮质激素替代的需求差异很大。人工合成的盐皮质激素氟氢可的松的初始剂量应为 100 μg/d（通常分次服用），并逐渐调整剂量使 PRA 保持在 1 ～ 3 ng/（ml·h）。

在轻微疾病（如恶心、呕吐、发热 > 38℃）的应激下，氢化可的松剂量应在尽可能短的时间内加倍。如果无法吞服氢化可的松药片，则有必要肠外给药。正在经历重大应激事件（如需要全身麻醉的手术、重大创伤）的患者应肠外应用 150 ～ 300 mg/d 氢化可的松（分次使用），并在恢复期间迅速减量至正常剂量。所有患者均应佩戴医疗信息手环，并指导患者使用紧急氢化可的松肌内注射或氢化可的松栓剂。

低肾素性低醛固酮血症

肾脏分泌的肾素减少会引起盐皮质激素缺乏。由此引起的低血管紧张素血症会导致低醛固酮血症，伴有高钾血症和高氯性代谢性酸中毒。患者的血浆钠浓度通常正常，但总血浆容量往往不足。PRA 和醛固酮水平偏低，且对低钾血症等刺激无反应。糖尿病和慢性肾小管间质性疾病是球旁器损害最常见的原因。低肾素性低醛固酮血症的一个亚型是由自主神经功能不全引起，且是体位性低血压的常见原因。由压力感受器介导的刺激（如直立姿势或血容量不足）不能引起正常的肾素反应。部分药物（如非甾体抗炎药、血管紧张素转换酶抑制剂和 β 受体阻滞剂）也可导致低醛固酮血症。补充盐并通常联用氟氢可的松和 α_1 受体激动剂米多君可有效纠正由低醛固酮血症引起的体位性低血压和电解质异常。

先天性肾上腺皮质增生症

先天性肾上腺皮质增生症（CAH）是一种肾上腺皮质类固醇生物合成障碍的常染色体隐性遗传病，可导致糖皮质激素和盐皮质激素缺乏，以及代偿性 ACTH 分泌增加（图 3.2）。CAH 包括 5 种主要类型，每种类型的临床表现取决于过量和缺乏的类固醇类型。CYP21A2 缺乏症是这些疾病中最常见的一种，约占 CAH 患者的 95%。在这种情况下，17- 羟孕酮和孕酮不能通过 21- 羟化酶分别转化为 11- 脱氧皮质醇和 11- 脱氧皮质酮，导致皮质醇和醛固酮分泌不足。皮质醇缺乏会导致 ACTH 释放增加，导致肾上腺增生、17- 羟孕酮和孕酮分泌过多。ACTH 分泌增加还会导致雄烯二酮和 DHEA 的生物合成增加，而这两种物质可转化为睾酮。CYP21A2 缺乏症患者可分为两种临床表型：经典型 21- 羟化酶缺乏症，通常在出生时或儿童期被诊断；迟发型 21- 羟化酶缺乏症，在青春期或青春期后发病。2/3 的经典型 CYP21A2 缺乏症患者有不同程度的盐皮质激素缺乏症（失盐型），其余 1/3 的患者为非失盐型（单纯男性化型）。醛固酮的生成减少和盐皮质激素拮抗剂前体物质（孕酮和 17- 羟基孕酮）堆积共同导致失盐。

迟发型 21- 羟化酶缺乏症是经典型 21- 羟化酶缺乏症的等位基因变型，其特点是轻度酶缺乏。这种缺乏是人类最常见的常染色体隐性遗传病，高发于阿什肯纳兹犹太人。患者通常在青春期发病，表现为男性化（多毛和痤疮）、闭经或月经稀发。如果女性出现不明原因的多毛和月经失调，则应考虑诊断该病。

经典型 21- 羟化酶缺乏症最有效的初步检测方法是血浆 17- 羟孕酮，其数值 > 200 ng/dl 支持该诊断。迟发型 21- 羟化酶缺乏症的诊断依据是在注射人工合成 ACTH（1-24）0.25 mg 后 30 min 血浆 17- 羟孕酮水平升高（> 1500 ng/dl）。

经典型 21- 羟化酶缺乏症的治疗目标是糖皮质激素和盐皮质激素替代，抑制 ACTH 和雄激素过度分泌，使儿童患者正常生长发育和性成熟。建议所有经典型 21- 羟化酶缺乏症患者使用氢化可的松和氟氢可的松进

TABLE 3.2   Syndromes of Adrenocortical Hypofunction

Primary Adrenal Disorders

Combined Glucocorticoid and Mineralocorticoid Deficiency

Autoimmune
  Isolated autoimmune disease (Addison's disease)
  Polyglandular autoimmune syndrome, type I
  Polyglandular autoimmune syndrome, type II
Infectious
  Tuberculosis
  Fungal
  Cytomegalovirus
  Human immunodeficiency virus
Vascular
  Bilateral adrenal hemorrhage
  Sepsis
  Coagulopathy
  Thrombosis, embolism
  Adrenal infarction
Infiltration
  Metastatic carcinoma and lymphoma
  Sarcoidosis
  Amyloidosis
  Hemochromatosis
Congenital
  Congenital adrenal hyperplasia
  21-Hydroxylase deficiency
  3β-ol Dehydrogenase deficiency
  20,22-Desmolase deficiency
  Adrenal unresponsiveness to ACTH
  Congenital adrenal hypoplasia
  Adrenoleukodystrophy
  Adrenomyeloneuropathy
Iatrogenic
  Bilateral adrenalectomy
  Drugs and supplements: See Table 3.3

Mineralocorticoid Deficiency Without Glucocorticoid Deficiency

  Corticosterone methyl oxidase deficiency
  Isolated zona glomerulosa defect
  Heparin therapy
  Critical illness
  Angiotensin-converting enzyme inhibitors

Secondary Adrenal Disorders

Secondary Adrenal Insufficiency

Hypothalamic-pituitary dysfunction
Exogenous glucocorticoids
After removal of an ACTH-secreting tumor

Hyporeninemic Hypoaldosteronism

Diabetic nephropathy
Tubulointerstitial diseases
Obstructive uropathy
Autonomic neuropathy
Nonsteroidal anti-inflammatory drugs
β-Adrenergic drugs

ACTH, Adrenocorticotropic hormone.

sexual maturation in children. A proposed approach to treating classic 21-hydroxylase deficiency recommends physiologic replacement with hydrocortisone and fludrocortisone in all affected patients. Virilizing effects can be prevented by the use of an antiandrogen (spironolactone or flutamide). Although the traditional treatment for late-onset 21-hydroxylase deficiency is dexamethasone (0.5 mg/day), the use of an antiandrogen such as spironolactone (100 to 200 mg/day) or flutamide (125 mg/day) is probably equally effective and has fewer side effects. Mineralocorticoid replacement is not needed in late-onset 21-hydroxylase deficiency.

11β-Hydroxylase (CYP11B1) deficiency accounts for about 5% of patients with CAH. In this condition, the conversions of 11-deoxycortisol to cortisol and 11-deoxycorticosterone to corticosterone (the precursor to aldosterone) are blocked. Affected patients usually have hypertension and hypokalemia because of increased amounts of precursors with mineralocorticoid activity. Virilization occurs, as with 21-hydroxylase deficiency, and a late-onset form manifesting as androgen excess also occurs. The diagnosis is made from the finding of elevated plasma 11-deoxycortisol levels, either basally or after ACTH stimulation.

Rare forms of CAH are 3β-HSD type II deficiency, 17α-hydroxylase (CYP17) deficiency, and steroidogenic acute regulatory protein (StAR) deficiency. Patients previously diagnosed with 3β-HSD type II deficiency most likely had polycystic ovarian syndrome (PCOS), which is associated with high DHEAS levels.

SYNDROMES OF ADRENOCORTICAL HYPERFUNCTION

Hypersecretion of the glucocorticoid hormone cortisol results in Cushing's syndrome, a metabolic disorder that affects carbohydrate, protein, and lipid metabolism (see Table 3.1). Hypersecretion of mineralocorticoids such as aldosterone results in a syndrome of hypertension and electrolyte disturbances.

Cushing's Syndrome
Pathophysiology

Cushing's syndrome refers to any condition of endogenous glucocorticoid excess, while Cushing's disease refers to an ACTH-secreting pituitary tumor leading to glucocorticoid excess. Increased production of cortisol is seen in both physiologic and pathologic states (Table 3.4). Physiologic hypercortisolism occurs with stress, during the last trimester of pregnancy, and in persons who regularly perform strenuous exercise. Pathologic conditions of elevated cortisol levels include exogenous or endogenous Cushing's syndrome and several psychiatric states, such as depression, alcoholism, anorexia nervosa, panic disorder, and alcohol or narcotic withdrawal.

Cushing's syndrome may be caused by exogenous administration of ACTH or glucocorticoid or by endogenous overproduction of these hormones. Endogenous Cushing's syndrome is either ACTH dependent or ACTH independent. ACTH dependency accounts for 85% of patients and includes pituitary sources of ACTH (Cushing's disease) and ectopic sources of ACTH. Pituitary Cushing's disease accounts for 90% of patients with ACTH-dependent Cushing's syndrome. Ectopic secretion of ACTH occurs most commonly in patients with small cell lung carcinoma. These patients are older, usually have a history of smoking, and primarily exhibit signs and symptoms of lung cancer rather than those of Cushing's syndrome. Patients with the clinically apparent ectopic ACTH syndrome, in contrast, have mostly lung, thymic or pancreatic carcinoid tumors. ACTH-independent causes account for 15% of patients with Cushing's syndrome and include adrenal adenomas, adrenal carcinomas, micronodular adrenal disease, and autonomous macronodular adrenal disease. The female-to-male ratio for noncancerous forms of Cushing's syndrome is 4:1.

表 3.2　肾上腺皮质功能减退综合征
原发性肾上腺疾病
糖皮质激素和盐皮质激素联合缺乏症
自身免疫
孤立性自身免疫病（Addison 病）
自身免疫性多内分泌腺综合征 I 型
自身免疫性多内分泌腺综合征 II 型
感染性
结核
真菌
巨细胞病毒
人类免疫缺陷病毒
血管
双侧肾上腺出血
感染中毒症
凝血功能障碍
血栓形成、栓塞
肾上腺梗死
浸润
转移癌和淋巴瘤
结节病
淀粉样变性
血色病
先天性
先天性肾上腺皮质增生症
21- 羟化酶缺乏症
3β- 羟脱氢酶缺乏症
20,22- 碳链裂解酶缺乏症
肾上腺对 ACTH 无反应
先天性肾上腺发育不全
肾上腺脑白质营养不良
肾上腺脊髓神经病
医源性
双侧肾上腺切除术
药物和补充剂：见表 3.3
无糖皮质激素缺乏症的盐皮质激素缺乏症
皮质酮甲基氧化酶缺乏症
孤立性球状带缺陷
肝素治疗
危重症疾病
血管紧张素转换酶抑制剂
继发性肾上腺疾病
继发性肾上腺皮质功能不全
下丘脑-垂体功能障碍
外源性糖皮质激素
切除 ACTH 分泌瘤术后
低肾素性低醛固酮血症
糖尿病肾病
肾小管间质性疾病
梗阻性尿路病
自主神经病变
非甾体抗炎药
β- 肾上腺素能药物

行生理性替代。男性化表现可通过使用抗雄激素药物（螺内酯或氟他胺）控制。尽管迟发型 21- 羟化酶缺乏症的传统治疗是使用地塞米松（0.5 mg/d），但抗雄激素药物［如螺内酯（100 ～ 200 mg/d）或氟他胺（125 mg/d）］可能同样有效，且副作用较少。迟发型 21- 羟化酶缺乏者不需要补充盐皮质激素。

11β- 羟化酶（CYP11B1）缺乏症约占 CAH 的 5%。在这种情况下，11- 脱氧皮质醇转化为皮质醇及 11- 脱氧皮质酮转化为皮质酮（醛固酮的前体）受阻。由于堆积大量具有盐皮质激素活性的前体，患者通常出现高血压和低钾血症。与 21- 羟化酶缺乏症类似，11β- 羟化酶缺乏症患者也会出现男性化，且迟发型也会出现雄激素过多的表现。其诊断依据是血浆 11- 脱氧皮质醇水平升高，无论是基础水平还是 ACTH 刺激后。

罕见的 CAH 类型包括 3β-HSD II 型缺乏症、17α- 羟化酶（CYP17）缺乏症和类固醇生成急性调节蛋白（StAR）缺乏症。既往被诊断为 3β-HSD II 型缺乏症的患者很可能患有多囊卵巢综合征（PCOS），而 PCOS 可伴随高硫酸脱氢表雄酮（DHEAS）水平。

肾上腺皮质功能亢进

皮质醇分泌过多会导致库欣综合征，这是一种会影响碳水化合物、蛋白质和脂质代谢的代谢性疾病（表 3.1）。盐皮质激素（如醛固酮）分泌过多会导致高血压和电解质紊乱。

库欣综合征

病理生理学

库欣综合征是指所有内源性糖皮质激素过多的情况，而库欣病是指由垂体 ACTH 分泌瘤导致的糖皮质激素过多。皮质醇生成增多可见于生理情况和病理情况（表 3.4）。生理性皮质醇增多症可见于应激状态下，如妊娠晚期、经常剧烈运动。病理性皮质醇增多症可见于外源性或内源性库欣综合征及多种精神疾病，如抑郁症、酗酒、神经性厌食症、惊恐障碍、酒精或麻醉药品戒断。

库欣综合征可由外源性应用 ACTH 或糖皮质激素或内源性过度分泌引起。内源性库欣综合征可分为 ACTH 依赖性和 ACTH 非依赖性。85% 的患者为 ACTH 依赖性，包括垂体性 ACTH（库欣病）和异位 ACTH 综合征。垂体性库欣病占 ACTH 依赖性库欣综合征患者的 90%。小细胞肺癌是异位分泌 ACTH 最常见的病因。这些患者年龄较大，通常有吸烟史，主要表现为肺癌的体征和症状，而不是库欣综合征的症状。相比之下，临床表现明显的异位 ACTH 综合征患者多患有肺、胸腺或胰腺类癌。ACTH 非依赖性库欣综合征占库欣综合征患者的 15%，包括肾上腺腺瘤、肾上腺癌、肾上腺小结节增生和肾上腺大结节增生。非癌症类型的库欣综合征的男女比例为 4:1。

TABLE 3.3   Medications and Supplements Affecting Cortisol Levels

Type of Drugs	Generic Name	Brand Name	Effect on Cortisol	Comments
Cushing's drugs	**Ketoconazole**	**Nizoral**	↓	Decreases cortisol biosynthesis
	Mifepristone	**Korlym**	↑	Blocks cortisol at the receptor
	Somatostatin analogues (octreotide, lanreotide, pasireotide)	**Sandostatin, Somatuline, Signifor**	↓	Lowers cortisol mildly
	Metyrapone	**Metopirone**	↓	High rate of adrenal insufficiency
	Etomidate	**Amidate**	↓	Can be given IV
	Mitotane	**Lysodren**	↓	Adrenolytic
Antidepressant	**Citalopram**	**Celexa**	↑	
	Sertraline	**Zoloft**	↑	
	Fluoxetine	Prozac	–	
	Imipramine	Tofranil	↓	
	Desipramine	Norpramin	↓	
	Trazodone	Desyrel	↓	
	Mirtazapine	Remeron	↓	
Antipsychotic	Olanzapine	Zyprexa	↓	
	Quetiapine	Seroquel	↓	
Anti-anxiety	Temazepam	Restoril	↓	
	Alprazolam	**Xanax**	↓	
	Lorazepam	Ativan	↓/–	Anecdotal-lowers cortisol, literature no effect
Dopamine agents	Cabergoline	Dostinex	↓	Variable effect
	Bromocriptine	Parlodel	↓	Variable effect
	Metoclopramide	Reglan	↑	
	Methylphenidate	Ritalin	↑	Found in one study but not another study
Antihypertensives	**Clonidine**	**Catapres**	↓	
Opioids/anti-opioids	Loperamide	Imodium	↓	
	Morphine, Methadone, Codeine	**Various**	↓	
	Buprenorphine	Buprenex	↓	
	Naloxone	**Narcan**	↑	
	Naltrexone	**Revia**	↑	Unclear if low-dose naltrexone (LDN) has the same effect
Drugs of abuse	**Heroin**		↓	
	Cocaine		↑	
	Alcohol		↑	
	Tobacco/nicotine		↑	
Hormones	Progesterone	Provera, Prometrium	↓	Binds to the cortisol receptor, so Cushingoid features could occur, even though cortisol levels are decreased
	Megestrol	**Megace**	↓	Used for weight gain
	Growth hormone	Various	↓	Increase catabolism of cortisol
	Thyroid hormone	Synthroid, Levoxyl, Cytomel Armour, etc.	↓	Increase catabolism of cortisol
	Raloxifene	Evista	↓	Used for osteoporosis
	Estrogens, birth control pills		–	Raises cortisol-binding protein and raises total cortisol, does not affect free cortisol
	DHEA		↓	
	Desmopressin	DDAVP	↑	
	Oxytocin		↓	Anecdotal reports of lowering cortisol

表 3.3　影响皮质醇水平的药物和补充剂

药物类型	通用名	商品名	对皮质醇的影响	备注
治疗库欣综合征的药物	酮康唑	里素劳	↓	减少皮质醇的生物合成
	米非司酮	Korlym	↑	在受体水平阻断皮质醇作用
	生长抑素类似物（奥曲肽、兰曲肽、帕瑞肽）	善宁、索马杜林、Signifor	↓	轻度降低皮质醇水平
	美替拉酮	Metopirone	↓	肾上腺皮质功能不全的发生率高
	依托咪酯	Amidate	↓	可静脉注射
	米托坦	Lysodren	↓	肾上腺破坏
抗抑郁药	西酞普兰	喜普妙	↑	
	舍曲林	左洛复	↑	
	氟西汀	百忧解	—	
	丙咪嗪	Tofranil	↓	
	地昔帕明	Norpramin	↓	
	曲唑酮	Desyrel	↓	
	米氮平	瑞美隆	↓	
抗精神病药	奥氮平	再普乐	↓	
	喹硫平	思瑞康	↓	
抗焦虑药	替马西泮	Restoril	↓	
	阿普唑仑	Xanax	↓	
	劳拉西泮	Ativan	↓ / —	个案报道可降低皮质醇水平，但研究显示无效果
多巴胺激动剂	卡麦角林	Dostinex	↓	效果不一致
	溴隐亭	Parlodel	↓	效果不一致
	甲氧氯普胺	Reglan	↑	
	哌甲酯	利他林	↑	仅在一项研究中发现
抗高血压药	可乐定	Catapres	↓	
阿片类 / 抗阿片类药物	洛哌丁胺	易蒙停	↓	
	吗啡、美沙酮、可待因	多种名称	↓	
	丁丙诺啡	Buprenex	↓	
	纳洛酮	Narcan	↑	
	纳曲酮	Revia	↑	尚不清楚低剂量纳曲酮（LDN）是否有同样的效果
滥用药物	海洛因		↓	
	可卡因		↑	
	酒精		↑	
	烟草 / 尼古丁		↑	
激素	孕酮	普维拉、Prometrium	↓	与皮质醇受体结合，故可出现库欣样外貌，即使皮质醇水平降低
	甲地孕酮	梅格施	↓	用于增加体重
	生长激素	多种名称	↓	增加皮质醇的分解代谢
	甲状腺激素	Synthroid、Levoxyl、Cytomel、Armour 等	↓	增加皮质醇的分解代谢
	雷洛昔芬	易维特	↓	用于治疗骨质疏松症
	雌激素、避孕药		—	提高皮质醇结合球蛋白和总皮质醇水平，但不会影响游离皮质醇水平
	DHEA		↓	
	去氨加压素	DDAVP	↑	
	催产素		↓	个案报道可降低皮质醇水平

TABLE 3.3	Medications and Supplements Affecting Cortisol Levels—cont'd			
Type of Drugs	**Generic Name**	**Brand Name**	**Effect on Cortisol**	**Comments**
Diabetes medications	Rosiglitazone	Avandia	↓/–	Initial studies found a reduction in cortisol, not confirmed by additional studies
	Pioglitazone	Actos	↓/–	
Supplements	**Phosphatidyl serine**	**Seriphos**	↓	Effective at night, Seriphos and phosphatidyl serine are slightly different
	Gingko biloba		↓	
	St. John's wort		↑	
	Rhodiola		↓	

Bold indicates substantial effect.

Clinical Presentation

The clinical signs, symptoms, and common laboratory findings of hypercortisolism observed in patients with Cushing's syndrome are listed in Table 3.5. Patients with Cushing's syndrome often have some, but not all, of the signs and symptoms discussed here. Typically, the obesity is centripetal, with a wasting of the arms and legs, which is distinct from the generalized weight gain observed in idiopathic obesity. Rounding of the face (called *moon facies*) and a dorsocervical fat pad *(buffalo hump)* may occur in obesity not related to Cushing's syndrome, whereas facial plethora and supraclavicular filling are more specific for Cushing's syndrome. Patients with Cushing's syndrome may have proximal muscle weakness; consequently, the inability to stand up from a squat or to comb their own hair can be revealing. Sleep disturbances and insomnia, hyperarousal in the evening and night, mood swings, and other psychological abnormalities are frequently seen. Cognitive dysfunction and severe fatigue are often present. Menstrual irregularities often precede other Cushingoid symptoms in affected women. Patients of both sexes complain of a loss of libido, and affected men frequently complain of erectile dysfunction. Adult-onset acne or hirsutism in women could also suggest Cushing's syndrome. The skin striae observed in patients with Cushing's syndrome are often violaceous (i.e., purple or dark red, from hemorrhage into the striae) depending on the level of hypercortisolism. Thinning of the skin on the top of the hands is a specific sign in younger adults with Cushing's syndrome. Old pictures of patients are extremely helpful for evaluating the progression of the physical stigmata of Cushing's syndrome.

Associated laboratory findings in Cushing's syndrome include elevated plasma alkaline phosphatase levels, granulocytosis, thrombocytosis, hypercholesterolemia, hypertriglyceridemia, and glucose intolerance, and/or diabetes mellitus. Hypokalemia or alkalosis usually occurs in patients with severe hypercortisolism as a result of the ectopic ACTH syndrome.

Diagnosis

If the history and physical examination findings are suggestive of hypercortisolism, then the diagnosis of Cushing's syndrome can usually be established by collecting urine for 24 hours and measuring the urinary free cortisol (UFC). This test is extremely sensitive for diagnosis of Cushing's syndrome because in 90% of affected patients the initial UFC level is greater than 50 μg/24 hours (Fig. 3.5).

Cortisol is normally secreted in a diurnal manner: The plasma concentration is highest in the early morning (between 6:00 and 8:00 AM) and lowest around midnight. Most patients with Cushing's syndrome have blunted diurnal variation. Nighttime plasma cortisol values greater than 50% of the morning values are considered to be consistent with Cushing's syndrome. Because of the difficulty of obtaining nighttime plasma cortisol levels, measurement of late-night salivary cortisol has been developed to assess hypercortisolism. This test has a high degree of sensitivity and specificity for the diagnosis of Cushing's syndrome and is convenient for patients. Multiple measurements of UFC or salivary cortisol may be needed to either diagnose or exclude Cushing's syndrome, especially in subjects with convincing and progressive signs and symptoms of hypercortisolism.

The overnight dexamethasone suppression test has been widely used as a screening tool to evaluate patients who may have hypercortisolism. Dexamethasone, 1 mg, is given orally at 11:00 PM or midnight, and plasma cortisol is measured the following morning at 8:00 AM. A morning plasma cortisol level greater than 1.8 μg/dL suggests hypercortisolism. This test produces a significant number of both false-positive and false-negative results, but it is recommended in the 2008 Endocrine Society consensus guidelines.

Differential Diagnosis

Once the diagnosis of Cushing's syndrome is established, the cause of the hypercortisolism needs to be ascertained by biochemical studies that evaluate the HPA axis; this should be accompanied by imaging procedures and at times, venous sampling. The initial approach is to measure basal ACTH levels, which are normal or elevated in Cushing's disease and the ectopic ACTH syndrome but are suppressed in primary adrenal Cushing's syndrome. Patients with a suppressed ACTH level can proceed to adrenal imaging studies. To distinguish between Cushing's disease and the ectopic ACTH syndrome, the 2-day dexamethasone suppression test or 8-mg overnight dexamethasone suppression test and bilateral simultaneous inferior petrosal sinus sampling (IPSS) may be used.

In the dexamethasone suppression test (Liddle test), 0.5 mg of dexamethasone is given orally every 6 hours for 2 days (low dose), followed by 2 mg of dexamethasone every 6 hours for another 2 days (high dose). On the second day of high-dose dexamethasone, the UFC level will be suppressed to less than 10% of the baseline collection value in patients with pituitary adenomas but not in patients with the ectopic ACTH syndrome or adrenal cortisol-secreting tumors. The Liddle test has some methodologic drawbacks, and results should be interpreted cautiously; other confirmatory tests should be performed before surgery is recommended.

An overnight high-dose dexamethasone suppression test can be helpful in establishing the cause of Cushing's syndrome. In this test, a baseline cortisol level is measured at 8:00 AM, and then 8 mg of dexamethasone is given orally at 11:00 PM. At 8:00 AM the following morning, a plasma cortisol measurement is obtained. Suppression, which occurs in patients with pituitary Cushing's disease, is defined as a decrease in plasma cortisol to less than 50% of the baseline level.

表 3.3　影响皮质醇水平的药物和补充剂（续表）

药物类型	通用名	商品名	对皮质醇的影响	备注
治疗糖尿病的药物	罗格列酮	文迪雅	↓ / –	早期研究发现可降低皮质醇水平，但未被其他研究证实
	吡格列酮	艾可拓	↓ / –	
补充剂	**磷脂酰丝氨酸**	**Seriphos**	↓	在夜间有效，Seriphos 和磷脂酰丝氨酸略有不同
	银杏叶		↓	
	圣约翰草		↑	
	红景天		↑	

粗体表示效果显著。

临床表现

表 3.5 总结了库欣综合征患者皮质醇增多症的临床症状、体征和常见实验室检查结果。库欣综合征患者通常出现部分体征和症状，而并非全部。患者通常表现为向心性肥胖，上肢和下肢消瘦，这与特发性肥胖症的全身性体重增加不同。与库欣综合征无关的肥胖症也可能出现面部变圆（称为"满月脸"）和颈后脂肪垫（水牛背），而多血质面容和锁骨上脂肪垫则是库欣综合征更具特异性的表现。库欣综合征患者可能出现近端肌无力；因此，无法从蹲位站起或梳头对疾病有提示意义。患者还常出现睡眠障碍和失眠、傍晚和夜间过度觉醒、情绪波动和其他心理异常，以及认知功能障碍和严重疲劳。女性患者在出现其他库欣样症状之前通常存在月经失调。男女性患者均会出现性欲减退，男性患者常伴有勃起功能障碍。女性成年后出现痤疮或多毛症可提示库欣综合征。根据皮质醇增多症的程度，库欣综合征患者常出现皮肤紫纹（即紫红色或暗红色皮纹，由皮肤变薄显露出皮下血管所致）。手掌皮肤变薄是库欣综合征年轻患者的特殊体征。患者的既往照片对评估库欣综合征的体征进展非常有帮助。

库欣综合征的相关实验室检查结果包括血浆碱性磷酸酶水平升高、粒细胞增多、血栓形成、高胆固醇血症、高甘油三酯血症、糖耐量异常和（或）糖尿病。低钾血症或碱中毒通常见于由异位 ACTH 综合征导致的严重皮质醇增多症患者。

诊断

如果病史和体格检查结果均提示皮质醇增多症，通常可通过收集 24 h 尿液并测定尿游离皮质醇（UFC）来确诊库欣综合征。该检测对诊断库欣综合征极为敏感，因为 90% 的患者初始 UFC > 50 μg/24 h（图 3.5）。

皮质醇分泌通常具有昼夜节律：血浆皮质醇浓度在清晨（06:00 至 08:00）最高，午夜前后最低。大多数库欣综合征患者的昼夜节律减弱。夜间血浆皮质醇浓度超过清晨浓度的 50% 被认为是库欣综合征。由于获取夜间血浆皮质醇样本较为困难，夜间唾液皮质醇已被用于评估皮质醇增多症。该检测具有很高的敏感性和特异性，且方便患者应用。诊断或排除库欣综合征需要多次检测 UFC 或唾液皮质醇，尤其是对于具有高度提示皮质醇增多症的症状和体征的患者。

过夜地塞米松抑制试验已被广泛用于可疑皮质醇增多症患者的筛查。在 23:00 或午夜口服地塞米松 1 mg，次日 08:00 测量血浆皮质醇。清晨血浆皮质醇 > 1.8 μg/dl 提示皮质醇增多症。该检查会产生大量的假阳性和假阴性结果，但是被 2008 年美国内分泌学会共识指南推荐。

鉴别诊断

一旦确诊库欣综合征，需进行评估 HPA 轴的生化检测、影像学检查及必要时进行静脉采血，以明确皮质醇增多症的原因。初步检测是测定基础 ACTH 水平，库欣病和异位 ACTH 综合征患者的基础 ACTH 水平通常正常或升高，而由肾上腺病因导致的库欣综合征患者的基础 ACTH 水平被抑制。ACTH 水平被抑制的患者可进行肾上腺影像学检查。为区分库欣病与异位 ACTH 综合征，可使用两日法地塞米松抑制试验或 8 mg 过夜地塞米松抑制试验及双侧岩下窦取血（IPSS）。

在地塞米松抑制试验（Liddle 试验）中，每 6 h 给予口服地塞米松 0.5 mg，共 2 天（小剂量），然后每 6 h 给予口服地塞米松 2 mg，共 2 天（大剂量）。对于垂体腺瘤患者（而非异位 ACTH 综合征或肾上腺皮质醇分泌瘤患者），在大剂量地塞米松服药的第 2 天，其 UFC < 基线水平的 10%。Liddle 试验存在方法学上的局限性，应谨慎解释结果；建议在手术前进行其他确诊性检查。

过夜大剂量地塞米松抑制试验有助于确定库欣综合征的病因。在该试验中，于 08:00 测定基础皮质醇水平，然后在 23:00 口服地塞米松 8 mg。次日 08:00 测定血浆皮质醇水平。如果皮质醇水平 < 基线水平的 50%，则提示为库欣病。

TABLE 3.4   Syndromes of Adrenocortical Hyperfunction

States of Glucocorticoid Excess

Physiologic States

Stress

Strenuous exercise

Last trimester of pregnancy

Pathologic States

Psychiatric conditions (pseudo-Cushing's disorders)

Depression

Alcoholism

Anorexia nervosa

Panic disorders

Alcohol and drug withdrawal

ACTH-dependent states

   Pituitary adenoma (Cushing's disease)

   Ectopic ACTH syndrome

   Bronchial carcinoid

   Thymic carcinoid

   Islet cell tumor

   Small cell lung carcinoma

   Ectopic CRH secretion

ACTH-independent states

   Adrenal adenoma

   Adrenal carcinoma

   Micronodular adrenal disease

Exogenous Sources

Glucocorticoid intake

ACTH intake

States of Mineralocorticoid Excess

Primary Aldosteronism

Aldosterone-secreting adenoma

Bilateral adrenal hyperplasia

Aldosterone-secreting carcinoma

Glucocorticoid-suppressible hyperaldosteronism

Adrenal Enzyme Deficiencies

11β-Hydroxylase deficiency

17α-Hydroxylase deficiency

11β-Hydroxysteroid dehydrogenase type II deficiency

Exogenous Mineralocorticoids

Licorice

Carbenoxolone

Fludrocortisone

Secondary Hyperaldosteronism

Associated with hypertension

   Accelerated hypertension

   Renovascular hypertension

   Estrogen administration

   Renin-secreting tumors

Without hypertension

   Bartter syndrome

   Sodium-wasting nephropathy

   Renal tubular acidosis

   Diuretic and laxative abuse

   Edematous states (cirrhosis, nephrosis, congestive heart failure)

ACTH, Adrenocorticotropin hormone; *CRH,* corticotropin-releasing hormone.

Bilateral IPSS is an accurate and safe procedure for distinguishing pituitary Cushing's disease from the ectopic ACTH syndrome.

Venous blood from the anterior lobe of the pituitary gland empties into the cavernous sinuses and then into the superior and inferior petrosal sinuses. Venous plasma samples for ACTH determination are obtained from both inferior petrosal sinuses, along with a simultaneous peripheral sample, both before and after intravenous bolus administration of ovine corticotropin-releasing hormone (oCRH). Significant gradients at baseline and after oCRH stimulation between petrosal sinus and peripheral samples suggest pituitary Cushing's disease. In baseline measurements, an ACTH concentration gradient of 1.6 or more between a sample from either of the petrosal sinuses and the peripheral sample is strongly suggestive of pituitary Cushing's disease, whereas patients with the ectopic ACTH syndrome or adrenal adenomas have no ACTH gradient between their petrosal and peripheral samples. After oCRH administration, a central-to-peripheral gradient of more than 3.2 is consistent with pituitary Cushing's disease. An ACTH gradient ipsilateral to the side of the tumor is found in 70% to 80% of pituitary Cushing's disease patients sampled. Although this procedure requires a radiologist who is experienced in IPSS, it is available at many tertiary care facilities. The test cannot be done to distinguish patients with Cushing's syndrome from those without the condition, and the test needs to be done when the patient is hypercortisolemic, making it less helpful in those with episodic cortisol secretion.

Magnetic resonance imaging (MRI) with gadolinium is the preferred procedure for localizing a pituitary adenoma. In many centers, a *dynamic* MRI is performed; the pituitary is visualized as the gadolinium enters and leaves the gland. Because about 10% of normal individuals are found to have a nonfunctioning pituitary adenoma on pituitary MRI, pituitary imaging should not be the sole criterion for the diagnosis of pituitary Cushing's disease.

Treatment

The preferred treatment for all forms of Cushing's syndrome is appropriate surgery or, in some cases, radiation therapy (see Chapter 1). A more appealing option for many patients with Cushing's disease who remain hypercortisolemic after pituitary surgery is bilateral adrenalectomy followed by lifelong glucocorticoid and mineralocorticoid replacement therapy.

In patients with the ectopic ACTH syndrome, the goal is to localize the tumor by appropriate scans so it can be removed surgically. A unilateral adrenalectomy is the treatment of choice in patients with a cortisol-secreting adrenal adenoma. Cortisol-secreting adrenal carcinomas initially should also be managed surgically; however, the prognosis is poor, with only 20% of patients surviving more than 1 year after diagnosis.

Medical treatment for hypercortisolism may be needed to prepare patients who are undergoing or have undergone pituitary irradiation and are awaiting its effects before surgery; it may also be needed for those who are not surgical candidates or elect not to have surgery. Ketoconazole, *o,p′*-DDD (mitotane), metyrapone, aminoglutethimide, mifepristone (FDA approved for Cushing's syndrome if accompanied by hypertension or glucose intolerance/diabetes), and trilostane are the most commonly used agents for adrenal blockade and can be used alone or in combination. The somatostatin analogue, pasireotide, which decreases ACTH and may decrease tumor size, is an FDA-approved drug for treating Cushing's disease.

Primary Mineralocorticoid Excess

Pathophysiology

The causes of primary aldosteronism (see Table 3.4) are aldosterone-producing adenoma (75%), bilateral adrenal hyperplasia (25%), adrenal carcinoma (1%), and glucocorticoid-remediable hyperaldosteronism (<1%). Adrenal enzyme defects (11β-HSD type II,

表 3.4　肾上腺皮质功能亢进综合征
糖皮质激素过量状态
生理状态
应激
剧烈运动
妊娠晚期
病理状态
精神疾病（假性库欣综合征）
抑郁症
酗酒
神经性厌食
惊恐障碍
戒酒和戒毒
ACTH 依赖性状态
垂体腺瘤（库欣病）
异位 ACTH 综合征
支气管类癌
胸腺类癌
胰岛细胞肿瘤
小细胞肺癌
异位 CRH 分泌
ACTH 非依赖性状态
肾上腺腺瘤
肾上腺癌
小结节性肾上腺疾病
外源性
应用糖皮质激素
应用 ACTH
盐皮质激素过量状态
原发性醛固酮增多症
醛固酮分泌瘤
双侧肾上腺增生
醛固酮分泌瘤
糖皮质激素可抑制性醛固酮增多症
肾上腺酶缺乏症
11β-羟化酶缺乏症
17α-羟化酶缺乏症
11β-羟基类固醇脱氢酶 II 型缺乏症
外源性盐皮质激素
甘草
甘珀酸
氟氢可的松
继发性醛固酮增多症
伴有高血压
急进性高血压
肾血管性高血压
使用雌激素
肾素分泌瘤
不伴有高血压
巴特综合征（Bartter 综合征）
失钠性肾病
肾小管性酸中毒
滥用利尿剂和泻药
水肿状态（肝硬化、肾病、充血性心力衰竭）

ACTH，促肾上腺皮质激素；CRH，促肾上腺皮质激素释放激素。

　　双侧 IPSS 是鉴别库欣病和异位 ACTH 综合征的准确而安全的方法。从垂体前叶流出的静脉血汇入海绵窦，然后进入岩上窦和岩下窦。测定 ACTH 浓度时，应在静脉注射绵羊 CRH（oCRH）之前和之后采集双侧岩下窦和外周血样本。在基线和 oCRH 刺激后，岩下窦和外周血样本之间存在明显梯度，提示存在垂体性库欣病。在基线检测中，若岩下窦样本与外周血样本的 ACTH 浓度梯度 ≥ 1.6（译者注：常规采用的临界值为 2.0），则强烈提示库欣病；异位 ACTH 综合征或肾上腺腺瘤患者的岩下窦样本和外周血样本之间没有 ACTH 浓度梯度。给予 oCRH 后，岩下窦样本与外周血样本的 ACTH 浓度梯度 > 3.2（译者注：常规采用的临界值为 3.0），则支持库欣病的诊断。在库欣病患者中，70% ~ 80% 存在肿瘤同侧的 ACTH 浓度梯度。虽然该检查操作需要由有 IPSS 经验的放射科医生进行，但在许多三级医院中均可实施。该检测无法区分库欣综合征患者与正常个体，且需要在患者处于皮质醇分泌过多时进行，因此不太适用于周期性皮质醇分泌增多的人群。

　　钆增强 MRI 是定位垂体腺瘤的首选方法。许多医学中心采用动态增强 MRI，当钆造影剂进入和离开腺体时，垂体可被成像。由于约 10% 的正常个体可能存在无功能垂体腺瘤，因此垂体影像学不应被作为诊断库欣病的唯一标准。

治疗

　　所有类型库欣综合征的首选治疗均为手术，或在某些情况下进行放疗（见第 1 章）。对于行垂体手术后仍存在皮质醇增多症的库欣病患者，更好的治疗选择是双侧肾上腺切除术，随后进行终身糖皮质激素和盐皮质激素替代治疗。

　　对于异位 ACTH 综合征患者，目标是通过合适的影像学检查定位肿瘤，以便进行外科切除。对于肾上腺皮质醇分泌瘤，单侧肾上腺切除是首选治疗方法。肾上腺皮质醇分泌癌首先应进行手术治疗，但预后较差，仅有约 20% 的患者在诊断后存活超过 1 年。

　　皮质醇增多症的药物治疗适用于即将或已经接受垂体放疗和等待手术的患者，以及无法手术或选择不手术的患者。酮康唑、米托坦、美替拉酮、氨鲁米特、米非司酮（FDA 批准用于治疗伴有高血压或糖耐量异常/糖尿病的库欣综合征）和曲洛司坦是常用的抑制肾上腺的药物，可单独使用或联合使用。帕瑞肽（一种生长抑素类似物）可降低 ACTH 水平并可能减小肿瘤体积，已获得 FDA 批准用于治疗库欣病。

原发性盐皮质激素过多
病理生理学

　　原发性醛固酮增多症（表 3.4）的主要病因是醛固酮分泌瘤（35%）、双侧肾上腺增生（即特发性醛固酮增多症，60%），其他少见病因包括原发性肾上腺皮质增生、家族性醛固酮增多症 I ~ IV 型、分泌醛固酮的肾上腺皮质癌、异位醛固酮分泌瘤（译者注：原比例现已更

TABLE 3.5	Signs, Symptoms, and Laboratory Abnormalities of Hypercortisolism
Feature	**Percentage of Patients**
Fat redistribution (dorsocervical and supraclavicular fat pads, temporal wasting, centripetal obesity, weight gain)	95
Menstrual irregularities	80 (of affected women)
Thin skin and plethora	80
Moon facies	75
Increased appetite	75
Sleep disturbances	75
Nocturnal hyperarousal	75
Hypertension	75
Hypercholesterolemia and hypertriglyceridemia	70
Altered mentation (poor concentration, decreased memory, euphoria)	70
Diabetes mellitus and glucose intolerance	65
Striae	65
Hirsutism	65 (of affected women)
Proximal muscle weakness	60
Psychological disturbances (emotional lability, depression, mania, psychosis)	50
Decreased libido and erectile dysfunction	50 (of affected men)
Acne	45
Osteoporosis and pathologic fractures	40
Easy bruisability	40
Poor wound healing	40
Virilization	20 (of affected women)
Edema	20
Increased infections	10
Cataracts	5

11β-hydroxylase, and 17α-hydroxylase deficiencies) and apparent mineralocorticoid excess (from ingestion of licorice or carbenoxolone, which inhibit 11β-HSD type II, or from a congenital defect in this enzyme) are also states of functional mineralocorticoid overactivity. Secondary aldosteronism (see Table 3.4) results from an overactive renin-angiotensin system.

Primary aldosteronism is usually recognized during evaluation of hypertension or hypokalemia and represents a potentially curable form of hypertension. Up to 5% of patients with hypertension have primary aldosteronism. These patients are usually between the ages of 30 and 50 years, and the female-to-male ratio is 2:1.

Clinical Presentation

Hypertension, hypokalemia, and metabolic alkalosis are the main clinical manifestations of hyperaldosteronism; most of the presenting symptoms are related to hypokalemia. Symptoms in patients with mild hypokalemia are fatigue, muscle weakness, nocturia, lassitude, and headaches. If more severe hypokalemia exists, polydipsia, polyuria, paresthesias, and even intermittent paralysis and tetany can occur. Blood pressure can range from minimally elevated to very high. A positive Trousseau or Chvostek sign may occur as a result of metabolic alkalosis.

Diagnosis and Treatment

Initially, hypokalemia in the presence of hypertension should be documented (Fig. 3.6), although mild cases of hyperaldosteronism without hypokalemia exist. The patient must have adequate salt intake and discontinue diuretics before potassium measurement. A morning plasma aldosterone level (measured in ng/dL) and a PRA value (in ng/mL/hour) should be obtained. A ratio of serum aldosterone to PRA greater than 20 with a serum aldosterone level greater than 15 ng/dL suggests the diagnosis of hyperaldosteronism.

Confirmatory tests for hyperaldosteronism should be performed, such as oral sodium loading, saline infusion, fludrocortisone suppression, or captopril challenge.

Once the diagnosis of primary aldosteronism has been demonstrated, it is important to distinguish between an aldosterone-producing adenoma and bilateral hyperplasia, because the former is treated with surgery and the latter is treated medically. A computed tomography (CT) scan of the adrenal glands should be performed to localize the tumor. Prior to surgery, imaging should be confirmed with adrenal venous sampling for cortisol due to the high degree of adrenal incidentalomas. The patient should undergo unilateral adrenalectomy if a discrete adenoma is observed in one adrenal gland, the contralateral gland is normal, and the adrenal venous sampling lateralizes to the side of the adenoma. Patients in whom biochemical and localization study findings are consistent with bilateral hyperplasia should be treated medically with a potassium-sparing diuretic, usually eplerenone or spironolactone. Hyperaldosteronism and hypertension secondary to activation of the renin-angiotensin system can occur in patients with accelerated hypertension, in those with renovascular hypertension, in those receiving estrogen therapies, and, rarely, in patients with renin-secreting tumors. Hyperaldosteronism without hypertension occurs in patients with Bartter syndrome, sodium-wasting nephropathy, or renal tubular acidosis, as well as those who abuse diuretics or laxatives.

ADRENAL MEDULLARY HYPERFUNCTION

The adrenal medulla synthesizes the catecholamines norepinephrine, epinephrine, and dopamine from the amino acid tyrosine. Norepinephrine, the major catecholamine produced by the adrenal medulla, has predominantly α-agonist actions, causing vasoconstriction. Epinephrine acts primarily on the β-receptors, having positive

表 3.5　皮质醇增多症的体征、症状和实验室检查异常

特征	患者比例（%）
脂肪重新分布（颈后和锁骨上脂肪垫、颞部消瘦、向心性肥胖、体重增加）	95
月经失调	80（女性患者）
皮肤菲薄、多血质	80
满月脸	75
食欲增加	75
睡眠障碍	75
夜间过度觉醒	75
高血压	75
高胆固醇血症和高甘油三酯血症	70
心智改变（注意力不集中、记忆力下降、欣快）	70
糖尿病和糖耐量异常	65
紫纹	65
多毛	65（女性患者）
近端肌无力	60
精神障碍（情绪不稳定、抑郁症、躁狂、精神病）	50
性欲减退和勃起功能障碍	50（男性患者）
痤疮	45
骨质疏松症和病理性骨折	40
易发瘀斑	40
伤口愈合不良	40
男性化	20（女性患者）
水肿	20
感染增加	10
白内障	5

新）。肾上腺酶缺乏（11β-HSD Ⅱ 型、11β-羟化酶和 17α-羟化酶缺乏症）和表观盐皮质激素增多（摄入甘草或甘珀酸抑制 11β-HSD Ⅱ 型或该酶先天性缺陷）也是功能性盐皮质激素过多的原因。继发性醛固酮增多症（表 3.4）由肾素-血管紧张素系统过度激活引起。

原发性醛固酮增多症通常在评估高血压或低钾血症时被发现，是一种潜在可治愈的高血压。5% 的高血压患者合并原发性醛固酮增多症，多见于 30～50 岁的患者，女性和男性比例为 2∶1（译者注：原文与临床不符，应为男女比例相当）。

临床表现

高血压、低钾血症和代谢性碱中毒是醛固酮增多症的主要临床表现；大多数症状与低钾血症有关。轻度低钾血症患者表现为疲劳、肌无力、夜尿和倦怠。严重低钾血症可出现多饮、多尿、感觉异常，甚至出现间断性麻痹和手足搐搦。血压可从轻微升高到非常高。代谢性碱中毒可导致低钙束臂征（Trousseau 征）或面神经叩击征（Chvostek 征）阳性。

诊断和治疗

高血压伴有低钾血症应在病历中记录（图 3.6），但轻度醛固酮增多症患者不伴有低钾血症。在测定血钾之前，患者必须充分摄入盐，并停用利尿剂。应检测清晨血浆醛固酮水平（ng/dl）和 PRA［ng/（ml·h）］。如果血浆醛固酮与 PRA 的比值 > 20，且血浆醛固

酮 > 15 ng/dl，则可诊断为醛固酮增多症。醛固酮增多症患者应行确诊试验，包括口服盐负荷试验、生理盐水输注试验、氟氢可的松抑制试验或卡托普利抑制试验。

一旦确诊原发性醛固酮增多症，鉴别醛固酮分泌瘤和双侧肾上腺增生非常重要，因为前者应进行手术治疗，而后者采用药物治疗。应进行肾上腺 CT，以确定肿瘤及其位置。由于肾上腺偶发瘤的高发生率，术前应通过肾上腺静脉取血检测皮质醇水平，以确认肿瘤的功能。如果单侧肾上腺出现肾上腺瘤，而对侧肾上腺正常，且肾上腺静脉取血支持单侧功能性腺瘤，则患者应接受单侧肾上腺切除术。如果生化和定位检查支持双侧肾上腺增生，则应使用保钾利尿剂进行药物治疗，常用依普利酮或螺内酯。肾素-血管紧张素系统激活导致的继发性醛固酮增多症和高血压可见于急进性高血压、肾血管性高血压及使用雌激素的患者中，极少数情况下可见于肾素分泌瘤患者。无高血压的醛固酮增多症可见于巴特综合征（Bartter 综合征）、失盐性肾病、肾小管性酸中毒及滥用利尿剂或泻药的患者。

肾上腺髓质功能亢进

肾上腺髓质通过酪氨酸合成儿茶酚胺（如去甲肾上腺素、肾上腺素和多巴胺）。去甲肾上腺素是肾上腺髓质分泌的主要儿茶酚胺。其主要激动 α 受体，引起血管收缩。肾上腺素主要作用于 β 受体，对心脏发挥

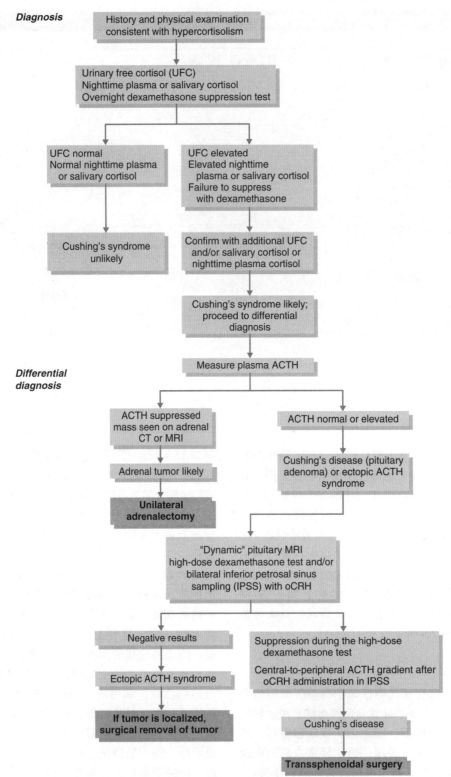

Fig. 3.5 Flowchart for evaluation of a patient with possible Cushing's syndrome. *ACTH,* Adrenocorticotropic hormone; *CT,* computed tomography; *MRI,* magnetic resonance imaging.

inotropic and chronotropic effects on the heart causing peripheral vasodilation and increasing plasma glucose concentrations in response to hypoglycemia. The action of circulating dopamine is unclear. Whereas norepinephrine is synthesized in the central nervous system and sympathetic postganglionic neurons, epinephrine is synthesized almost entirely in the adrenal medulla. The adrenal medullary contribution to total body norepinephrine secretion is relatively small. Hypofunction of the adrenal medulla has little physiologic effect, whereas hypersecretion of catecholamines produces the clinical syndrome of pheochromocytoma.

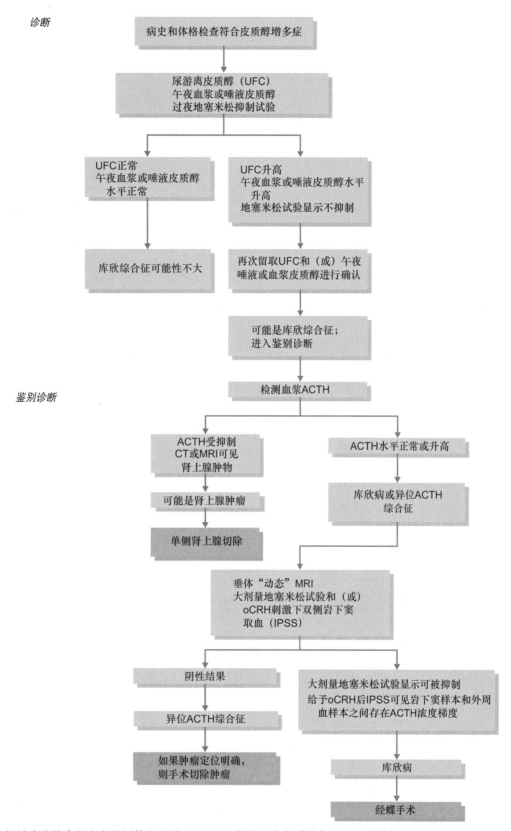

诊断

病史和体格检查符合皮质醇增多症

尿游离皮质醇（UFC）
午夜血浆或唾液皮质醇
过夜地塞米松抑制试验

UFC正常
午夜血浆或唾液皮质醇
水平正常

UFC升高
午夜血浆或唾液皮质醇水平
升高
地塞米松试验显示不抑制

库欣综合征可能性不大

再次留取UFC和（或）午夜
唾液或血浆皮质醇进行确认

可能是库欣综合征；
进入鉴别诊断

检测血浆ACTH

鉴别诊断

ACTH受抑制
CT或MRI可见
肾上腺肿物

ACTH水平正常或升高

可能是肾上腺肿瘤

库欣病或异位ACTH
综合征

单侧肾上腺切除

垂体"动态"MRI
大剂量地塞米松试验和（或）
oCRH刺激下双侧岩下窦
取血（IPSS）

阴性结果

大剂量地塞米松试验显示可被抑制
给予oCRH后IPSS可见岩下窦样本和外周
血样本之间存在ACTH浓度梯度

异位ACTH综合征

如果肿瘤定位明确，
则手术切除肿瘤

库欣病

经蝶手术

图 3.5 疑诊库欣综合征患者的评估流程图。ACTH，促肾上腺皮质激素；CT，计算机断层成像；MRI，磁共振成像

正性变力和正性变时作用，引起外周血管扩张，并在低血糖时增加血浆葡萄糖浓度。循环中多巴胺的作用尚不清楚。去甲肾上腺素在中枢神经系统和交感神经节后神经元中合成，而肾上腺素则几乎全部在肾上腺髓质内合成。肾上腺髓质分泌的去甲肾上腺素在全身去甲肾上腺素中的占比相对较小。肾上腺髓质功能减退对生理学功能的影响不大，而儿茶酚胺分泌过多会产生嗜铬细胞瘤的症状。

Pheochromocytoma

Pathophysiology

Although pheochromocytomas can occur in any sympathetic ganglion in the body, more than 90% arise from the adrenal medulla. Most extra-adrenal tumors occur in the mediastinum or abdomen. Bilateral adrenal pheochromocytomas are present in about 5% of the cases and may occur as part of familial syndromes. Pheochromocytoma occurs as part of multiple endocrine neoplasia type IIA or IIB. The former, type IIA, is also called Sipple syndrome and is marked by medullary carcinoma of the thyroid, hyperparathyroidism, and pheochromocytoma; the latter, type IIB, is characterized by medullary carcinoma of the thyroid, mucosal neuromas, intestinal ganglioneuromas, marfanoid habitus, and pheochromocytoma. Pheochromocytomas are also associated with neurofibromatosis, cerebelloretinal hemangioblastoma (von Hippel–Lindau disease), and tuberous sclerosis.

Clinical Presentation

Because most pheochromocytomas secrete norepinephrine as the principal catecholamine, hypertension (often paroxysmal) is the most common finding. Other symptoms include the triad of headache, palpitations, and sweating as well as skin blanching, diarrhea, anxiety, nausea, fatigue, weight loss, and abdominal and chest pain. Emotional stress, exercise, anesthesia, abdominal pressure, or intake of tyramine-containing foods may precipitate these symptoms. Orthostatic hypotension can also occur. Wide fluctuations in blood pressure are characteristic, and the hypertension associated with pheochromocytoma usually does not respond to standard antihypertensive medicines. Cardiac abnormalities, as well as idiosyncratic reactions to medications, may also occur.

Diagnosis and Treatment

Although measurements of fractionated catecholamine and metanephrine levels in the urine are often used as screening tests, plasma free metanephrine and normetanephrine levels are the best tests for confirming or excluding pheochromocytoma. A plasma free metanephrine level greater than 0.61 nmol/L and a plasma free normetanephrine level greater than 0.31 nmol/L are consistent with the diagnosis of a pheochromocytoma. If these levels are only mildly elevated, a clonidine suppression test can be performed. In patients with pheochromocytoma, levels are unchanged or increased. Once the diagnosis of pheochromocytoma is made, a CT scan of the adrenal glands should be performed. Most intra-adrenal pheochromocytomas are readily visible on this scan and enhance with contrast. If the CT scan is negative, then extra-adrenal pheochromocytomas can often be localized by iodine 131–labeled metaiodobenzylguanidine (^{131}I-MIBG), positron emission tomography, octreotide scan, or abdominal MRI. Pheochromocytomas show high signal intensity on MRI T2-weighted images.

The treatment of pheochromocytoma is surgical if the lesion can be localized. Patients should undergo preoperative α-blockade with phenoxybenzamine 1 to 2 weeks before surgery. About 5% to 10% of pheochromocytomas are malignant. ^{131}I-MIBG or chemotherapy may be useful, but the prognosis is poor. α-Methyl-*p*-tyrosine, an inhibitor of tyrosine hydroxylase, the rate-limiting enzyme in catecholamine biosynthesis, may be used to decrease catecholamine secretion from the tumor.

Incidental Adrenal Mass

Clinically inapparent adrenal masses may be discovered inadvertently in the course of diagnostic testing or treatment for other clinical conditions not related to the signs and symptoms of adrenal disease; they are commonly known as *incidentalomas*. Some of these

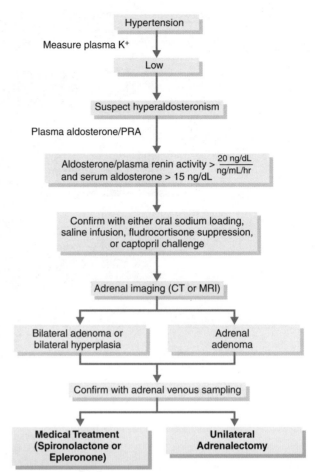

Fig. 3.6 Flowchart for evaluation of a patient with probable primary hyperaldosteronism. Plasma aldosterone is measured in ng/dL, and plasma renin activity (PRA) is measured in ng/mL/hour. *CT*, Computed tomography; *MRI*, magnetic resonance imaging.

tumors secrete a small amount of excess cortisol, leading to a condition that used to be called subclinical Cushing's syndrome and is now called *mild autonomous cortisol excess (MACE)* or *autonomous cortisol secretion*, a condition associated with comorbidities including hypertension, glucose intolerance/diabetes, obesity, dyslipidemia, osteoporosis, and increased cardiovascular events. This condition does not progress to overt Cushing's syndrome. An overnight 1-mg dexamethasone test is recommended for all patients with an adrenal mass seen on imaging. A morning cortisol post-dexamethasone of between 1.8 and 5 μg/dL suggests possible autonomous cortisol secretion that usually does not need surgery, whereas values greater than 5 μg/dL should be worked up for Cushing's syndrome as described previously. Under certain circumstances, surgical removal should be performed. Patients with hypertension should also undergo measurement of serum potassium, plasma aldosterone concentration, PRA, and plasma free metanephrines (only if the unenhanced CT attenuation value is greater than 10 Hounsfield units). Surgery should be considered for all patients with functional adrenal cortical tumors that are hormonally active or larger than 4 cm. Tumors not associated with hormonal secretion that are smaller than 4 cm and have benign imaging characteristics do not need follow-up.

Primary Adrenal Cancer

Primary adrenal carcinomas are rare, with an incidence of 1 to 5 per 1 million persons. The female-to-male ratio is 2.5:1, and the mean age at onset is 40 to 50 years. About 25% of patients have symptoms,

嗜铬细胞瘤

病理生理学

虽然嗜铬细胞瘤可发生于任何交感神经节，但80%～85%的嗜铬细胞瘤来自肾上腺髓质。大多数肾上腺外嗜铬细胞瘤发生于纵隔或腹部。双侧肾上腺嗜铬细胞瘤约占5%，可能是家族性综合征的一部分。嗜铬细胞瘤是多发性内分泌腺瘤病ⅡA/ⅡB型的一部分。前者（ⅡA型）又称Sipple综合征，以甲状腺髓样癌、甲状旁腺功能亢进症和嗜铬细胞瘤为特征；后者（ⅡB型）以甲状腺髓样癌、黏膜神经瘤、肠神经节瘤、类马方体型和嗜铬细胞瘤为特征。嗜铬细胞瘤还与神经纤维瘤病、脑视网膜血管母细胞瘤［希佩尔-林道病（von Hippel-Lindau病）］和结节性硬化症有关。

临床表现

由于大多数嗜铬细胞瘤分泌的主要儿茶酚胺类型是去甲肾上腺素，因此高血压（通常为阵发性）是最常见的症状。其他症状包括头痛、心悸和出汗三联征，以及皮肤苍白、腹泻、焦虑、恶心、疲劳、体重减轻、腹痛和胸痛。情绪应激、运动、麻醉、腹压增高或摄入含酪氨酸的食物可能会诱发这些症状。患者还可能出现体位性低血压。血压剧烈波动是其特征，标准的降压药物对嗜铬细胞瘤相关的高血压通常无效。患者可能出现心脏异常和对药物的特异质反应。

诊断和治疗

虽然尿液中的的儿茶酚胺组分和甲氧基肾上腺素水平测定通常被作为筛查试验，但血浆游离甲氧基肾上腺素和甲氧基去甲肾上腺素水平是确诊或排除嗜铬细胞瘤的最佳检查。如果血浆游离甲氧基肾上腺素＞0.61 nmol/L，血浆游离甲氧基去甲肾上腺素＞0.31 nmol/L，则支持诊断嗜铬细胞瘤。如果这些指标仅有轻度升高，则可进行可乐定抑制试验，嗜铬细胞瘤患者的上述指标应保持不变或升高。一旦确诊嗜铬细胞瘤，应进行肾上腺CT。大多数肾上腺嗜铬细胞瘤在CT中清晰可见，并在增强后强化。如果CT结果为阴性，肾上腺外的嗜铬细胞瘤通常可通过碘-131标记的间碘苄胍（[131]I-MIBG）显像、正电子发射断层成像（PET）、奥曲肽扫描或腹部MRI进行定位。嗜铬细胞瘤在MRI T2加权像上呈高信号。

如果病灶定位明确，嗜铬细胞瘤的治疗方法是手术。患者应在手术前1～2周（译者注：原文与临床实践不符，应为手术前至少2周）使用α受体阻滞剂酚苄明。5%～10%的嗜铬细胞瘤是恶性的。[131]I-MIBG或化疗可能有效，但预后较差。α-甲基酪氨酸是酪氨酸羟化酶（儿茶酚胺生物合成的限速酶）的抑制剂，可用于减少肿瘤分泌的儿茶酚胺。

肾上腺偶发瘤

无临床症状的肾上腺肿物可能是在与肾上腺疾病症

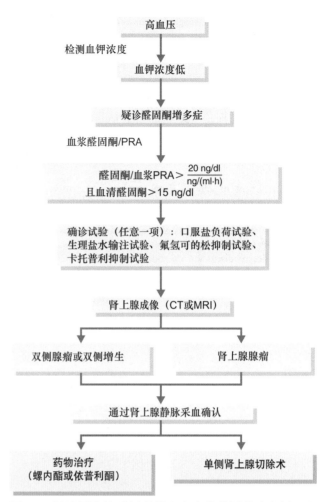

图3.6　疑诊原发性醛固酮增多症患者的评估流程图。血浆醛固酮的单位为ng/dl，血浆肾素活性（PRA）的单位为ng/（ml·h）。CT，计算机断层成像；MRI，磁共振成像

状和体征无关的其他临床情况的诊断性检查或治疗过程中被偶然发现，通常被称为偶发瘤。部分肾上腺偶发瘤会分泌少量皮质醇，导致亚临床库欣综合征［现在被称为轻度自主皮质醇过量（MACE）或自主皮质醇分泌］，这种情况会合并高血压、糖耐量异常/糖尿病、肥胖症、血脂异常、骨质疏松症和心血管事件，但不会进展至显性库欣综合征。建议所有在影像学检查中发现肾上腺肿物的患者进行过夜1 mg地塞米松抑制试验。服用地塞米松后的清晨皮质醇水平为1.8～5 μg/dl提示皮质醇可能存在自主分泌，但通常不需要进行手术，而皮质醇＞5 μg/dl时，则应进行库欣综合征相关检查。在某些情况下，应进行手术切除。伴随高血压的患者还应检测血钾、血浆醛固酮浓度、PRA和血浆游离甲氧基肾上腺素（仅在CT平扫值＞10 Hu时进行）。所有功能性肾上腺肿瘤或直径＞4 cm的肿瘤均应考虑手术治疗。无激素分泌功能且直径＜4 cm、影像学特征为良性的肿瘤，无须随访。

原发性肾上腺皮质癌

原发性肾上腺皮质癌非常罕见，发病率为（1～5）/1 000 000。女性与男性比例为2.5∶1，平均发病年龄为40～50岁。约25%的患者有症状，包括腹痛、体

including abdominal pain, weight loss, anorexia, and fever. Eighty percent of primary adrenal carcinomas are functional, with secretion of glucocorticoid alone (45%) or glucocorticoid plus androgens (45%) being most common.

At presentation, metastatic spread is evident in 75% of cases. An incidentally discovered adrenal mass that is large is more likely to be malignant. Resection is recommended for tumors larger than 6 cm and often for those larger than 4 cm. In patients who do not have a known cancer, most adrenal masses that turn out to be malignant are primary adrenocortical carcinomas, whereas in patients with a known malignancy, an adrenal mass is likely to be a metastasis in about 75% of cases.

The treatment of adrenocortical carcinomas is surgery. These cancers are usually resistant to radiation and chemotherapy, but the adrenolytic compound mitotane has been shown to improve survival. Adrenocortical carcinomas carry a poor prognosis, with overall 5-year survival rates of less than 20%.

❖　For a deeper discussion on this topic, please see Chapter 214, "Adrenal Cortex," in *Goldman-Cecil Medicine*, 26th Edition.

SUGGESTED READINGS

Annane D, Pastores SM, Rochwerg B, et al: Guidelines for the diagnosis and management of critical illness-related corticosteroid insufficiency (CIRCI) in critically ill patients (Part I): Society of Critical Care Medicine (SCCM) and European Society of Intensive Care Medicine (ESICM) 2017, Intensive Care Med 43:1751–1763, 2017.

Bornstein SR, Allolio B, Arlt W, et al: Diagnosis and treatment of primary adrenal insufficiency: an Endocrine Society clinical practice guideline, J Clin Endocrinol Metab 101:364–389, 2016.

Fassnacht M, Arlt W, Bancos I, et al: Management of adrenal incidentalomas: European Society of Endocrinology clinical practice guideline in collaboration with the European Network for the Study of Adrenal Tumors, Eur J Endocrinol 175:G1–G34, 2016.

Nieman LK, Biller BM, Findling JW, et al: The diagnosis of Cushing's syndrome: an Endocrine Society clinical practice guideline, J Clin Endocrinol Metab 93:1526–1540, 2008.

Rushworth RL, Torpy DJ, Falhammar H: Adrenal crisis, N Engl J Med 381:852–861, 2019.

Speiser PW, Arlt W, Auchus RJ, et al: Congenital adrenal hyperplasia due to steroid 21-hydroxylase deficiency: an Endocrine Society clinical practice guideline, J Clin Endocrinol Metab 103:4043–4088, 2018.

重减轻、厌食和发热。80% 的原发性肾上腺皮质癌为功能性，最常见的类型是单纯分泌皮质醇型（45%）或分泌皮质醇和雄激素型（45%）。

在就诊时，75% 的病例已发生转移。意外发现的巨大肾上腺肿物更有可能为恶性。直径＞ 6 cm 的肿瘤建议切除，直径＞ 4 cm 的肿瘤通常也建议进行切除。在没有已知癌症的患者中，若发现肾上腺恶性肿瘤，多为原发性肾上腺皮质癌，但如果患者有已知存在的恶性肿瘤，则其中约 75% 由肿瘤转移所致。

肾上腺皮质癌的治疗方法是手术。放疗和化疗通常疗效不佳，但肾上腺破坏剂米托坦已被证明可提高生存率。肾上腺皮质癌的预后较差，5 年总生存率不足 20%。

❖ 有关此专题的深入讨论，请参阅 *Goldman-Cecil Medicine* 第 26 版第 214 章 "肾上腺皮质"。

推荐阅读

Annane D, Pastores SM, Rochwerg B, et al: Guidelines for the diagnosis and management of critical illness-related corticosteroid insufficiency (CIRCI) in critically ill patients (Part I): Society of Critical Care Medicine (SCCM) and European Society of Intensive Care Medicine (ESICM) 2017, Intensive Care Med 43:1751–1763, 2017.

Bornstein SR, Allolio B, Arlt W, et al: Diagnosis and treatment of primary adrenal insufficiency: an Endocrine Society clinical practice guideline, J Clin Endocrinol Metab 101:364–389, 2016.

Fassnacht M, Arlt W, Bancos I, et al: Management of adrenal incidentalomas: European Society of Endocrinology clinical practice guideline in collaboration with the European Network for the Study of Adrenal Tumors, Eur J Endocrinol 175:G1–G34, 2016.

Nieman LK, Biller BM, Findling JW, et al: The diagnosis of Cushing's syndrome: an Endocrine Society clinical practice guideline, J Clin Endocrinol Metab 93:1526–1540, 2008.

Rushworth RL, Torpy DJ, Falhammar H: Adrenal crisis, N Engl J Med 381:852–861, 2019.

Speiser PW, Arlt W, Auchus RJ, et al: Congenital adrenal hyperplasia due to steroid 21-hydroxylase deficiency: an Endocrine Society clinical practice guideline, J Clin Endocrinol Metab 103:4043–4088, 2018.

4

Male Reproductive Endocrinology

Glenn D. Braunstein

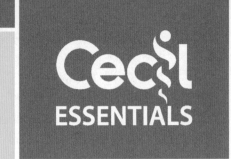

INTRODUCTION

The testes are composed of Leydig (interstitial) cells, which secrete testosterone and estradiol, and the seminiferous tubules, which produce sperm. They are regulated by the luteinizing hormone (LH) and follicle-stimulating hormone (FSH), which are secreted by the anterior pituitary under the influence of the hypothalamic decapeptide gonadotropin-releasing hormone (GnRH) (Fig. 4.1). LH stimulates the Leydig cells to secrete testosterone, which feeds back in a negative fashion at the level of the pituitary and hypothalamus to inhibit further LH production. FSH stimulates sperm production through interaction with the Sertoli cells in the seminiferous tubules. Feedback inhibition of FSH is through gonadal steroids, as well as through inhibin, a glycoprotein produced by Sertoli cells.

Biochemical evaluation of the hypothalamic-pituitary-Leydig axis is carried out by measurement of serum LH and testosterone concentrations, whereas a semen analysis and serum FSH determination provide an assessment of the hypothalamic-pituitary-seminiferous tubular axis. The ability of the pituitary to release gonadotropins can be tested dynamically through GnRH stimulation, and the ability of the testes to secrete testosterone can be evaluated through injections of human chorionic gonadotropin (HCG), a glycoprotein hormone that has biologic activity similar to that of LH.

HYPOGONADISM

Either testosterone deficiency or defective spermatogenesis constitutes *hypogonadism*. Often both disorders coexist. The clinical manifestations of androgen deficiency depend on the time of onset and the degree of deficiency. Testosterone is required for development of the Wolffian duct into the epididymis, vas deferens, seminal vesicles, and ejaculatory ducts, as well as for virilization of the external genitalia through the major intracellular testosterone metabolite, dihydrotestosterone (DHT). Consequently, early prenatal androgen deficiency leads to the formation of ambiguous genitalia and to male pseudohermaphroditism. Androgen deficiency occurring later during gestation may result in micropenis or *cryptorchidism*, the unilateral or bilateral absence of testes in the scrotum resulting from the failure of normal testicular descent.

During puberty, androgens are responsible for male sexual differentiation, which includes growth of the scrotum, epididymis, vas deferens, seminal vesicles, prostate, penis, skeletal muscle, and larynx. Additionally, androgens stimulate the growth of axillary, pubic, facial, and body hair and increase sebaceous gland activity. They are also responsible through conversion to estrogens for the growth and fusion of the epiphyseal cartilaginous plates, clinically seen as the *pubertal growth spurt*. Prepubertal androgen deficiency leads to poor muscle development, decreased strength and endurance, a high-pitched voice, sparse axillary and pubic hair, and the absence of facial and body hair. The long bones of the lower extremities and arms may continue to grow under the influence of growth hormone; this condition leads to eunuchoid proportions (i.e., arm span exceeding total height by ≥5 cm) and greater growth of the lower extremities relative to total height. Postpubertal androgen deficiency may result in a decrease in libido, impotence, low energy, fine wrinkling around the corners of the eyes and mouth, and diminished facial and body hair.

Male hypogonadism may be classified into three categories according to the level of the defect (Table 4.1). Diseases directly affecting the testes result in *primary* or *hypergonadotropic hypogonadism*, which is characterized by oligospermia or azoospermia and low testosterone levels but exhibits elevations of LH and FSH because of a decrease in the negative feedback regulation on the pituitary and hypothalamus by androgens, estrogens, and inhibin. In contrast, hypogonadism from lesions in the hypothalamus or pituitary gives rise to *secondary* or *hypogonadotropic hypogonadism*; the low testosterone level or ineffective spermatogenesis results from inadequate concentrations of the gonadotropins. The third category of hypogonadism is the result of defects in androgen action.

Hypothalamic-Pituitary Disorders

Panhypopituitarism occurs congenitally from structural defects or from inadequate production or release of the hypothalamic-releasing factors. The condition may also be acquired through replacement by tumors, infarction from vascular insufficiency, infiltrative disorders, autoimmune diseases, trauma, and infections.

Kallmann syndrome is a form of hypogonadotropic hypogonadism that is associated with problems in the ability to discriminate odors, either incompletely *(hyposmia)* or completely *(anosmia)*. This syndrome results from a defect in the migration of the GnRH neurons from the olfactory placode into the hypothalamus. Therefore, it represents a GnRH deficiency. Patients remain prepubertal, with small, rubbery testes, and they develop eunuchoidism.

Hyperprolactinemia may result in hypogonadotropic hypogonadism because prolactin elevation inhibits normal release of GnRH, decreases the effectiveness of LH at the Leydig cell level, and also inhibits some of the actions of testosterone at the level of the target organ. Normalization of prolactin levels through withdrawal of an offending drug, by surgical removal of the pituitary adenoma, or with the use of dopamine agonists reverses this form of hypogonadism.

Weight loss or systemic illness in male patients can cause another form of secondary hypogonadism, *hypothalamic dysfunction*. Weight loss or illness induces a defect in the hypothalamic release of GnRH and results in low levels of gonadotropin and testosterone. This condition is commonly observed in patients with cancer, AIDS, or chronic

男性生殖内分泌学

杜函泽 译 陈适 潘慧 审校 宁光 通审

引言

睾丸由分泌睾酮和雌二醇的间质细胞（Leydig 细胞）和产生精子的生精小管组成。它们受黄体生成素（LH）和卵泡刺激素（FSH）的调节，这两种激素是在下丘脑分泌促性腺激素释放激素（GnRH）的作用下由垂体前叶分泌的（图 4.1）。LH 刺激睾丸间质细胞分泌睾酮，而睾酮可通过负反馈抑制垂体和下丘脑的激素分泌，从而抑制 LH 的进一步产生。FSH 通过与输精管中的支持细胞相互作用而刺激产生精子。FSH 的负反馈抑制则是通过性腺类固醇和抑制素（一种由支持细胞产生的糖蛋白）来发挥作用。

下丘脑-垂体-性腺间质细胞轴可通过检测血清 LH 和睾酮水平进行评估，而下丘脑-垂体-生精小管轴的评估则可通过精液分析和监测血清 FSH 水平来完成。垂体分泌促性腺激素的能力可通过 GnRH 激发试验来评估；人绒毛膜促性腺激素（HCG）是一种与 LH 具有相似生物活性的糖蛋白激素，可用于评估睾丸分泌睾酮的功能。

性腺功能减退症

性腺功能减退症包括睾酮缺乏或精子发生障碍。这两种情况通常同时存在。雄激素缺乏的临床表现取决于起病年龄和激素缺乏的严重程度。睾酮是中肾管（Wolffian 管）发育为附睾、输精管、精囊和射精管所必需的，也是通过细胞内睾酮的主要代谢产物双氢睾酮（DHT）使外生殖器男性化的必要条件。因此，胚胎早期雄激素缺乏会导致外生殖器模糊和男性假两性畸形。妊娠后期雄激素缺乏可导致小阴茎或隐睾，即阴囊内单侧或双侧睾丸缺失，其由正常睾丸下降失败所致。

在青春期，雄激素负责男性性征的发育，包括阴囊、附睾、输精管、精囊、前列腺、阴茎、骨骼肌和喉结。此外，雄激素可刺激腋毛、阴毛、面部毛发和体毛，并增加皮脂腺活性。雄激素还通过转化为雌激素而促进骨骺软骨板的生长和融合，临床表现为青春期发育陡增。青春期前雄激素缺乏可导致肌肉发育不良、力量和耐力下降、声音尖细、腋毛和阴毛稀疏、

面部毛发和体毛缺失。在生长激素的持续作用下，此类患者下肢和手臂的长骨可能持续生长，并表现为类宦官体型（即臂展长度超过身高 ≥ 5 cm）、下肢增长速度明显快于身高增长等表现。青春期后雄激素缺乏则可能导致性欲减退、阳痿、精力不足、眼角和嘴角有细微皱纹、面部毛发和体毛减少。

根据病因，男性性腺功能减退症可分为 3 类（表 4.1）。直接影响睾丸的疾病可导致原发性或高促性腺激素性性腺功能减退症，其特征是少精子症或无精子症和睾酮水平低，但由于雄激素、雌激素和抑制素对垂体和下丘脑的负反馈调节减少，LH 和 FSH 水平升高。相反，下丘脑或垂体病变引起的性腺功能减退症可引起继发性或低促性腺激素性性腺功能减退症，即睾酮水平低或无效精子发生是由促性腺激素不足引起。第 3 类性腺功能减退症是由雄激素作用缺陷所致。

下丘脑-垂体疾病

全垂体功能减退症可由先天性因素（如结构缺陷、下丘脑激素生成或分泌障碍）导致。此外，该病也可能由获得性因素引起，如肿瘤压迫、血管功能障碍引起的梗死、浸润性疾病、自身免疫病、创伤和感染。

卡尔曼综合征（Kallmann 综合征）是一种低促性腺激素性性腺功能减退症，伴有不完全性（嗅觉减退）或完全性（嗅觉丧失）嗅觉异常。其发病机制是 GnRH 神经元从嗅板到下丘脑的迁移过程缺陷。因此，GnRH 水平低下导致患者无法进入青春期发育，睾丸小且质韧，最终表现为类宦官体型。

由于催乳素水平升高会抑制 GnRH 的正常释放，并降低间质细胞对 LH 的敏感性，从而抑制睾酮在靶器官水平上的作用，因此高催乳素血症可导致低促性腺激素性性腺功能减退症。通过停用致病药物、手术切除垂体腺瘤或使用多巴胺激动剂使催乳素水平恢复正常，可改善由高催乳素血症所致的性腺功能减退症。

男性患者体重减轻或全身性疾病可引起另一种形式的继发性性腺功能减退症，即下丘脑功能障碍。体重减轻或全身性疾病会影响下丘脑分泌 GnRH 水平，进而导致促性腺激素和睾丸激素水平下降。这种情况

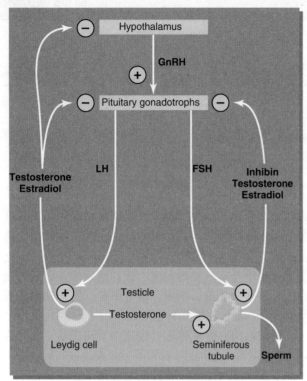

Fig. 4.1 Regulation of the hypothalamic-pituitary-testicular axis. The *plus (+)* and *minus (–)* symbols indicate positive and negative feedback, respectively. *FSH,* Follicle-stimulating hormone; *GnRH,* gonadotropin-releasing hormone; *LH,* luteinizing hormone.

TABLE 4.1 Classification of Male Hypogonadism
Hypothalamic-Pituitary Disorders (Secondary Hypogonadism)
Panhypopituitarism
Isolated gonadotropin deficiency
Complex congenital syndromes
Hyperprolactinemia
Hypothalamic dysfunction
Gonadal Disorders (Primary Hypogonadism)
Klinefelter's syndrome and associated chromosomal defects
Myotonic dystrophy
Cryptorchidism
Bilateral anorchia
Seminiferous tubular failure
Adult Leydig cell failure
Androgen biosynthesis enzyme deficiency
Defects in Androgen Action
Testicular feminization (complete androgen insensitivity)
Incomplete androgen insensitivity
5α-Reductase deficiency

inflammatory processes. Prolonged use of opioids and therapeutic doses of glucocorticoids may suppress gonadotropin production and cause secondary hypogonadism.

Primary Gonadal Abnormalities

The most common congenital cause of primary testicular failure is *Klinefelter's syndrome,* which occurs in about 1 of every 600 live male births and is usually caused by a maternal meiotic chromosomal nondisjunction that results in an XXY genotype. At puberty, clinical findings include the following: a variable degree of hypogonadism; gynecomastia; small, firm testes measuring less than 2 cm in the longest axis (normal testes, 3.5 cm or greater); azoospermia; eunuchoid skeletal proportions; and elevations of FSH and LH. Primary gonadal failure is also found in patients with another congenital condition, *myotonic dystrophy,* which is characterized by progressive weakness; atrophy of the facial, neck, hand, and lower extremity muscles; frontal baldness; and myotonia.

About 3% of full-term male infants have *cryptorchidism,* which spontaneously corrects during the first year of life in most cases; consequently, by 1 year of age, the incidence of this condition is about 0.8%. When the testes are maintained in the intra-abdominal position, the increased temperature leads to defective spermatogenesis and oligospermia. Leydig cell function usually remains normal, resulting in normal levels of adult testosterone.

Bilateral anorchia, also known as the vanishing testicle syndrome, is a rare condition in which the external genitalia are fully formed, indicating that ample quantities of testosterone and DHT were produced during early embryogenesis. However, the testicular tissue disappears before or shortly after birth, and the result is an empty scrotum. This condition is differentiated from cryptorchidism by an

HCG stimulation test. Patients with cryptorchidism have an increase in serum testosterone level after an injection of HCG, whereas patients with bilateral anorchia do not.

Acquired gonadal failure has numerous causes. The adult seminiferous tubules are susceptible to a variety of injuries, and seminiferous tubular failure is found after infections such as mumps, gonococcal or lepromatous orchitis, irradiation, vascular injury, trauma, alcohol ingestion, and use of chemotherapeutic drugs, especially alkylating agents. The serum FSH concentration may be normal or elevated, depending on the degree of damage to the seminiferous tubules. The Leydig cell compartment may also be damaged by these same conditions. In addition, some men experience a gradual decline in testicular function as they age, possibly because of microvascular insufficiency. Patients with decreased testosterone production may clinically exhibit lowered libido and potency, emotional lability, fatigue, and vasomotor symptoms such as hot flashes. The serum LH concentration is usually elevated in this situation.

Defects in Androgen Action

When either testosterone or its metabolite, DHT, binds to the androgen receptor in target cells, the receptor is activated and binds DNA; the resulting stimulation of transcription, protein synthesis, and cell growth collectively constitutes androgen action. An absence of androgen receptors causes the syndrome of *testicular feminization,* a form of male pseudohermaphroditism. These genetic males have cryptorchid testes but appear to be phenotypic females. Because androgens are inactive during embryogenesis, the labial-scrotal folds fail to fuse, and a short vagina results. The fallopian tubes, uterus, and upper portion of the vagina are absent because the fetal testicular Sertoli cells secrete Anti-Müllerian duct hormone (Müllerian duct inhibitory factor) during early fetal development. At puberty, these patients have breast enlargement because the testes secrete a small amount of estradiol and the peripheral tissues convert testosterone and adrenal androgens to estrogens. Axillary and pubic hair does not grow because androgen action is required for their development. The serum testosterone concentrations are elevated as a result of continuous stimulation by elevated concentrations of LH. LH is high because of the inability of the testosterone to act in a negative feedback fashion at

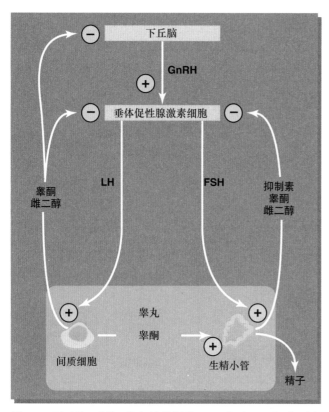

图 4.1 下丘脑-垂体-睾丸轴的调节。"＋"和"－"分别表示正反馈和负反馈。FSH，卵泡刺激素；GnRH，促性腺激素释放激素；LH，黄体生成素

常见于癌症、艾滋病或慢性炎症性疾病患者。长期使用阿片类药物和治疗剂量的糖皮质激素可抑制促性腺激素的生成，引起继发性性腺功能减退症。

原发性性腺功能异常

原发性睾丸功能衰竭最常见的先天性病因是 Klinefelter 综合征，其发生率为 1/600 例活产男婴，通常由母体减数分裂染色体不分离导致 XXY 基因型引起。Klinefelter 综合征的青春期临床表现包括：不同程度的性腺功能减退、男性乳房发育、睾丸小而质韧（睾丸长轴长度＜2 cm；正常睾丸长轴≥3.5 cm）、无精子症、类宦官体型、血清 FSH 和 LH 水平升高等。原发性性腺功能衰竭也可见于另一种先天性疾病——强直性肌营养不良，其临床特征是进行性肌无力（面部、颈部、手部、下肢肌肉萎缩），前额脱发和肌强直。

约 3% 的足月男婴患有隐睾，大多数患者在出生后第 1 年可自行恢复正常，因此 1 岁男婴的隐睾发生率约为 0.8%。当睾丸维持在腹内位置时，由于温度偏高会导致精子发生缺陷和无精症。患者的间质细胞功能通常正常，因此睾酮水平通常不受影响。

双侧无睾症又称睾丸消失综合征，是一种外生殖器完全形成的罕见情况，表明在胚胎发育早期产生了大量的睾酮和 DHT。然而，睾丸组织会在出生前或出生后不久消失，最终形成阴囊空虚的表现。该病可

通过 HCG 激发试验与隐睾进行鉴别。隐睾患者注射 HCG 后血清睾酮水平升高，而双侧无睾症患者通常没有反应。

继发性性腺功能衰竭有多种病因。成人生精小管易受多种损伤，感染性疾病（如腮腺炎、淋球菌性或麻风性睾丸炎），辐射，血管损伤，外伤，酒精摄入和应用化疗药物（尤其是烷化剂）等均可导致生精小管功能障碍。继发性性腺功能减退症患者血清 FSH 浓度可正常或升高，这取决于生精小管损伤的程度。上述疾病或理化因素也可损伤间质细胞。此外，随着年龄的增长，部分男性的睾丸功能会逐渐下降，这可能是因为微血管功能不全。睾酮生成减少的患者在临床上可能表现为性欲和性功能减退、情绪不稳定、疲劳和血管舒缩症状（如潮热）。在这种情况下，患者血清 LH 浓度通常升高。

雄激素作用缺陷

当睾酮或其代谢产物 DHT 与靶细胞中的雄激素受体结合时，受体被激活并结合 DNA；由此产生的刺激转录、蛋白质合成和细胞生长构成了雄激素的生物学作用。雄激素受体缺失可导致睾丸女性化综合征，这是男性假两性畸形的一种临床表现形式。这些患者的染色体为男性且有隐睾，但临床表型为女性。由于胚胎发育过程中雄激素活性缺乏，胚胎阴唇-阴囊褶皱无法融合，导致阴道缩短。由于胚胎睾丸支持细胞在胎儿发育早期分泌抗米勒管激素（米勒管抑制因子），可能导致输卵管缺失、子宫缺失和阴道上半部分缺失。在青春期，这些患者的睾丸分泌少量雌二醇，且外周组织将睾酮和肾上腺雄激素转化为雌激素，因此可能出现乳房增大。但是，腋毛和阴毛不生长，因其需要雄激素的作用。LH 水平持续升高可刺激血清睾酮浓度

表 4.1 男性性腺功能减退症的分类

下丘脑-垂体疾病（继发性性腺功能减退症）
全垂体功能减退症
孤立性促性腺激素缺乏症
复杂先天性综合征
高催乳素血症
下丘脑功能障碍

性腺功能障碍（原发性性腺功能减退症）
Klinefelter 综合征及相关染色体缺陷
强直性肌营养不良
隐睾
双侧无睾症
生精小管功能障碍
成人间质细胞功能障碍
雄激素生物合成酶缺乏

雄激素功能缺陷
睾丸女性化（完全性雄激素不敏感）
不完全性雄激素不敏感
5α-还原酶缺乏症

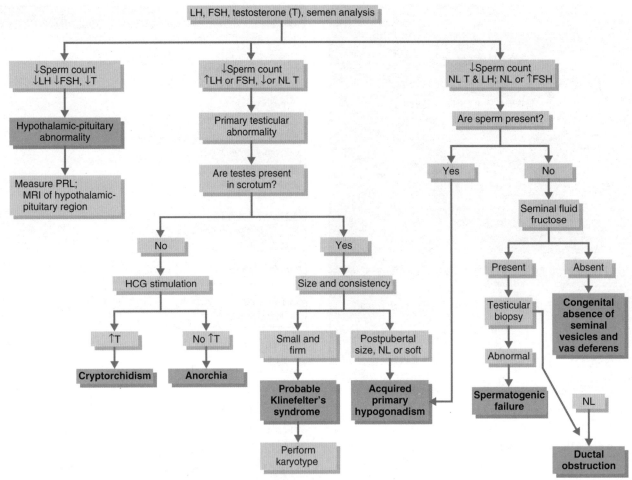

Fig. 4.2 Laboratory evaluation of hypogonadism. *↑,* Elevated; *↓,* decreased or low; *FSH,* follicle-stimulating hormone; *HCG,* human chorionic gonadotropin; *LH,* luteinizing hormone; *MRI,* magnetic resonance imaging; *NL,* normal; *PRL,* prolactin.

the hypothalamus. Patients may have incomplete forms of androgen insensitivity caused by point mutations affecting the androgen receptor gene, and clinically these patients show varying degrees of male pseudohermaphroditism.

Patients who lack the 5α-reductase enzyme that is required to convert testosterone to DHT are born with a *bifid scrotum,* which reflects abnormal fusion of the labial-scrotal folds, and *hypospadias,* in which the urethral opening is in the perineal area or in the shaft of the penis. At puberty, androgen production is sufficient to partially overcome the defect; the scrotum, phallus, and muscle mass enlarge, and these patients appear to develop into physiologically normal men.

Diagnosis

Fig. 4.2 illustrates an algorithm for the laboratory evaluation of hypogonadism in a phenotypic man. Serum concentrations of LH, FSH, and testosterone should be obtained, and a semen analysis should be performed. A low testosterone level with low concentrations of gonadotropins indicates a hypothalamic-pituitary abnormality, which needs to be evaluated with serum prolactin determination and radiographic examination. Elevated concentrations of gonadotropins with a normal or low testosterone level reflect a primary testicular abnormality. If no testes are palpable in the scrotum and careful *milking* of the patient's

lower abdomen does not bring retractile testes into the scrotum, an HCG stimulation test should be performed. A rise in serum testosterone concentrations indicates the presence of functional testicular tissue, and a diagnosis of cryptorchidism can be made. Absence of a rise in testosterone suggests bilateral anorchia. Small, firm testes in the scrotum are highly suggestive of Klinefelter's syndrome; this diagnosis needs to be confirmed with a chromosomal karyotype. Testes that are more than 3.5 cm in longest diameter and that are either of normal consistency or are soft indicate postpubertal acquired primary hypogonadism.

If the major abnormality is a deficient sperm count with or without an elevation of FSH, differentiation between a ductal problem and acquired primary hypogonadism must be made. If spermatozoa are present, at least the ducts emanating from one testicle are patent; this condition indicates an acquired testicular defect. If the patient has no sperm in the ejaculate, a primary testicular or ductal problem may be responsible. The seminal vesicles secrete fructose into the seminal fluid. Therefore, the presence of fructose in the ejaculate should be followed by a testicular biopsy to determine whether the defect results from spermatogenic failure or from an obstruction of the ducts leading from the testes to the seminal vesicles. Absence of seminal fluid fructose indicates a congenital absence of the seminal vesicles and vas deferens.

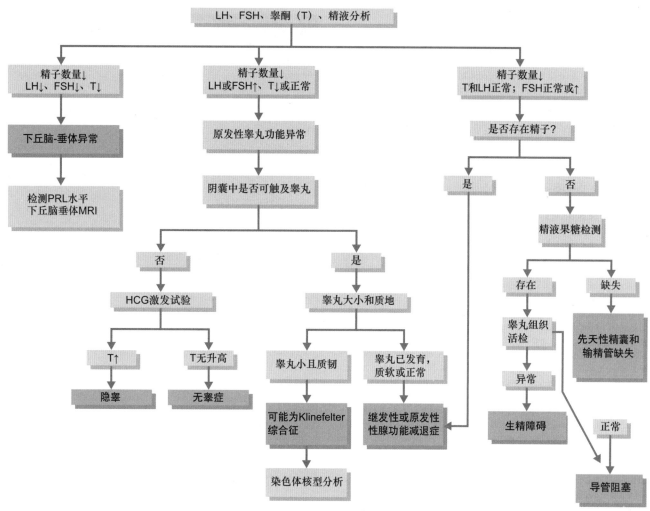

图 4.2　性腺功能减退症的实验室评估。↑，升高；↓，减少或降低；FSH，卵泡刺激素；HCG，人绒毛膜促性腺激素；LH，黄体生成素；MRI，磁共振成像；PRL，催乳素

升高。血清 LH 水平升高是由于睾酮无法在下丘脑以负反馈的方式发挥作用。患者可能由于雄激素受体基因的不同点突变位点而表现出不同程度的雄激素不敏感状态，临床上表现为不同程度的男性假两性畸形。

5α- 还原酶缺乏症患者由于胚胎时期无法将睾酮转化为 DHT，因此在出生时常表现为阴囊分裂，这反映了阴唇-阴囊褶皱的异常融合及尿道下裂（尿道开口位于会阴区或阴茎）。在青春期，由于雄激素的生成足以部分克服这种发育缺陷，患者可出现阴囊、阴茎发育及肌肉增加等表现，这些患者似乎可以发育成生理功能正常的男性。

诊断

图 4.2 展示了男性性腺功能减退症的实验室评估流程。应测定血清 LH、FSH 和睾酮浓度，并进行精液分析。低睾酮水平和低促性腺激素水平提示下丘脑-垂体异常，需要通过血清催乳素测定和影像学检查系统评估。促性腺激素浓度升高伴有睾酮水平正常或偏低，

提示患者可能存在原发性睾丸异常。如果在阴囊内无法触及睾丸，且缓慢推挤下腹部未触及睾丸进入阴囊，则应进行 HCG 激发试验。血清睾酮浓度升高表明存在功能性睾丸组织，可诊断为隐睾；睾酮浓度未升高则提示双侧无睾症。查体见睾丸小且质韧则高度提示 Klinefelter 综合征，但确诊需要完善染色体核型分析。睾丸最长直径 > 3.5 cm 且质地正常或质软，提示青春期后继发性或原发性性腺功能减退症。

如果精液分析提示精子数量不足，无论患者 FSH 水平是否升高，均需鉴别输精管异常和继发性或原发性性腺功能减退症。如果精液分析显示存在精子，则说明至少单侧睾丸的输精管通畅，这种情况通常提示患者可能为获得性睾丸功能障碍。如果患者无精，则可能是原发性睾丸功能异常或输精管异常。由于精囊可分泌果糖至精液中，因此若精液分析显示存在果糖成分，应进行睾丸组织活检，以确定病因是生精障碍还是由睾丸通往精囊的导管阻塞。若精液中无果糖成分，则提示患者可能存在先天性精囊和输精管缺失。

Male Infertility

The inability to conceive after 1 year of unprotected sexual intercourse affects about 15% of couples, and male factors appear to be responsible in about 20% of cases. Female factors account for close to 40%, and a couple factor is present in about 25% of cases with about 15% being undefined. In addition to the defects in spermatogenesis that occur in patients with hypothalamic, pituitary, testicular, or androgen action disorders, hyperthyroidism, hypothyroidism, adrenal abnormalities, and systemic illnesses can result in defective spermatogenesis, as can microdeletions of genetic material on the Y chromosome. Disorders of the vas deferens, seminal vesicles, and prostate may also lead to infertility, as may diseases affecting the bladder sphincter that result in *retrograde ejaculation*, in which the sperm passes into the bladder rather than through the penis. Anatomic defects of the penis (as observed in patients with hypospadias), poor coital technique, and the presence of antisperm antibodies in the male or female genital tract also are associated with infertility.

Therapy for Hypogonadism and Infertility

Treatment of androgen deficiency in patients who have hypothalamic-pituitary or primary testicular abnormalities is best accomplished with exogenous testosterone administration—either intramuscular injection of intermediate (1-3 weeks)- or long (3 months)-acting testosterone esters or transdermal testosterone patches or gel. Buccal, nasal, and subcutaneous testosterone pellets are also available but are less often used. Testosterone therapy increases libido, potency, muscle mass, strength, athletic endurance, hair growth on the face and body, and bone density. The most common side effect is erythrocytosis. Other side effects include acne, fluid retention, benign prostate hyperplasia, and, rarely, sleep apnea. This therapy is contraindicated in patients with cancer of the prostate.

If fertility is desired, patients with hypothalamic abnormalities may develop virilization and spermatogenesis with the use of GnRH delivered in a pulsatile fashion subcutaneously by an external pump. Direct stimulation of the testes in patients with hypothalamic or pituitary abnormalities may be accomplished with the use of exogenous gonadotropins, which increase testosterone and sperm production. If primary testicular failure is present and the patient has oligospermia, an attempt can be made to concentrate the sperm for intrauterine insemination or in vitro fertilization. If the azoospermia is caused by ductal obstruction, repair of the obstruction may be undertaken or aspiration of sperm from the epididymis may be accomplished for in vitro fertilization.

GYNECOMASTIA

Gynecomastia refers to a benign enlargement of the male breast that results from proliferation of the glandular component. This common condition is found in close to 70% of pubertal boys and in about one third of adults 50 to 80 years old. Estrogens stimulate and androgens inhibit breast glandular development; gynecomastia results from an imbalance between estrogen and androgen actions at the breast tissue level. This condition may result from an absolute increase in free estrogens, a decrease in endogenous free androgens, androgen insensitivity of the tissues, or enhanced sensitivity of the breast tissue to estrogens. Table 4.2 lists the common conditions associated with gynecomastia.

Gynecomastia must be differentiated from fatty enlargement of the breasts without glandular proliferation and from other disorders of the breasts, especially breast carcinoma. *Male breast cancer* usually manifests as a unilateral, eccentric, hard or firm mass that is fixed to the underlying tissues. It may be associated with skin dimpling or

TABLE 4.2   Conditions Associated With Gynecomastia
Physiologic Conditions
Neonatal
Pubertal
Involutional
Pathologic Conditions
Neoplasms
Testicular
Adrenal
Ectopic production of human chorionic gonadotropin
Primary gonadal failure
Secondary hypogonadism
Enzyme defects in testosterone production
Androgen insensitivity syndromes
Liver disease
Malnutrition with refeeding
Dialysis
Hyperthyroidism
Excessive extraglandular aromatase activity
Drugs
Estrogens and estrogen agonists
Gonadotropins
Antiandrogens or inhibitors of androgen synthesis
Cytotoxic agents
Highly active antiretroviral therapy (ART)
Spironolactone
Cimetidine
Growth hormone
Alcohol
Human immunodeficiency virus infection
Idiopathic

retraction or with crusting of the nipple or nipple discharge. In contrast, gynecomastia occurs concentrically around the nipple and is not fixed to the underlying structures. Although physical examination is usually sufficient to differentiate gynecomastia from breast carcinoma, mammography or ultrasonography may be required.

Painful and tender gynecomastia in a pubertal adolescent should be monitored with periodic examinations because, in most patients, pubertal gynecomastia disappears within 1 year. Incidentally discovered, asymptomatic gynecomastia in an adult requires a careful assessment for alcohol, drug, or medication use; liver, lung, or kidney dysfunction; and signs and symptoms of hypogonadism or hyperthyroidism. If these conditions are not present, only follow-up is required. In contrast, in an adult with recent onset of progressive painful gynecomastia, thyroid, liver, and renal function should be determined. If test results are normal, serum concentrations of HCG, LH, testosterone, and estradiol should be measured. Further evaluation should be carried out according to the schema outlined in Fig. 4.3.

Removal of the offending drug or correction of the underlying condition causing the gynecomastia may result in regression of the breast glandular tissue. If the gynecomastia persists, an off-label trial of antiestrogens (e.g., tamoxifen) may be given for 3 months to see whether regression occurs. Gynecomastia that has been present for longer than 1 year usually contains a fibrotic component that does not respond to medications. In these cases, correction usually requires surgical removal of the tissue.

For a deeper discussion on this topic, please see Chapter 223, "Reproductive Endocrinology and Infertility," in *Goldman-Cecil Medicine*, 26th Edition.

男性不育症

约 15% 的夫妻在未避孕的情况下性生活 1 年以上无法怀孕，其中男方因素约占 20%，女方因素约占 40%，双方共同因素约占 25%，其余约 15% 的病因无法确定。除下丘脑、垂体、睾丸或雄激素作用缺陷导致的男性生精障碍外，甲状腺功能亢进症、甲状腺功能减退症、肾上腺功能异常、全身性疾病和 Y 染色体基因序列微缺失也会导致生精障碍。同时，输精管、精囊和前列腺疾病也可能导致不育症，影响膀胱括约肌功能的疾病也可导致逆行射精，使精子进入膀胱而非由阴茎射出。此外，阴茎解剖缺陷（如尿道下裂）、不良的性交技术、男性或女性生殖道中存在抗精子抗体也与不育症相关。

性腺功能减退症和不育症的治疗

对于下丘脑-垂体功能障碍或原发性睾丸功能异常导致的雄激素缺乏，最有效的治疗方法是外源性睾酮替代治疗，即肌内注射中效睾酮（持续时间 1～3 周）、长效睾酮（持续时间 3 个月）、睾酮透皮贴片或凝胶。睾酮也可通过经口、鼻内给药或皮下微球给药，但通常较少应用。睾酮治疗可提高患者性欲、性功能、肌肉量、肌力、运动耐力，促进面部毛发和体毛生长并改善骨密度。最常见的副作用是红细胞增多症，其他副作用包括痤疮、体液潴留、良性前列腺增生、睡眠呼吸暂停（较罕见）。睾酮替代治疗的禁忌证是前列腺癌。

如果患者有生育需求，下丘脑功能异常患者可使用皮下脉冲泵入 GnRH 来促进男性化发育和精子发生。对于下丘脑或垂体功能异常的患者，可应用外源性促性腺激素直接刺激睾丸，增加雄激素分泌并促进精子生成。如果原发性睾丸功能衰竭患者合并少精子症，可尝试富集精子用于宫内人工授精或体外受精。如果无精子症是由导管阻塞所致，应治疗导管阻塞或从附睾抽取精子进行体外受精。

男性乳房发育

男性乳房发育是指男性乳房的良性肿大，由腺体增生引起。男性乳房发育可见于近 70% 的青春期男孩和约 1/3 的 50～80 岁的成人。雌激素可刺激乳腺发育，而雄激素抑制乳腺发育；男性乳房发育是由于乳房组织中雌激素和雄激素作用失衡。病因包括游离雌激素绝对增加、内源性游离雄激素减少、组织对雄激素不敏感或乳房组织对雌激素的敏感性增强。表 4.2 列出了与男性乳房发育相关的常见疾病。

男性乳房发育需要与无腺体增生的乳房脂肪组织增生及其他乳房疾病（尤其是乳腺癌）相鉴别。男性乳腺癌通常表现为单侧偏心性质韧或质硬的肿块，固定于基底层组织。此外，乳腺癌可表现为皮肤凹陷、

表 4.2　男性乳房发育的病因
生理情况
新生儿
青春期
更年期
病理情况
肿瘤
睾丸肿瘤
肾上腺肿瘤
异位产生人绒毛膜促性腺激素的肿瘤
原发性性腺功能减退症
继发性性腺功能减退症
酶缺陷影响睾酮生成
雄激素不敏感综合征
肝脏疾病
营养不良与再喂养
透析
甲状腺功能亢进症
腺体外芳香化酶活性升高
药物
雌激素及雌激素激动剂
促性腺激素
抗雄激素或雄激素合成抑制剂
细胞毒性药物
高效抗逆转录病毒治疗
螺内酯
西咪替丁
生长激素
酒精
人类免疫缺陷病毒感染
特发性

乳头结痂或乳头溢液。相反，男性乳房发育则常见于乳头周围，且不固定于基底层组织。虽然体格检查通常足以区分男性乳房发育和乳腺癌，但有时仍需要进一步行乳房 X 线检查或超声检查。

若青春期男性乳房发育伴有疼痛和压痛症状，需要定期检查，因为绝大多数青春期病例的症状可在 1 年内消失。偶然发现的无症状成人男性乳房发育需要仔细评估酒精、毒品及药物使用史，肝、肺及肾功能不全，性腺功能减退症或甲状腺功能亢进症的症状和体征。若未见上述情况，建议随诊观察。相反，对于新近出现进行性痛性男性乳房发育的成人，应评估甲状腺功能、肝功能和肾功能。如果上述检查未见明显异常，应检测血清 HCG、LH、睾酮和雌二醇水平以协助诊断。进一步的评估可参考图 4.3 所示的流程。

停用导致男性乳房发育的药物或纠正潜在诱因可能使已发育的乳腺组织退化。如果男性乳房发育持续存在，可超适应证试用抗雌激素（如他莫昔芬）3 个月，并观察乳腺组织是否退化。若男性乳房发育持续超过 1 年，则通常含有纤维性成分，对药物治疗反应不佳。在这种情况下，必要时可考虑行矫正手术切除乳腺组织。

有关此专题的深入讨论，请参阅 *Goldman-Cecil Medicine* 第 26 版第 223 章"生殖内分泌学和不育症"。

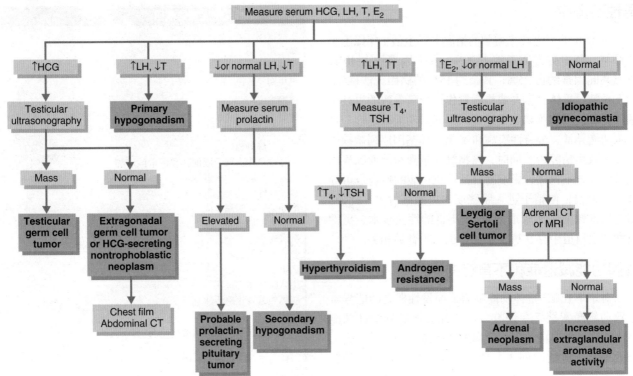

Fig. 4.3 Diagnostic evaluation for causes of gynecomastia based on measurements of serum human chorionic gonadotropin (HCG), luteinizing hormone (LH), testosterone (T), and estradiol (E_2). ↑, Increased; ↓, decreased; *CT*, computed tomography; *MRI*, magnetic resonance imaging; T_4, thyroxine; *TSH*, thyroid-stimulating hormone. (From Braunstein GD: Gynecomastia, N Engl J Med 328:490–495, 1993.)

SUGGESTED READINGS

Bhasin S, Brito J, Cunningham GR, et al: Testosterone therapy in men with hypogonadism: an Endocrine Society clinical practice guideline, J Clin Endocrinol Metab 103:1715–1744, 2018.

Gravholt CH, Chang S, Wallentin M, Fedder J, Moore P, Skakkebaek A: Klinefelter syndrome: integrating genetics, neuropsychology, and endocrinology, Endocr Rev 39:389–423, 2018.

Irwin GM: Erectile dysfunction, Clinics in Office Practice 46:249–255, 2019.

Pan MM, HGockenberry MS, Kirby EW, Lipshultz LI: Male infertility diagnosis and treatment in the era of in vitro fertilization and intracytoplasmic sperm injection, Med Clin N Amer 102:337–347, 2018.

Practice Committee of the American Society for Reproductive Medicine in collaboration with the Society for Male Reproduction and Urology: Evaluation of the azoospermic male: a committee opinion, Fertil Steril 109:777–782, 2018.

Sansone A, Romanelli F, Sansone M, Lenzi A, Luigi LD: Gynecomastia and hormones, Endocrine 55:37–44, 2017.

Shepard CL, Kraft KH: The nonpalpable testis: a narrative review, J Urol 198:1410–1417, 2017.

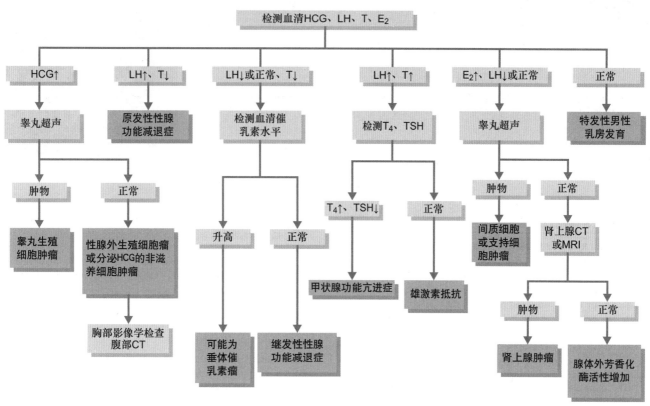

图 4.3 基于血清人绒毛膜促性腺激素（HCG）、黄体生成素（LH）、睾酮（T）和雌二醇（E₂）水平的男性乳房发育病因的诊断性评估。↑，升高；↓，降低；CT，计算机断层成像；MRI，磁共振成像；T₄，甲状腺素；TSH，促甲状腺激素（引自 Braunstein GD：Gynecomastia，N Engl J Med 328：490-495，1993.）

推荐阅读

Bhasin S, Brito J, Cunningham GR, et al: Testosterone therapy in men with hypogonadism: an Endocrine Society clinical practice guideline, J Clin Endocrinol Metab 103:1715–1744, 2018.

Gravholt CH, Chang S, Wallentin M, Fedder J, Moore P, Skakkebaek A: Klinefelter syndrome: integrating genetics, neuropsychology, and endocrinology, Endocr Rev 39:389–423, 2018.

Irwin GM: Erectile dysfunction, Clinics in Office Practice 46:249–255, 2019.

Pan MM, HGockenberry MS, Kirby EW, Lipshultz LI: Male infertility diagnosis and treatment in the era of in vitro fertilization and intracytoplasmic sperm injection, Med Clin N Amer 102:337–347, 2018.

Practice Committee of the American Society for Reproductive Medicine in collaboration with the Society for Male Reproduction and Urology: Evaluation of the azoospermic male: a committee opinion, Fertil Steril 109:777–782, 2018.

Sansone A, Romanelli F, Sansone M, Lenzi A, Luigi LD: Gynecomastia and hormones, Endocrine 55:37–44, 2017.

Shepard CL, Kraft KH: The nonpalpable testis: a narrative review, J Urol 198:1410–1417, 2017.

5

Diabetes Mellitus, Hypoglycemia

Robert J. Smith

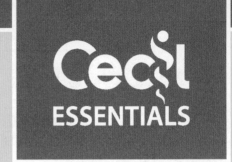

DIABETES MELLITUS

Definition and Diagnostic Criteria

Diabetes mellitus is not a single disease but a group of disorders that develop as a consequence of absolute or relative deficiency of the hormone insulin. Inadequate actions of insulin in stimulating the uptake of glucose by body tissues and regulating the metabolism of carbohydrate, fat, and protein result in *hyperglycemia*. Other metabolic disturbances in addition to hyperglycemia typically occur in uncontrolled diabetes, including altered lipoprotein dynamics and elevated free fatty acid levels. These abnormalities contribute to the acute and chronic clinical consequences of diabetes.

The criteria used to diagnose diabetes mellitus in nonpregnant individuals are summarized in Table 5.1 . The diagnosis can be made on the basis of a fasting blood glucose level of 126 mg/dL or higher, a random blood glucose concentration (i.e., determined at any time in association with meals or fasting) of 200 mg/dL or higher, or a 2-hour glucose level of 200 mg/dL or higher as part of a 75-g oral glucose tolerance test. Alternatively, diabetes can be diagnosed if the hemoglobin A_{1c} (HbA_{1c}) level is 6.5% or higher. HbA_{1c}, a measure of the percentage of hemoglobin in circulating erythrocytes that is glycosylated, correlates with mean circulating glucose levels. HbA_{1c} provides an index of the average blood glucose level over the preceding 2 to 3 months. Because HbA_{1c} accumulates progressively throughout the lifespan of an erythrocyte, spurious values may occur in states of altered erythrocyte turnover (e.g., with various anemias) or with certain hemoglobinopathies that increase or decrease the susceptibility of hemoglobin to glycosylation. In patients with marked elevations in blood glucose or HbA_{1c} and coincident symptoms typical for hyperglycemia (e.g., polyuria and polydipsia), the diagnosis can be made based on a single test result. With less marked glucose elevations in the absence of symptoms, the diagnosis should be confirmed by repeat testing on a separate day.

Patients who have mild elevations in plasma glucose levels that do not reach the threshold for diagnosis of diabetes (e.g., HbA_{1c} levels between 5.7% and 6.4%) are at increased risk for progression to diabetes and therefore are considered to have *prediabetes*. Prediabetes patients with fasting blood glucose levels between 100 and 125 mg/dL are more specifically labeled as having *impaired fasting glucose*, and those with 2-hour postprandial plasma glucose levels between 140 and 199 mg/dL (most reliably measured after a standardized 75-g oral glucose load) have *impaired glucose tolerance* (see Table 5.1). Although not all individuals with prediabetes will become diabetic, the mean progression rate to overt diabetes is approximately 6% per year. There also is evidence from observational studies that the prediabetic state is associated with an increased risk of cardiovascular disease.

Gestational diabetes mellitus (GDM) is a term applied to diabetes first recognized during pregnancy. The most widely accepted thresholds for diagnosis of GDM are a fasting plasma glucose level of 92 mg/dL or higher at any gestational stage and values on a 75-g oral glucose tolerance test at 24 to 28 weeks' gestation of 92 mg/dL or higher fasting, 180 mg/dL or higher at 1 hour, or 153 mg/dL or higher at 2 hours after glucose loading (Table 5.2). Untreated diabetes in pregnancy is associated with increased fetal malformations, problems in delivery, and possibly more frequent diabetes complications in the mother.

Etiologic Classification

Once the diagnosis is made based on elevated blood glucose or HbA_{1c} values, it is important to establish the specific subtype of diabetes based on a combination of clinical and molecular pathophysiologic features Table 5.3 .

Type 1 diabetes (T1DM) is characterized by extensive destruction of the insulin-producing beta cells within the islets of Langerhans in the pancreas and dependence on insulin therapy for survival. In previous medical literature, the terms *juvenile-onset diabetes* or *insulin-dependent diabetes* were used for T1DM. This terminology is no longer used, because T1DM not uncommonly has its onset in adulthood, and multiple other forms of diabetes often require treatment with insulin. T1DM accounts for 5% to 10% of all diabetes in the United States. In most patients, it involves autoimmune mechanisms leading to beta cell destruction (the *type 1A* form). Rare individuals have no markers for autoimmunity and are classified as having *type 1B (idiopathic) diabetes*. Most patients with T1DM progress to marked insulin deficiency over a period of several weeks to months after initial presentation. A smaller number of individuals with evidence of beta-cell autoimmunity but much slower disease progression have a variant form of T1DM that has been designated *latent autoimmune diabetes of adulthood* (LADA).

In patients with marked elevations in glucose and accompanying ketoacidosis, particularly if they are young and nonobese, the diagnosis of T1DM is highly probable. This can be confirmed by measuring autoantibodies against glutamic acid decarboxylase (GAD65), insulin, tyrosine phosphatases (IA-2 and IA2-beta), and zinc transporter 8 (ZnT8), with several of these often obtained as a panel, and also by a clinical course demonstrating an ongoing need for insulin to control hyperglycemia. A fasting C-peptide level can be measured later in the disease to confirm marked deficiency in insulin secretion. C-peptide is a fragment of the insulin precursor proinsulin, which is cleaved during the synthesis of insulin. It is secreted and circulates in proportion to endogenous insulin production but is absent from injected exogenous insulin preparations.

Type 2 diabetes (T2DM) is a heterogeneous, clinically defined subtype that accounts for more than 90% of all diabetes in the United States. It typically has a gradual onset with progression over multiple years or even decades. There is often prolonged preservation of at least partial insulin secretory capacity together with evidence

糖尿病与低血糖

袁涛 译 赵宇星 赵维纲 审校 宁光 通审

糖尿病

定义和诊断标准

糖尿病不是一种单一的疾病，而是由胰岛素绝对或相对缺乏引起的一组疾病。当胰岛素在促进机体组织摄取葡萄糖及调节碳水化合物、脂肪和蛋白质代谢中的作用不足时，可导致高血糖。除高血糖外，未控制的糖尿病通常还会导致其他代谢紊乱，包括脂蛋白代谢动力学改变和游离脂肪酸水平升高。这些异常会引起糖尿病的急性和慢性并发症。

非妊娠个体的糖尿病诊断标准见表 5.1。可根据空腹血糖 $\geqslant$ 126 mg/dl（1 mmol/L $=$ 18 mg/dl），随机血糖（即在餐后任意时间或空腹时测定）$\geqslant$ 200 mg/dl，或 75 g 口服葡萄糖耐量试验后 2 h 血糖 $\geqslant$ 200 mg/dl 来做出诊断。此外，糖化血红蛋白（HbA1c）$\geqslant$ 6.5% 也可用于诊断糖尿病。HbA1c 是循环红细胞中糖基化血红蛋白的百分比，与循环中平均血糖水平相关。HbA1c 是反映过去 2 ~ 3 个月平均血糖水平的指标。由于 HbA1c 在红细胞的整个生命周期中逐渐累积，因此在红细胞更新状态改变（如各种贫血）或改变血红蛋白对糖基化敏感性的血红蛋白病中，HbA1c 数值可能不准确。在血糖或 HbA1c 显著升高且伴有典型高血糖症状（如多尿和多饮）的患者中，可依据单项检测结果做出诊断。若患者无症状且血糖轻微升高，应择日进行重复检测以确认诊断。

血糖轻微升高但未达到糖尿病诊断阈值的患者（如 HbA1c 为 5.7% ~ 6.4%）发展为糖尿病的风险增加，因此被认为是糖尿病前期。糖尿病前期患者的空腹血糖为 100 ~ 125 mg/dl 被称为空腹血糖受损，而餐后 2 h 血糖为 140 ~ 199 mg/dl（最可靠的检测是在标准 75 g 口服葡萄糖负荷后）被称为糖耐量减低（表 5.1）。尽管并非所有糖尿病前期的个体都会进展为糖尿病，但平均每年约有 6% 的患者进展至显性糖尿病。观察性研究证据表明，糖尿病前期状态与心血管疾病风险增加有关。

妊娠期糖尿病（GDM）是指在妊娠期间首次被识别的糖尿病。诊断 GDM 最公认的阈值是妊娠期任意阶段的空腹血糖 $\geqslant$ 92 mg/dl，以及在妊娠第 24 ~ 28 周进行 75 g 口服葡萄糖耐量试验时空腹血糖 $\geqslant$ 92 mg/dl，1 h 血糖 $\geqslant$ 180 mg/dl，或 2 h 血糖 $\geqslant$ 153 mg/dl（表 5.2）。未治疗的 GDM 与胎儿畸形、分娩问题及母亲糖尿病并发症增加有关。

病因分类

基于血糖或 HbA1c 升高诊断糖尿病后，结合临床和分子病理生理学特征确定糖尿病的具体亚型非常重要（表 5.3）。

1 型糖尿病（T1DM）的特征是胰腺朗格汉斯胰岛中分泌胰岛素的 β 细胞被广泛破坏，患者需要依赖胰岛素治疗以维持生命。在既往文献中，T1DM 被称为幼年型糖尿病或胰岛素依赖型糖尿病。该术语已不再使用，因为 T1DM 在成年期发病并不罕见，而且许多其他类型的糖尿病通常也需要用胰岛素治疗。在美国，T1DM 占所有糖尿病的 5% ~ 10%。大多数患者涉及导致 β 细胞破坏的自身免疫机制（1A 型）。极少数患者没有自身免疫标志物，被归类为 1B 型（特发性）糖尿病。大多数 T1DM 患者在初次出现症状后的数周至数月会发展为明显的胰岛素缺乏。小部分患者有 β 细胞自身免疫的证据，但疾病进展缓慢，是一种变异型 T1DM，被称为成人晚发自身免疫性糖尿病（LADA）。

如果患者血糖显著升高且出现酮症酸中毒，尤其是非肥胖症的年轻患者，则诊断 T1DM 的可能性很大。这可以通过检测针对谷氨酸脱羧酶（GAD65）、胰岛素、酪氨酸磷酸酶（IA-2 和 IA2-β）和锌转运蛋白 8（ZnT8）的自身抗体来确认诊断，其中多种自身抗体通常作为组合检测；也可以通过临床病程需要持续胰岛素控制高血糖来验证 T1DM 的诊断。起病后可检测空腹 C 肽水平，以确认胰岛素分泌的显著缺乏。C 肽是胰岛素原（胰岛素前体）的一个片段，在胰岛素合成过程中被裂解。它与内源性胰岛素成比例分泌并进入循环，但注射的外源性胰岛素制剂中没有 C 肽。

2 型糖尿病（T2DM）是一个异质性、临床定义的亚型，在美国占所有糖尿病的 90% 以上。它通常起病缓慢，可能在数年甚至数十年中逐渐进展。T2DM 患者

TABLE 5.1 Criteria for the Diagnosis of Diabetes Mellitus

Measurement	Normal	Prediabetes	Diabetes Mellitus
Plasma glucose (mg/dL)			
Fasting[a]	<100	100-125[b]	≥126
2-hr Postload[c]	<140	140-199[d]	≥200
Random[e]			≥200
Hemoglobin A₁c (%)	≤5.6	5.7-6.4	≥6.5

[a]Fasting: no caloric intake for ≥8 hr.
[b]Impaired fasting glucose.
[c]Postload: Following a standardized 75-g oral glucose load or after a meal.
[d]Impaired glucose tolerance.
[e]Random: any time of day, unrelated to meals.
Data from the American Diabetes Association Standards of Medical Care in Diabetes 2019, Diabetes Care 42(Suppl 1):S13-S28, 2019.

TABLE 5.2 Criteria for the Diagnosis of Gestational Diabetes Mellitus

Measurement	Diagnostic Threshold (mg/dL)
Plasma glucose	
Fasting[a]	≥92
After 75-g oral glucose load	
1 hr	≥180
2 hr	<153

[a]Fasting: no caloric intake for ≥8 hr.
Data from the American Diabetes Association Standards of Medical Care in Diabetes 2019, Diabetes Care 42(Suppl 1):S13-S28, 2019.

TABLE 5.3 Etiologic Classification of Diabetes Mellitus

Type 1 Diabetes Mellitus
Immune-mediated (type 1A)
Idiopathic (type 1B)

Type 2 Diabetes Mellitus
Other Specific Types
Genetic defects of beta-cell function
    Maturity-onset diabetes of the young (MODY) and other disorders
Genetic defects in insulin action
    Insulin receptor mutations and other disorders
Diseases of the exocrine pancreas
Endocrinopathies
    Cushing's syndrome, acromegaly, and other disorders
Drug- or chemical-induced
    Glucocorticoids most common
Infections
Uncommon forms of immune-mediated diabetes
    Insulin receptor–blocking antibodies and other disorders
Other genetic syndromes sometimes associated with diabetes

Gestational Diabetes Mellitus

Classification consistent with the American Diabetes Association Standards of Medical Care in Diabetes 2019, Diabetes Care 42 (Suppl 1):S13-S28, 2019.

of insulin resistance. Most patients have associated obesity (80% to 90%), although a subset of patients with a clinical picture otherwise typical for T2DM are nonobese. T2DM usually can be presumptively distinguished from T1DM by its indolent course in the presence of risk factors such as obesity and by the milder hyperglycemia and absence of ketoacidosis due to residual insulin secretion. If there is clinical suspicion of T1DM based on earlier age at onset, degree of hyperglycemia, absence of obesity, or presence of ketoacidosis, an autoantibody panel (which should be negative) and a C-peptide level (which should be positive) can be measured.

An expanding number of diabetes etiologies distinct from T1DM and T2DM are classified under a broad category designated *other specific types*. Although these forms of diabetes are uncommon (<5% of all diabetes), it is important to recognize them in clinical practice. They include a group of inherited, monogenic, autosomal dominant disorders that previously were designated *maturity-onset diabetes of the young (MODY)*; many of these patients have clinical features similar to those of T2DM but onset typically before 25 years of age. Patients with hepatocyte nuclear factor-1alpha mutations (MODY3) are particularly sensitive to sulfonylureas, whereas those with glucokinase mutations (MODY2) have mild, nonprogressive blood glucose elevations and often require no treatment except during pregnancy. Because the genetic diagnosis can direct the treatment plan for these individuals, patients with early-onset diabetes, lack of autoimmune markers, and family histories suggestive of autosomal dominant inheritance should be considered for MODY gene sequencing.

Much less common monogenic causes include mutations in insulin receptors or various other genes involved in insulin action. Exocrine pancreatic disease from disorders such as chronic pancreatitis or surgery results in loss of the glucagon-producing islet alpha cells as well as the insulin-producing beta cells. These patients often exhibit greater sensitivity to insulin and more of a propensity for hypoglycemia than T1DM patients because of the absent insulin counter-regulatory effects of glucagon. Endocrine disorders with excess production of hormones that counteract insulin, such as growth hormone in acromegaly or cortisol in Cushing's syndrome, are important to recognize as causes of diabetes because removal of the source of excess hormone can lead to resolution of the diabetic state. Many drugs have been associated with diabetes, most notably glucocorticoids.

The category GDM includes any woman in whom diabetes is first recognized during pregnancy and usually represents T2DM.

Type 1 Diabetes
Epidemiology and Pathology
The principal features of T1DM, contrasted with T2DM, are summarized in Table 5.4. The peak incidence occurs between the ages of 6 and 14 years, but onset in approximately half of patients with T1DM occurs after the age of 20. The role of genetic factors in T1DM risk is supported by an observed increased incidence of T1DM among family members of affected patients: approximately 5% in siblings, 6% in offspring of a diabetic father, and 2% in offspring of a diabetic mother. It is hypothesized that the immune destruction of beta cells is predisposed by genetic risk factors and precipitated by environmental factors, the latter possibly including microbial, chemical, or dietary triggers (Fig. 5.1). The operation of a combination of genetic and environmental factors is thought to explain the high but not absolute concordance observed in monozygotic twins (30% to 50%).

The prevalence of T1DM varies substantially in different populations; for example, it is relatively high in northwestern Europe and much lower in parts of Asia. The overall prevalence in the United

表 5.1 糖尿病的诊断标准

检测	正常	糖尿病前期	糖尿病
血糖（mg/dl）			
空腹 [a]	< 100	100 ～ 125 [b]	≥ 126
2 h 负荷后 [c]	< 140	140 ～ 199 [d]	≥ 200
随机 [e]			≥ 200
糖化血红蛋白（%）	≤ 5.6	5.7 ～ 6.4	≥ 6.5

[a] 空腹：无热量摄入 ≥ 8 h。
[b] 空腹血糖受损。
[c] 负荷后：标准 75 g 口服葡萄糖负荷或进餐后。
[d] 糖耐量减低。
[e] 随机：全天的任意时间，与进餐无关。
引自 American Diabetes Association Standards of Medical Care in Diabetes 2019，Diabetes Care 42（Suppl 1）：S13-S28，2019.

表 5.2 妊娠期糖尿病的诊断标准

检测	诊断阈值（mg/dl）
血糖	
空腹 [a]	≥ 92
75 g 口服葡萄糖负荷后	
1 h	≥ 180
2 h	< 153

[a] 空腹：无热量摄入 ≥ 8 h。
引自 American Diabetes Association Standards of Medical Care in Diabetes 2019，Diabetes Care 42（Suppl 1）：S13-S28，2019.

通常至少保留部分胰岛素分泌功能，同时有胰岛素抵抗的证据。大多数患者伴有肥胖症（80% ～ 90%），少数患者虽然有典型的 T2DM 临床表现，但无肥胖症。T2DM 通常可与 T1DM 进行初步鉴别，因为 T2DM 患者在有危险因素（如肥胖症）的情况下病程进展缓慢，由于残留的胰岛素分泌，高血糖症状较轻且没有酮症酸中毒。如果根据发病较早、高血糖程度、无肥胖症或存在酮症酸中毒等表现临床怀疑 T1DM，可检测自身抗体谱（应为阴性）和 C 肽水平（应为阳性）。

越来越多与 T1DM 和 T2DM 病因不同的糖尿病被归类为其他特殊类型。尽管这些糖尿病类型不常见（在所有糖尿病中占比 < 5%），但在临床实践中识别它们很重要。它们包括一组遗传性、单基因、常染色体显性遗传病，既往被称为青少年起病的成人型糖尿病（MODY）；这些患者的临床表现多与 T2DM 相似，但通常在 25 岁之前发病。携带肝细胞核因子 -1α 突变（MODY3）的患者对磺酰脲类药物特别敏感，而携带葡萄糖激酶突变（MODY2）的患者有轻度、非进展性血糖升高，除在妊娠期外，通常不需要治疗。由于遗传学诊断可指导治疗方案，因此对于早期发病的糖尿病、缺乏自身免疫标志物、家族史提示常染色体显性遗传病的患者，应考虑进行 MODY 基因测序。

表 5.3 糖尿病的病因学分类

1 型糖尿病
免疫介导性（1A 型）
特发性（1B 型）

2 型糖尿病
其他特殊类型
胰岛 β 细胞功能的遗传缺陷
　青少年起病的成人型糖尿病（MODY）和其他疾病
胰岛素作用的遗传缺陷
　胰岛素受体基因突变和其他疾病
胰腺外分泌疾病
内分泌疾病
　库欣综合征、肢端肥大症和其他疾病
药物或化学品所致
　最常见于糖皮质激素所致
感染
免疫介导性糖尿病（少见）
　阻断胰岛素受体的抗体和其他疾病
其他与糖尿病相关的遗传综合征

妊娠期糖尿病

分类符合 American Diabetes Association Standards of Medical Care in Diabetes 2019，Diabetes Care 42（Suppl 1）：S13-S28，2019.

更少见的单基因病因包括胰岛素受体或参与胰岛素作用的其他基因的突变。胰腺外分泌疾病包括慢性胰腺炎或手术引起 α 细胞（生成胰高血糖素）和 β 细胞（生成胰岛素）丧失。这些患者通常比 T1DM 患者对胰岛素更敏感，更易出现低血糖，因为缺乏胰高血糖素的胰岛素拮抗效应。导致拮抗胰岛素作用的其他激素分泌过多的内分泌疾病（如肢端肥大症中的生长激素分泌过多或库欣综合征中的皮质醇分泌过多）也是糖尿病的重要病因，因为去除这些过量激素的来源可缓解糖尿病状态。许多药物与糖尿病有关，其中最常见的是糖皮质激素。

GDM 包括所有在妊娠期首次被诊断出患有糖尿病的女性，通常为 T2DM。

1 型糖尿病

流行病学和病理学

T1DM 与 T2DM 的主要区别见表 5.4。T1DM 的发病高峰年龄为 6 ～ 14 岁，但约有 1/2 的患者在 20 岁以后发病。T1DM 的风险与遗传因素有关，T1DM 患者亲属的 T1DM 发病率较高：亲兄弟姐妹的风险增加约 5%，糖尿病父亲的后代风险增加 6%，糖尿病母亲的后代风险增加 2%。据推测，遗传危险因素和环境因素可能导致 β 细胞易被免疫破坏，环境因素包括微生物、化学或饮食诱因（图 5.1）。遗传和环境因素的共同作用可以解释在同卵双胞胎中观察到的发病率高但并非绝对一致（30% ～ 50%）。

T1DM 在不同人群中的患病率差异很大；例如，欧洲西北部人群的患病率相对较高，而在亚洲部分地

TABLE 5.4	General Comparison of the Two Most Common Types of Diabetes Mellitus	
	Type 1	**Type 2**
Previous terminology	Insulin-dependent diabetes mellitus, type I; juvenile-onset diabetes	Non–insulin-dependent diabetes mellitus, type II; adult-onset diabetes
Age at onset	Usually <30 yr, particularly childhood and adolescence, but any age	Usually >40 yr, but increasingly at younger ages
Genetic predisposition	Moderate; environmental factors required for expression; 35-50% concordance in monozygotic twins; multiple candidate genes proposed	Strong; 60-90% concordance in monozygotic twins; many candidate genes proposed
Human leukocyte antigen associations	Linkage to DQA and DQB, influenced by DRB3 and DRB4 (DR2 protective)	None known
Other associations	Autoimmune; Graves' disease, Hashimoto thyroiditis, vitiligo, Addison's disease, pernicious anemia	Heterogeneous, ongoing subclassification based on identification of specific pathogenic processes and genetic defects
Precipitating and risk factors	Largely unknown; microbial, chemical, dietary, other	Age, obesity (central), sedentary lifestyle, previous gestational diabetes
Findings at diagnosis	85-90% of patients have one and usually more autoantibodies to GAD_{65}, insulin, IA-2, IA-2β, ZnT8	Possibly complications (microvascular and macrovascular) caused by significant hyperglycemia in the preceding asymptomatic period
Endogenous insulin levels	Low or absent	Usually present (relative deficiency), early hyperinsulinemia
Insulin resistance	Only with hyperglycemia or coincident obesity	Mostly present
Prolonged fast	Hyperglycemia, ketoacidosis	Euglycemia
Stress, withdrawal of insulin	Ketoacidosis	Nonketotic hyperglycemia, occasionally ketoacidosis

GAD, Glutamic acid decarboxylase; *IA-2,* IA-2β, insuloma-associated protein 2 and 2β (tyrosine phosphatases); *ZnT8,* zinc transporter 8.

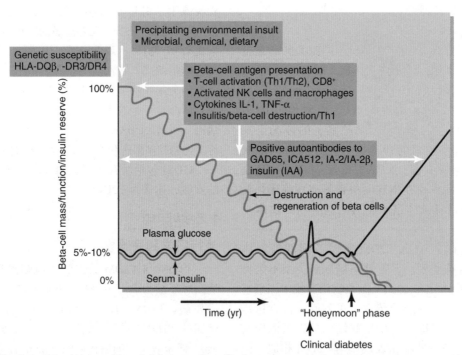

Fig. 5.1 Natural history of type 1 diabetes mellitus. The honeymoon period with temporary improvement in beta-cell function occurs with the initiation of insulin therapy at the time of clinical diagnosis. *GAD,* Glutamic acid decarboxylase; *HLA,* human leukocyte antigen; *IA-2,* IA-2β, tyrosine phosphatases; *ICA,* islet cell antibody; *ICA512,* islet cell autoantigen 512 (fragment of IA-2); *IL-1,* interleukin-1; *NK,* natural killer; *Th1,* subset of CD4+ helper T cells responsible for cell-mediated immunity; *Th2,* subset of CD4+ helper T cells responsible for humoral immunity; *TNF-α,* tumor necrosis factor-α.

表5.4 两种常见糖尿病类型的比较

	1 型糖尿病	2 型糖尿病
曾用名	胰岛素依赖型糖尿病，Ⅰ型；幼年型糖尿病	非胰岛素依赖型糖尿病，Ⅱ型；成人型糖尿病
发病年龄	通常＜30岁，尤其常见于儿童和青少年，但任何年龄均可见	通常＞40岁，但年轻人中越来越多见
遗传倾向	弱；表达需要环境因素；同卵双胞胎一致性为35%～50%；已有多个候选基因	强；同卵双胞胎一致性为60%～90%；已有很多候选基因
人类白细胞抗原关联	与DQA和DQB连锁，受DRB3和DRB4影响（DR2保护性）	未知
其他相关因素	自身免疫病；Graves病、桥本甲状腺炎、白癜风、Addison病、恶性贫血	异质性，目前基于特定致病过程和遗传缺陷持续进行分型
诱发和危险因素	很大程度上未知；微生物、化学、饮食、其他	年龄、肥胖症（向心性）、久坐的生活方式、妊娠期糖尿病史
诊断时发现	85%～90%患者有1种或多种（常见）自身抗体，如针对GAD65、胰岛素、IA-2、IA-2β、ZnT8的自身抗体	在无症状期出现显著高血糖可能导致并发症（微血管和大血管并发症）
内源性胰岛素水平	低或无	通常存在（胰岛素相对缺乏），早期高胰岛素血症
胰岛素抵抗	仅见于高血糖或合并肥胖症者	大多数存在
长期禁食	高血糖、酮症酸中毒	正常血糖
应激、停用胰岛素	酮症酸中毒	非酮症性高血糖，偶有酮症酸中毒

GAD，谷氨酸脱羧酶；IA-2 和 IA-2β，胰岛细胞瘤相关蛋白 2 和 2β（酪氨酸磷酸酶）；ZnT8，锌转运蛋白 8。

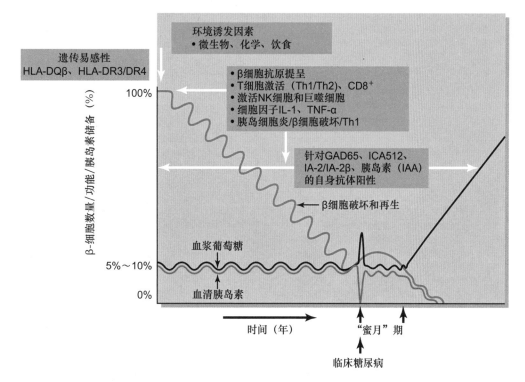

图5.1 T1DM 的自然病程。在临床诊断后开始胰岛素治疗后可发生 β 细胞功能暂时改善的蜜月期。GAD，谷氨酸脱羧酶；HLA，人类白细胞抗原；IA-2 和 IA-2β，酪氨酸磷酸酶；ICA，胰岛细胞抗体；ICA512，胰岛细胞自身抗原 512（IA-2 的片段）；IL-1，白介素 -1；NK，自然杀伤；Th1，负责细胞免疫的 CD4[+]辅助 T 细胞亚群；Th2，负责体液免疫的 CD4[+]辅助 T 细胞亚群；TNF-α，肿瘤坏死因子 -α

States is approximately 2.4 cases per 1000 individuals. The frequent onset before age 20 makes T1DM one of the most common chronic, serious childhood diseases. It is the most common subtype of diabetes in childhood, accounting for approximately 70% of all cases, with T2DM accounting for most of the remainder. LADA, an uncommon variant form of autoimmune T1DM, is characterized by onset in adulthood and a more prolonged waxing and waning course than is typical for T1DM.

The onset of overt T1DM follows a preclinical phase of variable duration (typically extending from months to years) during which there is destruction of beta cells resulting predominantly from cell-mediated immune mechanisms (mononuclear cells; mainly CD8+ T lymphocytes). It is believed that the autoantibodies (against glutamic acid decarboxylase, insulin, tyrosine phosphatases, and zinc transporter 8) are generated for the most part in response to exposure of beta-cell and islet antigens and do not function as primary mediators of the destructive process. Nevertheless, demonstration of one or more autoantibodies represents the most sensitive and useful way to establish preclinical disease in patients at risk (e.g., first-degree relatives of patients with T1DM).

The complement of beta cells in a healthy individual normally provides enough excess insulin secretory capacity to maintain blood glucose levels until 80% to 90% of beta cells have been lost. In some patients, the subclinical loss of beta cells may be unmasked, resulting in hyperglycemia and possibly diabetic ketoacidosis (DKA) during the course of an intercurrent illness such as an incidental upper respiratory tract infection. This reflects a lack of adequate insulin reserve to compensate for stress-induced insulin resistance. After institution of insulin and other therapy, stress-induced insulin resistance resolves, and there may be an improvement in beta-cell function. Some patients then revert to a state in which no insulin is required. This phenomenon, designated the *honeymoon* period, can last for several weeks to as long as 1 year. Patients generally should continue insulin administration at doses low enough to be tolerated during this interval, because progressive beta-cell function can be expected eventually to result in recurrent hyperglycemia and, potentially, DKA.

Screening for T1DM is not a part of standard medical care. Autoantibody determinations in individuals with a family history of T1DM can help to define risk but do not reliably predict time of onset or otherwise guide clinical care. Screening for thyroid, adrenal, or other associated autoimmune disorders should be considered in patients with T1DM on an individual basis.

Clinical Presentation

T1DM most often manifests clinically with symptoms resulting from hyperglycemia and consequent osmotic diuresis. Patients typically have a history extending over days to weeks of worsening polyuria, plus polydipsia (as a compensatory response to hypovolemia and increased serum osmolality). The polyuria may be evident as bed wetting or daytime incontinence in children and as nocturia in adults. There typically also is weight loss, and patients often describe low energy and lethargy. Approximately 25% of patients with T1DM have progressed to DKA by the time of clinical presentation.

Treatment

The management of T1DM involves immediate treatment at the outset to correct hyperglycemia, fluid deficits, and DKA, if present, plus attention to possible precipitating or complicating factors such as infection. The initial treatment of T1DM should be coupled with education of patients and their family members (appropriate to the patient's age) concerning the needed skills to manage insulin administration, blood glucose testing, nutrition, and exercise. This often is best accomplished by a team involving the physician, educators (typically specially trained nurses or pharmacists), and a dietician. Medical advice, patient education, and psychological support should be provided on an ongoing, long-term, individualized basis. The primary goal of glucose management is to minimize the degree of hyperglycemia and its attendant risks of long-term complications of diabetes, while avoiding the acute and chronic risks of hypoglycemia. Medical care should include attention to control of lipid levels, blood pressure, and other factors that affect the risks of long-term diabetes complications. Routine assessments of foot care, peripheral nerve function, retinal status, and renal function should be used to detect incipient diabetes complications and enable early treatment interventions. Other sources should be consulted for information on specific issues related to T1DM management in children and adolescents.

Blood glucose control. Patients with T1DM have an absolute requirement for exogenous insulin. The Diabetes Control and Complications Trial (DCCT) and other studies have established that improved glycemic control in patients with T1DM decreases long-term microvascular complications (retinopathy, nephropathy, and neuropathy). A follow-up study of the same patients (the Epidemiology of Diabetes Interventions and Complications [EDIC] study) further demonstrated lower cardiovascular morbidity and mortality with intensive insulin management. Based on these and other studies, the most generally accepted target goal for HbA$_{1c}$ in T1DM is 7.0%, although selected individuals may safely target HbA$_{1c}$ of 6.5%. For patients who have difficulty sensing hypoglycemia or who have other factors complicating blood glucose management (e.g., renal failure), it is appropriate to set an individualized HbA$_{1c}$ goal of 8.0% or even higher.

Many preparations of insulin are available. They differ in rapidity of absorption, degree of peaking of blood levels, and duration of action after subcutaneous injection (Table 5.5). The different kinetics of recombinant human insulin preparations derive from their specific complexing with proteins and zinc. Additionally, multiple analogues of human insulin are available that have rapid or slow kinetics as a consequence of altered solubility at subcutaneous injection sites. Most insulin preparations are provided at a concentration of 100 U/mL (U-100), with some available at higher concentrations (200 or 500 U/mL). Self-monitoring of blood glucose (SMBG) by patients using glucose meters is critical to the implementation of an effective insulin regimen. Ideally, SMBG should be performed as frequently as practicable: fasting, preprandial, 2 hours postprandial, at bedtime, and occasionally at 2:00 to 3:00 AM. Values and times are saved in most meters for subsequent review. It is helpful for patients to manually record these data on a flowchart, and it is also possible to download meter data to a computer. SMBG records are most useful when annotated with relevant details on food intake, exercise, or the occurrence of symptoms. HbA$_{1c}$ determinations generally should be obtained every 3 months.

Most cases of T1DM should be managed with an *intensive insulin therapy regimen* involving multiple (three or more) daily subcutaneous injections or continuous subcutaneous insulin infusion (CSII) using an insulin pump. Multiple-injection regimens, also termed *basal-bolus therapy*, typically involve injections of a long-acting insulin analogue (glargine, detemir, or degludec) once or twice daily to establish a stable basal insulin level. Regular insulin or a rapid-acting insulin analogue is additionally injected three or more times daily (before each meal and sometimes before snacks) to provide appropriate post-meal peaks in insulin levels. Usually, once glucose levels are stabilized on a regimen, the doses of long-acting insulin are kept constant from day to day. The rapid-acting insulin doses can be kept constant with efforts to ingest a fixed amount of carbohydrate and total calories at each meal. Alternatively, better control and greater flexibility can be achieved if

区人群则低得多。美国的整体患病率约为 2.4/1000。由于常在 20 岁之前发病，T1DM 成为常见的慢性、严重儿童疾病之一。它是儿童期最常见的糖尿病亚型，约占所有儿童病例的 70%，其余大多数为 T2DM。LADA 是一种少见的自身免疫性 T1DM 变异型，其特点是成年期发病，且病程比典型 T1DM 更长。

典型的 T1DM 发病前有一个持续时间不一的临床前期（通常从数月到数年），其间主要由细胞介导的免疫机制（单核细胞；主要是 CD8$^+$ T 淋巴细胞）导致 β 细胞破坏。自身抗体（针对谷氨酸脱羧酶、胰岛素、酪氨酸磷酸酶和锌转运蛋白 8）被认为主要是在 β 细胞和胰岛抗原暴露后产生，并不是破坏过程的主要介质。尽管如此，检测到 1 个或多个自身抗体是确定风险患者（如 T1DM 患者的一级亲属）临床前期最敏感和有效的方法。

健康个体的 β 细胞通常能提供足够的额外胰岛素分泌能力，以维持血糖水平，除非 β 细胞功能丧失达 80%～90%。在一些患者中，β 细胞功能的亚临床丧失可能被显露，导致在偶然的上呼吸道感染等突发疾病过程中出现高血糖，甚至发生糖尿病酮症酸中毒（DKA）。这反映了缺乏足够的胰岛素储备来代偿应激引起的胰岛素抵抗。在开始胰岛素和其他治疗后，应激引起的胰岛素抵抗可得到解决，β 细胞功能可能有所改善。部分患者随后可能恢复到不需要使用胰岛素的状态。这种现象被称为蜜月期，可持续数周至 1 年。患者通常应在这一阶段以可耐受的低剂量继续使用胰岛素，因为可预见 β 细胞功能最终会逐渐丧失，导致复发性高血糖和潜在的 DKA。

T1DM 筛查不是标准医疗保健的一部分。对有 T1DM 家族史的个体进行自身抗体测定有助于确定风险，但不能可靠地预测发病时间或指导临床照护。应在个体化基础上考虑对 T1DM 患者进行甲状腺、肾上腺或其他自身免疫病的筛查。

临床表现

T1DM 最常见的临床表现为高血糖及其导致的渗透性利尿症状。患者通常有数天到数周的多尿加重期和多饮（对低血容量和血清渗透压增高的代偿反应）。多尿可能表现为儿童尿床或白天尿失禁、成人夜尿。患者常出现体重减轻，并常主诉精力不足和嗜睡。约 25% 的 T1DM 患者在出现临床表现时已发展为 DKA。

治疗

T1DM 的管理包括起病时立即治疗以纠正高血糖、液体丢失和 DKA（如果存在），以及注意可能的诱发或合并因素，如感染。T1DM 的初始治疗应与患者及其家属（根据患者年龄）教育相结合，让他们了解管理胰岛素注射、血糖监测、营养和运动所需的技能。这通常需

要由包括医生、宣教人员（通常是经专业培训的护士或药剂师）和营养师在内的医疗团队来完成。应持续、长期、个体化地提供医疗建议、患者教育和心理支持。血糖管理的主要目标是使高血糖程度及其伴随的糖尿病长期并发症的风险最小化，同时避免急性和慢性低血糖风险。医疗护理应包括控制血脂水平、血压和其他影响糖尿病长期并发症风险的因素。应常规评估足部护理、周围神经功能、视网膜状况和肾功能，以发现初期糖尿病并发症并实现早期治疗干预。有关儿童和青少年 T1DM 管理的具体问题，应参考其他来源的信息。

血糖控制 T1DM 患者需要外源性胰岛素。糖尿病控制和并发症试验（DCCT）和其他研究表明，改善 T1DM 患者的血糖控制可减少长期微血管并发症（视网膜病变、肾病和神经病变）。对相同患者进行的随访研究［糖尿病干预和并发症流行病学（EDIC）试验］进一步证明，强化胰岛素治疗可降低心血管疾病的发病率和死亡率。基于现有研究结果，最公认的 T1DM 患者 HbA1c 目标值为 7.0%，尽管部分患者可以安全地将 HbA1c 目标值设定为 6.5%。对于难以感知低血糖或其他因素导致血糖管理困难的患者（如肾衰竭），应将个体化的 HbA1c 目标设定为 8.0% 或更高。

目前有许多种胰岛素制剂可供选择。它们经皮下注射后的吸收速度、血药浓度达峰时间及作用持续时间有所不同（表 5.5）。重组人胰岛素制剂的不同药动学源自它们与蛋白质和锌的特异性结合。此外，还有多种人胰岛素类似物可供选择，由于在皮下注射部位的溶解度不同，其药动学也有所不同。大多数胰岛素制剂的浓度为 100 U/ml（U-100），部分可提供更高浓度（200 U/ml 或 500 U/ml）。患者使用血糖仪进行自我血糖监测（SMBG）对于实施有效的胰岛素治疗方案至关重要。理想情况下，SMBG 应尽可能频繁地进行，包括：空腹、餐前、餐后 2 h、睡前监测，偶尔在 02:00 至 03:00 监测。大多数血糖仪能存储检测值和时间，以供后续回顾。患者手动纸质记录这些数据很有帮助，也可以将检测数据下载到计算机。SMBG 记录在标注有关食物摄入、运动或症状发生的相关详细信息时最有用。HbA1c 检测通常应每 3 个月进行 1 次。

大多数 T1DM 患者应通过强化胰岛素治疗方案进行管理，包括每日多次（≥ 3 次）皮下注射或使用胰岛素泵进行持续皮下胰岛素输注（CSII）。多次注射方案（又称基础-餐时治疗）通常是指每天注射 1 次或 2 次长效胰岛素类似物（甘精胰岛素、地特胰岛素或德谷胰岛素），以建立稳定的基础胰岛素水平。此外，还需要每天注射 ≥ 3 次（每餐前，有时在加餐前）常规胰岛素或速效胰岛素类似物，以提供适当的餐后胰岛素高峰。通常情况下，一旦血糖水平在治疗过程中稳定下来，长效胰岛素的剂量应每天保持稳定。通过尽量在每餐摄入固定量的碳水化合物和总热量，可以

TABLE 5.5	Types of Insulin[a]					
Insulin Type	Generic Name	Preprandial Injection Timing (hr)	Onset (hr)	Peak (hr)	Duration (hr)	Bg Nadir (hr)
Rapid-acting	Lispro[b]	0-0.2	0.1-0.5	0.5-2	<5	2-4
	Aspart[c]	0-0.2	0.1-0.3	0.6-3	3-5	1-3
	Glulisine[d]	0-0.25 (15 min before a meal or within 20 min after starting a meal)	0.15-0.3	0.5-1.5	1-5.3	2-4
Short-acting	Regular	0.5-1	0.3-1	2-6	4-8	3-7
Intermediate-acting	NPH	0.5-1	1-3	6-15	16-26	6-13
Long-acting	Glargine[e,f]	Once daily[g] or twice daily (approx 12 hourly)	1-4	Little or no peak	10.8->24	Before next dose
	Detemir[f]	Once daily[g] or twice daily (approx 12 hourly)	1-4	Little or no peak	12-24	Before next dose
	Degludec	Once daily	0.5-1.5	Little or no peak	42	Before next dose
Human Premixed						
NPH/regular	70/30	0.5-1	0.5-1	2-12	14-24	3-12
NPH/regular	50/50	0.5-1	0.5-1	2-5	14-24	3-12
Insulin Analogue Premixed						
NPL/lispro	75/25	0.25	0.15-0.25	1	14-24	—
NPA/aspart	70/30	0.25	0.15-0.3	2-4	24	—
NPL/lispro	50/50	0.25	0.15-0.25	1	14-24	—

BG, Blood glucose; *NPA,* neutral protamine aspart; *NPH,* neutral protamine Hagedorn; *NPL,* neutral protamine lispro.
[a]Time profiles depend on several factors, including dose, anatomic site of injection, method (profiles in this table are for subcutaneous injections), duration of diabetes, type of diabetes, degree of insulin resistance, level of physical activity, presence of obesity, and body temperature. Preprandial injection timing depends on premeal BG values and insulin type.
[b]Insulin analogue with reversal of lysine and proline at positions 28 and 29 on the B chain of the insulin molecule.
[c]Insulin analogue with substitution of aspartic acid for proline at position 28 on the B chain of the insulin molecule.
[d]Insulin analogue with substitution of lysine for asparagine at position 3 on the B chain and glutamic acid for lysine at position 29 on the B chain of the insulin molecule.
[e]Insulin analogue with substitution of glycine for asparagine at position 21 on the A chain and addition of two arginines to the carboxyl terminus of the B chain of the insulin molecule.
[f]Do not mix glargine or detemir in the same syringe with other insulins.
[g]Administer at same time each day, unrelated to meals. Morning administration may result in greater glucose lowering and less nocturnal hypoglycemia.

rapid-acting insulin doses are adjusted according to the blood glucose level (measured before each meal) and the carbohydrate calories ingested with the meal. The long-acting insulin glargine and detemir analogues cannot be mixed in a single syringe with other insulins; for this reason, basal-bolus regimens often require four or more daily injections.

For patients newly diagnosed with T1DM, a typical starting dose of insulin is a total of 0.2 to 0.4 U/kg/day, with the expectation that this will be increased to 0.6 to 0.7 U/kg/day over time. Approximately half of the total dose should be given as basal insulin. Basal glargine or detemir insulin may be administered as a single daily dose (in the morning or at bedtime), or two equally divided doses may be required, depending on individual patient blood glucose responses. Degludec normally requires only once daily injection. For a basal regimen using intermediate acting insulin (NPH), two thirds of the dose typically is given in the morning and one third at bedtime. This decreases the risk of nocturnal hypoglycemia and times the maximum NPH peak to approximately match the midday meal. The rapid-acting component of the daily insulin dose is distributed before meals according to meal size and content.

An insulin pump (continuous subcutaneous insulin infusion, CSII) represents the preferred method of insulin administration for many T1DM patients. These small, wearable devices contain a reservoir of rapid-acting insulin that is infused via an easily placed subcutaneous catheter. A microprocessor-controlled pump provides the basal insulin infusion and can be programmed to adjust basal rates at multiple points during the day according to predetermined patient needs. The patient further instructs the pump to make bolus insulin injections to cover meals, snacks, or needed corrections in hyperglycemia. Controlled studies have shown that modestly better blood glucose control can be achieved with CSII, compared to basal-bolus regimens with multiple daily injections. When used appropriately, CSII represents the most flexible means of managing insulin doses, with options for dose adjustments and supplementation that do not require separate injections. Limitations include need for greater patient involvement, lack of a protective, long-acting subcutaneous insulin reservoir, and pump failure. Newly diagnosed T1DM should be managed for a period of time (at least 6 to 12 months) with intermittently injected insulin before transition to a pump is considered. During the transition from intermittent insulin injections to CSII in a patient with well-controlled blood glucose levels (HbA$_{1c}$ ≤7.0%), the total daily insulin dose typically is decreased by 10% to 20% initially.

Many CSII patients require a slightly higher basal infusion rate in the early morning hours to accommodate the *dawn phenomenon,* a period of decreased insulin sensitivity secondary to circadian changes in secretion of insulin counter-regulatory hormones such as growth

表 5.5　胰岛素类型[a]

胰岛素类型	通用名	餐前注射时间（h）	起效时间（h）	达峰时间（h）	持续时间（h）	血糖谷值（h）
速效	赖脯胰岛素[b]	0～0.2	0.1～0.5	0.5～2	＜5	2～4
	门冬胰岛素[c]	0～0.2	0.1～0.3	0.6～3	3～5	1～3
	谷赖胰岛素[d]	0～0.25（餐前 15 min 或开始进餐后 20 min 以内）	0.15～0.3	0.5～1.5	1～5.3	2～4
短效	常规型	0.5～1	0.3～1	2～6	4～8	3～7
中效	NPH	0.5～1	1～3	6～15	16～26	6～13
长效	甘精胰岛素[e, f]	1 次 / 日[g] 或 2 次 / 日（约 12 h 1 次）	1～4	很少或无峰	10.8～＞24	在下一个剂量前
	地特胰岛素[f]	1 次 / 日[g] 或 2 次 / 日（约 12 h 1 次）	1～4	很少或无峰	12～24	在下一个剂量前
	德谷胰岛素	1 次 / 日	0.5～1.5	很少或无峰	42	在下一个剂量前
预混人胰岛素						
NPH/ 常规型	70/30	0.5～1	0.5～1	2～12	14～24	3～12
NPH/ 常规型	50/50	0.5～1	0.5～1	2～5	14～24	3～12
预混胰岛素类似物						
NPL/ 赖脯胰岛素	75/25	0.25	0.15～0.25	1	14～24	—
NPA/ 门冬胰岛素	70/30	0.25	0.15～0.3	2～4	24	—
NPL/ 赖脯胰岛素	50/50	0.25	0.15～0.25	1	14～24	—

NPA，中性鱼精蛋白门冬胰岛素；NPH，中性鱼精蛋白锌胰岛素；NPL，中性鱼精蛋白赖脯胰岛素。
[a] 时间谱取决于多个因素，包括剂量、注射部位解剖学、方法（本表中的时间谱为皮下注射）、糖尿病病程、糖尿病类型、胰岛素抵抗程度、体力活动水平、是否有肥胖症和体温。餐前注射时间取决于餐前血糖值和胰岛素类型。
[b] 将胰岛素分子 B 链位置 28 和 29 上的赖氨酸和脯氨酸互换的胰岛素类似物。
[c] 将胰岛素分子 B 链位置 28 上的脯氨酸替换为门冬氨酸的胰岛素类似物。
[d] 将胰岛素分子 B 链位置 3 的天冬酰胺替换为赖氨酸、位置 29 的赖氨酸替换为谷氨酸的胰岛素类似物。
[e] 将胰岛素分子 A 链位置 21 的门冬酰胺替换为甘氨酸，并在 B 链羧基端增加 2 个精氨酸的胰岛素类似物。
[f] 请勿将甘精胰岛素或地特胰岛素与其他胰岛素制剂混合在一个注射器中。
[g] 在每天相同时间注射，与进餐无关。早上注射的降糖效果可能更好且夜间低血糖更少。

保持速效胰岛素剂量稳定。此外，根据餐前血糖水平（每餐前检测）和餐中摄入的碳水化合物热量调整速效胰岛素剂量，可以实现更好的控制和更大的灵活性。长效胰岛素甘精胰岛素和地特胰岛素不能与其他胰岛素混合在一个注射器中；因此，基础-餐时方案通常需要每天注射 ≥ 4 次。

对于新诊断的 T1DM 患者，胰岛素的起始剂量通常为 0.2 ～ 0.4 U/（kg·d），预计将随时间增加至 0.6 ～ 0.7 U/（kg·d）。总剂量的约 1/2 应作为基础胰岛素给予。基础甘精胰岛素或地特胰岛素可每日给予 1 次（早上或睡前），可能需要等分为 2 次剂量给予，应根据患者个体化的血糖反应。德谷胰岛素通常只需要每天注射 1 次。对于使用中效胰岛素（NPH）的基础方案，通常早上给予 2/3 剂量，晚上睡前给予 1/3 剂量，这可降低夜间低血糖的风险，并将 NPH 的峰值时间大约与午餐时间相匹配。每日胰岛素剂量中的速效胰岛素部分应根据进餐量和具体食物在餐前设定。

胰岛素泵［持续皮下胰岛素输注（CSII）］是许多 T1DM 患者的首选胰岛素给药方法。这些小型可穿戴设备包含 1 个速效胰岛素的储药器，其通过皮下导管输注。微处理器控制的泵可提供基础胰岛素输注，并能根据预设的患者需求而在一天中的多个时间点调整基础输注速率。患者可进一步设定泵进行大剂量胰岛素注射，以覆盖进餐、加餐或需要纠正的高血糖。对照研究表明，与每日多次注射的基础-餐时方案相比，CSII 可以更好地控制血糖。如果使用恰当，CSII 是调整胰岛素剂量的最灵活方式，可用于剂量调整和补充，而不需要单独注射。CSII 的局限性包括需要患者更多参与、缺乏具有保护性的长效皮下胰岛素储药器、泵故障。新诊断的 T1DM 应在考虑转换到胰岛素泵之前使用间歇性注射胰岛素进行管理（至少 6 ～ 12 个月）。在从间歇性胰岛素注射过渡到 CSII 的患者中，如果血糖水平控制良好（HbA1c ≤ 7.0%），通常最初将每日胰岛素总剂量减少 10% ～ 20%。

许多使用 CSII 的患者需要在清晨稍微加快基础输注率，以适应黎明现象，这是由于胰岛素反调节激素（如生长激素和皮质醇）分泌的昼夜节律变化，导致胰岛素敏感性降低。由于胰岛素敏感性的变化（如运动

hormone and cortisol. Adjustments in the basal rate may also be needed at other times of day because of changes in insulin sensitivity (e.g., in response to exercise). Premeal insulin boluses are calculated to include a correction dose if needed, based on the premeal blood glucose level, plus a meal coverage dose calculated from the patient's predetermined individual carbohydrate/insulin ratio. It often is most effective for a patient to be seen in a specialty setting during transition to CSII, so that an experienced educator (often a specially trained RN) can assist with needed patient education. Devices are available that provide continuous glucose monitoring (CGM), either as a separate device or integrated into a sensor-augmented insulin pump. Some of the latter devices have the capacity to automatically interrupt insulin delivery for a proscribed period in response to low blood glucose levels as a protection against hypoglycemia (especially useful for nocturnal hypoglycemia). One approved sensor-augmented insulin pump can adjust the basal insulin infusion rate based on the CGM data but still requires manual control of premeal insulin boluses and periodic confirmation of blood glucose levels by fingerstick testing.

Intensive insulin therapy is not appropriate for all T1DM patients. Some patients are unwilling or unable to manage the required frequent glucose monitoring, diet adherence, and multiple insulin boluses. In other patients, the tight blood glucose control and low HbA$_{1c}$ targets that are the goals of intensive insulin therapy may not be feasible. For example, there may be an increased risk of hypoglycemia because of autonomic neuropathy and inability to sense hypoglycemia, or gastrointestinal neuropathy may cause gastroparesis resulting in unpredictable variations in nutrient digestion and absorption. Under such circumstances, simpler approaches to insulin therapy and blood glucose management, previously termed *conventional insulin therapy*, may be appropriate. Such a regimen may be based, for example, on two injections per day of intermediate-acting insulin with or without short- or rapid-acting insulin. As one example, a *split-mixed regimen* uses NPH/regular or NPH/lispro (or aspart or glulisine) formulations twice daily. Initially, two thirds of the estimated total daily dose is given before breakfast and one third before dinner; at each of these times, two thirds of the insulin is given as NPH and one third as regular or rapid-acting insulin. The amount of each insulin type at each of the injection times is then adjusted according to measured blood glucose levels, with the expectation that the peak of the morning NPH will cover lunch, the rapid-acting insulins will cover the other meals, and the NPH will otherwise ensure adequate basal blood glucose control. Two daily injections are made possible by mixing the intermediate- and rapid-acting insulins in a single syringe. Premixed insulin preparations, such as 70% NPH plus 30% rapid-acting insulin or 50% NPH plus 50% regular insulin, also are available for injection with syringes or with preloaded insulin pens. Premixed insulins provide greater ease of use but are less likely to achieve good glycemic control.

Hypoglycemia management. Irrespective of the specific treatment regimen, patients with T1DM need to learn how to manage hypoglycemia. Patients usually experience adrenergic symptoms (e.g., sweating, anxiety, tremulousness) as blood glucose levels decrease below the normal range (<50 to 70 mg/dL). If a patient is taking β-blockers, symptoms such as tachycardia and tremulousness might be blunted or absent. If glucose levels decrease markedly enough, patients may experience central nervous system (CNS) symptoms ranging from difficulty thinking clearly to confusion, obtundation, and loss of consciousness. If low blood glucose is confirmed (e.g., <70 mg/ dL), 10 to 15 g of rapidly absorbed carbohydrate should be ingested. For a glucose level lower than 50 mg/dL, 20 to 30 g of carbohydrate is advisable. This can be provided as orange juice or crackers, or patients can carry glucose tablets or squeeze tubes of glucose solution (obtainable over the counter from pharmacies) for use in treating hypoglycemia.

The blood glucose level should be retested after 15 minutes, and the treatment should be repeated as needed until hypoglycemia is resolved. An alternative is to inject glucagon. For patients who have a history of hypoglycemia severe enough (including loss of consciousness) to require assistance from others, it often is helpful for a family member to be trained in glucagon injection. With severe hypoglycemia, there is a risk of injury, such as from a fall or automobile accident, as well as neurologic damage if hypoglycemia is sustained.

Nutritional management. Appropriate nutritional management is an essential component of an effective T1DM treatment program, both to facilitate blood glucose control and reduce risks of long-term diabetes complications. Patients should work with a medical professional who is trained in diabetes care to establish nutritional goals. Rather than target specific percentages or sources of dietary carbohydrate, protein, and fat, the diet should be individualized to the patient's lifestyle, exercise regimen, eating habits, culture, and financial resources.

Most diets focus on measuring and controlling the amounts rather than the sources of carbohydrates. Patients can learn how to estimate the grams of carbohydrate in a meal *(carbohydrate counting)* as a means of ensuring that a consistent amount of carbohydrate is ingested. Alternatively, they can use carbohydrate counting with each meal as part of a strategy that enables day-to-day variations in consumption with adjustments of mealtime insulin doses according to a predetermined, patient-specific *insulin/carbohydrate ratio.*

Because of the contribution of excess body weight to increased cardiovascular risk, a fundamental goal of nutritional management should be to maintain normal body weight or to achieve weight reduction in overweight or obese patients. Eating disorders including binge eating, anorexia nervosa, and bulimia are relatively common in T1DM, especially among younger female patients.

Exercise. Regular physical exercise should be encouraged for its beneficial effects on weight control, risks of long-term complications, and overall quality of life. The general recommendation of several expert panels is 30 minutes or more of moderate-intensity physical exercise on at least 5 days per week. Physical exercise burns calories in proportion to its duration and intensity and also may result in increased insulin sensitivity after exercise (sometimes lasting for many hours). It often is most effective for patients to schedule exercise periods with a consistent temporal relationship to meals and insulin injections. Blood glucose should be tested before and after exercise, and exercise should not be undertaken if the initial blood glucose level is low (because of increased risk of hypoglycemia) or if it is higher than 250 mg/dL (because of risk of inducing further blood glucose elevation and development of ketosis). Patients with T1DM should be encouraged to pursue age- and overall health-appropriate athletic interests, including competitive sports, but this should be done only with careful attention to blood glucose monitoring and appropriate adjustments in insulin regimen and diet.

Type 2 Diabetes
Epidemiology and Pathology
T2DM is an extraordinarily common disorder, affecting nearly 10% of the population in the United States and with a similar prevalence in most other developed or developing countries. Many additional individuals (approximately 8% of the US population) have a prediabetic state. T2DM is characterized by varying degrees of insulin resistance and insulin deficiency, which are believed to result from the impact of environmental factors on a background of genetic risk. The principal features of T2DM, contrasted with T1DM, are summarized in Table 5.4. The prevalence of T2DM has increased more than 10-fold over the past 50 years, driven primarily by population-wide increased

时的反应），可能还需要在一天中的其他时间调整基础速率。计算餐前胰岛素大剂量常需要校正，基于餐前血糖水平和患者预先确定的个体化的碳水化合物 / 胰岛素比值计算的进餐剂量。在过渡到 CSII 期间，最有效的方法通常是专科住院治疗，以便于有经验的宣教人员（通常是经专业培训的执业护士）协助进行必要的患者教育。能提供连续血糖监测（CGM）的设备可单独使用或集成到传感器增强型胰岛素泵中。部分传感器增强型胰岛素泵具有在低血糖时自动中断胰岛素输送的能力，以防止低血糖（特别是夜间低血糖）。目前已获得批准的一种传感器增强型胰岛素泵可根据 CGM 数据调整基础胰岛素输注率，但仍需要手动控制餐前胰岛素大剂量，并定期通过检测指血确认血糖水平。

强化胰岛素治疗并不适用于所有 T1DM 患者。部分患者不愿意或无法很好地管理所需的频繁血糖监测、饮食依从性和多次胰岛素大剂量注射。在其他患者中，强化胰岛素治疗的目标——严格控制血糖和 HbA1c 低目标值，可能并不可行。例如，由于自主神经病变和无法感知低血糖，低血糖的风险可能会增加，或者胃肠神经病变可能引起胃轻瘫，从而导致营养物质消化和吸收发生不可预测的变化。在这种情况下，可能适合采用更简单的胰岛素治疗和血糖管理方法，既往被称为传统胰岛素治疗。该方案可能基于每天注射 2 次中效胰岛素，联用或不联用短效或速效胰岛素。例如，每天注射 2 次 NPH/ 常规型胰岛素或 NPH/ 赖脯胰岛素（或门冬胰岛素或谷赖胰岛素）制剂的分次-混合方案。最初，每日总剂量的 2/3 在早餐前给予，1/3 在晚餐前给予；在每个时间点，胰岛素的 2/3 为 NPH，1/3 为常规型或速效胰岛素。然后，根据测量的血糖水平调整每次注射的每种胰岛素剂量，目标是早上注射的 NPH 峰值将覆盖午餐，速效胰岛素将覆盖其他餐食，NPH 将确保充分的基础血糖控制。通过在同一注射器中混合中效和速效胰岛素，可以实现每日注射 2 次。预混胰岛素制剂（如 70%NPH + 30% 速效胰岛素，或 50%NPH + 50% 常规型胰岛素）也可用注射器或预填充胰岛素笔注射。预混胰岛素提供了更大的使用便利性，但不太可能实现良好的血糖控制。

低血糖管理 无论具体的治疗方案如何，T1DM 患者均需要学会如何处理低血糖。当血糖降至正常范围以下（< 50 ～ 70 mg/dl）时，患者通常会经历肾上腺素能症状（如出汗、焦虑、震颤）。如果患者正在服用 β 受体阻滞剂，则心动过速和震颤等症状可能减弱或缺失。如果血糖水平显著降低，患者可能出现中枢神经系统（CNS）症状，从思维混乱到意识错乱、反应迟钝，甚至意识丧失。如果确认低血糖（如 < 70 mg/dl），应摄入 10 ～ 15 g 快速吸收的碳水化合物。若血糖 < 50 mg/dl，建议摄入 20 ～ 30 g 碳水化合物。可选择橙汁、饼干，患者可携带葡萄糖片剂或挤压管装葡萄糖溶液（可在

药店柜台购买）用于治疗低血糖。15 min 后应重新检测血糖水平，并根据需要重复治疗，直至低血糖得到纠正。另一种选择是注射胰高血糖素。对于有严重低血糖病史（包括意识丧失）并需要他人帮助的患者，通常有必要对患者家属进行胰高血糖素注射培训。在严重低血糖的情况下，存在受伤的风险（如跌倒或车祸），如果低血糖持续存在，可能导致神经损伤。

营养管理 适当的营养管理是有效的 T1DM 治疗计划的重要组成部分，其旨在促进血糖控制并降低长期糖尿病并发症的风险。患者应与接受过糖尿病护理培训的医疗专业人员共同制定营养目标。饮食管理应针对患者的生活方式、运动计划、饮食习惯、文化和经济状况进行个体化设定，而不是制订特定比例或来源的膳食碳水化合物、蛋白质和脂肪方案。

大多数饮食专注于测量和控制碳水化合物的量，而不是来源。患者可以学习如何估计一餐中的碳水化合物克数（碳水化合物计算），以确保碳水化合物的摄入量保持一致。此外，可将每餐的碳水化合物计算作为治疗的一部分，根据预先确定的患者特定的胰岛素 / 碳水化合物比值调整餐时胰岛素剂量，以适应每日摄入量的变异。

由于超重会增加心血管风险，营养管理的基本目标应是保持正常体重或实现超重或肥胖患者的减重。进食障碍（包括暴食症、神经性厌食症和神经性贪食症）在 T1DM 患者中相对常见，特别是在年轻的女性患者中。

运动 应鼓励定期运动，因其有益于控制体重，降低长期并发症的风险和提高整体生活质量。多个专家小组普遍建议每周至少运动 5 天，每天进行 ≥ 30 min 的中等强度运动。运动消耗的热量与持续时间和强度成正比，且运动后可能增加胰岛素敏感性（有时持续数小时）。对患者来说，最有效的方法通常是将运动时间与进餐和注射胰岛素的时间相匹配。运动前后应检测血糖，如果初始血糖水平低（有增加低血糖的风险）或 > 250 mg/dl（有进一步升高血糖和发生酮症的风险），则不应进行运动。应鼓励 T1DM 患者进行适合其年龄和整体健康状况的运动，包括竞技体育项目，但必须仔细监测血糖并适当调整胰岛素方案和饮食。

2 型糖尿病

流行病学和病理学

T2DM 是一种极其常见的疾病，几乎影响美国近 10% 的人口，大多数其他发达国家或发展中国家人群的患病率相似。还有许多人（约 8% 的美国人口）处于糖尿病前期状态。T2DM 的特征是不同程度的胰岛素抵抗和胰岛素缺乏，这被认为是环境因素在遗传风险背景下作用的结果。T2DM 与 T1DM 的主要特点对比见表 5.4。过去 50 年来，T2DM 的患病率增加了

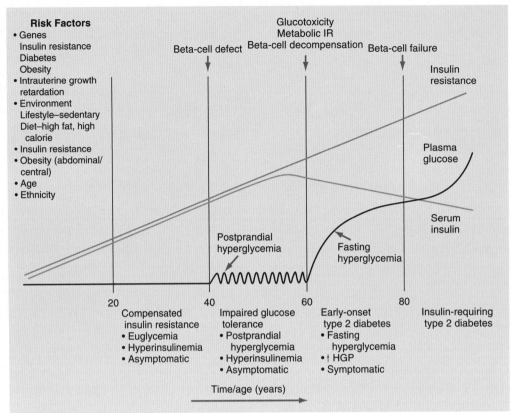

Fig. 5.2 Natural history of type 2 diabetes mellitus. The numbers for time/age markers in years for the different phases of beta-cell decompensation toward overt diabetes and an insulin-requiring state are approximate guides. Certain groups are more insulin sensitive and require a greater loss of beta-cell function to precipitate diabetes, compared with obese insulin-resistant people, who develop diabetes after small declines in beta-cell function. Use of insulin in patients with type 2 diabetes varies considerably and is not age dependent. *HGP*, Hepatic glucose production; *IR*, insulin resistance.

calorie intake, decreased exercise, and resulting obesity. More than 80% of patients with T2DM are obese. The peak incidence of T2DM occurs in the fifth and sixth decades; however, T2DM now accounts for up to 30% of childhood diabetes in some populations. The lifetime risk of developing T2DM is approximately 40% among the offspring of a single affected parent, and approximately 70% if both parents are affected. The incidence of T2DM in the United States is higher in Hispanic/Latino populations, among African Americans, and in some east Asian populations, compared to populations of northern and western European ancestry. This is thought to result in part from effects of socioeconomic and cultural factors (e.g., differences in consumption of low-cost, calorie-dense foods) and also from genetic differences among these populations. The genetic predisposition is thought to reflect the combined influence of more than 100 genes. No single gene or small group of genes with dominant influence on diabetes risk in any population has been identified.

T2DM is typically preceded by a prolonged preclinical or prediabetic phase during which there is a gradual deterioration in glucose tolerance (Fig. 5.2). This process occurs over a decade or more on average, with marked individual variation in the rate of progression. Most patients are insulin resistant during the preclinical phase but are able to compensate by producing enough insulin to maintain euglycemia. With time, there is progressive deterioration in the capacity to compensate for the insulin resistance. This is associated with a decrease in beta cell-mass during the preclinical phase of T2DM, but substantial

residual beta cells (typically 40% to 50% of the normal complement) are still present at the time that overt hyperglycemia develops. Therefore, there is compromised function as well as a reduced number of beta cells in T2DM. As blood glucose levels rise, the hyperglycemia itself may contribute to progression of the diabetic state by further decreasing insulin secretion and insulin resistance through mechanisms that are not well understood (referred to as *glucotoxicity*).

Screening of certain high-risk populations for T2DM and prediabetes by determination of a fasting or random plasma glucose measurement is considered cost-effective. Approximately 25% of people with T2DM and an even higher percentage of those with prediabetes are undiagnosed. Expert panel recommendations from the ADA for screening based on age, lifestyle factors, family history, and ethnicity are summarized in Table 5.6. Because of the insidious nature of T2DM, patients have a high risk for development of complications by the time of clinical diagnosis (see later discussion).

Clinical Presentation

Many patients are asymptomatic and are diagnosed on routine blood glucose testing. Blood glucose levels that rise high enough to exceed the renal threshold for glucose reabsorption (>170 mg/dL) induce an osmotic diuresis, resulting in the typical presenting symptoms of polyuria and polydipsia, as well as blurred vision secondary to osmotic shifts in the lens. Patients may also have weight loss or bacterial urinary tract or cutaneous fungal infections at presentation. Osmotic diuresis

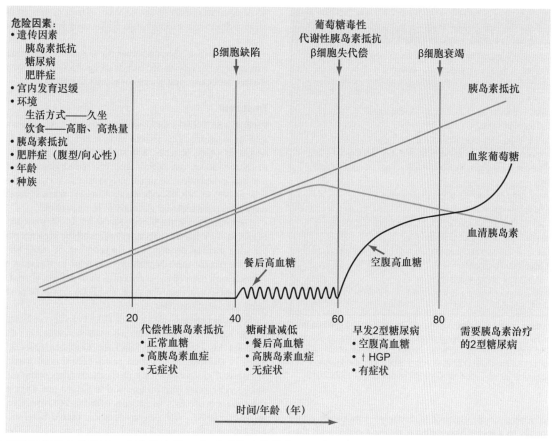

图 5.2　2 型糖尿病的自然病程。大致描述了 β 细胞功能失代偿向显性糖尿病和需要胰岛素状态发展的不同阶段的时间 / 年龄节点（以年为单位）。某些人群对胰岛素更敏感，需要更多的 β 细胞功能丧失才能诱发糖尿病，而伴有肥胖症的胰岛素抵抗人群在 β 细胞功能轻微下降时即可发展成糖尿病。2 型糖尿病患者中胰岛素的使用差异很大，且不依赖于年龄。HGP，肝脏葡萄糖生成

10 倍以上，主要原因是全民热量摄入增加、运动量减少及由此导致的肥胖症。超过 80% 的 T2DM 患者伴有肥胖症。T2DM 的发病高峰年龄为 40 ～ 60 岁；然而，T2DM 在某些人群中占儿童糖尿病的 30%。单亲患病的后代发生 T2DM 的终身风险约为 40%，双亲患病的后代约为 70%。在美国，与北欧和西欧血统的人群相比，西班牙裔 / 拉丁美洲裔人群、非裔美国人和一些东亚人群的 T2DM 发病率较高。部分原因是社会经济和文化因素的影响（如购买低价格高热量食物的差异）及这些人群的遗传差异。遗传倾向反映的是 100 多个基因的联合影响。在任何人群中均未发现对糖尿病风险有主导影响的单一基因或小组基因。

在 T2DM 发病之前，通常有一个长期的临床前期或糖尿病前期，糖耐量在此期间逐渐恶化（图 5.2）。该过程平均为 10 年或更长时间，进展速度有显著的个体差异。大多数患者在临床前期存在胰岛素抵抗，但能够通过代偿产生足够的胰岛素来维持正常血糖。随着时间的推移，胰岛素抵抗的代偿能力逐渐恶化。这与 T2DM 临床前期的 β 细胞数量减少有关，但在出现明显的高血糖时仍然存在大量的残留 β 细胞（通常为

正常的 40% ～ 50%）。因此，在 T2DM 中，虽然 β 细胞数量减少，但仍有一定功能。随着血糖水平的升高，高血糖本身可通过进一步减少胰岛素分泌和增加胰岛素抵抗来促进糖尿病状态的进展，这些机制目前尚不清楚（被称为葡萄糖毒性）。

通过测定空腹或随机血糖对高风险人群进行 T2DM 和糖尿病前期的筛查被认为具有成本效益。约 25% 的 T2DM 患者和更高比例的糖尿病前期患者未被诊断。美国糖尿病协会（ADA）专家小组对根据年龄、生活方式因素、家族史和种族进行筛查的建议见表 5.6。由于 T2DM 的隐匿性，患者在临床诊断时发生并发症的风险很高（见下文）。

临床表现

许多患者无症状，通常在常规血糖检测中被诊断。血糖水平升高至超过肾对葡萄糖重吸收的阈值（＞ 170 mg/dl）时，会引发渗透性利尿，导致典型症状多尿和多饮，以及由于晶状体渗透压变化而引起的视物模糊。患者还可能在发病时出现体重减轻或有细菌性尿路感染或皮肤真菌感染。高血糖引起的渗透性

TABLE 5.6 Screening Criteria for Diabetes in Asymptomatic Adults

1. Testing for diabetes should be considered in all persons ≥45 yr of age; if normal, the test should be repeated at 3-yr intervals.
2. Testing should be considered at a younger age (<30 yr) or performed more frequently in individuals who
   a. Have BMI ≥ 25 kg/m² (≥ 23 kg/m² in Asian Americans)
   b. Have a sedentary lifestyle
   c. Have a first-degree relative with diabetes (i.e., parent or sibling)
   d. Are members of a high-risk ethnic population (e.g., African American, Latino/Hispanic American, Native American, Asian American, Pacific Islander)
   e. Have been diagnosed with gestational diabetes
   f. Are hypertensive (≥140/90 mm Hg)
   g. Have an HDL cholesterol level <35 mg/dL (0.9 mmol/L) and/or a triglyceride level >250 mg/dL (2.82 mmol/L)
   h. Have other clinical conditions associated with insulin resistance (e.g., PCOS, acanthosis nigricans)
   i. Have a history of cardiovascular disease
   j. Had prediabetes on previous testing (see criteria in Table 5.1); should be tested annually

BMI, Body mass index (weight [kg]/height [m²]); *HbA₁C*, glycosylated hemoglobin; *HDL*, high-density lipoprotein; *PCOS*, polycystic ovary syndrome; *T1DM*, type 1 diabetes mellitus; *T2DM*, type 2 diabetes mellitus. Modified from the American Diabetes Association Clinical Practice Recommendations 2013, Diabetes Care 36(Suppl 1):S11-S66, 2013.

secondary to hyperglycemia may lead to electrolyte abnormalities and even occasionally to a severe hyperosmolar state associated with clinical symptoms and signs including fatigue, weakness, and ultimately compromised mental status that can range from confusion to coma (see later discussion). This most frequently occurs in elderly patients who may have compromised baseline renal function. In contrast to patients with T1DM, those with T2DM usually have enough residual insulin activity to partially suppress lipolysis, and this protects them from developing DKA. In a subset of T2DM patients, DKA can develop, possibly reflecting individual variations in the degree of suppression of insulin secretion by glucotoxicity.

As a consequence of prolonged exposure to hyperglycemia and associated metabolic disturbances, patients with T2DM may already have developed long-term microvascular or macrovascular complications of diabetes by the time of diagnosis. Therefore, patients may experience a cardiovascular event, such as acute myocardial infarction, and then incidentally be found to have T2DM.

The metabolic syndrome. Susceptibility to cardiovascular disease is further increased by the frequent association of insulin resistance, prediabetes, and T2DM with other cardiovascular risk factors, including abdominal or visceral obesity, dyslipidemia, and hypertension. The term *metabolic syndrome* has been applied to patients who have a combination of these risk factors. Different but overlapping diagnostic criteria for the metabolic syndrome have been proposed by various expert panels. The National Cholesterol Education Program Adult Treatment Panel III (ATP III) defines this syndrome as the presence of any three of the following five characteristics:

1. Fasting blood glucose level ≥100 mg/dL or drug treatment for elevated blood glucose
2. High-density lipoprotein (HDL)-cholesterol <40 mg/dL in men or <50 mg/dL in women or drug treatment for low HDL-cholesterol
3. Plasma triglycerides ≥150 mg/dL or drug treatment for elevated triglycerides

4. Abdominal obesity (waist ≥102 cm in men or ≥88 cm in women
5. Blood pressure ≥130/85 mm Hg or drug treatment for hypertension.

There is debate about whether the metabolic syndrome represents a discrete pathologic entity, but its recognition does draw attention to the frequent clustering of cardiovascular risk factors.

Treatment

Patients with T2DM should receive nutrition counseling starting at the time of diagnosis. This should include efforts at weight loss in overweight or obese patients. Adjustments in diet, especially reductions in calorie intake, can rapidly improve blood glucose levels in many patients independent of other interventions. Weight reduction by as little as 10% to 20% of body weight can have marked beneficial effects on insulin resistance and glycemia in some patients.

Depending on initial blood glucose levels, the presence or absence of symptoms related to hyperglycemia, and the presence of other complicating medical conditions, a decision can be made on whether to treat the patient initially with diet alone or to also start medication. Patients with marked hyperglycemia, fluid deficits, altered mental status related to hyperosmolar state, and DKA should be hospitalized for acute treatment (see later discussion).

For most patients, treatment of T2DM can be conducted on an outpatient basis. Useful guidelines are available online from the American Diabetes Association (ADA) and the European Association for the Study of Diabetes. Most expert panels recommend starting with one or two oral glucose-lowering medications (depending on the degree of hyperglycemia) with progression to a third oral agent or insulin if this proves ineffective. In patients with marked hyperglycemia (≥300 mg/dL or HbA₁c >10%), consideration should be given to starting insulin from the outset. There typically is gradually progressive loss of beta-cell function in T2DM, extending sometimes over many years, and this results in a need over time for increased doses or additional glucose-lowering agents and often, ultimately, the use of insulin. As for T1DM, the overall management of T2DM should include not only the treatment of hyperglycemia but also interventions that assess, decrease the risks for, and treat long-term microvascular and macrovascular complications.

Blood glucose control. The United Kingdom Prevention of Diabetes Study (UKPDS) and other randomized, controlled trials have established that improved blood glucose control lowers the risk of microvascular long-term complications (retinopathy, nephropathy, and neuropathy) in T2DM. The risk appears to increase progressively, starting with any increment above normoglycemia. Randomized clinical trial data have not convincingly demonstrated improved macrovascular (i.e., cardiovascular disease) outcomes in response to improved blood glucose control in T2DM. T2DM patients, particularly those who are older or have complicating comorbid conditions, may have limited capacity to manage a tight blood glucose control regimen and also increased susceptibility to adverse effects of hypoglycemia. HbA₁c goals therefore should be developed on an individualized basis, such that the benefits of improving microvascular complications are balanced against the risks of hypoglycemia. Whereas HbA₁c of 7% or less is an appropriate target for younger T2DM patients, 8% or less may be an acceptable and safer target for older patients with complicating medical conditions and limited life expectancy. HbA₁c should be measured every 6 months, or at intervals of 3 months if glucose control is unstable or the treatment regimen is being adjusted. SMBG should be performed on a regular basis if patients are being treated with agents that can cause hypoglycemia (sulfonylureas, meglitinides, and insulin). Regular SMBG is not generally needed for patients on agents that do not cause hypoglycemia, although testing during intercurrent

表5.6　无症状成人糖尿病的筛查标准
1. 所有 ≥ 45 岁的个体应考虑进行糖尿病相关检查；如果检查结果正常，应每 3 年复查 1 次
2. 对于年龄较小（≤ 30 岁）的个体，存在以下情况时应考虑进行更频繁的检测：
a. BMI ≥ 25 kg/m² （亚洲裔美国人 ≥ 23 kg/m²）
b. 久坐的生活方式
c. 一级亲属中有糖尿病患者（即父母或亲兄弟姐妹）
d. 高风险种族人群（如非裔美国人、拉丁裔 / 西班牙裔美国人、美国原住民、亚洲裔美国人、太平洋岛民）
e. 曾被诊断为妊娠糖尿病
f. 高血压（≥ 140/90 mmHg）
g. HDL 胆固醇 < 35 mg/dl（0.9 mmol/L）和（或）甘油三酯 > 250 mg/dl（2.82 mmol/L）
h. 其他与胰岛素抵抗相关的临床表现（如 PCOS、黑棘皮症）
i. 有心血管疾病史
j. 既往检测出糖尿病前期（见表 5.1 中的标准）；应每年检测 1 次

BMI，体重指数［体重（kg）/ 身高的平方（m²）］；HDL，高密度脂蛋白；PCOS，多囊卵巢综合征。

改编自 American Diabetes Association Clinical Practice Recommendations 2013, Diabetes Care 36（Suppl 1）：S11-S66, 2013.

利尿可能导致电解质异常，甚至偶尔会导致严重高渗状态，表现为疲劳、虚弱，最终可能导致从意识模糊到昏迷的精神状况受损（见下文）。这种情况最常见于基线肾功能不全的老年患者。与 T1DM 患者不同，T2DM 患者通常有足够的残余胰岛素活性来部分抑制脂肪分解，这可以防止他们发生糖尿病酮症酸中毒（DKA）。部分 T2DM 患者仍会发生 DKA，可能反映了胰岛素分泌受葡萄糖毒性抑制程度的个体差异的影响。

由于长期暴露于高血糖和相关的代谢紊乱，T2DM 患者在诊断时可能已经出现糖尿病的长期微血管或大血管并发症。因此，患者可能发生心血管事件（如急性心肌梗死），然后偶然被发现患有 T2DM。

代谢综合征　胰岛素抵抗、糖尿病前期和 T2DM 常伴随其他心血管危险因素，包括腹型或内脏肥胖、血脂异常和高血压，这进一步增加了心血管疾病的易感性。代谢综合征这一术语用于指具有这些危险因素组合的患者。不同的专家小组提出了不同但有重叠的代谢综合征诊断标准。美国国家胆固醇教育计划成人治疗小组 Ⅲ（ATP Ⅲ）将代谢综合征定义为以下 5 项特征中存在任何 3 项：

1. 空腹血糖 ≥ 100 mg/dl 或已用药物治疗高血糖

2. 男性高密度脂蛋白（HDL）胆固醇 < 40 mg/dl，女性 < 50 mg/dl，或已用药物治疗低 HDL 胆固醇

3. 血浆甘油三酯 ≥ 150 mg/dl 或已用药物治疗高甘油三酯血症

4. 腹型肥胖（男性腰围 ≥ 102 cm 或女性腰围 ≥ 88 cm）

5. 血压 ≥ 130/85 mmHg 或已用药物治疗高血压

关于代谢综合征是否是一个独立的实体疾病仍存在争议，但对它的认识确实引起了人们对心血管危险因素的关注。

治疗

T2DM 患者应在诊断时开始接受营养咨询，包括超重或肥胖患者的减重。饮食调整（特别是减少热量摄入）可使许多患者的血糖水平迅速改善，而无须其他干预措施。部分患者体重减轻 10% ～ 20% 即可对胰岛素抵抗和血糖产生显著的有益效果。

根据初始血糖水平、有无高血糖相关症状及是否存在其他并发症，可以决定初始治疗仅采用饮食干预还是同时开始药物治疗。有明显高血糖、液体丢失、与高渗状态相关的精神状况改变和 DKA 的患者，应住院接受紧急治疗（见下文）。

对于大多数 T2DM 患者，可在门诊进行治疗。可在线获取 ADA 和欧洲糖尿病研究协会的指南。大多数专家小组建议从 1 种或 2 种口服降糖药开始治疗（取决于高血糖的程度），如果效果不佳，则加用第 3 种口服药物或胰岛素。对于明显高血糖（≥ 300 mg/dl 或 HbA1c > 10%）的患者，应考虑在起病时就开始使用胰岛素。在 T2DM 中，β 细胞功能通常逐渐丧失，有时持续多年，这导致需要随时间而增加剂量或额外的降糖药物，最终通常需要使用胰岛素。与 T1DM 一样，T2DM 的总体管理不仅应包括治疗高血糖，干预措施还应包括评估、降低风险和治疗长期微血管和大血管并发症。

血糖控制　英国糖尿病预防研究（UKPDS）和其他随机对照试验证实，改善血糖控制可降低 T2DM 患者微血管长期并发症（视网膜病变、肾病和神经病变）的风险。并发症风险从超过正常血糖的任何增量开始逐渐增加。随机临床试验尚未证实优化 T2DM 患者的血糖控制可以改善大血管并发症（即心血管疾病）的结局。T2DM 患者（特别是年龄较大或有合并症的患者）在管理严格血糖控制方案方面的能力可能有限，且对低血糖不良反应的易感性增加。因此，应个体化制定 HbA1c 目标，以平衡改善微血管并发症的获益与低血糖的风险。对于较年轻的 T2DM 患者，HbA1c ≤ 7% 是适当的目标，而对于年龄较大、有并发症和预期寿命有限的患者，HbA1c ≤ 8% 可能是一个可接受且更安全的目标。应每 6 个月检测 1 次 HbA1c，如果血糖控制不稳定或正在调整治疗方案，则应每 3 个月检测 1 次。如果患者正在接受可能引起低血糖的药物（磺酰脲类、格列奈类和胰岛素）治疗，则应定期进行 SMBG。对于使用不会引起低血糖的药物的患

TABLE 5.7	Non-Insulin Antidiabetic Agents by Drug Class[a]		
Drug Class	**Available Agents (Generic Name)**	**Route of Administration**	**Mode of Action**
Biguanide	Metformin	Oral	Insulin sensitizer
SGLT2 inhibitors	Canagliflozin, dapagliflozin, empagliflozin, ertugliflozin	Oral	Increase urinary glucose excretion
GLP-1 receptor agonists	Dulaglutide, exenatide, liraglutide, lixisenatide, semaglutide	Subcutaneous injection, semaglutide oral	Incretin mimetic
DPP-4 inhibitors	Alogliptin, linagliptin, saxagliptin, sitagliptin	Oral	Incretin amplifier
Thiazolidinediones	Pioglitazone, rosiglitazone	Oral	Insulin sensitizer
Sulfonylureas	Glipizide, glyburide, glimeperide, gliclazide, chlorpro-pamide, tolazamide	Oral	Insulin secretagogue
Meglitinides	Repaglinide, nateglinide	Oral	Insulin secretagogue
α-Glucosidase inhibitors	Acarbose, miglitol	Oral	Delay carbohydrate digestion/absorption
Amylin mimetics	Pramlintide	Subcutaneous injection	Delay gastric emptying, suppress glucagon

DPP-4, Dipeptidyl peptidase-4; *GLP-1,* glucagon-like peptide-1; *SGLT2,* sodium glucose co-transporter 2.
[a]Consult current manufacturer information for details on available combinations, prescribing, and safety.

illnesses or with occurrence of symptoms suggestive of hyperglycemia is advisable.

Non-insulin pharmacologic (antidiabetic) agents in T2DM. Non-insulin pharmacologic agents from many different drug classes are available for treatment of T2DM, some taken orally and others by injection (Table 5.7). When non-insulin pharmacologic agents are appropriate, metformin is generally preferred as first-line therapy because of its glucose-lowering efficacy, absence of weight gain and hypoglycemia, favorable safety and tolerability profile based on many years of clinical experience, and low cost. For patients who are unable to tolerate metformin, the choice of an alternative drug may be influenced by considerations such as glucose-lowering efficacy, patient preference for an oral versus an injectable agent, potential adverse effects (e.g., hypoglycemia, weight gain, or fluid retention), the presence of comorbidities (cardiovascular disease, heart failure, or chronic renal insufficiency), and cost. For patients with established atherosclerotic cardiovascular disease or chronic kidney disease (CKD), a sodium glucose cotransporter (SGLT2) inhibitor or glucagon-like peptide-1 (GLP-1) receptor agonist with established cardiovascular disease or CKD benefit should be considered. For patients with atherosclerotic heart disease and heart failure or high risk of heart failure, an SGLT2 inhibitor might be most appropriate. Dipeptidyl peptidase-4 (DPP-4) inhibitors represent another reasonable option as well-tolerated agents with established cardiovascular safety. When drug cost is a critical issue, a sulfonylurea is a reasonable choice, although these drugs have the disadvantages of inducing modest weight gain and causing hypoglycemia. Pioglitazone is another low-cost agent that is effective in lowering blood glucose, but it is associated with increased risk of fluid retention and heart failure.

If a single drug is tolerated but does not adequately control blood glucose levels, the usual practice is to continue that drug and add a second from a distinct drug class with choice of agent influenced by the factors stated previously. In patients with marked hyperglycemia (e.g., with $HbA_{1c} \geq 1.5\%$ above target) that is not judged severe enough to merit insulin treatment, two agents may be started from the outset. This has the potential advantage of more rapidly achieving blood glucose control but the disadvantage of exposing patients to the potential side effects of taking two drugs simultaneously. Many combination preparations are available for administration of more than one drug; these are more convenient for patients and sometimes less expensive than taking the multiple drugs separately.

Available non-insulin antidiabetic agents are summarized here and in Table 5.7. Current manufacturer information should be consulted before prescribing these drugs to ensure updated and adequately detailed information on available single and combination agents and their effective and safe use.

Metformin. Metformin is an oral agent in the biguanide class that produces its most prominent effects by decreasing gluconeogenesis and thus reducing hepatic glucose production. This insulin-sensitizing effect is associated with a low risk of hypoglycemia. It has been in use for more than 30 years and is available in inexpensive generic form. The usual starting dose is 500 mg once or twice daily with incremental advancement at several-week intervals to a usual maximum of 2000 mg daily in two or three divided doses. Metformin typically decreases HbA_{1c} by up to 1.5%. Further benefits include modest weight loss (approximately 3 kg on average) and a small improvement in plasma lipid profile (decrease in low-density lipoprotein [LDL]-cholesterol and triglycerides and increase in HDL). Adverse reactions include gastrointestinal effects and, rarely, lactic acidosis. The drug should be avoided in patients with an estimated glomerular filtration rate (eGFR) of <30 mL/min/1.73m^2 and used at decreased dosage with an eGFR of 30 to 45 mL/min/1.73m^2.

SGLT2 inhibitors. Canagliflozin, dapagliflozin, empagliflozin, and ertugliflozin function by inhibiting SGLT2. SGLT2 mediates more than 90% of glucose reabsorption in the proximal renal tubule, and the drug lowers blood glucose levels by promoting excretion of glucose in the urine. This typically results in a decrease in HbA_{1c} in the range of 0.5% to 1.0%, plus modest weight loss (2-3 kg on average) and decrease in blood pressure. The mechanism of action is independent of insulin, and this class of drugs does not cause hypoglycemia. Large-scale, prospective, randomized clinical trials have shown decreased major cardiovascular events in T2DM patients with established cardiovascular disease with canagliflozin and empagliflozin. These studies, plus a similar trial with dapagliflozin in T2DM patients with milder cardiovascular disease history, have shown decreases in hospitalization for heart failure and progression of diabetic nephropathy. As a result, drugs in this class appear to be a favorable choice in patients with established cardiovascular disease or diabetic nephropathy. Concerns about potential side effects include urinary and genital infections, hypotension, acute renal injury, fractures in the context of low bone mineral density, increased lower extremity amputations, and DKA. Further studies will be needed to validate the benefits and potential adverse effects of these drugs and determine whether some of these responses are specific to individual members of the drug class. They are taken orally once daily, with dosage specific to each drug.

Glucagon-like peptide-1 receptor agonists. GLP-1 is one of several hormones produced in the small intestine (designated *incretins*) that modify gastrointestinal motility and insulin secretion. The GLP-1 receptor agonists, dulaglutide, exenatide, liraglutide, lixisenatide, and

表 5.7 非胰岛素抗糖尿病药物的分类 [a]

药物分类	药物（通用名）	给药途径	作用机制
双胍类	二甲双胍	口服	胰岛素增敏剂
SGLT2 抑制剂	卡格列净、达格列净、恩格列净、艾托格列净	口服	增加尿液葡萄糖排泄
GLP-1 受体激动剂	度拉糖肽、艾塞那肽、利拉鲁肽、利西那肽、司美格鲁肽	皮下注射，司美格鲁肽口服	肠降血糖素模拟剂
DPP-4 抑制剂	阿格列汀、利格列汀、沙格列汀、西格列汀	口服	肠降血糖素放大剂
噻唑烷二酮类	吡格列酮、罗格列酮	口服	胰岛素增敏剂
磺酰脲类	格列吡嗪、格列本脲、格列美脲、格列齐特、氯磺丙脲、妥拉磺脲	口服	胰岛素促泌剂
格列奈类	瑞格列奈、那格列奈	口服	胰岛素促泌剂
α-葡萄糖苷酶抑制剂	阿卡波糖、米格列醇	口服	延缓碳水化合物消化/吸收
胰岛淀粉素模拟剂	普兰林肽	皮下注射	延缓胃排空，抑制胰高血糖素

DPP-4，二肽基肽酶 -4；GLP-1，胰高血糖素样肽 -1；SGLT2，钠-葡萄糖耦联转运体 2。
[a] 有关可用组合、处方和安全性的详细信息，请查阅生产商的最新信息。

者，通常不需要定期 SMBG，但是建议在出现并发症或提示高血糖的症状时进行检测。

治疗 T2DM 的非胰岛素（抗糖尿病）药物 多种类型的非胰岛素药物可用于治疗 T2DM，其中部分为口服剂型，部分为注射剂型（表 5.7）。当患者适用非胰岛素药物时，通常首选二甲双胍作为一线治疗，因其降糖效果好，不会导致体重增加和低血糖，多年临床经验显示其安全性和耐受性良好，且价格低廉。对于不能耐受二甲双胍的患者，选择替代药物时可能受到降糖效果，患者对口服与注射的偏好，潜在不良反应（如低血糖、体重增加或液体潴留），合并症（心血管疾病、心力衰竭或慢性肾功能不全）和成本等因素的影响。对于已经确诊动脉粥样硬化性心血管疾病或慢性肾脏病（CKD）的患者，应考虑使用已证明具有心血管疾病或 CKD 获益的钠-葡萄糖耦联转运体 2（SGLT2）抑制剂或胰高血糖素样肽 -1（GLP-1）受体激动剂。对于动脉粥样硬化性心脏病和心力衰竭或心力衰竭高风险的患者，SGLT2 抑制剂可能是最佳选择。二肽基肽酶 -4（DPP-4）抑制剂是另一个合理的选择，其耐受性良好，已被证明具有心血管安全性。当药物成本是一个关键问题时，磺酰脲类药物是合理的选择，尽管这些药物有导致体重增加和引起低血糖的缺点。吡格列酮是另一种低成本药物，能有效降低血糖，但它与液体潴留和心力衰竭风险增加相关。

如果单一药物可耐受但不能完全控制血糖，通常的做法是继续使用该药物并添加第 2 种不同类别的药物，选择药物需考虑的因素如前所述。在明显高血糖的患者中（如 HbA1c 超过目标值 ≥ 1.5%），如果认为尚未严重到需要胰岛素治疗，则可以从一开始就使用两种药物。这具有更快实现血糖控制的潜在优势，但缺点是使患者暴露于同时服用两种药物的潜在副作用。目前有多种组合制剂可供使用；这些复方制剂对患者来说更方便，有时比单独服用多种药物更便宜。

非胰岛素抗糖尿病药物见表 5.7。在开具这些药物处方之前，应查阅生产商的最新信息，以确保获得关于现有单药和复方制剂及其有效性和安全性的最新详细信息。

二甲双胍 二甲双胍是一种口服双胍类药物，其最显著的作用是通过减少糖异生来降低肝脏葡萄糖生成。这种胰岛素增敏作用与低血糖风险低相关。二甲双胍已上市 30 多年，并有廉价的仿制药。通常起始剂量为 500 mg，1～2 次/日，每隔数周递增 1 次，通常最大剂量为 2000 mg/d，分 2～3 次服用。二甲双胍通常可使 HbA1c 降低 1.5%。其他益处包括适度减重（平均约 3 kg）和轻度改善血脂水平［降低低密度脂蛋白（LDL）胆固醇和甘油三酯，升高 HDL］。不良反应包括胃肠道反应及罕见的乳酸性酸中毒。估算的肾小球滤过率（eGFR）< 30 ml/（min·1.73 m²）的患者应避免使用二甲双胍，eGFR 为 30～45 ml/（min·1.73 m²）的患者应减量使用。

SGLT2 抑制剂 卡格列净、达格列净、恩格列净和艾托格列净可通过抑制 SGLT2 来发挥作用。SGLT2 介导近曲小管中超过 90% 的葡萄糖重吸收，该药物通过促进葡萄糖在尿液中的排泄来降低血糖水平。使用 SGLT2 抑制剂通常可使 HbA1c 降低 0.5%～1.0%、适度减重（平均 2～3 kg）和血压降低。其作用机制独立于胰岛素，且该类药物不会引起低血糖。大型前瞻性随机临床试验表明，卡格列净和恩格列净在已确诊心血管疾病的 T2DM 患者中可减少主要心血管事件。这些研究和一项针对达格列净治疗心血管疾病病史较轻的 T2DM 患者的类似试验显示，患者的心力衰竭住院率和糖尿病肾病进展率均有所下降。因此，SGLT2 抑制剂似乎是心血管疾病或糖尿病肾病患者的首选。潜在副作用包括泌尿和生殖系统感染、低血压、急性肾损伤、低骨密度骨折、增加下肢截肢和 DKA 的风险。尚需要进一步的研究来验证这些药物的益处和潜在不良反应，并确定其中一些反应是否是该类药物的个别成员所特有的。使用方法为每天口服 1 次，具体剂量应基于每种药物而定。

GLP-1 受体激动剂 GLP-1 是小肠产生的一种激素（被称为肠降血糖素），能够调节胃肠动力和胰岛素分泌。GLP-1 受体激动剂（度拉糖肽、艾塞那肽、利

semaglutide, bind to GLP-1 receptors and improve blood glucose control by enhancing glucose-dependent insulin secretion, slowing gastric emptying, suppressing postprandial glucagon production, and decreasing food intake through enhanced satiety. This results in decreases in HbA_{1c} by 0.5% to 1.5% and modest weight loss (in the range of 3 kg). There is evidence for improved cardiovascular outcomes for several of these agents in patients with established cardiovascular disease and possibly an improvement in CKD outcomes. They may be a favorable choice as a second-line drug for glycemia management if weight loss is a goal and in patients with established cardiovascular disease, with attention to the data available for specific agents. Because of their relatively high efficacy, GLP-1 receptor agonists are a reasonable option to consider before starting insulin in patients not adequately controlled on other agents. Most members of this drug class are administered via injection with prefilled pens, twice daily, once daily, or once weekly depending on the specific drug, and semaglutide also is available in an orally administered form. The most common side effects are nausea and sometimes diarrhea, likely related to effects on gastrointestinal motility, and these agents should not be used in patients with a history of pancreatitis or in combination with DPP-4 inhibitors.

Dipeptidyl peptidase-4 inhibitors. DPP-4 inhibitors (alogliptin, linagliptin, saxagliptin, and sitagliptin) block the deactivation of GLP-1 and glucose-dependent insulinotropic peptide (GIP), peptide hormones that are important in the regulation of glucose homeostasis. DPP-4 inhibitors are taken orally and result in decreased HbA_{1c} in the range of 0.5% to 1.0%. They have a low risk of causing hypoglycemia, have neutral effects on cardiovascular disease outcomes and body weight, and can be used in the context of CKD with agent-specific dose reductions. They have generally favorable side effect profiles, although there is concern that some members of the class may increase heart failure risk. They should not be used in combination with GLP-1 receptor agonists.

Pioglitazone. The thiazolidinedione, pioglitazone, activates the nuclear peroxisome proliferator-activated receptor-γ, which leads to changes in transcription rates of multiple genes. The net effect is reduced insulin resistance, resulting in increased glucose uptake in peripheral tissues and reduced hepatic glucose production. Pioglitazone typically lowers HbA_{1c} by 0.5% to 1.4% and is available as a low-cost drug. It carries a low risk of hypoglycemia, but potential side effects include weight gain, fluid retention and heart failure, hepatoxicity, concerns about increased fracture risk in the setting of low bone density, and a potential link to bladder cancer. Another member of this drug class, rosiglitazone, is little used because of its potential link to increased cardiovascular events.

Sulfonylureas. Sulfonylureas stimulate endogenous insulin secretion by binding and activating potassium channels in beta cells. In patients with adequate residual beta-cell function, they can lower HbA_{1c} levels by 1% to 2%. Drugs in this class have been in clinical use for more than 40 years, and many inexpensive, generic sulfonylureas are available that differ in duration of action, metabolism, and mode of clearance. Because they can increase insulin secretion even in the absence of hyperglycemia, they have significant potential to cause hypoglycemia. Patients need to be instructed how to recognize and treat hypoglycemia before starting a sulfonylurea. Factors that increase the risk for hypoglycemia with sulfonylureas include advanced age, poor nutrition, alcohol ingestion, and hepatic and renal insufficiency. Other disadvantages of this drug class are a tendency to cause weight gain and a yet unresolved concern about increased risk for cardiovascular events.

Meglitinides. Repaglinide and nateglinide activate beta cell potassium channels and thus stimulate endogenous insulin secretion through a mechanism similar to that of sulfonylureas, although they generally result in less reduction in blood glucose than sulfonylureas. They have rapid action and have less tendency to cause hypoglycemia than sulfonylureas. Their use has been limited by high cost and lack of advantage over the sulfonylureas.

α-Glucosidase inhibitors. The α-glucosidase inhibitors, acarbose and miglitol, are oral agents that improve glycemia by inhibiting the enzymatic breakdown of complex carbohydrates within the lumen of the small intestine. They have modest glucose-lowering effects, decreasing HbA_{1c} in the range of 0.5% to 0.8%. Their use is limited by the frequent occurrence of flatulence and diarrhea as a consequence of undigested carbohydrates reaching lower intestinal regions.

Pramlintide. Pramlintide is a stable analogue of the beta-cell peptide, amylin, which has actions that include slowing of gastric emptying, satiety effects that decrease food intake, and decrease in postmeal glucagon. It is not widely used because of required multiple injections and limited efficacy in lowering HbA1c.

Insulin treatment in T2DM. For patients who have inadequate glycemic control with oral agents, insulin may be started as a basal supplement to the oral regimen. Frequently used choices include glargine or detemir (once or twice daily), degludec (once daily), or NPH (once daily at bedtime) (see later discussion and Table 5.5 for more details on different types of insulin). Starting doses are typically in the range of 10 U (or can be more specifically calculated as 0.2 U/kg), with increases of 2 to 4 U at intervals of 3 days or longer based on blood glucose response. Oral agent regimens commonly are simplified at the time of starting insulin (e.g., shifting from multiple agents to a single oral agent). For patients who do not achieve adequate control with basal insulin, mealtime coverage is provided by a rapid-acting insulin. Often, under this circumstance, all oral agents are discontinued, and blood glucose control is achieved with the use of exogenous insulin alone. Compared to patients with T1DM, those with T2DM may not require as tight a match of carbohydrate to insulin doses at meals, perhaps because of some residual insulin secretion. For this reason, insulin pumps are less frequently used in T2DM.

Nutritional and weight management. Patients should receive counseling from a dietician and be assisted in developing a nutritional plan that is individualized to their lifestyle, exercise, culture, and financial resources. Guidelines from many current expert panels allow flexibility in the relative amounts of carbohydrate, fat, and protein. Nutritional management in T2DM often has a major focus on achieving reductions in calorie intake and weight loss. Achieving weight loss may be made more difficult by a tendency of some oral antidiabetic agents and also insulin to induce a degree of weight gain.

An important goal of nutritional management should be to balance the timing and quantities of ingested macronutrients with medications and exercise to help achieve targets for blood glucose control without periods of hypoglycemia.

For overweight or obese patients, it often is practical to set an initial goal of losing 5% to 10% of body weight. This may significantly improve diabetes control and increase the patient's motivation to then set goals for further weight loss (see Chapter 6).

Bariatric surgical procedures represent a method for achieving weight loss and potentially dramatic improvements in glycemia and risk factors for long-term complications in T2DM. Patients typically have improvements in glycemic control and lower requirements for antidiabetic medications within days after undergoing the Roux-en-Y gastric bypass procedure. This is thought to reflect changes in gut hormones and metabolic factors independent of weight loss. Beneficial effects on glucose control develop more gradually after the placement of an adjustable gastric band, sleeve gastrectomy, or other device.

拉鲁肽、利西那肽和司美格鲁肽）与 GLP-1 受体结合，并通过增强葡萄糖依赖性胰岛素分泌、减慢胃排空、抑制餐后胰高血糖素生成及通过增强饱腹感减少食物摄入，从而改善血糖控制。这可导致 HbA1c 水平下降 0.5% ～ 1.5%，并有适度的体重减轻（约 3 kg）。有证据表明，多种 GLP-1 受体激动剂可改善已确诊心血管疾病患者的心血管结局，并可能改善 CKD 结局。对于已确诊心血管疾病的患者，如果目标是减重，则 GLP-1 受体激动剂可能是血糖管理首选的二线药物，具体取决于特定药物的数据。由于疗效相对较好，GLP-1 受体激动剂是其他药物控制不佳的患者在开始使用胰岛素之前的合理选择。大多数 GLP-1 受体激动剂可通过预填充笔注射给药，可 2 次 / 日、1 次 / 日或 1 次 / 周，具体取决于特定的药物，司美格鲁肽还有口服剂型。最常见的副作用是恶心和偶尔腹泻，可能与对胃肠动力的影响有关，这些药物不应用于有胰腺炎病史的患者或与 DPP-4 抑制剂联合使用。

DPP-4 抑制剂　DPP-4 抑制剂（阿格列汀、利格列汀、沙格列汀和西格列汀）可阻断 GLP-1 和葡萄糖依赖性促胰岛素肽（GIP）的失活，这些肽激素在调节葡萄糖稳态中很重要。DPP-4 抑制剂为口服给药，可使 HbA1c 水平下降 0.5% ～ 1.0%，引起低血糖的风险低，对心血管疾病预后和体重影响不大，且 CKD 患者可以使用，但特定药物需要减少剂量。DPP-4 抑制剂的副作用较少，但部分药物仍有可能增加心力衰竭的风险。DPP-4 抑制剂不应与 GLP-1 受体激动剂联合使用。

吡格列酮　噻唑烷二酮类药物吡格列酮可激活核过氧化物酶体增殖物激活受体 -γ，导致多个基因的转录速率发生变化，其总体作用是减轻胰岛素抵抗，增加外周组织对葡萄糖的摄取，并减少肝脏产生葡萄糖。吡格列酮通常可使 HbA1c 降低 0.5% ～ 1.4%，且价格低廉。它引起低血糖的风险低，潜在的副作用包括体重增加、液体潴留和心力衰竭、肝毒性、增加低骨密度患者的骨折风险，以及与膀胱癌潜在相关。由于可能增加心血管事件，这类药物的另一个成员罗格列酮很少被使用。

磺酰脲类药物　磺酰脲类药物通过结合并激活 β 细胞中的钾通道来刺激内源性胰岛素分泌。在有足够残余 β 细胞功能的患者中，它们可使 HbA1c 降低 1% ～ 2%。这类药物已在临床使用超过 40 年，且有多种作用持续时间、代谢和清除方式不同的价格低廉的仿制磺酰脲类药物。由于它们在没有高血糖的情况下也能增加胰岛素分泌，因此会显著增加低血糖风险。在使用磺酰脲类药物之前，需要指导患者如何识别和治疗低血糖。增加用药后低血糖风险的因素包括高龄、营养不良、饮酒和肝肾功能不全。这类药物的其他缺点是可能导致体重增加和心血管事件的风险增加。

格列奈类　瑞格列奈和那格列奈可激活 β 细胞钾通道，从而刺激内源性胰岛素分泌，这与磺酰脲类药物的作用机制类似，但它们降低血糖的幅度通常小于磺酰脲类药物。这类药物起效迅速，引起低血糖的风险小于磺酰脲类药物。比磺酰脲类药物相比，格列奈类药物的成本高且缺乏优势，因此其应用受到限制。

α - 葡萄糖苷酶抑制剂　α - 葡萄糖苷酶抑制剂阿卡波糖和米格列醇为口服药物，可通过抑制小肠内多糖碳水化合物的酶解作用来改善血糖。它们有适度的降血糖效果，可使 HbA1c 降低 0.5% ～ 0.8%。这类药物的使用受到频繁发生腹胀和腹泻的限制，这是由于未消化的碳水化合物到达小肠下部区域。

普兰林肽　普兰林肽是一种 β 细胞肽——胰岛淀粉素的稳定类似物，其作用包括减慢胃排空、增加饱腹感，从而减少食物摄入，降低餐后胰高血糖素水平。由于需要多次注射且在降低 HbA1c 方面的疗效有限，其未被广泛使用。

T2DM 的胰岛素治疗　对于使用口服药物后血糖控制不佳的患者，可在口服治疗方案的基础上开始基础胰岛素补充治疗。常用的选择包括甘精胰岛素或地特胰岛素（1 次 / 日或 2 次 / 日）、德谷胰岛素（1 次 / 日）或 NPH（每晚 1 次）（不同类型胰岛素的详细信息见下文和表 5.5）。起始剂量通常为 10 U（或按 0.2 U/kg 计算），根据血糖反应，在 3 天或更长间隔后增加 2 ～ 4 U。在起始胰岛素治疗时，通常会简化口服药物方案（如由多种药物转变为单一口服药物）。对于使用基础胰岛素无法达到充分控制的患者，可通过速效胰岛素提供餐时覆盖。在这种情况下，通常会停用所有口服药物，仅通过外源性胰岛素来进行血糖控制。与 T1DM 患者相比，T2DM 患者可能不需要在餐时将碳水化合物与胰岛素剂量严格匹配，这可能是因为还有部分残余的胰岛素分泌。因此，T2DM 患者较少使用胰岛素泵。

营养和体重管理　患者应进行营养咨询，并在营养师的帮助下制订适应其生活方式、运动、文化和经济状况的个体化营养计划。当前许多专家小组的指南允许灵活控制碳水化合物、脂肪和蛋白质的相对摄入量。T2DM 的营养管理通常主要关注减少热量摄入和减重。部分口服降糖药和胰岛素可导致一定程度的体重增加，使得实现减重变得更加困难。

营养管理的一个重要目标应是在摄入宏量营养素的时机和数量与药物和运动之间达到平衡，以帮助实现血糖控制目标，同时避免低血糖。

对于超重或肥胖症患者，最初设定的目标通常是减重 5% ～ 10%。这可能显著改善糖尿病控制，并增加患者设定进一步减重目标的动力（见第 6 章）。

减重术是实现减重的一种方法，可能显著改善 T2DM 的血糖控制和长期并发症风险。患者在接受 Roux-en-Y 胃旁路手术后的数天内通常能获得血糖控制的改善，且对降糖药物的需求降低。这反映了与减重无关的胃肠激素和代谢因素的变化。在放置可调节胃

Randomized trials comparing bariatric surgery with medical nutrition therapy alone for weight loss have shown greater efficacy in achieving HbA$_{1c}$ goals with surgery, and some studies have shown dramatic rates of remission, with 75% of patients or more becoming normoglycemic off all antidiabetic agents (see Chapter 6).

Exercise. Physical exercise should be encouraged in T2DM as an important component of weight loss regimens and also for its beneficial effects in decreasing the risks of long-term complications. The general recommendation of several expert panels is 30 minutes or more of moderate-intensity physical exercise on at least 5 days per week, but the regimen needs to be highly individualized according to a patient's capabilities and limitations imposed by other medical conditions such as cardiovascular disease. Patients who are unwilling or unable to undertake significant aerobic exercise should be encouraged to do daily walking or other physical activities within their limitations.

Standards of Care in T1DM and T2DM in Addition to Blood Glucose Control

A number of assessments and interventions should be performed at intervals in patients with T1DM or T2DM. These include blood pressure measurement and examination of the feet at each physician visit. Patients who smoke should receive counseling at each visit about the importance of and strategies for discontinuing. A dilated eye examination should be performed annually, or more often in patients with diabetic eye disease. A dental examination also should be performed at least annually. Starting 5 years after disease onset in T1DM and at the time of diagnosis in T2DM, patients should have annual measurement of their urinary albumin/creatinine ratio with confirmation if elevated (>30 mg albumin per gram of creatinine). A fasting lipid profile should be obtained annually. Aspirin (75 to 162 mg daily) is usually recommended for secondary prevention of cardiovascular disease (supported by clinical trial evidence) or for primary prevention in patients with a 10-year cardiovascular risk greater than 10% (based on expert opinion). Influenza vaccination should be provided yearly; pneumococcal immunization should be given once and then repeated after age 65 (see latest CDC recommendations).

Management of Diabetes During Intercurrent Illness

Diabetes often requires changes in the blood glucose management regimen during an intercurrent illness to accommodate potential decreases in nutrient intake and increases in insulin resistance secondary to disease-related release of stress hormones. Patients with T1DM require exogenous insulin administration at all times to prevent marked hyperglycemia and DKA, even if they are unable to consume nutrients during an illness (e.g., with gastroenteritis). Depending on the degree and duration of interruption of food intake, they may require a transient, partial reduction in insulin dosage as well as more frequent glucose monitoring. Alternatively, if they are consuming a normal diet, they may require a modest increase in insulin dose because of insulin resistance related to the stress of illness. T2DM patients taking oral agents who are undergoing surgical procedures or are hospitalized for serious illness often require discontinuation of the oral agents and use of insulin to control blood glucose until normal eating patterns are resumed.

For hospitalized patients, blood glucose target goals are adjusted to prevent marked hyperglycemia and at the same time protect against hypoglycemia. For noncritical illness, typical blood glucose targets include lowest levels of 90 to 100 mg/dL, premeal levels lower than 140 mg/dL, and random levels lower than 180 mg/dL. For critically ill patients, intravenous insulin infusion may be needed to allow for rapid adjustments in dosage, and the blood glucose range recommended by most expert panels is 140 to 180 mg/dL.

Gestational Diabetes Mellitus

The hormonal environment of pregnancy results in insulin resistance and therefore predisposes to the development or unmasking of diabetes during pregnancy. GDM occurs in 2% to 5% of all pregnancies and is associated with consequences for both mother and fetus if untreated. For this reason, screening for GDM is routinely performed between 24 and 28 weeks of gestation in women older than 25 years of age and in younger women who fulfill one or more of the risk criteria in Table 5.6 (2a through 2d and 2g). Women who are at high risk (i.e., those who are obese, have a personal history of GDM, glycosuria, or have a first-degree relative with diabetes) should be screened at their initial obstetric or prenatal visit. A broadly accepted approach to screening is a 2-hour 75-g oral glucose tolerance test with cutoff values as specified in Table 5.2.

A detailed discussion of the approach to managing GDM and also preexisting diabetes during pregnancy is beyond the scope of this chapter. The fundamental principles include diet, exercise, and glucose-lowering oral agents or insulin as needed. Blood glucose goals are set lower than in nonpregnant individuals because of the importance of minimizing exposure of the fetus to hyperglycemia: fasting, 95 mg/dL (5.3 mmol/L) or lower; 1-hour postprandial, 140 mg/dL (7.8 mmol/L) or lower; and 2-hours postprandial, 120 mg/dL (6.7 mmol/L) or lower. HbA$_{1c}$ levels may be useful in establishing the presence of hyperglycemia before its discovery during pregnancy, but they have limited value in managing GDM. Women with GDM should be reevaluated with a 75-g glucose tolerance test 6 to 12 weeks after delivery, at which point approximately 10% will still have overt diabetes. Up to 40% of women with GDM go on to develop diabetes in the subsequent 20 years, with this risk varying substantially depending on ethnic background and obesity. Pregnancy serves as a provocative test and not as a risk factor for the future development of diabetes.

Management of Severe Metabolic Decompensation in Diabetes
Diabetic Ketoacidosis

DKA develops most commonly in patients with T1DM (approximately 2.5 cases per 100 T1DM patients per year). It also can occur in those with T2DM, especially during acute illness (severe infection, medical illness, or trauma), and in a subset of *ketosis-prone* T2DM patients. DKA is present in approximately 25% of T1DM patients at diagnosis and otherwise most often develops when patients with known T1DM stop taking prescribed insulin. It is a potentially life-threatening condition that has an overall mortality rate of approximately 1% to 2%, with most deaths resulting from complicating or precipitating medical conditions rather than the metabolic disturbances of DKA itself.

The pathophysiology of DKA results from the combined effects of insulin deficiency and increased levels of *insulin counter-regulatory (stress) hormones*. With insulin deficiency, glucose levels rise as a consequence of decreased uptake and metabolism by body tissues, the breakdown of hepatic glycogen stores (*glycogenolysis*), and net glucose production by the liver and kidney (*gluconeogenesis*). Catabolism of muscle proteins as a result of low insulin levels leads to the release of amino acids, which provide substrate that further drives gluconeogenesis. Because glucose is being synthesized endogenously, blood glucose levels rise markedly, even in the fasted state. Blood glucose levels greater than 170 mg/dL result in glycosuria. Excretion of glucose in the urine necessitates the co-excretion of large amounts of water and electrolytes (Na$^+$ and K$^+$). Patients experience polyuria but cannot

束带、袖状胃切除术或其他装置后，对血糖控制的有益效果会逐渐显现。比较减重术和单纯医学营养治疗的随机试验表明，手术在实现 HbA1c 达标方面更有效，一些研究显示，≥ 75% 的患者在停用所有降糖药物后血糖恢复正常（见第 6 章）。

运动 应鼓励 T2DM 患者运动，并将其作为减重方案的重要组成部分，这有助于降低长期并发症的风险。多个专家小组的一般建议是每周至少运动 5 天，每天进行 ≥ 30 min 的中等强度运动，但该方案需要根据患者的体能和其他医疗状况（如心血管疾病）的限制来制订高度个体化的方案。对于不愿意或无法进行大量有氧运动的患者，应鼓励他们在能力范围内每天散步或进行其他运动。

除血糖控制外的 T1DM 和 T2DM 管理标准

在 T1DM 或 T2DM 患者中，应定期进行多项评估和干预。包括每次就诊时测量血压和检查足部。吸烟患者应在每次就诊时接受关于戒烟重要性和策略的咨询。患者应每年进行 1 次散瞳眼底检查，糖尿病眼病患者应提高检查频率。患者还应每年至少进行 1 次口腔科检查。在 T1DM 发病后 5 年和诊断 T2DM 后，患者应每年检测尿白蛋白 / 肌酐比值，并在比值升高（> 30 mg/g）时进行确认。应每年检测 1 次空腹血脂谱。通常推荐使用阿司匹林（75 ～ 162 mg/d）进行心血管疾病的二级预防（已得到临床试验证据的支持）或用于 10 年心血管风险 > 10% 的患者（基于专家意见）的一级预防。患者应每年接种流感疫苗，并应接种 1 次肺炎球菌疫苗，然后在 65 岁以后再接种 1 次（参见最新的 CDC 建议）。

并发症期间的糖尿病管理

在出现并发症期间，糖尿病患者通常需要改变血糖管理方案，以适应因疾病相关的营养摄入减少和应激激素释放而导致的胰岛素抵抗增加。T1DM 患者需要始终接受外源性胰岛素治疗，以防止明显的高血糖和 DKA，即使是在并发症期间（如胃肠炎）无法摄取营养时。根据食物摄入中断的程度和持续时间，患者可能需要暂时部分减少胰岛素剂量及进行更频繁的血糖监测。此外，如果能正常饮食，患者可能需要适当增加胰岛素剂量，因为疾病应激会增加胰岛素抵抗。对于应用口服降糖药的 T2DM 患者，需要接受手术治疗或因严重疾病住院时通常需要停用口服药物，并用胰岛素控制血糖，直到恢复正常的饮食模式。

对于住院患者，需要调整血糖目标值，以防止明显的高血糖，同时预防低血糖。对于非危重症患者，通常最低血糖目标值为 90 ～ 100 mg/dl，餐前血糖 < 140 mg/dl，随机血糖 < 180 mg/dl。对于危重症患者，可能需要静脉注射胰岛素以利于迅速调整剂量，

大多数专家小组推荐的血糖范围为 140 ～ 180 ml/dl。

妊娠期糖尿病

妊娠期间的激素环境会导致胰岛素抵抗，因此妊娠期间易发生糖尿病或进展为显性糖尿病。妊娠期糖尿病（GDM）在全部妊娠患者中的发生率为 2% ～ 5%，如果不治疗，GDM 会对母亲和胎儿产生不良后果。因此，对于 25 岁以上女性和符合表 5.6 中 ≥ 1 个危险因素（2a ～ 2d 和 2g）的年轻女性，通常在妊娠第 24 ～ 28 周进行 GDM 常规筛查。处于高风险的女性（如肥胖症、有 GDM 病史、尿糖阳性或一级亲属患有糖尿病）应在初次产科或产前就诊时进行筛查。普遍接受的筛查方法是进行 2 h 75 g 口服葡萄糖耐量试验，诊断阈值见表 5.2。

有关 GDM 及妊娠期间原有糖尿病的管理方法，本章不进行详细讨论。基本原则包括饮食、运动和必要时使用口服降糖药物或胰岛素。由于尽量减少胎儿暴露于高血糖非常重要，因此血糖目标值应低于非妊娠患者：空腹血糖 ≤ 95 mg/dl（5.3 mmol/L）；餐后 1 h 血糖 ≤ 140 mg/dl（7.8 mmol/L）；餐后 2 h 血糖 ≤ 120 mg/dl（6.7 mmol/L）。HbA1c 水平可能有助于在妊娠期间发现高血糖之前确定高血糖的存在，但在管理 GDM 方面的价值有限。GDM 患者应在分娩后第 6 ～ 12 周进行 75 g 口服葡萄糖耐量试验重新评估，此时约有 10% 的患者仍有显性糖尿病。多达 40% 的 GDM 患者在未来 20 年中会发展为糖尿病，该风险因种族背景和肥胖症程度而有显著差异。妊娠是一种激发性试验，而不是未来发生糖尿病的危险因素。

糖尿病严重代谢紊乱的管理
糖尿病酮症酸中毒

DKA 最常见于 T1DM 患者（每年每 100 名 T1DM 患者中约有 2.5 例发生 DKA）。它也可能见于 T2DM 患者，特别是在急性疾病期间（严重感染、内科疾病或创伤），以及易发生酮症的 T2DM 患者亚组。约 25% 的 T1DM 患者在诊断时存在 DKA，且最常见于 T1DM 患者停用胰岛素时。DKA 是一种可危及生命的状态，总死亡率为 1% ～ 2%，大多数死亡是由于并发症或诱发疾病，而不是 DKA 本身的代谢紊乱。

DKA 的病理生理学机制是胰岛素缺乏和胰岛素反调节（应激）激素水平增加的综合效应。由于胰岛素缺乏，葡萄糖水平升高，这是由于机体组织摄取和代谢葡萄糖减少、肝储备糖原的分解（糖原分解），以及肝和肾的净葡萄糖产生（糖异生）。由于低胰岛素水平导致肌肉蛋白质的分解，导致氨基酸释放，而这些氨基酸为进一步糖异生提供了底物。由于葡萄糖的内源性合成，即使在禁食状态下，患者的血糖水平也会显著升高。血糖 > 170 mg/dl 可导致尿糖阳性。尿液中葡萄糖的排出需要伴随大量水分和电解质（Na^+ 和 K^+）的共同排出。

compensate adequately and become progressively more fluid and electrolyte depleted. The osmotic diuresis is characterized by greater losses of water than electrolytes, and this leads to progressively increasing hyperosmolality. Because of insulin deficiency, there is decreased *lipogenesis* and accelerated *lipolysis* leading to increased levels of circulating free fatty acids, which serve as a substrate for the hepatic synthesis of ketone bodies (β-hydroxybutyrate, acetoacetate, and acetone). β-Hydroxybutyrate and acetoacetate are acids, and their rising plasma levels contribute to the development of a metabolic acidosis.

These processes can result from simple insulin deficiency, but often they are exacerbated by an underlying or precipitating illness, such as an infection. Infection results in insulin resistance secondary to increased levels of *stress hormones* (cortisol, catecholamines, glucagon, and growth hormone). A series of positive feedback loops are thus generated and lead to ever-accelerating hyperglycemia, fluid and electrolyte depletion, ketosis, and metabolic acidosis. More than simple restoration of insulin dosing is required, and patients usually need hospital admission and multicomponent interventions.

Common presenting symptoms in DKA include polyuria, thirst and polydipsia, recent weight loss (especially in new-onset diabetes), blurred vision, weakness, anorexia, nausea and vomiting, abdominal pain (which can mimic acute abdomen), and mental status changes varying from somnolence to coma. DKA and these associated symptoms usually evolve over 2 to 4 days but can have an onset of less than 12 hours in patients using insulin pumps. On physical examination, patients typically have evidence of dehydration, especially intravascular volume depletion, including decreased skin turgor, hypotension, and tachycardia (best assessed in skin overlying the sternum and forehead). The skin may be warm and dry from the vasodilating effects of acidosis, and marked hypotension should generate concern for impending vascular collapse. Patients often have deep, rapid respirations (Kussmaul breathing) as respiratory compensation for the metabolic acidosis, together with a characteristic fruity odor on their breath from exhaled acetone. The diagnosis is made in patients who have (1) a high blood glucose concentration (>250 mg/dL), (2) moderate to severe ketonemia (β-hydroxybutyrate >5 mmol/L or positive ketone levels by Ketostix at a serum dilution of 1:2 or higher), and (3) acidosis (pH <7.3 or plasma bicarbonate ≤15 mEq/L). Measurements of urine ketones may be misleading, because urinary ketones can be positive during fasting in the absence of DKA.

Additional evaluation besides the diagnostic tests already mentioned should include electrolytes, blood urea nitrogen, creatinine, phosphate, liver function tests, and amylase; arterial or mixed venous blood gases (including pH); complete blood count; urinalysis; electrocardiogram; and chest radiographs. The serum anion gap, which is usually greater than 12 mEq/L in DKA, should be calculated (anion gap = $[Na^+] - [Cl^- + HCO_3^-]$). Serum osmolality should be measured directly or calculated: estimated osmolality = $(2 \times [Na^+]) + ([glucose in mg/dL]/18)$.

Precipitating causes of DKA include infection (most common), myocardial infarction (including silent infarction), inflammatory processes (appendicitis, pancreatitis), and medications (especially glucocorticoids).

Treatment of DKA should start promptly with institution of measures to correct life-threatening abnormalities, including insulin deficiency, fluid and electrolyte depletion, potassium (K^+) depletion, and metabolic acidosis. In a typical regimen, regular insulin or a rapid-acting insulin analog is administered as a bolus (0.1 U/kg) followed by a continuous intravenous infusion at 0.1 U/kg/hour. Plasma glucose is monitored hourly until it is less than 250 mg/dL, and the rate of insulin infusion is adjusted as needed to target a rate of blood glucose

decline of 75 to 100 mg/dL/hour to avoid potential complications of rapid shifts in osmolality.

At the time of starting insulin, it is essential to begin fluid and electrolyte replacement. The initial fluid deficit should be estimated based on the magnitude of weight loss (if known), mucous membrane dryness, skin turgor, and whether or not there is postural hypotension, with the knowledge that losses in DKA usually range from 3 to 8 L. A typical program for intravenous fluid replacement starts with 1 L of normal saline in the first hour. Normal saline may then be continued at 15 mL/minute for a second hour depending on the estimated severity of initial fluid depletion. This then may be changed to 0.45% (half-normal) saline at 7.5 mL/minute for the next 2 hours and gradually tapered thereafter to achieve full replacement of the estimated fluid deficit in approximately 8 hours. During that time, there should be frequent monitoring for jugular venous distention and chest auscultation to ensure early detection of fluid overload. Central venous pressure should be monitored in patients who are at risk for congestive heart failure.

Potassium repletion is needed in all patients, and there should be careful monitoring and replacement to ensure that patients do not develop potentially harmful hypokalemia or hyperkalemia. Urine output should be verified with the use of a Foley catheter if necessary before K^+ replacement is started. Unless patients are anuric, K^+ replacement should be initiated within 1 to 2 hours after starting insulin. A key goal is to maintain serum K^+ at all times higher than 3.5 mEq/L, and it is especially important to administer K^+ early in the course of treatment if there is initial hypokalemia or if bicarbonate is administered to correct acidosis, because the latter action promotes a shift of extracellular K^+ into cells. Potassium typically is withheld if the serum K^+ is 5 mEq/L or higher; otherwise, it is administered as part of the intravenous fluid regimen at 10 to 40 mEq/hour depending on the measured serum level. Serum K^+ should be monitored every 2 hours if it is less than 4 or greater than 5 mEq/L.

Bicarbonate infusion in general should be avoided but needs to be considered for patients who have a pH lower than 7, a serum bicarbonate level lower than 5.0 mEq/L, a K^+ concentration greater than 6.5 mEq/L, hypotension unresponsive to fluid replacement, severe left ventricular failure, or respiratory depression. Under these circumstances, 50 to 100 mEq (1 to 2 ampules) of bicarbonate may be infused intravenously over 2 hours. Serum phosphate should be measured, and phosphate repletion should be considered if the level falls below 1 mg/dL, especially if there is coincident heart failure, respiratory depression, or hemolytic anemia. Under these circumstances, 20 to 30/L potassium or sodium phosphate can be added to IV fluids. Phosphate repletion is not recommended with less marked decreases in serum levels, because this has not been shown to improve outcomes in DKA and may lead to hypocalcemia or hypomagnesemia.

As DKA resolves, it is important to continue providing adequate insulin to effectively resolve the ketosis, which may correct more slowly than the other abnormalities. This can be accomplished by adding glucose to the intravenous regimen (e.g., 5% glucose in half-normal saline) when blood glucose levels decrease to less than 200 to 250 mg/dL and continuing insulin infusion at 1 to 2 U/hour.

In patients with resolved DKA, transition to subcutaneous insulin can be made when the patient is clinically stable with normal vital signs, the acidosis is fully corrected, the patient is able take fluids orally without nausea or vomiting, and any precipitating conditions (e.g., infection) are controlled.

Hyperglycemic Hyperosmolar State

A hyperglycemic hyperosmolar state (HHS) occurs almost exclusively in patients with T2DM, one third of whom have not been previously

患者会出现多尿，但无法得到充分代偿，液体和电解质消耗逐渐增加。渗透性利尿的特点是水分丢失大于电解质丢失，导致渗透压不断增加。由于胰岛素缺乏，脂质生成减少和脂肪分解加速，导致循环中游离脂肪酸水平增加，这些脂肪酸为肝脏合成酮体（β-羟丁酸、乙酰乙酸和丙酮）提供了底物。β-羟丁酸和乙酰乙酸是酸性物质，其血浆水平升高可导致代谢性酸中毒。

这些过程可能由单纯胰岛素缺乏引起，但通常会因潜在疾病或诱发疾病（如感染）而加剧。感染会导致应激激素（皮质醇、儿茶酚胺、胰高血糖素和生长激素）水平升高，进而引起胰岛素抵抗。因此，这会产生一系列正反馈循环，导致高血糖、液体和电解质丢失、酮症和代谢性酸中毒不断加剧。患者通常需要住院治疗并接受多方面的干预，而不仅是恢复胰岛素剂量。

DKA 的常见症状包括多尿、口渴和多饮、近期体重减轻（特别是新发糖尿病患者）、视物模糊、乏力、厌食、恶心和呕吐、腹痛（可能类似于急腹症），以及从嗜睡到昏迷的精神状况变化。DKA 及其相关症状通常在 2 ～ 4 天出现，但使用胰岛素泵的患者可能在 12 h 内即会发生。体格检查时，患者通常有脱水表现，特别是血管内容量减少，包括皮肤弹性下降、低血压和心动过速（胸骨和前额皮肤的评估效果最佳）。皮肤可能因酸中毒的血管舒张效应而温暖、干燥，严重低血压应考虑即将发生血管收缩功能衰竭。患者通常出现深快呼吸（Kussmaul 呼吸）以作为代谢性酸中毒的呼吸代偿，伴呼气带有丙酮的特征性烂苹果味。符合下列标准的患者可诊断 DKA：①高血糖（> 250 mg/dl）；②中重度酮症（β-羟丁酸 > 5 mmol/L，或在 1∶2 或更高的血清稀释倍数下尿酮体试纸结果呈阳性）；③酸中毒（pH 值 < 7.3 或血浆碳酸氢盐 ≤ 15 mmol/L）。检测尿酮体可能产生误导作用，因为在没有 DKA 的情况下，禁食期间尿酮体也可能呈阳性。

除上述诊断性检测外，其他评估应包括电解质、血尿素氮、肌酐、磷酸盐、肝功能检查和淀粉酶；动脉或混合静脉血气分析（包括 pH 值）；全血细胞计数；尿液分析；心电图；胸部 X 线检查。应计算血清阴离子间隙，阴离子间隙 = $[Na^+] - [Cl^- + HCO_3^-]$，DKA 患者的血清阴离子间隙通常 > 12 mmol/L。此外，应直接检测或计算血清渗透压：估计的渗透压 = 2× $[Na^+]$ + $[$葡萄糖（mg/dl）$]$ /18。

DKA 的诱发因素包括感染（最常见）、心肌梗死（包括无症状心肌梗死），炎症过程（阑尾炎、胰腺炎）和药物（特别是糖皮质激素）。

应立即开始治疗 DKA，采取措施纠正危及生命的异常，包括胰岛素缺乏、液体和电解质丢失、K^+ 丢失和代谢性酸中毒。经典治疗方案是先给予普通胰岛素或速效胰岛素类似物冲击量（0.1 U/kg），然后以 0.1 U/（kg·h）的速度进行持续静脉输注。每小时监测血糖，直至血糖 < 250 mg/dl，根据需要调整胰岛素的输注速率，使

血糖下降速率达到 75 ～ 100 mg/（dl·h），以避免渗透压快速变化的潜在并发症。

开始胰岛素治疗时，必须同时补充液体和电解质。初始液体丢失量应根据体重下降的程度（如果已知）、黏膜干燥度、皮肤弹性及是否有体位性低血压来估计，通常 DKA 患者的失液量为 3 ～ 8 L。静脉补液的经典方案是第 1 个小时先给予 1 L 生理盐水，然后根据最初液体丢失的严重程度，第 2 个小时可继续以 15 ml/min 的速率给予生理盐水。随后，可能在接下来的 2 h 内改为 0.45%（半张）盐水以 7.5 ml/min 的速率输注，并逐渐调整，以便在约 8 h 内完全补足估计的液体丢失量。在此期间，应频繁监测颈静脉扩张和胸部听诊，以确保早期发现补液过量。有充血性心力衰竭风险的患者应监测中心静脉压。

所有 DKA 患者均需要补钾，并应仔细监测，以避免出现严重的低钾血症或高钾血症。在开始补钾前，必要时应使用 Foley 导尿管确认尿量。除非患者无尿，否则补钾治疗应在使用胰岛素后 1 ～ 2 h 开始。补钾的关键目标是在治疗过程中始终维持血清 K^+ > 3.5 mmol/L，如果初始存在低钾血症或使用碳酸氢盐纠正酸中毒，则在治疗早期补钾尤为重要，因为碳酸氢盐会促进细胞外 K^+ 进入细胞内。如果血清 K^+ ≥ 5 mmol/L，通常无须补钾；否则，应根据血清 K^+ 水平以 10 ～ 40 mmol/h 的速率补钾。如果血清 K^+ < 4 mmol/L 或 > 5 mmol/L，应每 2 h 监测 1 次。

通常应避免输注碳酸氢盐，但对于 pH 值 < 7、血清 HCO_3^- < 5.0 mmol/L、血清 K^+ > 6.5 mmol/L、对补液无反应的低血压、严重左心衰竭或呼吸抑制的患者，应考虑使用碳酸氢盐。在这些情况下，可在 2 h 内静脉输注 50 ～ 100 mmol（1 ～ 2 安瓿）碳酸氢盐。应检测血清磷酸盐，< 1 mg/dl 时应考虑补充磷酸盐，特别是合并心力衰竭、呼吸抑制或溶血性贫血的患者。在这些情况下，可在静脉补液中加入 20 ～ 30 mmol/L 磷酸钾或磷酸钠。不推荐在血清磷水平下降不明显时补充磷酸盐，因为尚未证明其可以改善 DKA 患者的结局，并可能导致低钙血症或低镁血症。

随着 DKA 的纠正，继续给予足量胰岛素以有效缓解酮症非常重要，因为酮症的缓解可能比纠正其他异常更慢。当血糖降至 < 200 ～ 250 mg/dl 时，可在静脉输液方案中添加葡萄糖（如在半张盐水中加入 5% 葡萄糖），并继续以 1 ～ 2 U/h 的速度输注胰岛素。

在 DKA 已纠正的患者中，若病情稳定，生命体征正常，酸中毒完全纠正，患者能够口服液体而不感到恶心或呕吐，且诱发病因（如感染）均已得到控制时，可以过渡到皮下注射胰岛素。

高血糖高渗状态

高血糖高渗状态（HHS）几乎只发生在 T2DM 患者中，其中 1/3 的患者既往未被诊断。HHS 患者通常

diagnosed. Patients often are elderly and frequently have compromised renal function. Insulin deficiency, often exacerbated by insulin resistance resulting from the stress of an intercurrent illness, leads to hyperglycemia, glucosuria, and an osmotic diuresis. However, the presence of some endogenous insulin secretion suppresses lipolysis and ketogenesis enough to prevent ketoacidosis. Patients with HHS typically develop more marked hyperglycemia, fluid and electrolyte deficits, and hyperosmolality compared to those with DKA. HHS usually develops insidiously over days to weeks, and patients may be vulnerable to development of more severe hyperglycemia and volume deficits over this extended period.

HHS is associated with infections (40%), diuretic use (35% to 40%), and residency in nursing homes (25% to 30%). Other precipitating and complicating factors may include intestinal obstruction, mesenteric thrombosis, pulmonary embolism, peritoneal dialysis, subdural hematoma, and an extensive list of medications. The overall mortality rate exceeds that of DKA (10% to 40%), with higher mortality rates associated with age older than 70 years, nursing home residency, and higher osmolality or serum Na^+ concentration. Clinically, patients have evidence of the marked fluid and electrolyte deficits and tend to have more prominent neurologic abnormalities than those with DKA, including confusion, obtundation, and coma.

Therapy for HHS follows the same general principles as that for DKA, with a greater volume replacement required (typically 8 to 12 L in fully developed HHS). Restoration of the fluid and electrolyte deficits should proceed more slowly than in DKA (e.g., over 36 to 72 hours). Insulin therapy should be started only after rehydration is in progress. There is a need for K^+ replacement, but less than in DKA. Patients with HHS may be more sensitive to insulin than those with DKA and may require lower insulin doses. In view of the severe dehydration and predisposition to vascular thrombosis, heparin prophylaxis usually should be provided. Despite the very marked hyperglycemia of HHS, patients may be able to ultimately return to oral medications.

Chronic Complications of Diabetes

Chronic complications of T1DM and T2DM are similar and include microvascular complications (nephropathy, retinopathy, and neuropathy) and macrovascular or cardiovascular complications (coronary artery disease, peripheral vascular disease, and cerebrovascular disease). The long-term complications of diabetes result in substantial morbidity and shorten average lifespan by approximately 10 years. Candidate mechanisms for microvascular and macrovascular complications include activation of the polyol pathway (with accumulation of sorbitol), formation of glycated proteins and advanced glycation end products (cross-linked glycated proteins), abnormalities in lipid metabolism, increased oxidative damage, hyperinsulinemia, hyperperfusion of certain tissues, hyperviscosity, platelet dysfunction (increased aggregation), endothelial dysfunction, and activation of various growth factors.

Microvascular Complications

Retinopathy. Diabetic retinopathy affects almost all patients with T1DM and 60% to 80% of those with T2DM by 20 years after the diagnosis of diabetes. It is the most common cause of blindness in persons between the ages of 20 and 74 years in the developed world. The incidence and progression of diabetic retinopathy increase with duration of diabetes, poor glycemic control, the type of diabetes (T1DM more than T2DM), and the presence of hypertension, smoking, dyslipidemia, nephropathy, and pregnancy.

Early interventions often are beneficial in slowing or sometimes reversing diabetic retinopathy, but most patients have no symptoms until the lesions are advanced. Therefore, annual ophthalmologic screening is recommended starting at 5 years after diagnosis in T1DM and at the time of diagnosis in T2DM.

In nonproliferative retinopathy, the progression to visual loss in patients with clinically significant macular edema is improved by focal laser photocoagulation. Panretinal photocoagulation improves outcomes in patients with proliferative retinopathy and also in the subset of T2DM patients with severe nonproliferative diabetic retinopathy. Patients who have had vitreous hemorrhage and resulting visual loss may have significant restoration of vision with vitrectomy. Patients with macular edema also may benefit from intravitreous anti–vascular endothelial factor (VEGF) pharmacotherapy. In addition to diabetic retinopathy, patients with diabetes are at increased risk for development of cataracts.

Nephropathy. Diabetic nephropathy is the most common cause of end-stage renal disease (ESRD) in developed countries (about 30% of cases). However, the risk of progression to ESRD has been markedly decreasing over the last several decades. ESRD now appears to affect fewer than 10% of patients. The risk of developing advanced renal disease in diabetes is increased by poor glycemic control, hypertension, smoking, and possibly use of oral contraceptives, obesity, dyslipidemia, and more advanced age.

Diabetic nephropathy is primarily a glomerulopathy, with pathologic features that include mesangial expansion, glomerular basement membrane thickening, and glomerular sclerosis. Many but not all patients develop albuminuria early in the course, and the level of albumin correlates with the rate of progression and the degree of renal injury. For this reason, patients should be monitored annually for albuminuria starting 5 years after diagnosis in T1DM and at the time of diagnosis in T2DM. Measurement of the ratio of microalbumin to creatinine in a random urine sample is adequate, because this ratio correlates well with results from 24-hour collections. Albumin excretion of 30 to 300 mg per gram of creatinine (designated *moderately increased albuminuria*) indicates probable diabetic nephropathy. Albumin excretion of greater than 300 mg per gram of creatinine (designated *severely increased albuminuria*) indicates high risk for progression to nephrotic-range proteinuria and ESRD.

Efforts to achieve blood glucose targets and rigorously control blood pressure (appropriate to age and overall risk profile) should be part of the strategy for primary prevention of nephropathy in all patients with diabetes. For patients with greater than 300 mg protein per gram creatinine and an eGFR greater than 30 mL/min/1.73m², canagliflozin should be considered for blood glucose management, since it has been shown to delay progression to ESRD. Blood pressure should be maintained lower than 140/90 mm Hg unless otherwise contraindicated. In patients with high risk for adverse cardiovascular events, a target of 130/80 mm Hg should be considered. Angiotensin-converting enzyme (ACE) inhibitors or angiotensin receptor blockers (ARBs) are preferable first-line agents. The calcium-channel blockers diltiazem and verapamil can be used as alternatives in patients who are unable to tolerate ACE inhibitors or ARBs, or as additive therapy in patients who need multiple drugs to control blood pressure. Diuretics and moderate Na^+ restriction also frequently are needed to reach blood pressure goals.

Neuropathy. The likelihood of development of diabetic neuropathy increases with duration of disease and is influenced by the degree of glycemic control (occurring overall in up to 70% of people with diabetes). Any part of the peripheral or autonomic nervous system may be affected. *Peripheral polyneuropathy* occurs most commonly, usually manifesting as a bilaterally symmetrical, distal, primarily sensory polyneuropathy (with or without motor involvement) in a *glove-and-stocking* distribution. Pain, numbness, hyperesthesias, and paresthesias progress to sensory loss. This condition, together with loss of proprioception, can lead to

是老年人，且常合并肾功能不全。胰岛素缺乏（通常是由于伴随疾病应激加剧胰岛素抵抗）可导致高血糖、尿糖和渗透性利尿。然而，一些内源性胰岛素分泌的存在足以抑制脂肪分解和酮体生成，从而防止酮症酸中毒。与 DKA 患者相比，HHS 患者通常有更显著的高血糖、液体及电解质缺乏和高渗透压。HHS 通常在数天至数周内隐匿发展，患者可能在这段时期发生更严重的高血糖和液体丢失。

HHS 常与感染（40%）、利尿剂使用（35% ～ 40%）和在疗养院居住（25% ～ 30%）有关。其他诱发和并发症因素包括肠梗阻、肠系膜血栓形成、肺栓塞、腹膜透析、硬膜下血肿及药物使用。HHS 的总体死亡率超过 DKA（10% ～ 40%），死亡率较高与年龄 > 70 岁、在疗养院居住、渗透压或血清 Na^+ 浓度较高有关。临床上，患者有明显的液体和电解质缺乏症状，且神经系统异常通常比 DKA 患者更突出，包括意识错乱、迟钝和昏迷。

HHS 的治疗遵循与 DKA 相同的一般原则，但需要更大的补液量（通常需要 8 ～ 12 L）。液体和电解质的恢复速度慢于 DKA（如超过 36 ～ 72 h）。只有在补液时才可开始胰岛素治疗。HHS 患者需要补钾，但补钾量少于 DKA。与 DKA 患者相比，HHS 患者对胰岛素可能更敏感，可能需要更低剂量的胰岛素。考虑到严重脱水和血栓形成的倾向，通常应给予肝素预防。尽管 HHS 的高血糖非常显著，患者最终仍可能恢复口服药物治疗。

糖尿病的慢性并发症

T1DM 和 T2DM 的慢性并发症相似，包括微血管并发症（肾病、视网膜病变和神经病变）和大血管或心血管并发症（冠状动脉疾病、周围血管疾病和脑血管疾病）。糖尿病的长期并发症可导致死亡率升高，并使平均寿命缩短约 10 年。微血管和大血管并发症的可能机制包括多元醇通路激活（伴有山梨醇堆积）、糖基化蛋白和糖基化终末产物（交联糖基化蛋白）的形成、脂代谢异常、氧化损伤增加、高胰岛素血症、某些组织的过度灌注、高黏滞综合征、血小板功能障碍（聚集增加）、内皮功能障碍和多种生长因子激活。

微血管并发症

视网膜病变　糖尿病视网膜病变几乎影响所有 T1DM 患者，并在 T2DM 诊断后 20 年内影响 60% ～ 80% 的 T2DM 患者。它是发达国家 20 ～ 74 岁人群失明的最常见原因。可影响糖尿病视网膜病变发生和进展的因素包括糖尿病的病程、血糖控制不良、糖尿病类型（T1DM 多于 T2DM）、高血压、吸烟、血脂异常、肾病和妊娠。

早期干预通常有助于减缓或逆转糖尿病视网膜病变，但大多数患者在病变晚期之前没有症状。因此，建议从诊断 T1DM 后 5 年和诊断 T2DM 时开始每年进行眼科筛查。

在非增殖性视网膜病变中，局部激光光凝治疗可改善临床症状明显的黄斑水肿患者视力丧失的进展。全视网膜光凝治疗可改善增殖性视网膜病变患者和伴有严重非增殖性糖尿病视网膜病变的 T2DM 患者的预后。玻璃体出血并导致视力丧失的患者可能通过玻璃体切除术显著恢复视力。黄斑水肿患者可能获益于玻璃体内注射抗血管内皮生长因子（VEGF）药物治疗。除糖尿病视网膜病变外，糖尿病患者患白内障的风险也会增加。

肾病　糖尿病肾病是发达国家终末期肾病（ESRD）的最常见原因（约占 30%）。然而，在过去几十年中，发展至 ESRD 的风险显著降低。目前 ESRD 似乎仅发生于不足 10% 的患者。糖尿病发展为晚期肾病的危险因素包括血糖控制不良、高血压、吸烟、口服避孕药（可能）、肥胖症、血脂异常和高龄。

糖尿病肾病主要是肾小球病变，其病理学特征包括系膜扩张、肾小球基底膜增厚和肾小球硬化。许多（但不是所有）患者在病程早期就会出现白蛋白尿，且白蛋白尿水平与肾病进展速度和肾损伤程度相关。因此，建议从诊断 T1DM 后 5 年和诊断 T2DM 时开始每年监测白蛋白尿。检测随机尿样本中微量白蛋白与肌酐的比值即可，因为该比值与 24 h 尿样本检测结果的相关性良好。微量白蛋白 / 肌酐比值为 30 ～ 300 mg/g（白蛋白尿中度增加）提示糖尿病肾病可能。微量白蛋白 / 肌酐比值 > 300 mg/g（白蛋白尿重度增加）提示发展为肾病范围蛋白尿和 ESRD 的风险高。

实现血糖达标和严格血压控制（适应于年龄和整体风险状况）应作为所有糖尿病患者肾病一级预防策略的一部分。对于微量白蛋白 / 肌酐比值 > 300 mg/g 且 eGFR > 30 ml/（min·1.73m²）的患者，应考虑使用卡格列净进行血糖管理，因为研究证明卡格列净可延缓 ESRD 的进展。血压应保持在 140/90 mmHg 以下，除非有其他禁忌证。在有不良心血管事件高风险的患者中，血压目标值应考虑为 130/80 mmHg。血管紧张素转换酶抑制剂（ACEI）或血管紧张素受体阻滞剂（ARB）是首选的一线药物。钙通道阻滞剂地尔硫䓬和维拉帕米可作为不能耐受 ACEI 或 ARB 患者的替代药物，或作为需要多种药物控制血压患者的附加治疗。患者通常需要应用利尿剂和适度限钠来使血压达标。

神经病变　糖尿病神经病变发生的风险随病程的延长而增加，并受血糖控制程度的影响（总体上 70% 的糖尿病患者会发生神经病变）。周围神经系统或自主神经系统的任何部分均可能受累。多发性周围神经病变最为常见，通常表现为双侧对称、远端、以感觉性多神经病变为主（伴或不伴运动神经参与）、呈手套和袜子样分布。疼痛、麻木、过敏和感觉异常可逐渐

an abnormal gait with repeated trauma and potential for fractures of the tarsal bones, sometimes resulting in the development of Charcot joints. These changes lead to abnormal pressures in the feet that, together with the soft tissue atrophy related to peripheral arterial insufficiency, result in foot ulcers that may progress to osteomyelitis and gangrene. Detailed, regular neurologic examination of all patients is essential to elicit the early loss of light touch (using a size 5.07/10-g monofilament), reflexes, and vibratory sensation.

A second common form of diabetic neuropathy is autonomic neuropathy, which may develop in concert with or separate from distal polyneuropathy. Resulting symptoms can be debilitating, including postural hypotension leading to falls or syncope, gastroparesis, enteropathy with constipation or diarrhea, and bladder outflow obstruction with urinary retention. Diabetic autonomic neuropathy together with vascular disease is a contributor to erectile dysfunction in males. Gastrointestinal dysfunction with autonomic neuropathy can complicate efforts to achieve blood glucose control by causing variable absorption of food. A suspected diagnosis of autonomic neuropathy can be strengthened by demonstrating loss of normal variability in heart rate with deep respirations or the Valsalva maneuver.

Other, less common manifestations of diabetic neuropathy include thoracic and lumbar nerve root *polyradiculopathies*, individual peripheral and cranial nerve *mononeuropathies*, and asymmetrical neuropathies of multiple peripheral nerves (mononeuropathy multiplex). Diabetic amyotrophy causing muscle atrophy and weakness most often involving the anterior thigh muscles and pelvic girdle is an uncommon form of diabetic neuropathy that often resolves after several months.

The primary approach to all diabetic neuropathies consists of efforts to improve blood glucose control. Clinical trials have shown decreased development of distal polyneuropathy with improved glycemia in T1DM. It also is particularly important for patients with neuropathies to receive regular foot care, including daily self-inspection of the feet, regular physician examinations, and early interventions for developing calloses, infections, or other foot lesions. Painful polyneuropathies cause substantial morbidity and are difficult to treat. First-line drugs include amitriptyline, venlafaxine, duloxetine, and pregabalin. For patients who do not respond adequately to one drug, combination therapy with two drugs of different classes can be tested. Alternative treatments that may be effective in some patients include topical capsaicin cream, lidocaine patch, α-lipoic acid, isosorbide dinitrate topical spray, and transcutaneous electrical nerve stimulation (TENS). *Gastroparesis* secondary to autonomic neuropathy may improve symptomatically with metoclopramide or domperidone (dopamine D2 antagonists), erythromycin (motilin agonist) for bacterial overgrowth, cisapride (cholinergic agonist), or mosapride (selective serotonin 5-HT4 receptor agonist). Diarrhea may respond to loperamide or diphenoxylate and atropine. Orthostatic hypotension can be treated by attention to mechanical factors such as elevation of the head of the bed, gradual rising from a lying to standing position, use of support stockings, and sometimes use of the mineralocorticoid fludrocortisone.

Macrovascular Complications

The risk of macrovascular disease including cardiovascular disease, transient ischemic attacks and strokes, and peripheral vascular disease is increased 2-fold to 4-fold and accounts for 70% to 80% of deaths in patients with diabetes. This increased risk is believed to result from the altered metabolism in diabetes and also from the frequent occurrence of associated risk factors in diabetic patients, including hypertension and dyslipidemia. Screening for macrovascular disease and predisposing factors were discussed earlier. Approaches to decreasing the risk of macrovascular disease should include optimization of blood glucose control (including consideration of specific drugs for T2DM that may decrease cardiovascular event risk as discussed previously), weight loss for overweight and obese patients, smoking cessation, control of blood pressure, and treatment of dyslipidemia. (See Chapter 8 for details on the management of dyslipidemia.)

HYPOGLYCEMIA

Definition

Hypoglycemia most often occurs in patients with T1DM or T2DM under circumstances in which insulin or other antidiabetic therapies result in blood glucose levels decreasing below the lower limit of normal (<50 to 60 mg/dL for most laboratories). This may be caused by overtreatment with glucose-lowering agents, failure to take in anticipated calories, or the combination of increased glucose utilization and increased insulin sensitivity induced by exercise.

Hypoglycemia much less commonly occurs as a primary disorder in patients who do not have drug-treated diabetes. Under these circumstances, clinically significant hypoglycemia can be difficult to identify based on blood glucose measurements alone, because the normal lower limit of blood glucose varies in individuals and is influenced by duration of fasting and gender. Plasma glucose levels during a fast in men decrease to approximately 55 mg/dL at 24 hours and 50 mg/dL at 48 and 72 hours, whereas in premenopausal women they may be as low as 35 mg/dL at 24 hours without symptoms of hypoglycemia. In evaluating glucose determinations, it is important to recognize that plasma levels are approximately 15% higher than glucose levels in whole blood. Clinically significant hypoglycemia can be most readily established if patients manifest *Whipple triad*, which refers to the combination of: (1) symptoms suggestive of hypoglycemia, (2) documented low plasma glucose levels (<50 to 60 mg/dL), and (3) prompt resolution of symptoms when the low blood glucose is corrected.

Signs and Symptoms

Typical signs and symptoms of hypoglycemia are listed in Table 5.8. *Autonomic* symptoms result from sympathetic neural outflow that occurs as part of the counter-regulatory response to hypoglycemia. Although most patients appear to fully recover CNS function after a neuroglycopenic episode, there is a risk of irreversible brain damage or death with sustained or repeated episodes of severe neuroglycopenia.

Pathology

Hypoglycemic disorders can result when there is overproduction of hormones that lower glucose concentrations, underproduction of hormones that serve to elevate glucose levels, deficiency of substrates for endogenous glucose synthesis, or changes in cells and tissues that result in their increased consumption of glucose.

Etiologic Classification

Causes of hypoglycemia by etiologic categories are listed in Table 5.9.

Drug-Induced

The most common causes of hypoglycemia are excess insulin or insulin secretagogues (especially sulfonylureas) administered in the treatment of diabetes. Ethanol can cause hypoglycemia, most often in the context of chronic alcoholism in an individual who is nutritionally depleted after binge drinking for several days or longer. Under these circumstances, hepatic glycogen stores become depleted, and the process of alcohol metabolism blocks gluconeogenesis by depriving the liver of nicotinamide adenine dinucleotide (NAD+). Commonly used pharmacologic agents that have been associated with hypoglycemia include β-blockers (especially nonselective β₂-adrenergic antagonists), ACE

发展为感觉丧失。这种情况和本体感觉丧失可能导致步态异常、反复创伤和蹠骨骨折，有时可导致沙尔科（Charcot）关节。这些变化会导致足部压力异常，再加上与外周动脉供血不足相关的软组织萎缩，进而引起足部溃疡，可能发展为骨髓炎和坏疽。对所有患者定期进行详细的神经系统检查至关重要，以发现早期轻触觉（使用 5.07/10 g 单丝）、腱反射和振动觉丧失。

糖尿病神经病变的第二种常见形式是自主神经病变，它可能与远端多神经病变并存或单独存在。自主神经病变导致的症状可使人虚弱，包括体位性低血压导致跌倒或晕厥、胃轻瘫、肠病伴便秘或腹泻，以及膀胱排尿梗阻导致尿潴留。糖尿病自主神经病变伴血管疾病是男性勃起功能障碍的原因之一。自主神经病变伴胃肠功能障碍可引起食物吸收的改变，从而使血糖控制复杂化。深呼吸或 Valsalva 动作时心率丧失正常变异性，可强化对自主神经病变的疑似诊断。

糖尿病神经病变的其他少见表现包括胸腰椎神经根多发性神经根病变、周围神经和颅神经单神经病变，以及多根周围神经的非对称性神经病变（多发性单神经病变）。糖尿病肌萎缩可导致肌肉萎缩和肌无力，最常累及大腿前部和骨盆带肌肉，是一种少见的糖尿病神经病变形式，通常在数月后自行缓解。

所有糖尿病神经病变的主要治疗方法均包括改善血糖控制。临床试验表明，在 T1DM 患者中，改善血糖控制可减少远端多神经病变。对于神经病变患者，接受定期足部管理非常重要，包括每日自我检查足部、定期医生检查，以及对已经出现的肿胀、感染或其他足部病变进行早期干预。痛性多神经病变的并发症发病率高，且难以治疗。一线治疗药物包括阿米替林、文拉法辛、度洛西汀和普瑞巴林。对于单药治疗效果不佳的患者，可尝试两种不同类别药物的联合治疗。其他治疗包括局部辣椒素霜、利多卡因贴片、α-硫辛酸、硝酸异山梨酯局部喷雾和经皮神经电刺激（TENS），可能对部分患者有效。由自主神经病变引起的胃轻瘫可能通过甲氧氯普胺或多潘立酮（多巴胺 D$_2$ 拮抗剂）、红霉素（胃动素激动剂；治疗细菌过度生长）、西沙必利（胆碱能激动剂）或莫沙必利（选择性 5-HT$_4$ 受体激动剂）改善症状。腹泻患者可能对洛哌丁胺或地芬诺酯和阿托品有治疗反应。体位性低血压可通过抬高床头、从卧位缓慢起身至站立位、使用弹力袜来治疗，有时需要使用盐皮质激素氟氢可的松。

大血管并发症

糖尿病患者出现心血管疾病、短暂性脑缺血发作、卒中，以及周围血管疾病等大血管疾病的风险可增加 2～4 倍，占糖尿病患者死亡原因的 70%～80%。这种风险增加是由糖尿病代谢改变和糖尿病患者常见的相关危险因素（包括高血压和血脂异常）所致。筛查大血管疾病和易感因素的内容见上文。降低大血管疾病风险的方法应包括优化血糖控制（包括考虑使用特定药物降低 T2DM 患者的心血管事件风险，见上文）、超重和肥胖症患者减重、戒烟、控制血压和治疗血脂异常（有关血脂异常管理的详细信息见第 8 章）。

低血糖

定义

低血糖最常发生在 T1DM 或 T2DM 患者中，由于胰岛素或其他降糖治疗导致血糖水平降至正常值下限以下［＜50～60 mg/dl（大多数实验室）］。这可能是由于降糖药物的过度治疗、未能摄入预期的热量，以及运动引起的葡萄糖利用率增加和胰岛素敏感性增加。

在未接受药物治疗的糖尿病患者中，低血糖很少作为原发性疾病发生。在这些情况下，仅凭血糖检测很难确定临床显著的低血糖，因为血糖的正常值下限存在个体差异，并受禁食持续时间和性别的影响。男性血浆葡萄糖水平在禁食 24 h 降至约 55 mg/dl，禁食 48 h 和 72 h 降至 50 mg/dl，而绝经前女性可能在禁食 24 h 血糖降至 35 mg/dl 而没有低血糖症状。在评估血糖测定值时，应认识到血浆葡萄糖水平约比全血中的葡萄糖水平高 15%。如果患者表现出 Whipple 三联症，则更容易确定具有临床意义的低血糖，其特征包括：①有提示低血糖的症状；②发作时的血浆葡萄糖水平低（＜50～60 mg/dl）；③纠正低血糖后症状迅速缓解。

症状和体征

低血糖的典型症状和体征见表 5.8。自主神经症状是由低血糖反调节反应引起交感神经兴奋所致。尽管大多数患者在神经性低血糖发作后中枢神经系统功能可完全恢复，但如果发生持续或反复的严重神经性低血糖发作，仍有出现不可逆性脑损伤或死亡的风险。

病理学

当降低葡萄糖水平的激素生成过多、升高葡萄糖水平的激素生成不足、内源性葡萄糖合成的底物缺乏、细胞和组织改变导致葡萄糖消耗增加时，可出现低血糖性疾病。

病因分类

低血糖的病因见表 5.9。

药物诱导

低血糖最常见的原因是糖尿病治疗中使用过量胰岛素或胰岛素促泌剂（特别是磺酰脲类药物）。乙醇也可能导致低血糖，最常见于连续狂饮数天后营养耗竭的长期酗酒个体。在这些情况下，肝脏的糖原储备被耗尽，酒精代谢过程通过消耗肝脏的烟酰胺腺嘌呤二核苷酸（NAD$^+$）来阻断糖异生。与低血糖相关的常用药物包括 β 受体阻滞剂（特别是非选择性 β$_2$ 受体阻

TABLE 5.8 Signs and Symptoms of Hypoglycemia

Autonomic		
Sweating	Palpitations	Hunger
Pallor	Tachycardia	Nausea
Anxiety	Hypertension	Vomiting
Tremor	Irritability	Paresthesias
Neuroglycopenic		
Difficulty thinking	Dizziness	Seizures
Fatigue, weakness	Visual blurring	Loss of consciousness
Somnolence	Confusion	Coma
Headache	Abnormal behavior	Death

TABLE 5.9 Etiologic Classification of Hypoglycemic Disorders Manifesting in Adults

Drug-Induced
Antidiabetic agents (insulin, sulfonylureas, meglitinides)
Alcohol
Other pharmacologic agents (β-blockers, ACE inhibitors, pentamidine, quinine, quinolones and many others)

Altered Gastrointestinal Function
Alimentary hypoglycemia

Beta-Cell Insulin Oversecretion
Insulinoma
Non-insulinoma pancreatogenous hypoglycemia (without or with bariatric surgery)

Non–Islet Cell Neoplasms
Tumor insulin-like growth factor-II secretion
Tumor glucose consumption

Autoimmune
Circulating insulin antibodies
Insulin receptor activating antibodies

Endocrine Deficiencies
Glucocorticoids (adrenal insufficiency), growth hormone, catecholamines, glucagon

Severe Illness
Sepsis
Hepatic failure
Renal failure

Malnutrition
Anorexia nervosa

ACE, Angiotensin-converting enzyme.

inhibitors, pentamidine (through toxic effects on beta cells), quinine, and quinolones.

Excess Endogenous Insulin or Insulin-like Hormones

Alimentary hypoglycemia is a disorder in which low blood glucose levels occur typically 90 to 180 minutes after meals in patients who have undergone gastric outlet surgery with resulting accelerated gastric emptying. This is distinct from the more common *dumping syndrome*, which results from rapid entry of an osmotic load into the small intestine and associated fluid shifts and autonomic responses and is not associated with hypoglycemia. "Reactive hypoglycemia" is a now outmoded term that previously was applied to adrenergic symptoms occurring 2 to 4 hours after a meal in patients who are not hypoglycemic; these individuals may experience decreased symptoms with frequent feedings and avoidance of high-carbohydrate meals.

Tumors of islet beta cells *(insulinomas)* can cause hypoglycemia by producing excess insulin in an unregulated manner. They are uncommon (1 in 250,000 patient-years) but important to recognize when they do occur. Insulinomas usually are small (1 to 2 cm), benign (>90%), solitary (>90%), and confined to the endocrine pancreas (99%). Some patients have an indolent course extending over many years before diagnosis, but insulinomas can produce profound hypoglycemia. There is a tendency for adrenergic symptoms to become suppressed as a consequence of repeated exposures to hypoglycemia, and neuroglycopenic symptoms may predominate, including sometimes bizarre behavioral abnormalities. Patients may eat frequently in response to the hypoglycemia and exhibit moderate weight gain.

Non-insulinoma pancreatogenous hypoglycemia is a disorder that may manifest with symptoms similar to those of insulinomas, but the pathology involves beta-cell hypertrophy and hyperplasia rather than the presence of a discrete tumor. More recently, the development of hypoglycemia with similar beta-cell hyperplasia has been described in some patients months to years after Roux-en-Y gastric bypass surgery.

Non–islet cell neoplasms are a rare cause of hypoglycemia; they produce an insulin-like growth factor (IGF), usually a partially processed form of IGF-II designated *big IGF-II*, that can have insulin-like effects. The tumors typically are large and malignant and are most often located in the retroperitoneal space, abdomen, or thoracic cavity. Tumor types include hemangiopericytomas, hepatocellular carcinomas, lymphomas, adrenocortical carcinomas, gastrointestinal carcinoids, and mesenchymal tumors. Some large tumors cause hypoglycemia in the absence of detectable insulin-like factors.

Hormone Deficiencies

Deficiencies of insulin counter-regulatory hormones, which normally function to raise glucose levels, can result in or contribute to hypoglycemia. An example is low levels of corticosteroids caused by primary or secondary adrenocorticoid insufficiency. Deficiencies of other hormones, including catecholamines, glucagon, and growth hormone, also can cause hypoglycemia.

Severe Illness

Hypoglycemia can occur during severe illness through a number of different mechanisms in association with sepsis, hepatic insufficiency, and renal failure. Patients with severe illness appear to be particularly vulnerable to hypoglycemia when they are poorly nourished, although malnutrition alone is rarely associated with hypoglycemia.

Approach to the Diagnosis

For patients who have well-documented hypoglycemia, the diagnosis often is evident or strongly suggested by the clinical setting, history, and physical examination findings. Hypoglycemia induced by insulin or other glucose-lowering agents in diabetic patients often is immediately apparent from the medical history. Alcohol-induced hypoglycemia may be suspected in a patient with a known or suspected history of alcohol use and binge drinking. Identification of other candidate drugs as a cause of hypoglycemia requires a thorough medical history, and the condition can be expected to resolve if the suspect medication is stopped. The patient may have a known diagnosis of adrenal

表5.8	低血糖的症状和体征	
自主神经症状		
出汗	心悸	饥饿感
苍白	心动过速	恶心
焦虑	高血压	呕吐
震颤	易激惹	感觉异常
神经性低血糖症状		
思维混乱	头晕	癫痫发作
疲劳、乏力	视物模糊	意识丧失
嗜睡	意识错乱	昏迷
头痛	行为异常	死亡

表5.9	成人低血糖性疾病的病因分类
药物诱导	
抗糖尿病药物（胰岛素、磺酰脲类、格列奈类）	
酒精	
其他药物（β 受体阻滞剂、ACEI、喷他脒、奎宁、喹诺酮类和其他药物）	
胃肠道功能改变	
营养性低血糖	
β 细胞胰岛素过量分泌	
胰岛素瘤	
非胰岛素瘤胰源性低血糖（接受或未接受减重术）	
非胰岛细胞肿瘤	
胰岛素样生长因子 - Ⅱ分泌瘤	
消耗葡萄糖的肿瘤	
自身免疫性	
循环胰岛素抗体	
胰岛素受体激活抗体	
内分泌激素缺乏	
糖皮质激素（肾上腺功能不全）、生长激素、儿茶酚胺、胰高血糖素	
严重疾病	
感染中毒症	
肝衰竭	
肾衰竭	
营养不良	
神经性厌食症	

ACEI，血管紧张素转换酶抑制剂。

滞剂）、ACEI、喷他脒（对 β 细胞具有毒性作用）、奎宁和喹诺酮类药物。

内源性胰岛素或胰岛素样激素过多

营养性低血糖是指接受胃出口手术导致胃排空加速的患者在餐后 90 ～ 180 min 发生的低血糖。这与更常见的倾倒综合征不同，后者是由高渗性食物快速进入小肠、相关的液体转移和自主神经反应引起，不伴有低血糖。"反应性低血糖"这一术语目前已被弃用，既往被用于描述未患低血糖的个体在餐后 2 ～ 4 h 出现的肾上腺素能症状；这些个体可通过频繁进食和避免高碳水化合物饮食来减少症状。

胰岛 β 细胞肿瘤（胰岛素瘤）可通过不受控制地产生过量胰岛素而引起低血糖。胰岛素瘤较少见（1/250 000 患者-年），但发生时必须加以识别。胰岛素瘤通常为小的（1 ～ 2 cm）、良性（＞ 90%）、单发（＞ 90%）肿瘤，且局限于胰腺内分泌部位（99%）。一些患者在诊断前有长达多年的隐匿病程，但胰岛素瘤也可导致严重的低血糖。由于反复暴露于低血糖，肾上腺素能症状有被抑制的倾向，神经性低血糖症状可能占主导地位，包括行为异常。患者可能会频繁进食以应对低血糖，并表现为中度体重增加。

非胰岛素瘤胰源性低血糖是一种可能表现出与胰岛素瘤相似症状的疾病，但病理学机制为 β 细胞肥大和增生，而不是实体瘤。近期报道显示，在行 Roux-en-Y 胃旁路手术后数月至数年的患者中，部分会出现低血糖伴有类似的 β 细胞增生。

非胰岛细胞肿瘤是低血糖的罕见原因；肿瘤可产生胰岛素样生长因子（IGF），通常是 IGF- Ⅱ 的部分加工形式，被称为大 IGF- Ⅱ，具有胰岛素样作用。肿瘤通常为巨大的恶性肿瘤，最常见于腹膜后间隙、腹部或胸腔。肿瘤类型包括血管外皮细胞瘤、肝细胞癌、淋巴瘤、肾上腺皮质癌、胃肠道类癌和间充质肿瘤。一些巨大肿瘤在没有检测到胰岛素样因子的情况下会引起低血糖。

激素缺乏

胰岛素反调节激素（正常功能是升高血糖）缺乏可能导致或促进低血糖。一个例子是由原发性或继发性肾上腺皮质功能不全引起的皮质类固醇缺乏。儿茶酚胺、胰高血糖素和生长激素等其他激素缺乏也可能导致低血糖。

严重疾病

在严重疾病期间，与感染中毒症、肝功能不全和肾衰竭相关的多种机制均可导致低血糖。当重症患者营养不足时，特别容易发生低血糖，尽管单纯营养不良很少引起低血糖。

诊断

对于有充分证据证明患有低血糖的患者，临床情况、病史和体格检查结果通常可诊断或强烈提示诊断。糖尿病患者由胰岛素或其他降糖药物引起的低血糖，通常可从病史中立即明确诊断。对于有已知或疑似饮酒过量史的患者，应疑诊酒精引起的低血糖。确定导致低血糖的其他候选药物需要详细了解病史，停用可疑药物后病情可得到预期缓解。患者还可能合并肾上腺皮质功能不全，或通过其他临床表现（如体位性低血压、皮肤色素沉着）提示有肾上腺皮质功能不全，

insufficiency, or this may be suggested by other clinical findings (e.g., orthostatic hypotension, increased skin pigmentation) or the development of markedly increased insulin sensitivity in a patient with T1DM. The patient may have a known tumor, suggesting the possibility of a non–islet cell neoplasm as a cause of hypoglycemia. There may be a history of Roux-en-Y bypass surgery, raising the possibility of beta-cell hyperplasia. The co-occurrence of sepsis, hepatic failure, renal failure, profound malnutrition, or a diagnosis of anorexia nervosa may suggest one of these potential underlying causes.

A number of algorithms have been developed to guide the evaluation of documented or potential hypoglycemia, including a recommended approach from an expert panel published by the Endocrine Society. If there is an opportunity to observe the patient during a symptomatic episode of presumed hypoglycemia, plasma should be obtained, if possible before treatment, for measurement of glucose, insulin, proinsulin, C-peptide, β-hydroxybutyrate, and screening for sulfonylureas and meglitinides. Hypoglycemia can be rapidly, provisionally confirmed with a test meter and later confirmed by laboratory analysis. After blood samples have been obtained for the tests described, glucose should be administered orally (15 to 30 g) or intravenously (25 g, or 1 ampule of 50% dextrose), and recovery of glucose levels and symptoms should be observed.

For patients with suspected or confirmed hypoglycemia developing specifically in the fasted state, it may be possible to replicate the condition by observing during several hours of daytime fasting, with or without a preceding overnight fast. The same laboratory testing panel as described earlier then can be obtained if symptoms suggestive of hypoglycemia occur. For patients who describe postprandial hypoglycemic symptoms (within 5 hours after a meal), a mixed meal (not a pure glucose load) should be provided, with blood sampling at baseline and every 30 minutes thereafter for 5 hours.

For patients who do not manifest hypoglycemia with the testing procedures described despite a strong suspicion of hypoglycemia, the most frequently utilized approach is a 72-hour fast according to a protocol developed at the Mayo Clinic. Blood is obtained every 6 hours and at test termination. The test is ended at 72 hours or at an earlier time point if the plasma glucose level decreases (by glucose meter testing) with associated symptoms to 45 mg/dL (2.5 mmol/L) or lower or to less than 55 mg/dL (3 mmol/L) in a patient with prior documentation of Whipple triad. At the end of the 72-hour test period, the patient is given 1 mg of glucagon intravenously, and blood is obtained at 10, 20, and 30 minutes, after which the patient is given a meal. The final blood sample obtained at the end of the fast (before glucagon administration) is analyzed additionally for β-hydroxybutyrate and a sulfonylurea/meglitinide panel.

For any of these test protocols, elevations of insulin, proinsulin, and C-peptide associated with hypoglycemia at the same time point are consistent with an insulinoma, beta-cell hyperplasia, the effects of an insulin secretagogue (sulfonylurea or meglitinide), or the presence of insulin antibodies. An elevation in these three hormones during a meal test in a patient who has had gastric surgery is suggestive of alimentary hypoglycemia. Plasma insulin, proinsulin, and C-peptide are not elevated in patients with hypoglycemia secondary to extrapancreatic neoplasms. This diagnosis usually can be further confirmed by evidence of a large tumor with various imaging techniques. High insulin levels, together with low proinsulin and C-peptide concentrations in the presence of hypoglycemia, are indicative of exogenous insulin administration. Factitious hypoglycemia secondary to insulin or insulin secretagogue administration is uncommon and has been observed in individuals with or without diabetes.

Treatment

The most important therapeutic step in hypoglycemia is to identify and treat the underlying causes, including drugs, alcohol, serious infection, tumors, and hypoadrenalism. The occurrence of hypoglycemia usually can be substantially improved in patients with alimentary hypoglycemia by a modified feeding regimen with frequent, small meals and avoidance of concentrated sources of rapidly digested and absorbed carbohydrate.

Non–islet cell tumor hypoglycemia is treated by tumor resection if possible. For nonresectable tumors, a debulking procedure may be effective in reducing hypoglycemia. Hypoglycemia in patients with insulinomas can be cured by resection. Persistent hypoglycemia secondary to nonresectable insulinoma can sometimes be treated effectively with diazoxide, long-acting somatostatin analogues (octreotide or lanreotide), verapamil, or phenytoin. For patients with beta-cell hyperplasia after bariatric surgery, first-line treatment includes diet modifications with more frequent, small meals and avoidance of concentrated sources of carbohydrate to decrease meal-induced insulin secretion.

For a deeper discussion of this topic, please see Chapter 216, ❖ "Diabetes Mellitus," and Chapter 217, "Hypoglycemia and Pancreatic Islet Cell Disorders," in *Goldman-Cecil Medicine*, 26th Edition.

SUGGESTED READINGS

ACOG Practice Bulletin No. 190: Gestational diabetes mellitus. Committee on practice bulletins—obstetrics, Obstet Gynecol 131:e49–e64, 2018.

American Diabetes Association Standards of Medical Care in Diabetes 2019: Diabetes Care 42(Suppl 1):S1–S193, 2019.

Cryer PE, Axelrod L, Grossman AB, et al: Evaluation and management of adult hypoglycemic disorders: an Endocrine Society clinical practice guideline, J Clin Endocrinol Metab 94:709–728, 2009.

Davies MJ, D'Alessio DA, Fradkin J, et al: Management of hyperglycemia in type 2 diabetes, 2018. A consensus report by the American Diabetes Association (ADA) and the European Association for the Study of Diabetes (EASD), Diabetes Care 41:2669–2701, 2018.

Eckel RH, Grundy SM, Zimmet PZ: The metabolic syndrome, Lancet 365:1415–1428, 2005.

Forbes JM, Cooper ME: Mechanisms of diabetic complications, Physiol Rev 93:137–188, 2013.

Nathan DM, Cleary PA, Backlund JY, et al: Intensive diabetes treatment and cardiovascular disease in patients with type 1 diabetes. Diabetes Control and Complications Trial/Epidemiology of Diabetes Interventions and Complications (DCCT/EDIC) Study Research Group, N Engl J Med 353:2643–2653, 2005.

Pathak V, Pathak NM, O'Neill CL, et al: Therapies for type 1 diabetes: current scenario and future perspectives, Clin Med Insights Endocrinol Diabetes 12:1179551419844521, 2019.

Pop-Busu R, Boulton AJM, Feldman EL, et al: Diabetic neuropathy: a position statement by the American Diabetes Association, Diabetes Care 40:136–154, 2017.

Sanyoura M, Philipson LH, Naylor R: Monogenic diabetes in children and adolescents: recognition and treatment options, Curr Diab Rep 18:58, 2018. https://doi.org/10.1007/s11892-018-1024-2.

Seaquist ER, Anderson J, Childs B, et al: Hypoglycemia and diabetes: a report of a workgroup of the American Diabetes Association and the Endocrine Society, J Clin Endocrinol Metab 98:1845–1859, 2013.

Tauschmann M, Hovorka R: Technology in the management of type 1 diabetes mellitus—current status and future prospects, Nat Rev Endocrinol 14:464–475, 2018.

Torres JM, Cox NJ, Philipson LH: Genome wide association studies for diabetes: perspective on results and challenges, Pediatr Diabetes 14:90–96, 2013.

Warren AM, Knudsen ST, Cooper ME: Diabetic nephropathy: an insight into molecular mechanisms and emerging therapies, Expert Opin Ther Targets 23:579–591, 2019.

或 T1DM 患者出现胰岛素敏感性显著增加。患者可能患有已知肿瘤，提示非胰岛细胞肿瘤可能是低血糖的原因。既往接受过 Roux-en-Y 旁路手术可增加 β 细胞增生的可能性。合并感染中毒症、肝衰竭、肾衰竭、严重营养不良或神经性厌食症时，提示这些疾病可能是低血糖的潜在原因。

目前已有多种流程用于指导低血糖的评估，包括美国内分泌学会发布的专家小组推荐方案。如果有机会在推测的低血糖症状发作期间观察患者，应尽可能在治疗前获取血浆，用于检测葡萄糖、胰岛素、胰岛素原、C 肽、β - 羟丁酸，以及筛查磺酰脲类药物和格列奈类药物。低血糖可通过血糖仪迅速初步确定，然后通过实验室检测确认。获取上述用于检测的血液样本后，应给予口服葡萄糖（15 ～ 30 g）或静脉注射葡萄糖（25 g 或 1 安瓿 50% 葡萄糖），并观察血糖水平和症状的恢复。

对于疑诊或已确诊空腹低血糖的患者，可通过日间禁食数小时或前一晚开始禁食来诱发低血糖症状。如果出现提示低血糖的症状，可进行上述实验室检测。对于有餐后低血糖症状（进餐后 5 h 内）的患者，应提供混合餐（不是纯葡萄糖负荷），并从基线开始每 30 min 采血 1 次，持续 5 h。

对于强烈怀疑低血糖但通过上述检测流程未表现出低血糖的患者，最常用的方法是根据梅奥诊所制定的流程进行 72 h 禁食试验。每 6 h 检测 1 次，并在试验结束时检测 1 次。试验在 72 h 后结束，当血糖（采用血糖仪检测）≤ 45 mg/dl（2.5 mmol/L）且伴有低血糖症状或 Whipple 三联症患者血糖≤ 55 mg/dl（3 mmol/L）时，则试验提前结束。在试验结束时，给予患者静脉注射 1 mg 胰高血糖素，并在 10 min、20 min 和 30 min 后采血，之后给予患者进食。在禁食结束时（胰高血糖素给药前）获取的最终血液样本还可用于检测 β - 羟丁酸和磺酰脲类药物 / 格列奈类药物。

在低血糖发作时检测到胰岛素、胰岛素原和 C 肽任一指标的升高，考虑诊断胰岛素瘤、β 细胞增生、应用胰岛素促泌剂（磺酰脲类药物或格列奈类药物）或存在胰岛素抗体。在有胃手术史的患者中，进餐混合餐后低血糖发作时若上述 3 种激素水平升高，则提示营养性低血糖。在继发于胰腺外肿瘤的低血糖患者中，血浆胰岛素、胰岛素原和 C 肽水平不升高。胰腺外肿瘤的诊断通常可通过影像学检查证明有巨大肿瘤来进一步确认。在低血糖的情况下，胰岛素水平升高、胰岛素原水平降低和 C 肽水平降低提示给予了外源性胰岛素。给予胰岛素或胰岛素促泌剂引起的人为性低血糖并不常见，但在有或无糖尿病的个体中均有报道。

治疗

低血糖最重要的治疗步骤是识别和治疗潜在病因，包括药物、酒精、严重感染、肿瘤和肾上腺功能减退。通过调整进食方案（少食多餐、避免摄入快速消化和吸收的高升糖指数碳水化合物），通常可显著减少营养性低血糖。

手术切除肿瘤可治疗非胰岛细胞肿瘤引起的低血糖。对于无法切除的肿瘤，减瘤手术可能在减少低血糖方面有效。胰岛素瘤患者的低血糖可通过切除肿瘤而治愈。对于无法切除的胰岛素瘤引起的持续性低血糖，有时可使用二氮嗪、长效生长抑素类似物（奥曲肽或兰瑞肽）、维拉帕米或苯妥英治疗。对于减重术后 β 细胞增生的患者，一线治疗包括饮食调整（少食多餐，避免摄入高升糖指数碳水化合物），以减少餐后胰岛素分泌。

有关此专题的深入讨论，请参阅 *Goldman-Cecil Medicine* 第 26 版第 216 章 "糖尿病" 和第 217 章 "低血糖和胰岛细胞疾病"。 ❖

推荐阅读

ACOG Practice Bulletin No. 190: Gestational diabetes mellitus. Committee on practice bulletins—obstetrics, Obstet Gynecol 131:e49–e64, 2018.

American Diabetes Association Standards of Medical Care in Diabetes 2019: Diabetes Care 42(Suppl 1):S1–S193, 2019.

Cryer PE, Axelrod L, Grossman AB, et al: Evaluation and management of adult hypoglycemic disorders: an Endocrine Society clinical practice guideline, J Clin Endocrinol Metab 94:709–728, 2009.

Davies MJ, D'Alessio DA, Fradkin J, et al: Management of hyperglycemia in type 2 diabetes, 2018. A consensus report by the American Diabetes Association (ADA) and the European Association for the Study of Diabetes (EASD), Diabetes Care 41:2669–2701, 2018.

Eckel RH, Grundy SM, Zimmet PZ: The metabolic syndrome, Lancet 365:1415–1428, 2005.

Forbes JM, Cooper ME: Mechanisms of diabetic complications, Physiol Rev 93:137–188, 2013.

Nathan DM, Cleary PA, Backlund JY, et al: Intensive diabetes treatment and cardiovascular disease in patients with type 1 diabetes. Diabetes Control and Complications Trial/Epidemiology of Diabetes Interventions and Complications (DCCT/EDIC) Study Research Group, N Engl J Med 353:2643–2653, 2005.

Pathak V, Pathak NM, O'Neill CL, et al: Therapies for type 1 diabetes: current scenario and future perspectives, Clin Med Insights Endocrinol Diabetes 12:1179551419844521, 2019.

Pop-Busu R, Boulton AJM, Feldman EL, et al: Diabetic neuropathy: a position statement by the American Diabetes Association, Diabetes Care 40:136–154, 2017.

Sanyoura M, Philipson LH, Naylor R: Monogenic diabetes in children and adolescents: recognition and treatment options, Curr Diab Rep 18:58, 2018. https://doi.org/10.1007/s11892-018-1024-2.

Seaquist ER, Anderson J, Childs B, et al: Hypoglycemia and diabetes: a report of a workgroup of the American Diabetes Association and the Endocrine Society, J Clin Endocrinol Metab 98:1845–1859, 2013.

Tauschmann M, Hovorka R: Technology in the management of type 1 diabetes mellitus—current status and future prospects, Nat Rev Endocrinol 14:464–475, 2018.

Torres JM, Cox NJ, Philipson LH: Genome wide association studies for diabetes: perspective on results and challenges, Pediatr Diabetes 14:90–96, 2013.

Warren AM, Knudsen ST, Cooper ME: Diabetic nephropathy: an insight into molecular mechanisms and emerging therapies, Expert Opin Ther Targets 23:579–591, 2019.

6

Obesity

Osama Hamdy, Marwa Al-Badri

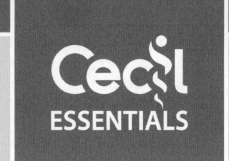

DEFINITION AND EPIDEMIOLOGY

Obesity is a disease that is usually defined as a body mass index (BMI) greater than or equal to 30 kg/m^2 (weight [kg]/(height [m])^2). A BMI of 30 to 34.9 is considered class 1 obesity, 35 to 39.9 is class 2 obesity, and 40 or higher is class 3 or severe obesity. The term "morbid obesity" previously was applied to individuals weighing at least 45 kg (100 lb) more than, or typically about 60% more than, desirable body weight; the term also has been applied to any individual with BMI greater than or equal to 40 kg/m^2.

There is increasing recognition of limitations to defining obesity based on BMI resulting from the variable correlation between BMI and amount of body fat in different ethnic (genetic) populations or in individuals with different degrees of muscularity. Many investigators and clinicians are moving toward a definition that defines obesity as an excess of body fat sufficient to confer risk. According to the percentage of body fat, obesity is defined in men as percentage of body fat greater than 25%, with 21% to 25% being borderline, and in women as percentage of body fat greater than 33%, with 31% to 33% being borderline.

Linking obesity to cardiometabolic risk, body fat distribution, and waist circumference is more important than measuring percentage body fat or BMI alone. People who accumulate abdominal visceral fat and clinically have higher waist circumference (metabolic obesity) are at much higher risk for cardiovascular disease and diabetes than those with the same BMI or the same percentage of body fat but with lower waist circumference. The National Cholesterol Education Program Adult Treatment Panel III (ATP III) considered a waist circumference greater than 40 inches (102 cm) in American men or 35 inches (88 cm) in American women to be among the five criteria that define the cardiometabolic syndrome. In spite of its limitations, BMI remains a simple measurement with utility in estimating a person's health risks and comparing outcomes between trials.

During the last 30 years, there has been a dramatic increase in the percentage of both adults and children in the United States who are overweight (defined as BMI of 25 to 30) or obese. According to the 2015-2016 National Health and Nutrition Examination Survey (NHANES) conducted by the Centers for Disease Control and Prevention (CDC), 39.8% of US adults were obese, including 7.6% with severe obesity, and an additional 31.8% are overweight. This was more than double the prevalence in the 1976-1980 NHANES data (15.0%). Mexican Americans had the highest age-adjusted percentage of obesity (49.25%), followed by all Hispanic individuals (46.85%), non-Hispanic black (45.8%), and non-Hispanic white individuals (37.95%). More recently, there appears to have been a slowing in the rate of obesity increase or even a leveling off. In 2017, obesity prevalence seemed to vary significantly across states, from 20% or less in Colorado, Hawaii, and District of Columbia to 35% or more in seven states (Alabama, Arkansas, Iowa, Louisiana, Mississippi, Oklahoma, and West Virginia). In general, higher prevalence of adult obesity was found in the south (32.4%) and the midwest (32.3%) and lower prevalence in the northeast (27.7%) and the west (26.1%). The percentage of children and adolescents who are overweight or obese has almost tripled since 1980. Currently, 18.5% of children and adolescents aged 2 to 19 years are obese, including 5.6% with severe obesity, and another 16.6% are overweight. NHANES data from 1976-1980 and from 2015-2016 show that the prevalence of obesity increased from 5.0% to 13.9% for children aged 2 to 5 years and from 5.0% to 20.6% for those aged 12 to 19 years. Among low-income preschool children, the prevalence of obesity increased between 1998 and 2016 from 13.0% to 13.9% and severe obesity from 1.8% to 2.1%.

Overweight and obesity and their associated health problems have a significant economic impact on the US health care system through direct medical expenses and indirect costs (e.g., loss of work time and productivity). Medical costs of obesity and their associated health problems account for an estimated 10% of total US medical expenditures.

PATHOLOGY OF OBESITY

Obesity develops as a consequence of genetic-environmental interactions, such that genetically prone individuals who lead a sedentary lifestyle and consume larger amounts of dietary calories are at higher risk. For example, children of obese parents are 80% more likely to become obese, and it is believed that this results from a combination of genetic and environmental influences.

The genetic contributions to obesity are most commonly considered to reflect the combined effects of variations in multiple genes and only rarely appear to result from a defect in a single powerful gene. Single-gene defects identified in experimental animals have been useful to demonstrate appetite and satiety mechanisms. Mutations in some of these same genes have subsequently been identified in rare human forms of genetic obesity. For example, loss-of-function mutations in the leptin gene and in the cellular receptor for leptin were first identified as a cause of obesity in laboratory mice (*ob/ob* and *db/db* mice, respectively). Leptin is a hormone that is produced in fat cells, mostly in subcutaneous fat. It is a potent satiety factor that acts in the arcuate nucleus of the hypothalamus to reduce the production of neuropeptide Y, a stimulator of food intake. After its discovery in mice, leptin gene mutations were identified as a cause of a rare form of heritable human obesity. Affected individuals develop marked obesity in childhood as a consequence of increased food intake. Leptin secretion normally follows a circadian pattern, with higher levels during evening and night hours. Loss of leptin secretion has particularly marked effects during these hours, resulting in a phenomenon known as the night-eating syndrome, in which patients tend to consume large amounts of food during the night.

肥胖症

赵宇星 译 王林杰 朱惠娟 审校 宁光 通审

定义和流行病学

肥胖症通常被定义为体重指数（BMI）≥ 30 kg/m²［体重（kg）/身高（m）的平方］的疾病。BMI 为 30 ～ 34.9 kg/m² 为 1 级肥胖症，35 ～ 39.9 kg/m² 为 2 级肥胖症，≥ 40 kg/m² 为 3 级或重度肥胖症。术语"病态肥胖症"曾被定义为体重超过理想体重 ≥ 45 kg 或超过理想体重 ≥ 60% 的个体；该术语也适用于 BMI ≥ 40 kg/m² 的个体。

人们越来越认识到基于 BMI 定义肥胖的局限性，因为不同种族（遗传）人群或肌肉含量的个体，其 BMI 与身体脂肪量的相关性不同。许多研究者和临床医生逐渐倾向于将肥胖定义为可引发健康风险的体内脂肪过量。男性体脂百分比 > 25% 被定义为肥胖症，21% ～ 25% 为临界范围，女性体脂百分比 > 33% 被定义为肥胖症，31% ～ 33% 为临界范围。

将肥胖症与心脏代谢风险、体脂分布和腰围联系起来比单独测量体脂百分比或 BMI 更为重要。腹部内脏脂肪堆积和腰围较大者（代谢性肥胖）罹患心血管疾病和糖尿病的风险远高于相同 BMI 或相同体脂百分比但腰围较小者。美国国家胆固醇教育计划成人治疗小组 Ⅲ（ATP Ⅲ）认为，美国男性腰围 > 102 cm 或女性腰围 > 88 cm 是心脏代谢综合征的 5 项标准之一。尽管存在局限性，BMI 仍然是评估个人健康风险和临床试验中用于结果比较的简便方法。

在过去 30 年中，美国成人和儿童的超重（BMI 为 25 ～ 30 kg/m²）率和肥胖率显著升高。根据美国疾病预防控制中心（CDC）于 2015—2016 年进行的美国全国健康与营养调查（NHANES）显示，39.8% 的美国成人患有肥胖症，其中 7.6% 为重度肥胖症，另有 31.8% 为超重，比 1976—1980 年 NHANES 统计的肥胖症患病率（15.0%）高出 1 倍以上。墨西哥裔美国人的年龄调整后肥胖率最高（49.25%），其次是所有西班牙裔人群（46.85%）、非西班牙裔黑人（45.8%）和非西班牙裔白人（37.95%）。近期，肥胖率升高的速度似乎有所放缓，甚至出现趋于稳定的迹象。2017 年，肥胖率在美国各州之间存在显著差异，如科罗拉多州、夏威夷州和哥伦比亚特区的肥胖率 ≤ 20%，而另外 7 个州（阿拉巴马州、阿肯色州、爱荷华州、路易斯安那州、密西西比

州、俄克拉荷马州和西弗吉尼亚州）则 ≥ 35%。总体而言，美国成人肥胖率较高的地区为南部（32.4%）和中西部（32.3%），而东北部（27.7%）和西部（26.1%）的肥胖率较低。自 1980 年以来，儿童和青少年的超重率和肥胖率几乎增长了 2 倍。目前，在 2 ～ 19 岁的儿童及青少年中，18.5% 患有肥胖症，其中 5.6% 为重度肥胖症，另有 16.6% 为超重。1976—1980 年和 2015—2016 年的 NHANES 数据显示，2 ～ 5 岁儿童的肥胖症患病率从 5.0% 升至 13.9%，12 ～ 19 岁青少年的肥胖症患病率从 5.0% 升至 20.6%。根据 1998—2016 年的统计，在低收入家庭的学龄前儿童中，肥胖症患病率从 13.0% 升至 13.9%，重度肥胖症患病率从 1.8% 升至 2.1%。

超重和肥胖症及其相关健康问题对美国医疗保健系统产生了严重的经济影响，包括直接医疗费用和间接成本（如工作时间和生产力损失）。肥胖症及其相关健康问题的医疗费用估计占美国总医疗支出的 10%。

肥胖症的病理学

肥胖症是遗传和环境相互作用的结果，因此，久坐不动、摄入较多热量的遗传易感人群患肥胖症的风险更高。例如，父母患有肥胖症的个体患肥胖症的可能性高达 80%，这被认为是遗传因素和环境因素综合作用的结果。

肥胖症的遗传因素通常是多个基因变异的综合效应，只有极少数情况下是由单一基因缺陷造成。在实验动物中鉴定的单基因缺陷已被证实与食欲和饱腹感机制相关。随后，这些基因中的部分基因突变在罕见的遗传性肥胖症患者中被鉴定出来。例如，瘦素及瘦素细胞受体基因的功能缺失突变首次被确定为肥胖症实验小鼠（分别为 ob/ob 和 db/db 小鼠）的病因。瘦素主要由皮下脂肪细胞分泌。它是一种强效的饱腹感因子，作用于下丘脑弓状核，使神经肽 Y（促进食物摄入的因子）生成减少。继小鼠动物实验后，瘦素基因突变也被证实为人类罕见的遗传性肥胖症的原因之一。瘦素基因突变的个体由于食物摄入量增加而在童年期出现明显肥胖。瘦素分泌通常具有昼夜节律，傍晚和夜间分泌水平较高。瘦素分泌减少在这些时段的影响尤为明显，导致"夜食症"，患者通常在夜间摄入大量食物。

Other single-gene defects identified as rare causes of human obesity include loss-of-function mutations in genes encoding carboxypeptidase E, melanocortin-4 or melanocortin-3 receptors, and serotonin-2C or serotonin-1B receptors. Obesity is also a feature of many other genetic disorders in which the specific mechanisms of the obesity are less well understood. These different syndromes may have autosomal dominant, autosomal recessive or X-linked inheritance patterns, consistent with multiple different genetic causes. Among the best known of these disorders is the Bardet-Biedl syndrome, which is an autosomal recessive disorder characterized by obesity and other abnormalities, including hypogonadism in men, mental retardation, retinal dystrophy, polydactyly, and renal malformations. In Prader-Willi syndrome, loss of portions of the long arm of chromosome 15 (q11-13) is associated with obesity, poor muscle tone in infancy, defects in cognition, behavioral abnormalities (irritability), short stature, and hypogonadotropic hypogonadism.

Although known single-gene mutations account for only a small percentage of human obesity, there is evidence for widespread heritable influences in more common forms of human obesity. For example, in twin and adoptee studies, both members of identical twin pairs tend to become obese in concordance with the same weight pattern as their biologic parents, even when raised apart. Metabolic rate, spontaneous physical activity, and thermic response to food seem to be heritable to a variable extent, but the specific genes that contribute to prevalent forms of human obesity have not yet been identified. Genomic analyses in large populations have identified multiple genes or genetic regions in which polymorphisms are associated with obesity risk. These include polymorphisms in or near genes for the melanocortin-4 receptor (a protein involved in appetite suppression pathways in the hypothalamus), brain-derived neurotrophic factor (role in energy balance), the β_3-adrenergic receptor (role in visceral fat accumulation), and peroxisome proliferator-activated receptor-$\gamma2$ (PPAR-$\gamma2$), a transcription factor involved in adipocyte differentiation. Multiple other sites of genetic variation associated with increased obesity risk have been identified for which potential mechanistic links to obesity are not yet apparent. It is hypothesized that the heritable component of common forms of human obesity derives from the effects of variations in these and many yet unidentified genes acting both additively and synergistically.

Important environmental factors driving the recent increased prevalence of obesity include increased caloric intake (reflecting greater availability of high-calorie, low-cost foods) and decreased energy expenditure (as a consequence of decreased physical activity). Lower socioeconomic status, lower education level, cessation of smoking, and high consumption of carbohydrates with a high glycemic index have been identified as specific confounders of obesity. Additional factors that may influence obesity risk include intrauterine growth, weight gain during pregnancy, hormonal changes during menopause, history of depression, use of major antipsychotic medications, and factors that may alter the feedback between energy intake and expenditure.

Many hormones affect appetite and food intake. Ghrelin, which is secreted from the stomach fundus, is a major hunger hormone. Endocannabinoids, through their effects on endocannabinoid receptors in the brain, increase appetite, promote nutrient absorption, and promote lipogenesis. Melanocortin hormone, through its effects on various melanocortin receptors in the brain, modifies appetite. Meanwhile, several gut hormones play significant roles in influencing satiety, including glucagon-like peptide-1 (GLP-1), neuropeptide YY (PYY), and cholecystokinin. Leptin and pancreatic amylin are other potent satiety hormones. Ultimately, an increase in total body fat results from an increase in energy intake that exceeds energy expenditure.

This occurs through the operation of genetic and environmental influences, together with individual behavioral characteristics.

PATHOLOGY OF OBESITY-ASSOCIATED HEALTH RISKS

Adipose tissue is not just a passive depot for lipids. Adipocytes also function as a complex and active endocrine organ with metabolic and secretory products (hormones, prohormones, cytokines, and enzymes) that play a major role in whole-body metabolism. Relationships between obesity and both insulin resistance and endothelial dysfunction (the early stage of atherosclerosis) are mediated through the release of several hormones from adipose tissue. These hormones, designated adipocytokines or adipokines, comprise a group of pharmacologically active low- and medium-molecular-weight proteins that possess autocrine and paracrine effects and are known products of the inflammatory and immune systems. They play an important role in adipose tissue physiology and in initiating metabolic and cardiovascular abnormalities, not only in overweight and obese individuals, but also in lean persons with higher visceral fat mass. These adipokines include adiponectin, leptin, tumor necrosis factor-α (TNF-α), interleukin-6 (IL-6), resistin, plasminogen activator inhibitor-1 (PAI-1), angiotensinogen, and monocyte chemoattractant protein-1 (MCP-1). An increased amount of adipose tissue or its disproportionate distribution between central and peripheral body regions is related to altered serum levels of these factors. With the exceptions of leptin and adiponectin, the adipokines are produced both from fat cells and from adipose tissue–resident macrophages in the stromal tissues surrounding fat cells. For unknown reasons, an increase in the amount of body fat is associated with increases in the number of adipose tissue macrophages and their production of cytokines.

Human adiponectin is a relatively abundant, 244-amino-acid polypeptide in plasma, accounting for 0.01% of total plasma proteins. Adiponectin gene expression in adipose tissue is associated with obesity, insulin resistance, and type 2 diabetes (T2DM). Hypoadiponectinemia is more strongly related to the degree of insulin resistance than to the degree of adiposity or glucose intolerance. Genetic polymorphisms may influence the regulation of adiponectin and lead to variations in its levels among different individuals. Several human studies have shown that high adiponectin levels protect against development of T2DM and point to the possible future use of adiponectin as an indicator of diabetes risk. Low plasma concentrations of adiponectin are observed in patients with coronary artery disease (CAD), and lower adiponectin levels have been found in patients with diabetes and CAD than in those without CAD. In obesity, a 10% reduction in body weight leads to a significant increase in adiponectin (40% to 60%) in both patients with and without diabetes. Adiponectin is also involved in the modulation of inflammatory responses through attenuation of TNF-α–mediated inflammatory effects, regulation of endothelial function, and inhibition of growth factor–induced proliferation of vascular smooth muscle cells.

Leptin is a 167-amino-acid adipocyte-derived hormone that circulates in the plasma in free and bound forms. It affects energy balance by activating specific centers in the hypothalamus to decrease food intake, increase energy expenditure, modulate glucose and fat metabolism, and alter neuroendocrine function. Leptin plasma levels increase exponentially with increased fat mass (4-fold higher in obese compared with lean individuals in one study), and this is thought to reflect resistance to leptin in obesity. Leptin therapy in lipodystrophic patients has been shown to lower blood glucose, improve insulin-stimulated hepatic and peripheral glucose metabolism, and reduce hepatic and muscle triglyceride content, suggesting that leptin acts as a signal that

被确定为人类肥胖症罕见病因的其他单基因缺陷包括编码羧肽酶 E、促黑素细胞激素 -4 或促黑素细胞激素 -3 受体，以及 5- 羟色胺 2C 受体或 5- 羟色胺 1B 受体的基因的功能缺失突变。肥胖症也是许多遗传性疾病的特征之一，这些疾病导致肥胖症的具体机制尚不清楚。与多种遗传学病因一样，这些综合征可呈常染色体显性遗传、常染色体隐性遗传或 X 连锁遗传。其中最为人所熟知的疾病之一是巴尔得－别德尔综合征（Bardet-Biedl 综合征），这是一种以肥胖症和其他器官异常（包括男性性腺功能减退症、智力低下、视网膜萎缩、多指、肾畸形）为特征的常染色体隐性遗传病。在普拉德－威利综合征（Prader-Willi 综合征）中，15 号染色体长臂（q11-13）部分缺失与肥胖症、婴儿期肌张力下降、认知障碍、行为异常（易激惹）、身材矮小和低促性腺激素性性腺功能减退症有关。

虽然已知的单基因突变仅占人类肥胖症的一小部分，但有证据表明，在更常见的人类肥胖症形式中，遗传因素的影响普遍存在。例如，在双胞胎和领养者研究中发现，同卵双胞胎会逐渐发展为与亲生父母体重模式一致的肥胖症，即使是在不同的环境中长大。代谢率、自发运动和食物热效应似乎在一定程度上是可遗传的，但目前尚未确定导致人类常见肥胖症形式的具体基因。大规模人群基因组分析已经确定了多个与肥胖症风险相关的基因或基因区域的多态性。包括编码促黑素细胞激素 -4 受体（一种参与下丘脑食欲抑制通路的蛋白质）、脑源性神经营养因子（参与能量平衡）、β_3 受体（参与内脏脂肪积聚）和过氧化物酶体增殖物激活受体 - $\gamma 2$（PPAR- $\gamma 2$；一种参与脂肪细胞分化的转录因子）的基因或附近基因的多态性。多个其他遗传变异位点与肥胖症风险增加相关，但其相关性的潜在机制尚不明确。据推测，人类常见肥胖症形式的遗传因素来源于这些已确定和许多尚未确定的基因变异的叠加和协同作用。

导致近年来肥胖症患病率升高的重要环境因素包括热量摄入增加（反映出高热量、低成本食品的供应量增加）和能量消耗减少（运动减少的结果）。社会经济地位较低、教育水平较低、戒烟、大量摄入高升糖指数的碳水化合物等因素已被确定为肥胖症的特异性混杂因素。可能影响肥胖症风险的其他因素包括子宫内发育、妊娠期体重增加、绝经期激素变化、抑郁症病史、使用抗精神病药，以及可能改变能量摄入与消耗之间反馈机制的因素。

许多激素会影响食欲和食物摄入。胃底部分泌的胃生长激素释放素是主要的饥饿激素。内源性大麻素可通过对大脑内源性大麻素受体的作用而增加食欲，促进营养吸收，并促进脂肪合成。促黑素细胞激素可通过对大脑中多种促黑素细胞激素受体的作用而调节食欲。同时，多种肠道激素在影响饱腹感方面也发挥着重要作用，包括胰高血糖素样肽 -1（GLP-1）、神经肽 YY（PYY）和胆囊收缩素。瘦素和胰岛淀粉素是强效的饱腹感激素。总体脂的增加是由能量摄入超过能量消耗所致。这是通过遗传影响、环境影响及个体行为特征的共同作用来实现。

肥胖症相关健康风险的病理学

脂肪组织不仅是脂质的被动储存库。脂肪细胞也是一个复杂而活跃的内分泌器官，可参与代谢且具有分泌功能（可分泌激素、激素原、细胞因子和酶），并在全身代谢中发挥重要作用。肥胖症与胰岛素抵抗和内皮功能障碍（动脉粥样硬化的早期阶段）之间的关系是通过脂肪组织释放多种激素介导的。这些激素被称为脂肪细胞因子或脂肪因子，包括一组具有药理学活性的低分子量和中分子量蛋白质，具有自分泌和旁分泌作用，是炎症和免疫系统的产物。它们在脂肪组织生理代谢及促发代谢异常和心血管异常方面发挥重要作用，不仅在超重和肥胖症个体中，在腹部脂肪过多的非肥胖症人群中也是如此。这些脂肪因子包括脂联素、瘦素、肿瘤坏死因子 - α（TNF- α）、白介素 -6（IL-6）、抵抗素、纤溶酶原激活物抑制剂 -1（PAI-1）、血管紧张素原和单核细胞趋化蛋白 -1（MCP-1）。脂肪组织量增加或脂肪组织在躯干和四肢区域的不均匀分布与这些因子的血清水平异常相关。除瘦素和脂联素外，其他脂肪因子既可由脂肪细胞产生，也可由环绕在脂肪细胞周围的基质组织中的巨噬细胞产生。体脂含量增加与脂肪组织巨噬细胞数量的增加及其产生的细胞因子相关，但其原因尚不明确。

人类脂联素是一种在血浆中含量相对丰富的多肽，由 244 个氨基酸组成，占血浆蛋白总量的 0.01%。脂肪组织中的脂联素基因表达与肥胖症、胰岛素抵抗和 2 型糖尿病（T2DM）有关。相比于与脂肪过多或糖耐量异常程度的关联，低脂联素血症与胰岛素抵抗程度的关联更为密切。基因多态性可能影响脂联素的调节，并导致个体之间脂联素水平的差异。多项人类研究表明，高脂联素水平可预防 T2DM 的发生，且脂联素未来可能成为糖尿病风险的潜在预测指标。在冠心病（CAD）患者中可观察到血浆脂联素浓度降低，且合并 CAD 的糖尿病患者的脂联素水平低于不合并 CAD 的患者。在肥胖症患者中，体重减轻 10% 可使脂联素显著增加（40% ～ 60%），无论是否患有糖尿病。脂联素还可减轻 TNF- α 介导的炎症效应、调节内皮功能和抑制生长因子诱导的血管平滑肌细胞增殖，从而参与炎症反应的调节。

瘦素是一种由脂肪细胞生成的含有 167 个氨基酸的激素，在血浆中以游离和结合形式循环。它通过激活下丘脑中的特定中枢来减少摄食、增加能量消耗、调节葡萄糖和脂肪代谢、改变神经内分泌功能，从而影响能量平衡。血浆瘦素水平随脂肪量的增加呈指数增长（在一项研究中，肥胖症患者的血清瘦素水平较瘦者高 4 倍），这与肥胖症患者存在瘦素抵抗相关。研究表明，给予脂肪营养不良患者瘦素治疗可降低血糖，改善胰岛素介导的肝脏和外周葡萄糖代谢，并减少肝脏和肌肉的甘油三

contributes to regulation of total body sensitivity to insulin. It has also been found that leptin is independently associated with cardiovascular mortality. Although both adiponectin and leptin are integrally related to insulin resistance, adiponectin is more strongly related to visceral abdominal fat stores, whereas leptin is more closely related to subcutaneous fat.

Adipose tissue, especially visceral fat and intermuscular fat, serves as a major source of TNF-α and substantial amounts of IL-6. Levels of these two proinflammatory cytokines correlate with obesity and are strongly related to insulin resistance. Several studies have demonstrated a strong link between TNF-α and cardiovascular disease. Plasma levels of TNF-α are increased in individuals with premature cardiovascular disease independent of insulin sensitivity. Conversely, circulating levels of TNF-α decrease after weight reduction in parallel with the improvement in endothelial function.

Resistin is an adipocyte-derived, cysteine-rich signaling protein that is expressed predominantly in white adipose tissue and is also detectable in serum. Resistin is thought to act at sites remote from adipose tissue, similar to other adipokines, and to contribute to insulin resistance in obesity. *PAI-1* is another bioactive peptide produced by subcutaneous and visceral fat. Its circulating levels correlate better with visceral than with subcutaneous adiposity and are strong predictors of CAD. High PAI-1 levels are associated with increased blood coagulability. Improvement in insulin sensitivity by either weight reduction or medication lowers circulating levels of PAI-1. This decrease in PAI-1 correlates with the amount of weight loss and the decline in serum triglycerides.

Visceral, subcutaneous, and intermuscular fat differ in their production of specific adipokines, pointing to differences in endocrine function between these three adipose depots. Removal of a significant amount of only subcutaneous fat by liposuction in obese individuals with and without diabetes resulted in reduction in serum leptin but did not change the serum levels of other cytokines or any other metabolic parameters. It also did not improve insulin sensitivity or decrease the high serum insulin level observed initially in those individuals. In animal models, removal of subcutaneous fat resulted in an increase in mesenteric fat volume and increased production of TNF-α by visceral fat. Although surgical removal of visceral fat has not been attempted in humans, two studies of aging in rodent models showed that removal of visceral fat reduces the production of inflammatory adipokines and improves glucose tolerance and insulin sensitivity. More recently, it was shown that inflammatory adipokines are also secreted from intermuscular and subfascial fat and in excess of those secreted from abdominal visceral fat. Excess accumulation of intermuscular and subfascial fat (myosteatosis) is seen with ageing in both men and women and is strongly associated with insulin resistance.

Risks Associated With Obesity

Individuals who are overweight or obese are at increased risk for the following health conditions:
- Cardiometabolic syndrome
- T2DM
- Hypertension
- Dyslipidemia
- Coronary heart disease
- Congestive heart failure
- Atrial fibrillation
- Osteoarthritis
- Stroke
- Gallbladder disease
- Hepatic steatosis and nonalcoholic steatohepatitis (NASH)
- Obstructive sleep apnea

- Asthma
- Gastroesophageal reflux (GERD)
- Some cancers (endometrial, breast, and colon)
- Gynecologic disorders (abnormal menses, infertility, polycystic ovarian syndrome)
- Erectile dysfunction
- Depression

Weight loss of 7% to 10% is associated with reduced risk for many if not all of these disorders. Recent studies have shown that significant weight reduction (15% to 25% of initial body weight) after bariatric surgery in class 2 and class 3 obese patients with T2DM may result in partial or complete remission of diabetes, especially in patients with recent history of diabetes.

DIAGNOSIS AND ASSESSMENT OF OBESITY

The form of obesity that characteristically occurs in men—android or abdominal obesity (apple-shaped body configuration)—is closely associated with metabolic complications such as insulin resistance, hypertension, dyslipidemia, and hyperuricemia. By contrast, the typical female or gynecoid obesity (pear-shaped body configuration), in which fat accumulates in the hips and gluteal and femoral regions, has milder metabolic complications. The waist-to-hip circumference ratio (WHR) has been used to distinguish these forms of obesity. A ratio greater than 1.0 in men or greater than 0.8 in women, indicative of visceral fat deposition and abdominal obesity, correlates with increased health risks.

Standard laboratory studies in the evaluation of obesity should include the following:
- Fasting lipid panel
- Liver function tests
- Thyroid function tests
- Fasting plasma glucose
- Hemoglobin A1c (A1C)

Previously, the "gold standard" technique for measuring total body fat was *hydrodensitometry* (underwater weighing). This is based on the principle that fatty tissue is less dense than muscle. Currently, *dual-energy x-ray absorptiometry (DXA)* scanning is used to accurately measure body composition, particularly fat mass and fat-free mass. It has an additional advantage of measuring regional fat distribution. DXA is more accurate than anthropometric measures and is more cost-effective than computerized tomography (CT) or magnetic resonance imaging (MRI) scans. However, DXA cannot distinguish between subcutaneous and visceral abdominal fat depots, or between subcutaneous and intramuscular peripheral fat depots. Bioelectric impedance is a simpler and less expensive method for measuring total body fat, but it is greatly affected by the hydration state of the body and is less accurate than DXA.

BMI is widely used as a measure of obesity. It is calculated by dividing a person's body weight in kilograms by the square of the person's height in meters; alternatively, weight in pounds multiplied by 703 is divided by the square of the height in inches). A BMI between 19 and 27 has little association with cardiometabolic risk in white individuals. Adverse health consequences occur with a BMI of 27 or more and increase with increasing levels of BMI. Risks associated with increased BMI are more pronounced in older patients.

Waist circumference or *WHR* or both are often used to indirectly estimate intra-abdominal fat volume in epidemiologic studies. Although these measures show good correlation with intra-abdominal fat volume as measured by CT, they are less accurate than CT. At present, waist circumference is the easiest anthropometric measurement for routine use by health care professionals to estimate visceral adiposity and monitor changes in visceral fat volume.

酯含量，这表明瘦素参与调节全身对胰岛素的敏感性。研究发现，瘦素与心血管死亡率独立相关。虽然脂联素和瘦素均与胰岛素抵抗密切相关，但脂联素与内脏脂肪储存的关系更密切，而瘦素与皮下脂肪更为相关。

脂肪组织（尤其是内脏脂肪和肌间脂肪）是 TNF-α 和大量 IL-6 的主要来源。这两种促炎性细胞因子的水平与肥胖症相关，并与胰岛素抵抗密切相关。多项研究表明，TNF-α 与心血管疾病密切相关。无论胰岛素敏感性如何，早发心血管疾病患者的血浆 TNF-α 水平均会升高。相反，减重后，TNF-α 循环水平下降，同时内皮功能得到改善。

抵抗素是一种由脂肪细胞产生的富含半胱氨酸的信号蛋白，主要在白色脂肪组织中表达，在血清中也可检测到。与其他脂肪因子相似，抵抗素在远离脂肪组织的部位发挥作用，促进肥胖症患者发生胰岛素抵抗。PAI-1 是另一种由皮下脂肪和内脏脂肪产生的生物活性肽。相比于皮下脂肪，循环 PAI-1 水平与内脏脂肪的相关性更强，且是 CAD 的强预测因子。高水平 PAI-1 与血液高凝相关。通过减重或药物改善胰岛素敏感性会降低 PAI-1 的循环水平。PAI-1 水平下降与体重减轻和血清甘油三酯水平下降相关。

内脏脂肪、皮下脂肪和肌间脂肪在分泌特定脂肪因子方面存在差异，表明这 3 种脂肪库的内分泌功能也存在差异。对肥胖症患者（伴或不伴糖尿病）行吸脂术抽取大量皮下脂肪会导致血清瘦素水平下降，但不会改变其他细胞因子或代谢指标的血清水平，也没有改善患者的胰岛素敏感性或降低最初观察到的血清高胰岛素水平。在动物模型中，去除皮下脂肪会导致肠系膜脂肪体积增加，并使内脏脂肪分泌 TNF-α 增多。虽然尚未在临床试验中尝试手术切除内脏脂肪，但两项关于衰老的啮齿类动物模型研究表明，切除内脏脂肪可减少炎性脂肪因子的产生，并改善糖耐量和胰岛素敏感性。近期研究表明，肌间脂肪和筋膜下脂肪也会分泌炎性脂肪因子，且比腹部内脏脂肪分泌得更多。随着年龄的增长，男性和女性中均会出现肌间脂肪和筋膜下脂肪（肌肉脂肪浸润）的过度堆积，且与胰岛素抵抗密切相关。

肥胖症的相关风险

超重或肥胖症患者合并以下健康问题的风险会增加：
- 心脏代谢综合征
- T2DM
- 高血压
- 血脂异常
- 冠心病
- 充血性心力衰竭
- 心房颤动
- 骨关节炎
- 卒中
- 胆囊疾病
- 肝脏脂肪变性和非酒精性脂肪性肝炎（NASH）
- 阻塞性睡眠呼吸暂停

- 哮喘
- 胃食管反流（GERD）
- 某些癌症（子宫内膜癌、乳腺癌和结肠癌）
- 妇科疾病（月经异常、不孕症、多囊卵巢综合征）
- 勃起功能障碍
- 抑郁症

体重减轻 7% ～ 10% 可降低上述多种疾病（并非所有疾病）的发生风险。近期研究表明，在接受减重术的 2 级和 3 级肥胖症合并糖尿病的患者（尤其是近期诊断糖尿病）中，体重显著减轻（初始体重的 15% ～ 25%）可使糖尿病部分或完全缓解。

肥胖症的诊断和评估

男性的特征性肥胖类型——男性型或腹型肥胖（苹果型身材），与代谢性并发症密切相关，如胰岛素抵抗、高血压、血脂异常和高尿酸血症。相反，典型的女性型肥胖（梨形身材；即脂肪在臀部和大腿区域积聚）的代谢性并发症较轻。腰臀比（WHR）已被用于区分这些肥胖类型。当男性 WHR > 1.0 或女性 WHR > 0.8 时，表明内脏脂肪堆积和腹型肥胖，与健康风险增加相关。

在评估肥胖症时，标准的实验室检查应包括以下内容：
- 空腹血脂检查
- 肝功能检查
- 甲状腺功能检查
- 空腹血糖
- 糖化血红蛋白（HbA1c）

既往用于测量全身脂肪的“金标准”技术是水下称重法。这是基于脂肪组织比肌肉组织密度小的原理。目前，双能 X 射线吸收法（DXA）扫描可用于准确测量体成分，特别是脂肪量和非脂肪量。它还具有测量区域脂肪分布的额外优势。DXA 比身体形态测量更准确，比 CT 或 MRI 更具成本效益。然而，DXA 无法区分皮下脂肪和内脏脂肪堆积，也无法区分皮下脂肪和肌内周围脂肪堆积。生物电阻抗是一种更简便、成本更低的全身脂肪测量方法，但它受机体水合状态的影响很大，准确度低于 DXA。

BMI 被广泛用作肥胖症的衡量标准。它的计算方法是体重（kg）除以身高（m）的平方；或将体重（磅）乘以 703，再除以身高（英寸）的平方。在白种人中，BMI 为 19 ～ 27 kg/m^2 与心脑血管风险几乎没有关联。当 BMI ≥ 27 kg/m^2 时，可导致不良健康结果，且发生率随着 BMI 的增大而升高。与 BMI 增大相关的风险在年龄较大的患者中更为显著。

腰围和（或）WHR 在流行病学研究中常被用于间接估计腹腔内脂肪体积。尽管这些测量值与 CT 测量的腹腔内脂肪体积有很好的相关性，但准确性低于 CT。目前，腰围是医疗保健专业人员常规使用的最简单的身体形态测量，用于估算内脏脂肪量，并监测内脏脂肪体积的变化。

The current gold standard techniques for measuring visceral fat volume are abdominal CT (at the L4-L5 vertebral level) and MRI. These methods are not widely used because of high cost. In contrast to CT, MRI requires additional definition of adipose tissue by adjusting settings on the MRI scanner. Several commercial software packages are available for calculation of visceral fat volume, and it is possible to further subdivide body fat into at least three separate and measurable compartments; subcutaneous, intramuscular, and visceral fat.

Visceral fat volume determination by abdominal ultrasonography has been investigated for use in research and clinical settings. Several studies found good correlation between intra-abdominal fat volume measured by abdominal ultrasound and that measured by abdominal CT scanning. Measurements should be performed with the patient in the supine position at the end of a quiet inspiration with compression of the transducer against the abdomen. Intra-abdominal fat is quantified based on the distance between the peritoneum and the lumbar spine. Studies have shown that intra-abdominal fat measured by ultrasound has a stronger association with metabolic risk factors for CAD than does waist circumference or WHR. Recently, visceral fat has been measured using *bioelectric impedance*, but this technique is less accurate than CT. Determinations of intrahepatic fat by ultrasonography, CT and *vibration controlled transient elastography* (VCTE) are of significant clinical value. Determination of intermuscular and subfascial fat volume by CT has been investigated for use in research but not used yet in routine clinical setting.

TREATMENT OF OBESITY

Current guidelines for treatment of obesity are summarized in Table 6.1. The preferred intervention varies with the obesity level based on five BMI categories. The major four therapeutic options are lifestyle modification (diet and exercise), behavior modification, pharmacologic intervention, and bariatric surgery. In general, better results are obtained with a combination of different interventions rather than a single modality.

Lifestyle Modification

Key components of effective lifestyle modification most often include structured dietary interventions and individualized physical activity programs. Behavior modification strategies and patient education are also critical for achievement and maintenance of target weight loss. Evidence-based dietary guidelines should be used to design individualized patient plans in consultation with a registered dietitian or qualified health care provider. First, daily caloric intake should be reduced by a modest 250 to 500 calories. Reasonable and paced reductions can help patients continue on the recommended dietary plan for a longer time. Daily calories from carbohydrate should be reduced to

approximately 40% to 45% of intake, with a total daily carbohydrate intake of no less than 130 g/day. Except in patients with renal impairment (creatinine clearance <60 mL/min) or significant microalbuminuria, protein intake should not be less than 1.2 g/kg of adjusted body weight (adjusted body weight = ideal body weight + 0.25 [current weight − ideal body weight]). This typically accounts for 20% to 30% of total calorie intake and is intended to minimize loss of lean body mass during weight reduction. The remaining 30% to 35% of calorie intake should come from fat. *Trans*-fats should be eliminated, and saturated fat, especially from meat and meat-products, should be reduced. Meal plans should also include substantial soluble fiber (e.g., from fresh fruits) and insoluble fiber (e.g., from vegetables) and consumption of healthy carbohydrates, especially foods that have a low glycemic index and high fiber content. Approximately 14 g of fiber per 1000 calories (20 to 35 g of fiber) per day is recommended.

Caloric intake should be adjusted downward over time until weight loss is achieved. Underlying all of these steps should be the goal of designing an individualized plan that can be maintained over the long term. Many patients find it helpful to receive a structured dietary intervention that includes specific suggestions for daily meals and snacks. Such structured diets may increase adherence and can be easier to follow than a list of general guidelines. Nutritionally complete meal replacement (e.g., in the form of shakes or bars) can be useful for some patients, especially at the start of a weight reduction program. If meal replacement is used, 100- to 200-calorie snacks (e.g., fruits and nuts) may be added at breakfast, lunch, or between meals. A recent study showed that a structured meal plan that includes menus, snack lists, and meal replacements in obese patients with T2DM resulted in 2.7 to 3.5 kg weight loss over 16 weeks in comparison to individualized meal plans.

Each patient should meet with an exercise physiologist to construct an individualized plan that is responsive to his or her lifestyle, capabilities, and potential cardiovascular risks. Because obese individuals frequently have difficulty exercising, this process requires careful attention. A balanced exercise plan incorporates a mix of cardiovascular, stretching, and strength exercises and should be graded to increase gradually in both duration and intensity. Patients can start with 10 to 20 minutes of daily stretching and aerobic exercise (e.g., moderate-intensity walking) with subsequent progressive increases. Any exercise should be preceded by a warm-up period to minimize injuries.

Long-term lifestyle modification trials, such as the Diabetes Prevention Program, have targeted 150 minutes of exercise per week. Newer guidelines recommend 60 to 90 minutes of daily exercise, with a minimum of 150 to 175 minutes per week needed to obtain weight loss benefit. Emphasis should be placed on moderate-intensity exercise, such as walking 20-minute miles, rather than strenuous exercise. Because patients who are not used to exercising may find it difficult

TABLE 6.1	Guide to Selecting Treatment Based on BMI Category[a]				
	BMI CATEGORY				
Treatment	25-26.9	27-29.9	30-34.9	35-39.9	≥40
Diet, physical activity, behavior therapy	Yes with comorbidities	Yes with comorbidities	Yes	Yes	Yes
Pharmacotherapy	No	Yes with comorbidities	Yes	Yes	Yes
Weight-loss surgery	No	No	Yes with comorbidities	Yes with comorbidities	Yes with comorbidities

[a]"Yes" indicates that the treatment is indicated regardless of comorbidities.
From National Institutes of Health (NIH), National Heart, Lung, and Blood Institute (NHLBI), North American Association for the Study of Obesity (NAASO): The practical guide to the identification, evaluation, and treatment of overweight and obesity in adults. NIH Publication No. 00-4084, Bethesda, Md., October 2000, NIH. http://www.nhlbi.nih.gov/files/docs/guidelines/prctgd_c.pdf. Accessed November 2014.

目前用于测量内脏脂肪体积的金标准技术是腹部 CT（L4～L5 椎体水平）和 MRI。由于费用高昂，这些方法并未得到广泛应用。与 CT 不同，MRI 需要额外调整 MRI 扫描仪的设置来确定脂肪组织。多种市售软件包可用于计算内脏脂肪体积，还可进一步将身体脂肪分成至少 3 个独立且可测量的区域：皮下脂肪、肌内脂肪和内脏脂肪。

通过腹部超声检查测量内脏脂肪体积已被用于研究和临床。多项研究显示，腹部超声检查测得的腹腔内脂肪量与腹部 CT 测得的腹腔内脂肪体积之间存在良好的相关性。测量时，患者应取仰卧位，在安静吸气末将探头压向腹部。腹腔内脂肪是基于腹膜与腰椎之间的距离来量化。研究表明，通过超声检查测得的腹腔内脂肪与 CAD 的代谢性危险因素的相关性比腰围或 WHR 更密切。近期，人们开始使用生物电阻抗测量内脏脂肪，但这种技术的准确性不如 CT。通过超声、CT 和振动控制瞬态弹性成像（VCTE）测定肝内脂肪具有重要的临床价值。通过 CT 测定肌间脂肪和筋膜下脂肪体积已被用于研究，但尚未常规用于临床。

肥胖症的治疗

表 6.1 中总结了目前治疗肥胖症的指南。首选的干预措施因肥胖症程度（BMI 的 5 个级别）而异。4 种主要治疗方案包括改变生活方式（饮食和运动）、行为调整、药物干预和减重术。总体来说，综合使用不同的干预方法比使用单一的方法效果更好。

生活方式调整

有效调整生活方式的关键包括结构化的膳食干预和个体化的运动计划。行为调整策略和患者教育对于实现和保持目标体重同样重要。应在咨询注册营养师或有资质的医疗保健人员后，根据循证饮食指南来设计个体化的计划。每日热量摄入应适度减少 250～500 卡路里。合理和逐步减少有助于患者长时间坚持推荐的饮食计划。碳水化合物的每日热量应减少至总摄入量的 40%～45%，不应 < 130 g/d。除非患者存在肾功能

受损（肌酐清除率 < 60 ml/min）或明显的微量白蛋白尿，蛋白质摄入量应≥ 1.2 g/kg 调整体重 [调整体重＝理想体重＋0.25×（当前体重－理想体重）]，通常占总热量摄入的 20%～30%，旨在减少体重减轻过程中的瘦体重丢失。剩余 30%～35% 的热量摄入应来自脂肪。应避免摄入反式脂肪，减少饱和脂肪（特别是来自肉类和肉制品的脂肪）的摄入。饮食计划中还应包括大量可溶性纤维（如来自新鲜水果）和不溶性纤维（如来自蔬菜），以及摄入健康的碳水化合物，特别是低升糖指数和高纤维含量的食物。建议每 1000 卡路里摄入约 14 g 纤维（每天 20～35 g 纤维）。

摄入的热量应随时间逐渐下调，直至达到目标体重。设计一个能够长期坚持的个体化方案是饮食调整的基础目标。许多患者发现，接受结构化的饮食干预很有帮助，其中包括对每日膳食和零食的具体建议。这种结构化饮食可能会增加依从性，比常规的指南更容易遵循。营养均衡的餐食替代品（如奶昔或能量棒）对部分患者（尤其是在减重计划的初始阶段）有效。如果使用代餐，可在早餐、午餐或餐间添加 100～200 卡路里的零食（如水果和坚果）。近期的一项研究表明，在合并 T2DM 的肥胖症患者中，与个体化饮食计划相比，使用包括菜单、零食清单和代餐在内的结构化饮食计划坚持 16 周后体重下降 2.7～3.5 kg。

每位患者均应咨询运动生理学专家，根据生活方式、运动能力和潜在心血管风险制订个体化的运动计划。由于肥胖症患者在运动时经常存在困难，因此运动过程中需要特别关注。均衡的运动计划应包括心肺功能锻炼、伸展运动和力量练习，并应逐渐增加持续时间和强度。患者可从每天 10～20 min 的伸展和有氧运动（如中等强度的步行）开始，然后逐渐增加。所有运动均应在热身之后进行，以减少受伤风险。

长期生活方式调整试验（如糖尿病预防计划）设定了每周 150 min 的运动目标。更新的指南建议每天进行 60～90 min 运动，每周至少需要 150～175 min 才能达到减重获益。重点在于进行中等强度的运动，如步行 20 min，而不是剧烈运动。由于不习惯运动的患者可能

表 6.1　基于 BMI 的治疗选择指南 [a]

治疗	BMI 分级（kg/cm²）				
	25～26.9	27～29.9	30～34.9	30～34.9	≥ 40
饮食、运动、行为治疗	是，有合并症	是，有合并症	是	是	是
药物治疗	否	是，有合并症	是	是	是
减重术	否	否	是，有合并症	是，有合并症	是，有合并症

[a] "是"表示无论是否有合并症，均有治疗指征。

引自 National Institutes of Health（NIH），National Heart, Lung, and Blood Institute（NHLBI），North American Association for the Study of Obesity（NAASO）：The practical guide to the identification, evaluation, and treatment of overweight and obesity in adults. NIH Publication No. 00-4084, Bethesda, Md., October 2000, NIH. http://www.nhlbi.nih.gov/files/docs/guidelines/prctgd_c.pdf. Accessed November 2014.

to incorporate physical activity into daily practice, it is also important to use a variety of exercises to maintain interest. Increasing exercise duration to 300 minutes/week was found to help in long-term maintenance of weight reduction. Frequent short bouts of exercise as brief as 10 minutes each can increase adherence to an exercise regimen and increase overall duration of exercise.

Behavior Modification and Patient Education

Cognitive-behavioral intervention and patient education are important components of successful weight loss programs. Whenever possible, cognitive-behavioral intervention should be conducted by an experienced psychologist. The fundamental principles of intervention typically include behavioral goal setting, stimulus control techniques, cognitive restructuring, assertive communication skills, stress management, and relapse prevention. Cognitive-behavioral support conducted in a group setting with weekly meetings is frequently successful. Patients should learn how to set *SMART* goals (*s*pecific, *m*easurable, *a*ction-oriented, *r*ealistic, *t*ime-limited). It can be helpful to emphasize real-life examples (e.g., success stories, logbook learning, recommitting to progress). The behavioral modification strategy should assist patients in identifying precipitants for deviations from a diet (e.g., timing, types of food or exercise, situations, feelings), overcoming challenges (planning ahead, delay and distraction, problem solving), managing automatic negative thinking ("detour thoughts"), coping with cravings through mindful strategic eating, preventing relapses using logbook learning, navigating social eating, and setting personal weight maintenance plans.

Pharmacologic Treatment of Obesity

Several anti-obesity drugs are currently approved by the US Food and Drug Administration (FDA) for use in the United States. These drugs include orlistat, phentermine, lorcaserin, a combination of phentermine and long-acting topiramate, liraglutide, and a combination of bupropion and naltrexone. Generally, all these medications are indicated for patients with a BMI of 30 kg/m^2 or more or with BMI of 27 kg/m^2 or more with other weight-related comorbidities (e.g., diabetes, hypertension, dyslipidemia, obstructive sleep apnea) in combination with caloric restriction, increased physical activity, and behavioral modifications.

Orlistat

Orlistat limits caloric intake through inhibition of the lipase-mediated breakdown of fat in the gastrointestinal tract. This mechanism results in an approximately 30% reduction of fat absorption and an increase in fecal fat content. In addition to weight loss, orlistat use has been associated with decreased incidence of diabetes, improved concentrations of total cholesterol and low-density lipoprotein (LDL)-cholesterol, and improved blood pressure and glycemic control in patients with diabetes. However, high-density lipoprotein (HDL)-cholesterol has been found to be slightly lowered. Most people develop side effects with variable degrees of diarrhea, flatulence, oily stools, fecal urgency, and, rarely, fecal incontinence. There also is an increased risk of cholelithiasis. Gastrointestinal side events are usually proportional to the amount of fat intake. Supplemental fat-soluble vitamins A, D, E, and K must be taken to prevent possible deficiencies. The usual dose of orlistat is 120 mg before each meal. A 60 mg dose formulation is currently available over the counter. The lower dose is less effective but is associated with fewer side effects.

Phentermine

Phentermine is approved for short-term treatment of obesity (up to 6 months). Because phentermine has actions similar to amphetamines, it can elevate blood pressure, increase heart rate, and stimulate the central nervous system (frequently causing insomnia), in addition to suppressing the appetite. The recommended phentermine dose is 30 mg once daily. Combining phentermine with tricyclic antidepressants or monoamine oxidase inhibitors may result in substantial increases in blood pressure and other serious reactions because of elevated serotonin levels in the blood.

Lorcaserin

Lorcaserin is a selective serotonin (5-hydroxytryptamine) receptor agonist with specificity for the 5-HT2C receptor subtype. The activation of these receptors in the hypothalamus is thought to activate production of pro-opiomelanocortin (POMC) and, consequently, to promote weight loss through satiety signals. Lorcaserin has 100-fold higher selectivity for 5-HT2C versus the closely related 5-HT2B receptor. Activation of the 5-HT2B receptor by the less selective agents like fenfluramine and dexfenfluramine was linked to serious cardiac valvulopathy, but there is no evidence for this adverse effect with lorcaserin. Clinical trials showed that 47.5% of patients treated with lorcaserin lost at least 5% of their initial body weight, and 22.6% lost at least 10%, in 1 year. Lorcaserin treatment also resulted in significantly lower A_{1C} values in patients with T2DM and improved lipid profile and decreased blood pressure in clinical studies.

Lorcaserin is approved for use as an adjunct to a reduced-calorie diet and exercise for chronic weight management in patients with initial BMI values of 30 kg/m^2 or higher and in those with BMI values of 27 kg/m^2 or higher with at least one weight-related comorbid condition. It is given in a dose of 10 mg twice daily or 20 mg of extended release (XR) form once daily. Side effects usually are mild to moderate, with the most common being headache, upper respiratory tract infection, nasopharyngitis, sinusitis, dizziness, nausea, and fatigue. The US Drug Enforcement Administration has classified lorcaserin as a schedule IV drug because it has hallucinogenic properties that could lead to psychiatric complications.

Phentermine and Long-Acting Topiramate

Phentermine is an appetite suppressant and stimulant of the amphetamine and phenethylamine class (see earlier discussion for details on the use of phentermine alone for weight reduction). Topiramate is an anticonvulsant that was found to have weight loss side effects. The combination of phentermine plus low doses of topiramate has been shown to have synergistic effects on weight loss. As with lorcaserin, this combination tablet is indicated as an adjunct to a reduced-calorie diet and exercise for chronic weight management. Clinical trials showed that average weight loss after 1 year of 10.9% for patients receiving the maximum dose (phentermine/topiramate, 15 mg/92 mg) and 5.1% for those taking the recommended starting dose (3.75 mg/23 mg). The drug is taken once daily in the morning to avoid insomnia caused by the phentermine component. The initial dose of 3.75 mg/23 mg is given for 2 weeks before titration to 7.5 mg/46 mg for another 12 weeks. If a patient has not lost at least 3% of baseline body weight on the higher dosage, the drug may be discontinued or the dose may be escalated to 11.25 mg/69 mg for an additional 2 weeks before a further increase to the maximum dose of 15 mg/92 mg. If a patient has not lost at least 5% of baseline body weight after 12 weeks, the drug is discontinued gradually. Side effects include paresthesias, dry mouth, constipation, metabolic acidosis, nasopharyngitis, upper respiratory infection, and headache.

Data indicate that fetuses exposed during the first trimester to topiramate (when used alone as an anticonvulsant) have an increased risk (9.6%) of cleft lip with or without cleft palate. Therefore, the drug should not be given to women of childbearing age unless an effective method of contraception is used and a pregnancy test is conducted monthly during use. Phentermine/topiramate may increase resting heart rate up to 20 beats/minute, so the drug should be used cautiously in patients with a

很难将运动融入日常实践中，因此采用多种不同运动保持兴趣非常重要。将运动时长增加到每周 300 min 有利于长期保持体重减轻。经常进行短时间运动（每次 10 min）可以提高对运动计划的依从性，并延长总运动时间。

行为矫正和患者教育

认知行为干预和患者教育是成功的减重计划的重要组成部分。条件允许时，应由经验丰富的心理学专家进行认知行为干预。干预的基本原则通常包括行为目标设定、刺激控制技术、认知重构、自信沟通技巧、压力管理和复发预防。在每周会面的团体环境中提供认知行为支持通常会取得成功。患者应学习如何设定 SMART 目标 [具体的（**s**pecific）、可衡量的（**m**easurable）、以行动为导向的（**a**ction-oriented）、现实可行的（**r**ealistic）、有时限的（**t**ime-limited）]。强调现实生活中的实例（如成功故事、日志学习、再次承诺取得进步）可能有所帮助。行为矫正策略应协助患者识别偏离饮食习惯的诱因（如时间、食物或运动类型、情境、情绪），克服挑战（提前计划、延迟和转移注意力、解决问题），管理自动负面思维（"绕道思维"），通过有意识的策略性进食来应对食欲，利用日志学习预防复发，应对社交进餐，并制订个人体重维持计划。

肥胖症的药物治疗

目前 FDA 已批准多种减重药物在美国使用，包括奥利司他、芬特明、氯卡色林、芬特明与长效托吡酯的复方制剂、利拉鲁肽、安非他酮与纳曲酮的复方制剂。通常情况下，这些药物适用于 BMI ≥ 30 kg/m² 的患者，或 BMI ≥ 27 kg/m² 伴有其他肥胖症相关并发症（如糖尿病、高血压、血脂异常、阻塞性睡眠呼吸暂停）的患者，同时联合限制热量摄入、增加运动和行为矫正。

奥利司他

奥利司他通过抑制肠道脂肪酶介导的脂肪分解来限制热量摄入，使脂肪吸收减少约 30%，粪便中的脂肪含量增加。除减轻体重外，奥利司他还能降低糖尿病发病率，降低总胆固醇和低密度脂蛋白（LDL）胆固醇的浓度，改善糖尿病住院患者的血压和血糖控制。然而，奥利司他也会导致高密度脂蛋白（HDL）胆固醇水平略微降低。大多数患者会出现不同程度的副作用，如腹泻、胃肠胀气、大便油滴、排便急迫感，极少数人会出现大便失禁。此外，胆石症的发生风险也会增加。胃肠道副作用通常与脂肪摄入量成正比。此外，必须补充脂溶性维生素 A、D、E 和 K，以预防可能出现的相关维生素缺乏。奥利司他的常规剂量为每餐前 120 mg。目前有 60 mg 剂量的非处方药，低剂量奥利司他的效果相对较差，但副作用相对较少。

芬特明

芬特明被批准用于短期治疗肥胖症（最长 6 个月）。由于芬特明的作用类似于苯丙胺，因此除抑制食欲外，还可能升高血压，加快心率，兴奋中枢神经系统（通

常导致失眠）。芬特明的推荐剂量为 30 g，1 次 / 日。芬特明与三环类抗抑郁药或单胺氧化酶抑制剂联合使用时可使血液中的 5- 羟色胺水平升高，可能导致血压显著升高和其他严重不良反应。

氯卡色林

氯卡色林是一种选择性 5- 羟色胺受体激动剂，对 5-HT2C 受体具有特异性。目前认为，氯卡色林可激活位于下丘脑的 5-HT 受体，促进阿黑皮素原（POMC）的产生，通过饱信号通路促进体重减轻。氯卡色林对 5-HT2C 受体的选择性比对 5-HT2B 受体高 100 倍。通过非选择性药物（如芬氟拉明和右芬氟拉明）激活 5-HT2B 受体与严重的心脏瓣膜病有关，但没有证据表明氯卡色林会产生这种不良反应。临床试验显示，在接受氯卡色林治疗的患者中，47.5% 的患者在 1 年内体重减轻至少 5%，22.6% 的患者至少减轻 10%。在临床试验中，氯卡色林治疗可使糖尿病住院患者的糖化血红蛋白水平轻度下降，并改善血脂和降低血压。

氯卡色林被批准作为以饮食控制和运动为基础的减重治疗的辅助手段，用于治疗初始 BMI ≥ 30 kg/m² 的患者和 BMI ≥ 27 kg/m² 且患有至少 1 种肥胖症相关并发症的患者。剂量为 10 mg，2 次 / 日，或 20 mg 缓释（XR）剂型，1 次 / 日。副作用通常为轻中度，常见的副作用包括头痛、上呼吸道感染、鼻咽炎、鼻窦炎、头晕、恶心和疲劳。美国缉毒局将氯卡色林列为 Ⅳ 级药物，因为它具有致幻作用，可能导致精神并发症。

芬特明和长效托吡酯

芬特明是一种食欲抑制剂，属于苯丙胺和苯乙胺类兴奋剂（有关单用芬特明减轻体重的详细内容见上文）。托吡酯是一种抗惊厥药，在应用中发现它具有减轻体重的副作用。芬特明联合低剂量托吡酯已被证明对减重具有协同作用。与氯卡色林相同，这种复方制剂被作为以饮食控制和运动为基础的体重管理的辅助治疗。临床试验显示，接受最大剂量芬特明 / 托吡酯（15 mg/92 mg）的患者 1 年后平均体重减轻 10.9%，接受推荐起始剂量（3.75 mg/23 mg）的患者体重减轻 5.1%。建议每天早晨服用 1 次，以避免芬特明成分引起的失眠。初始剂量为 3.75 mg/23 mg，使用 2 周后可逐步增加剂量至 7.5 mg/46 mg 维持 12 周。如果患者在使用更高剂量药物后体重减轻幅度未达到基线体重的 3%，则可停药或将剂量升至 11.25 mg/69 mg，维持 2 周后进一步增加至最大剂量 15 mg/92 mg。如果患者在用药 12 周后体重减轻未达到基线体重的 5%，则可逐渐减停。副作用包括感觉异常、口干、便秘、代谢性酸中毒、鼻咽炎、上呼吸道感染和头痛。

研究数据表明，妊娠早期暴露于托吡酯（作为抗惊厥药单独用药时）的胎儿患唇裂（伴或不伴腭裂）的风险增加 9.6%。因此，除非采用有效的避孕方法并在使用期间每月进行孕检，否则育龄期女性不应使用该药物。芬特明 / 托吡酯可使静息心率增加 20 次 / 分，因此有

history of cardiac or cerebrovascular disease. Topiramate also increases the risk of suicidal thoughts or behaviors and mood disorders including depression, anxiety, and insomnia. It can also cause cognitive dysfunction, including impairment of concentration or attention, difficulty with memory, and speech or language problems, particularly word-finding difficulties. It is contraindicated in patients with closed-angle glaucoma because it increases intraocular pressure and the risk of permanent loss of vision.

Bupropion and Naltrexone

This combination is thought to cause a reduction in appetite and an increase in energy expenditure by increasing activity of POMC neurons. Bupropion is a dopamine and norepinephrine reuptake antagonist, which increases dopamine activity in the brain and in turns leads to reduction in appetite and increase in energy expenditure by increasing activity of POMC neurons. Naltrexone blocks opioid receptors on the POMC neurons, preventing feedback inhibition of these neurons and further increasing POMC activity.

The combination tablet of 8 mg of naltrexone and 90 mg of bupropion is initially taken once daily in the morning for 1 week then increased each week by one tablet until reaching the effective dose of two tablets taken twice daily. Average weight loss after 56 weeks of full dose of 32 naltrexone/360 bupropion was 8.4% of the initial body weight (6.4% in intention to treat analysis). The major side events include nausea, constipation, headache, vomiting, dizziness, and insomnia. Bupropion also increases the risk of suicidal thoughts similar to all other antidepressant medications.

Liraglutide

Liraglutide is a GLP-1 analog. GLP-1 is a physiologic regulator of appetite and calorie intake, and the GLP-1 receptor is present in several areas of the brain involved in appetite regulation. GLP-1 analogs, including liraglutide, are used for management of T2DM, but liraglutide dose for obesity indication is much higher, up to 3 mg/day by subcutaneous injection in comparison to a maximum dose of 1.8 mg/day for treatment of T2DM. The dose is escalated gradually every week from 0.6 mg/day to 1.2, 1.8, 2.4, and finally 3 mg/day to reduce nausea. Average weight loss with liraglutide 3 mg daily for 56 weeks is around 5.9%. Side effects include nausea, vomiting, constipation, diarrhea or, rarely, acute pancreatitis. There is an FDA warning about the possibility of developing medullary-cell carcinoma of the thyroid gland, which was seen in experimental animals during preclinical studies, but this is very rare in humans.

Other Drugs for Short-term Treatment of Obesity

Besides phentermine, three other FDA-approved drugs are available in the United States for the short-term (8-12 weeks) treatment of obesity:

diethylpropion, phendimetrazine, benzphetamine. Any of these drugs can be used as an adjunct in a regimen of weight reduction based on caloric restriction in patients with an initial BMI of 30 kg/m^2 or higher who have not responded to an appropriate weight-reduction regimen alone.

Bariatric Surgery

At present, there are three broad categories of bariatric surgical procedures: (1) pure gastric restriction; (2) gastric restriction with some malabsorption, as represented by the Roux-en-Y gastric bypass (RYGB) procedure; and (3) gastric restriction with significant intestinal malabsorption. The number of bariatric procedures performed in the United States increased from an estimated 13,365 in 1998 to almost 228,000 in 2017. Bariatric surgery is considered to be indicated for adults with class 3 obesity (BMI ≥40 kg/m^2). In patients with less severe obesity (BMI 35 to 40 kg/m^2), bariatric surgery can be considered if there are one or more high-risk comorbid conditions present, such as life-threatening cardiopulmonary disease (e.g., severe obstructive sleep apnea, obesity-related cardiomyopathy) or uncontrolled T2DM. Bariatric surgery is sometimes performed for patients with diabetes or metabolic syndrome and a BMI of 30 to 35 kg/m^2, although current evidence on benefit in this weight bracket is limited. For teenagers younger than 17 years old who have attained skeletal maturity (usually by 13 years for girls and 15 years for boys), bariatric surgery has been recommended with different guidelines: BMI 35 to 40 kg/m^2 with at least one serious comorbid condition (e.g., T2DM, obstructive sleep apnea, pseudotumor cerebri) or BMI 50 kg/m^2 or higher with less serious comorbidities. Contraindications for bariatric surgery include high operative risk (e.g., congestive heart failure, unstable angina), active substance abuse, and significant psychopathology.

The three most common bariatric procedures are RYGB, sleeve gastrectomy (SLG), and laparoscopic adjustable gastric banding (LAGB). Currently, the most common bariatric procedure in the United States is sleeve gastrectomy. Other procedures such as biliopancreatic diversion (BPD), biliopancreatic diversion with duodenal switch (BPD/DS), and staged bariatric surgical procedures are less commonly performed. Different types of commonly used bariatric procedures are shown in Fig. 6.1. Gastric restriction procedures induce weight loss by producing early satiety and limiting food intake.

LAGB carries a very low operative mortality rate (0.1%). However, it is associated with significantly lower loss of excess weight at 5 years and 10 years and with higher risk of weight regain compared with RYGB and sleeve gastrectomy. LAGB has been demonstrated to be safe in patients older than 55 years of age. Complications associated with the LAGB procedure include band slippage, band erosion, balloon failure, injection port malposition, band and port infections, and esophageal dilatation. Some of these problems have been decreased by

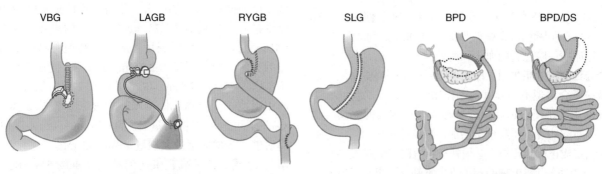

Fig. 6.1 Common bariatric procedures. *BPD*, Biliopancreatic diversion; *BPD/DS*, BPD with duodenal switch; *LAGB*, laparoscopic adjustable gastric band; *RYGB*, Roux-en-Y gastric bypass; *SLG*, sleeve gastrectomy; *VBG*, vertical banded gastroplasty.

心脏病或脑血管疾病病史的患者应慎用该药。托吡酯还会增加自杀倾向或行为障碍及心境障碍的风险，包括抑郁症、焦虑和失眠。它还可能导致认知功能障碍，包括注意力或专注力受损、记忆障碍、言语或语言问题，尤其是找词困难。由于托吡酯可增加眼内压和永久失明的风险，因此闭角型青光眼患者禁用该药。

安非他酮和纳曲酮

这种复方制剂可通过增加 POMC 神经元的活性来降低食欲并增加能量消耗。安非他酮是多巴胺和去甲肾上腺素再摄取抑制剂，可增加脑内多巴胺的活性，进而通过增加 POMC 神经元活性使食欲下降、能量消耗增多。纳曲酮可阻断 POMC 神经元上的阿片受体，阻止这些神经元受负反馈抑制，以进一步增加 POMC 的活性。

起始剂量为纳曲酮 8 mg 和安非他酮 90 mg，每天早上服用 1 次，持续 1 周，然后每周增加 1 片，直至达到有效剂量（每次 2 片，2 次／日）。在服用全剂量（纳曲酮 32 mg／安非他酮 360 mg）56 周后，体重平均可减轻 8.4%（意向性治疗分析显示为 6.4%）。主要的副作用包括恶心、便秘、头痛、呕吐、头晕和失眠。与其他抗抑郁药类似，安非他酮也会增加自杀倾向的风险。

利拉鲁肽

利拉鲁肽是一种 GLP-1 类似物。GLP-1 是食欲和热量摄入的生理调节剂，GLP-1 受体分布于脑内参与食欲调节的多个区域。利拉鲁肽等 GLP-1 类似物适用于 T2DM 患者的治疗，利拉鲁肽治疗 T2DM 的最大剂量为 1.8 mg/d，若用于肥胖症治疗，则需要更高剂量，可达 3 mg/d 皮下注射。为了减轻恶心，剂量可每周递增，从 0.6 mg/d 依次增至 1.2 mg/d、1.8 mg/d、2.4 mg/d，最终达到 3 mg/d。使用利拉鲁肽 3 mg/d 治疗 56 周后，患者体重平均减轻约 5.9%。副作用包括恶心、呕吐、便秘、腹泻，极少数情况下可出现急性胰腺炎。FDA 提出警告：在临床前研究中，实验动物使用 GLP-1 后可能罹患甲状腺髓样癌，但这种情况在人类中非常罕见。

其他用于短期减重治疗的药物

除芬特明外，还有 3 种经 FDA 批准用于短期

（8～12 周）治疗肥胖症的药物已在美国上市：安非拉酮、苯甲曲秦、苄非他明。这些药物均可作为减重治疗的辅助用药，适用于初始 BMI ≥ 30 kg/m² 且单用减重方案疗效不佳的患者。

减重术

目前，肥胖症的外科手术大致分为 3 类：①单纯胃容量限制；②胃容量限制联合部分吸收不良，如 Roux-en-Y 胃旁路术（RYGB）；③胃容量限制联合显著肠道吸收不良。在美国，减重术的数量已从 1998 年的 13 365 例增至 2017 年的近 228 000 例。减重术适用于 3 级肥胖症成人患者（BMI ≥ 40 kg/m²）。对于 BMI 为 35～40 kg/m² 的中度肥胖症患者，如果存在 1 种或多种高风险合并症，如危及生命的心肺疾病（如严重阻塞性睡眠呼吸暂停、肥胖症相关心肌病）或未控制的 T2DM，则考虑进行减重术。BMI 为 30～35 kg/m² 且合并糖尿病或代谢综合征的患者有时可进行减重术，但目前有关该体重范围患者手术获益的证据有限。对于未满 17 岁的青少年患者，若已达到骨骼成熟（通常女孩为 13 岁，男孩为 15 岁），不同指南建议符合以下情况的患者进行减重术：BMI 为 35～40 kg/m² 伴有至少 1 种严重合并症（如 T2DM、阻塞性睡眠呼吸暂停、特发性颅内压增高），或 BMI ≥ 50 kg/m² 伴有轻度合并症。减重术的禁忌证包括手术风险高（如充血性心力衰竭、不稳定型心绞痛），滥用药物及严重精神疾病。

目前，最常用的 3 种减重术包括 RYGB、袖状胃切除术（SLG）和腹腔镜可调节性胃束带术（LAGB）。美国目前最常用的减重术是 SLG。其他手术［如胆胰分流术（BPD）、胆胰分流与十二指肠切换术（BPD/DS）和分阶段减重术］相对少用。常用的减重术如图 6.1 所示。胃容量限制手术通过产生早饱和限制食物摄入来促进体重减轻。

LAGB 的手术死亡率非常低（0.1%）。然而，与 RYGB 和 SLG 相比，LAGB 在术后 5 年和 10 年时额外体重下降的比例更小，且体重反弹的风险更高。研究表明，55 岁以上的患者行 LAGB 是安全的。与 LAGB 相关的并发症包括束带滑移、束带侵蚀、球囊失效、

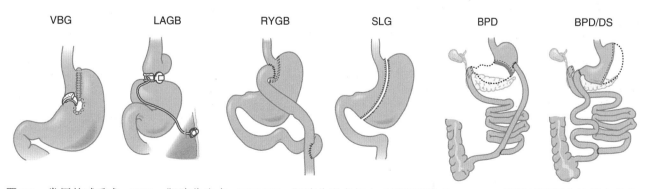

图 6.1 常用的减重术。BPD，胆胰分流术；BPD/DS，胆胰分流术与十二指肠切换术；LAGB，腹腔镜可调节性胃束带术；RYGB，Roux-en-Y 胃旁路术；SLG，袖状胃切除术；VBG，垂直捆绑胃成形术

use of a different method of band insertion and revision of the port connection. Because the absorptive surface of the entire small intestine remains intact, nutritional deficiencies are rare.

In RYGB, the upper stomach is transected, thereby creating a very small proximal gastric pouch measuring 10 to 30 mL. The gastric pouch is anastomosed to a Roux-en-Y proximal jejunal segment, bypassing the remaining stomach, duodenum, and a small portion of jejunum. The standard Roux (alimentary) limb length is about 50 to 100 cm, and the biliopancreatic limb is 15 to 50 cm. As a result, the RYGB serves to limit food intake and induces some nutritional deficiencies such as vitamin B_{12}, vitamin B_1 (thiamine), iron, calcium, copper and vitamin D, which can be corrected by supplementation. It may also lead to protein malnutrition. Dumping syndrome is another complication that occurs as a result of mechanical and hormonal changes that are commonly seen after any gastric restrictive procedure such as RYGB. The primary management of dumping syndrome is dietary modification for prevention of symptoms.

SLG is another popular restrictive surgery in which the stomach is reduced to about 25% of its original size by surgical removal of a large portion of the stomach fundus, resulting in a tube-like structure. Although the procedure permanently reduces stomach size, some dilatation of the stomach may occur later. The procedure is frequently performed by a laparoscopic technique. Sleeve gastrostomy is a similar procedure done by gastroenterologists through gastroscopy without surgical removal of the stomach fundus. Nutritional deficiencies are less common in SLG when compared to RYGB and include vitamin D, vitamin B_{12}, vitamin B_1, folic acid, and iron. Dumping syndrome may also occur but to a lesser extent than with RYGB. This could be caused by an increase in gastric motility consequent to the increase in intraluminal pressure within the remaining stomach.

Currently, most bariatric procedures are performed laparoscopically. This approach has the advantages of fewer wound complications, less postoperative pain, a shorter hospital stay, and more rapid postoperative recovery with comparable efficacy.

The Agency for Healthcare Research and Quality (AHRQ) identified a 0.19% in-hospital mortality rate for all bariatric discharges in the United States. One meta-analysis showed that the mortality rate from bariatric surgery within 30 days was 0.08% and the mortality rate after 30 days was 0.31%. Bariatric surgery is not uniformly a "low-risk" procedure, and judicious patient selection and diligent perioperative care are mandatory. Preoperative patient selection and education as well as careful postsurgical follow-up are important for successful outcomes.

The mortality rate associated with standard bariatric surgical procedures in an experienced center should not exceed 1.5% to 2%. The surgical mortality rate is less than 0.5% at centers specializing in bariatric surgery. Mortality rates exceeding 2% suggest a risk-to-benefit ratio that probably is unacceptable.

The benefits of bariatric surgery extend beyond calorie restriction and weight loss. Foregut bypass leads to improvement in the physiologic responses of gut hormones involved in glucose regulation and appetite control, including ghrelin, GLP-1, and peptide YY[3-36] (PYY). Mechanical improvements include less weight-bearing burden on joints, improved lung compliance, and reduced fatty tissue around the neck, which can relieve obstruction to breathing and sleep apnea.

In an extensive meta-analysis of 22,000 bariatric surgeries, patients lost on average 61% of excess body weight and exhibited improvements in T2DM, hypertension, sleep apnea, and dyslipidemia. The beneficial effect of bariatric surgery on T2DM is one of the most important outcomes observed, with RYGB, SLG, and malabsorptive procedures having the greatest impact. A shorter duration of diabetes and greater weight loss are independent predictors of diabetes partial or complete remission after bariatric surgery. Improvements in fasting blood glucose levels occur before significant weight loss is achieved. Insulin-treated patients experience significant decreases in insulin requirements, and most T2DM patients are able to discontinue insulin therapy by 6 weeks after surgery. Euglycemia is maintained in some patients for up to 5 years after RYGB and SLG. Two recent randomized controlled studies compared RYGB to intensive lifestyle intervention in moderately obese patients with T2DM and found RYGB to be superior in inducing diabetes remission and reducing use of antihyperglycemic medications.

Weight loss after malabsorptive bariatric surgery usually reaches a nadir after 12 to 18 months. Over the following decade, there is weight regain of approximately 10% of body weight. In purely restrictive procedures, failure to experience optimal weight loss has been associated with increased consumption of calorically dense liquids that can pass through the stoma without producing satiety.

Other FDA-approved procedures include *gastric pacing*. Gastric pacing achieved by using implantable electrodes induces weight loss. This outcome was initially discovered with the use of gastric pacemaker devices for gastroparesis in patients with diabetes. Currently, it is an FDA-approved procedure for obesity management.

Gastric aspiration system is an obesity management technique which consists of an endoscopically placed gastrostomy tube and siphon assembly that allows patients to aspirate gastric contents 20 min after meal consumption three times daily. Aspiration takes about 10 min to perform and removes approximately 30% of ingested calories. The side effects include pain, leakage or tube displacement, and stoma site–related problems.

Intra-gastric balloons are used to occupy space in the stomach. Each inflated balloon with air occupies approximately 250 mL volume. Up to three balloons can be placed over a 6-month treatment period, then deflated and removed with an endoscopic procedure.

PROGNOSIS

Although recent clinical data show that patients on average can maintain a 4% to 6.9% weight loss for 10 years with ongoing medically supervised intensive lifestyle intervention, many patients are subjected to less intensive intervention and regain their initial weight loss over months or years. Weight regain even after bariatric surgery is not uncommon and most often occurs after 2 years of peak weight loss. Loss of 10% to 20% of the initial body weight is associated with a decrease in total and resting energy expenditure, a change that retards further weight loss. Similarly, weight gain is associated with an increase in energy expenditure, which retards further weight gain. These observations suggest that the human body adopts a biologic set point or mechanism that tends to maintain body weight, and they lend support to the theory that behavior is not the sole determinant of obesity. Although long-term intensive lifestyle intervention in obese patients with T2DM resulting in approximately 5% body weight loss can significantly decrease the risks of chronic kidney disease and depression and further improve glucose control, blood pressure, physical fitness, and some lipid parameters in patients with T2DM and obesity, it has not been shown to reduce cardiovascular events or mortality. Further understanding of genetic and hormonal regulation of obesity may help researchers create more effective and long-lasting interventional tools.

For further discussion on this topic, please see Chapter 207, ❖ "Obesity," in *Goldman-Cecil Medicine*, 26th Edition.

注射端位置不当、束带和注射端感染，以及食管扩张。通过使用不同的束带置入方法和修改端口连接，可有效减少这些问题的出现。由于整个小肠的吸收表面保持完整，营养不良很少见。

在 RYGB 中，胃上部被切断，形成一个容量非常小（10～30 ml）的近端胃囊。胃囊与 Roux-en-Y 近端空肠段吻合，绕过剩余的胃、十二指肠和一小部分空肠。标准 Roux（营养支）肠袢长度为 50～100 cm，胆胰肠支为 15～50 cm。因此，RYGB 有助于限制食物摄入，并引起部分营养素缺乏，如维生素 B_{12}、维生素 B_1、铁、钙、铜和维生素 D，这些可通过营养补充来纠正。该手术还可能导致蛋白质营养不良。倾倒综合征是由胃限制性手术（如 RYGB）引起的一种并发症，由术后机械和激素变化导致。倾倒综合征主要通过饮食调整来预防症状。

SLG 是另一种流行的胃限制性手术，通过手术切除胃底部的大部分组织，将胃缩小至原始大小的 25%，形成类似管状的结构。虽然该手术永久性地缩小了胃容积，但后续可能会出现部分胃扩张。该手术通常采用腹腔镜进行。袖状胃造瘘术是一种类似的手术，可通过胃镜进行，而无须手术切除胃底部。与 RYGB 相比，SLG 术后营养缺乏相对少见，包括维生素 D、维生素 B_{12}、维生素 B_1、叶酸和铁。倾倒综合征也可能发生，但程度轻于 RYGB，其机制是剩余胃的腔内压力增大导致胃蠕动增加。

目前，大多数减重术均可通过腹腔镜进行。这种方式的切口并发症较少、术后疼痛较轻、住院时间较短、术后康复更快，且疗效相当。

据美国医疗保健研究与质量局（AHRQ）统计，美国进行减重术的肥胖症患者的总体住院死亡率为 0.19%。一项荟萃分析显示，减重术后 30 天内的死亡率为 0.08%，30 天后的死亡率为 0.31%。减重术并非都是"低风险"手术，因此必须审慎地选择患者，并做好围术期护理。术前对患者的选择和教育及术后的密切随访对于减重术成功及预后良好非常重要。

在经验丰富的中心进行标准减重术的死亡率不应超过 1.5%～2%。在专门进行减重术的中心，手术死亡率应＜ 0.5%。死亡率＞ 2% 表明风险效益比不可接受。

减重术的益处不仅限于能量限制和体重减轻。前肠的旁路术可改善参与葡萄糖调节和食欲控制的肠道激素的生理学反应，包括胃生长激素释放素、GLP-1 和肽 YY^{3-36}（PYY）。机械改善包括减轻关节负担、改善肺顺应性、减少颈部周围脂肪组织，这可以缓解呼吸困难和睡眠呼吸暂停。

一项纳入 2.2 万例接受减重术的肥胖症患者的大型荟萃分析显示，患者平均减少了 61% 的额外体重，T2DM、高血压、睡眠呼吸暂停和血脂异常方面均得到显著改善。减重术对 T2DM 的有益影响是最重要的结果之一，其中 RYGB、SLG 和吸收不良型减重术的影响最

大。减重术后糖尿病可部分或完全缓解的独立预测因子是糖尿病持续时间较短和体重减轻较多。空腹血糖水平的改善可出现在体重显著减轻之前。接受胰岛素治疗的患者术后的胰岛素用量大幅减少，大部分 T2DM 患者在术后 6 周能够停用胰岛素。部分患者在 RYGB 和 SLG 术后可维持正常血糖水平长达 5 年。近期的两项随机对照试验比较了 RYGB 与强化生活方式干预在中度肥胖症合并 T2DM 的患者中的疗效，结果显示，RYGB 在促进糖尿病缓解和减少降糖药物使用方面表现出优越性。

接受吸收不良型减重术后，患者体重通常在 12～18 个月后达到最低值。在随后的 10 年中，体重会增加约 10%。在单纯胃容量限制性手术中，未能达到最大限度体重减轻通常与摄入高热量浓缩液体有关，这些液体可通过胃通道但不产生饱腹感。

其他经 FDA 批准的手术包括胃起搏术。通过使用可植入电极的胃起搏术可使体重减轻。这一作用最初是在糖尿病患者使用胃起搏器设备治疗胃排空障碍时发现的。目前，FDA 已批准其用于肥胖症的治疗。

胃抽吸系统是一种肥胖症治疗技术，通过内镜放置胃造瘘管和虹吸装置，在患者进餐后 20 min 内进行胃内容物抽吸，3 次 / 日。抽吸约需要 10 min，可去除约 30% 的摄入热量。副作用包括疼痛、漏液或管道移位、瘘口相关问题。

胃内球囊可占据一定胃内空间。每个充气球囊约占据 250 ml 的胃容积。在为期 6 个月的治疗期间，最多可放置 3 个球囊，后续可通过内镜手术将其放气并取出。

预后

尽管近期临床数据显示，在持续医学监督的强化生活方式干预下，患者可在 10 年内保持体重减轻 4%～6.9%，但许多患者生活方式管理不严格，体重会在数月或数年内反弹。即使在减重术后，体重再次增加也并不罕见，常发生在体重减轻高峰期后 2 年。初始体重减轻 10%～20% 会伴随总能量和静息能量消耗减少，这种变化会减缓进一步的体重减轻。同样，体重增加后会伴随能量消耗增加，这会减缓进一步的体重增加。这些观察结果表明，人体通过生物学调定点或某些机制使体重维持稳定，这也支持了行为方式并非肥胖症的唯一决定因素的理论。虽然在肥胖症合并 T2DM 的患者中进行长期强化生活方式干预可使体重减轻 5%，并显著降低慢性肾脏病和抑郁症的发生风险，且能进一步改善血糖、血压、健康状况及脂代谢，但并未显示可减少心血管事件或降低死亡率。进一步理解肥胖症的遗传和激素调节可能有助于研究人员开发出更有效和持久的干预方法。

有关此专题的深入讨论，请参阅 *Goldman-Cecil Medicine* 第 26 版第 207 章"肥胖症"。

SUGGESTED READINGS

Aldahi W, Hamdy O: Adipokines, inflammation, and the endothelium in diabetes, Curr Diabetes Rep 3:293–298, 2003.

Angrisani L, Lorenzo M, Borrelli V: Laparoscopic adjustable gastric banding versus Roux-en-Y gastric bypass: 5-year results of a prospective randomized trial, Surg Obes Relat Dis 3:127–134, 2007.

Chang SH, Stoll CR, Song J, et al: The effectiveness and risks of bariatric surgery: an updated systematic review and meta-analysis, 2003-2012, JAMA Surg 149:275–287, 2014.

Després J-P, Moorjani S, Lupien PJ, et al: Regional distribution of body fat, plasma lipoproteins, and cardiovascular disease, Arteriosclerosis 10:497–511, 1990.

Hales CM, Carroll MD, Fryar CD: Ogden CL prevalence of obesity among adults and youth: United States, 2015–2016. NCHS data brief, no 288, Hyattsville, MD, 2017, National Center for Health Statistics.

Hamdy O: Obesity chapter. Medscape. https://emedicine.medscape.com/article/123702-overview. Updated: Mar 20, 2018.

Hamdy O: The role of adipose tissue as an endocrine gland, Curr Diabetes Rep 5:317–319, 2005.

Hamdy O, Carver C: The Why WAIT program: improving clinical outcomes through weight management in type 2 diabetes, Curr Diabetes Rep 8:413–420, 2008.

Hamdy O, Mottalib A, Morsi A, et al: Long-term effect of intensive lifestyle intervention on cardiovascular risk factors in patients with diabetes in real-world clinical practice: a 5-year longitudinal study, BMJ Open Diabetes Res Care 5(1):e000259, 2017.

Ikramuddin S, Korner J, Lee WJ, et al: Roux-en-Y gastric bypass vs intensive medical management for the control of type 2 diabetes, hypertension, and hyperlipidemia: the Diabetes Surgery Study randomized clinical trial, J Am Med Assoc 309:2240–2249, 2013.

Look AHEAD Research Group, Wing RR, Bolin P, et al: Cardiovascular effects of intensive lifestyle intervention in type 2 diabetes, N Engl J Med 369:145–154, 2013.

Maggard MA, Shugarman LR, Suttorp M, et al: Meta-analysis: surgical treatment of obesity, Ann Intern Med 142:547–559, 2005.

Mottalib A, Salsberg V, et al: Effects of nutrition therapy on HbA1c and cardiovascular disease risk factors in overweight and obese patients with type 2 diabetes, Nutr J 17(1):42, 2018.

Schauer PR, Bhatt DL, Kirwan JP, et al: Bariatric surgery versus intensive medical therapy for diabetes—5-year outcomes, N Engl J Med 376(7):641–651, 2017.

Schauer PR, Kashyap SR, Wolski K, et al: Bariatric surgery versus intensive medical therapy in obese patients with diabetes, N Engl J Med 366:1567–1576, 2012.

Sjostrom L, Lindroos AK, Peltonen M, et al: Swedish Obese Subjects Study Scientific Group. Lifestyle, diabetes, and cardiovascular risk factors 10 years after bariatric surgery, N Engl J Med 351:2683–2693, 2004.

Strauss RS, Bradley LJ, Brolin RE: Gastric bypass surgery in adolescents with morbid obesity, J Pediatr 138:499–504, 2001.

推荐阅读

Aldahi W, Hamdy O: Adipokines, inflammation, and the endothelium in diabetes, Curr Diabetes Rep 3:293–298, 2003.

Angrisani L, Lorenzo M, Borrelli V: Laparoscopic adjustable gastric banding versus Roux-en-Y gastric bypass: 5-year results of a prospective randomized trial, Surg Obes Relat Dis 3:127–134, 2007.

Chang SH, Stoll CR, Song J, et al: The effectiveness and risks of bariatric surgery: an updated systematic review and meta-analysis, 2003-2012, JAMA Surg 149:275–287, 2014.

Després J-P, Moorjani S, Lupien PJ, et al: Regional distribution of body fat, plasma lipoproteins, and cardiovascular disease, Arteriosclerosis 10:497–511, 1990.

Hales CM, Carroll MD, Fryar CD: Ogden CL prevalence of obesity among adults and youth: United States, 2015–2016. NCHS data brief, no 288, Hyattsville, MD, 2017, National Center for Health Statistics.

Hamdy O: Obesity chapter. Medscape. https://emedicine.medscape.com/article/123702-overview. Updated: Mar 20, 2018.

Hamdy O: The role of adipose tissue as an endocrine gland, Curr Diabetes Rep 5:317–319, 2005.

Hamdy O, Carver C: The Why WAIT program: improving clinical outcomes through weight management in type 2 diabetes, Curr Diabetes Rep 8:413–420, 2008.

Hamdy O, Mottalib A, Morsi A, et al: Long-term effect of intensive lifestyle intervention on cardiovascular risk factors in patients with diabetes in real-world clinical practice: a 5-year longitudinal study, BMJ Open Diabetes Res Care 5(1):e000259, 2017.

Ikramuddin S, Korner J, Lee WJ, et al: Roux-en-Y gastric bypass vs intensive medical management for the control of type 2 diabetes, hypertension, and hyperlipidemia: the Diabetes Surgery Study randomized clinical trial, J Am Med Assoc 309:2240–2249, 2013.

Look AHEAD Research Group, Wing RR, Bolin P, et al: Cardiovascular effects of intensive lifestyle intervention in type 2 diabetes, N Engl J Med 369:145–154, 2013.

Maggard MA, Shugarman LR, Suttorp M, et al: Meta-analysis: surgical treatment of obesity, Ann Intern Med 142:547–559, 2005.

Mottalib A, Salsberg V, et al: Effects of nutrition therapy on HbA1c and cardiovascular disease risk factors in overweight and obese patients with type 2 diabetes, Nutr J 17(1):42, 2018.

Schauer PR, Bhatt DL, Kirwan JP, et al: Bariatric surgery versus intensive medical therapy for diabetes—5-year outcomes, N Engl J Med 376(7):641–651, 2017.

Schauer PR, Kashyap SR, Wolski K, et al: Bariatric surgery versus intensive medical therapy in obese patients with diabetes, N Engl J Med 366:1567–1576, 2012.

Sjostrom L, Lindroos AK, Peltonen M, et al: Swedish Obese Subjects Study Scientific Group. Lifestyle, diabetes, and cardiovascular risk factors 10 years after bariatric surgery, N Engl J Med 351:2683–2693, 2004.

Strauss RS, Bradley LJ, Brolin RE: Gastric bypass surgery in adolescents with morbid obesity, J Pediatr 138:499–504, 2001.

7

Malnutrition, Nutritional Assessment, and Nutritional Support in Adult Patients

Thomas R. Ziegler

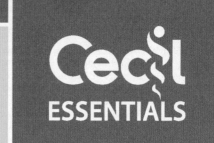

MALNUTRITION IN HOSPITALIZED PATIENTS

Numerous surveys conducted in developed countries in the 21st century continue to demonstrate the frequent rate of protein-energy malnutrition as well as depletion of specific micronutrients in hospitalized patients with chronic illnesses and those requiring elective or emergent hospital admission. Hospitalized patients commonly receive inadequate amounts of calories, protein, vitamins, and minerals during their stay, and ad libitum intake of prescribed diets is typically inadequate. Studies have shown that worsening of malnutrition during hospitalization is common. This is problematic because adequate intake of essential macronutrients (energy, carbohydrate, protein/amino acids, and fats) and micronutrients (vitamins, minerals, and electrolytes) is critical for optimal cellular and organ structure and function, muscle mass, tissue repair, immune function, ambulatory capacity, and patient recovery. Significant erosion of lean body mass (predominately derived from skeletal muscle) and deficiencies of specific vitamins and minerals are variously associated with weakness and fatigue, increased rates of infection, impaired wound healing, and delayed convalescence. This relationship is especially apparent in patients with chronic protein-energy malnutrition and body weight loss associated with illness.

Patients with acute or chronic illnesses typically have experienced several days to several months of continuous or intermittent decreased food intake due to anorexia, gastrointestinal symptoms, depression and anxiety, and other medical factors. They may also have had food intake restricted by surgical operations or diagnostic or therapeutic procedures and recovery from these. Some patients have abnormal nutrient losses due to diarrhea (e.g., with chronic malabsorptive and maldigestive disorders or infectious diarrhea), vomiting, polyuria (as in uncontrolled diabetes mellitus), wound drainage, dialysis, or other causes. Certain drugs, including corticosteroids, chemotherapeutic agents, antirejection drugs, and diuretics, are associated with skeletal muscle breakdown, gastrointestinal injury, or loss of electrolytes or water-soluble vitamins. Bedrest or markedly decreased ambulation are common in outpatient and inpatient settings and are associated with skeletal muscle wasting and impaired protein synthesis.

Catabolic and critical illnesses are associated with concomitantly increased blood concentrations of "counterregulatory" hormones derived from the adrenal glands and pancreas (e.g., cortisol, catecholamines, glucagon); release of pro-inflammatory cytokines from stimulated immune, endothelial, and epithelial cells, such as interleukins (e.g., IL-1, IL-6, IL-8) and tumor necrosis factor-α (TNF-α); and peripheral tissue resistance to anabolic hormones such as insulin and insulin-like growth factor-I (IGF-I). These hormonal and cytokine alterations increase the availability of endogenous metabolic substrates that are critical for cellular and organ function, wound healing, and host survival (e.g., glucose via glycogenolysis and gluconeogenesis, amino acids via skeletal muscle breakdown, and free fatty acids via lipolysis). This combination of decreased nutrient intake and increased tissue nutrient losses (from the actions of these hormones and cytokines), coupled with increased energy (calorie), protein, and micronutrient needs due to inflammation, infection, and cytokinemia, is responsible for the wasting and micronutrient depletion commonly observed in medical patients with acute and chronic illnesses. Common causes of protein-energy malnutrition and micronutrient depletion in medical patients are shown in Table 7.1. Obesity has become a widespread medical problem and is also a form of malnutrition; it is considered in detail in Chapter 6.

NUTRITIONAL ASSESSMENT

Serial assessment of nutritional status is a critically important component of routine medical care. The major objectives are to detect preexisting depletion of body protein, energy reserves, and micronutrients; to identify risk factors for malnutrition (see Table 7.1); and to take steps to prevent nutrient deficiencies, depletion of lean body mass, and loss of skeletal muscle. There are still no practical "gold standard" tests that can provide an index of general nutritional status. Blood concentrations of specific micronutrients (e.g., copper, zinc, thiamine, 25-hydroxyvitamin D, vitamin B_6, folate, vitamin B_{12}) and electrolytes (e.g., magnesium, potassium, phosphorus) are important to guide needs and repletion responses. Nutritional assessment involves an integration of multiple factors, including the patient's medical and surgical history, type and severity of the acute or chronic underlying illness and its anticipated medical and surgical course, fluid drainage sites and amounts, physical examination findings, history of body weight change (degree and temporal aspects), dietary intake pattern, use of nutritional supplements including prior administration of specialized enteral nutrition (EN) or parenteral nutrition (PN), evaluation of current organ function and fluid status, and determination of selected vitamin, mineral, and electrolyte concentrations in blood. In the intensive care unit (ICU) setting, measured body weight typically reflects recent intravenous fluid administration and is typically much higher than recent "dry" or preoperative body weight, which is the best parameter to use.

Patients who have experienced an involuntary body weight loss

成年患者的营养不良、营养评估和营养支持

周翔 译 陈伟 潘慧 审校 宁光 通审

住院患者的营养不良状况

发达国家在 21 世纪进行的大量调查均显示，在患有慢性疾病及需要择期或紧急入院的患者中，蛋白质-能量营养不良和特定微量营养素缺乏的情况十分普遍。患者在住院期间对能量、蛋白质、维生素和矿物质的摄入通常不足，且即使获得了膳食建议，其自主摄入也往往难以达到推荐量。研究表明，住院期间营养不良恶化很常见。这可能引起不良后果，因为摄入足够的必需宏量营养素（包括能量、碳水化合物、蛋白质/氨基酸和脂肪）和微量营养素（包括维生素、矿物质和电解质）对于维持细胞和器官的最佳结构与功能、肌肉质量、组织修复、免疫功能、行动能力和患者恢复至关重要。瘦体重显著下降（主要源于骨骼肌的衰减）和特定维生素及矿物质缺乏与乏力、疲劳、感染率升高、伤口愈合障碍及康复延迟有不同程度的关联。这种关联在患有慢性蛋白质-能量营养不良和疾病相关体重减轻的患者中尤为明显。

由于食欲减退、胃肠道症状、抑郁和焦虑及其他临床情况，急慢性疾病患者通常会经历数日至数月的连续性或间歇性食物摄入减少。他们也可能因外科手术、诊断性检查或治疗相关操作而被要求限制饮食。一些患者会出现由腹泻（如慢性吸收不良和消化不良性疾病或感染性腹泻）、呕吐、多尿（如未控制的糖尿病）、伤口引流、透析或其他原因导致的异常营养流失。皮质类固醇、化疗药物、抗排斥药物和利尿剂等药物则与骨骼肌分解、胃肠道损伤，以及电解质或水溶性维生素的流失有关。卧床或活动减少在门诊和住院环境中十分常见，这进一步加剧了骨骼肌衰减和蛋白质合成受损。

当处于分解代谢和危重疾病状态时，肾上腺和胰腺分泌的"反调节"激素（如皮质醇、儿茶酚胺、胰高血糖素）的血液浓度增加；被激活的免疫细胞、内皮细胞和上皮细胞释放促炎性细胞因子，如白介素（IL）（如 IL-1、IL-6、IL-8）和肿瘤坏死因子 -α（TNF-α）；外周组织对促合成的激素［如胰岛素、胰岛素样生长

因子 -Ⅰ（IGF-Ⅰ）］产生抵抗。上述激素和细胞因子的变化增加了内源性代谢底物的供给，这对维持细胞和器官功能、伤口愈合和宿主生存至关重要（如通过糖原分解和糖异生产生葡萄糖、通过骨骼肌分解产生氨基酸、通过脂肪分解产生游离脂肪酸）。营养摄入减少、组织营养损失增加（由上述激素和细胞因子介导），加之炎症、感染和细胞因子血症导致机体对能量（热量）、蛋白质和微量营养素的需求增加，均为急慢性疾病患者常出现消瘦和微量营养素缺乏的原因。患者发生蛋白质-能量营养不良和微量营养素缺乏的常见原因见表 7.1。肥胖症已成为一个普遍存在的医学问题，其也是一种营养不良的形式；相关内容见第 6 章。

营养评估

营养状况的连续评估是常规医疗照护中至关重要的一部分。主要目的是检测当前体内蛋白质、能量储备和微量营养素的缺乏情况，识别营养不良的危险因素（表 7.1），并采取措施预防营养缺乏、瘦体重丢失和骨骼肌流失。目前尚无实用的"金标准"检测能够提供反映一般营养状况的指数。特定微量营养素（如铜、锌、硫胺素、25- 羟维生素 D、维生素 B_6、叶酸、维生素 B_{12}）和电解质（如镁、钾、磷）的血液浓度对于指导评估机体对营养元素的需求和补充后的效果非常重要。营养评估需整合多种因素，包括：患者的疾病史和手术史、急慢性基础疾病的类型和严重程度及其预期的药物和手术治疗、体液引流的部位和量、体格检查结果、体重变化史（程度和时间）、膳食模式、营养补充剂的使用［含既往接受的特定肠内营养（EN）或肠外营养（PN）］、当前器官功能和液体状态评估，以及血液中特定维生素、矿物质和电解质浓度的测定结果。在重症监护病房（ICU）测得的体重通常反映了近期静脉输液的情况，且通常显著高于近期干体重或术前体重，而后者才是最佳参数。

应仔细评估在过去数周或数月内非自主体重下

TABLE 7.1 **Common Causes of Protein-Energy Malnutrition and Micronutrient Depletion in Medical Patients With Acute or Chronic Illnesses**

Decreased spontaneous food intake due to anorexia from chronic or acute illness, gastrointestinal symptoms (e.g., nausea, vomiting, abdominal pain), or depression and anxiety

Restricted food intake required for surgical operations or diagnostic or therapeutic procedures and gastrointestinal dysfunction after these procedures

Abnormal macronutrient and micronutrient losses from the body due to malabsorption (e.g., celiac sprue, short gut syndrome, inflammatory bowel disease, cystic fibrosis, diarrhea), maldigestion (e.g., pancreatitis), emesis, polyuria (e.g., in diabetes), wound drainage, or renal replacement therapy

Periods of increased energy expenditure (caloric needs), protein requirements, and micronutrient needs (e.g., critical illness, increased inflammation)

Catabolic effects of counterregulatory hormones (e.g., cortisol, catecholamines, glucagon), release of pro-inflammatory cytokines from stimulated immune cells and endothelial and epithelial cells such as interleukins (e.g., IL-1, IL-6, IL-8) and tumor necrosis factor-α (TNF-α), and peripheral tissue resistance to the anabolic hormones insulin and insulin-like growth factor-I (IGF-I)

Bedrest, decreased ambulation, and chemical paralysis during mechanical ventilation (skeletal muscle wasting due to impaired protein synthesis)

Administration of drugs that induce skeletal muscle breakdown, gastrointestinal injury, or loss of electrolytes and water-soluble vitamins (e.g., corticosteroids, chemotherapeutic agents, diuretics, antirejection regimens)

Socioeconomic deprivation, inadequate caregivers, ambulation difficulties in the home setting

Inadequate provision of calories, protein, and essential micronutrients (vitamins, minerals, trace elements) during hospitalization

of 5% to 10% or more of their usual body weight in the previous few weeks or months, those who weigh less than 90% of their ideal body weight (IBW), and those who have a body mass index (BMI) lower than 18.5 kg/m^2 should be carefully evaluated, because these individuals are likely to be malnourished.

Among hospitalized patients, especially those in the ICU, circulating concentrations of proteins (e.g., albumin, prealbumin) are often quite low and not useful as protein nutritional status biomarkers given their lack of specificity. Plasma concentrations of albumin and prealbumin typically fall during active inflammation or infection, in critical illness, and after traumatic injury (due to deceased synthesis by the liver and catabolism of blood proteins). They are markedly affected by non-nutritional factors, including fluid status, capillary leak, decreased hepatic synthesis, and increased clearance from blood. Because of the long circulating half-life of albumin (18 to 21 days), concentrations in blood remain low despite adequate feeding and are slow to respond to nutritional repletion, irrespective of other confounding factors. Prealbumin has a much shorter circulating half-life (several days), and serial blood levels can be used as a general indicator of protein status in clinically stable outpatients.

Energy requirements can be estimated with the use of standard equations, such as the Harris-Benedict equation, which incorporate the patient's age, gender, weight, and height to determine basal energy expenditure (BEE). Recently published European and American Clinical Practice Guidelines suggest that an adequate energy goal for most patients can be estimated at 20 to 25 kcal/kg/day (using the most

recent prehospital clinic dry body weight), which is approximately equivalent to measured or estimated BEE multiplied by 1.0 to 1.3. Ongoing RCTs are designed to better define caloric dosing guidelines in hospitalized general and ICU patients.

Typically, lower amounts of calories are now given to ICU patients (as discussed later). Use of data obtained from a bedside metabolic cart machine (indirect calorimeter), which measures expired breath to determine oxygen consumption and carbon dioxide production, provides accurate actual energy expenditure in most settings and can be very useful.

In ICU patients, even lower caloric doses (equivalent to 15-20 kcal/kg dry weight/day) have been advocated by some, based on known complications of overfeeding (see later discussion) and limited data on clinical outcome as a function of energy dose. In clinically stable, malnourished, non-ICU patients who require nutritional repletion, higher doses of calories (up to 35 kcal/kg/day) appear to be generally well tolerated if refeeding syndrome is avoided (see later discussion). In obese subjects (defined for these calculations as patients with body weight 20% to 25% greater than ideal), an adjusted body weight value should be used for calculation of energy and protein needs, as determined by the following equation:

$$\text{Adjusted body weight} = (\text{current weight} - \text{IBW}) \times 0.25 + \text{IBW}$$

Studies in nonburned ICU patients indicate that protein loads of more than 2.0 g/kg/day may not be efficiently utilized for protein synthesis, and the excess may be oxidized, contributing to azotemia. In most catabolic patients requiring specialized feeding, a recommended protein dose is 1.5 g/kg/day for individuals with normal renal function. This is about twice the recommended dietary allowance (RDA) for healthy adults of 0.8 g/kg/day. The administered protein dose should be adjusted downward as a function of the degree and tempo of azotemia (in the absence of dialysis therapy) and of hyperbilirubinemia. These strategies take into account the relative inability of catabolic patients to efficiently use exogenous nutrients and knowledge that most protein and lean tissue repletion occurs over a period of several weeks to months during posthospital convalescence. Adequate nonprotein energy is essential to allow amino acids to be effectively used for protein synthesis and not oxidized for production of energy (adenosine triphosphate, or ATP). The commonly recommended protein/amino acid dose range is 1.2 to 1.5 g/kg/day for most adults with normal renal and hepatic function (50% to 100% above the RDA of 0.8 g/kg/day); although some guidelines recommend higher doses (up to 2.0 to 2.5 g/kg/day) in specific conditions such as in patients requiring renal replacement therapy or burns.

NUTRITIONAL SUPPORT

Table 7.2 lists common clinical scenarios in which specialized oral/EN or PN support may be indicated. In these settings, consultation with a multidisciplinary nutrition support team, if available, has been shown to reduce complications and costs and to increase the appropriate use of EN and PN in both academic and community medical centers.

Oral Nutrition Support

Oral nutrition supplementation includes provision of balanced oral diets of usual foods supplemented with complete liquid (or solid) nutrient products, protein supplements (e.g., hydrolyzed whey or casein powder that can be mixed with dietary beverages), high-potency multivitamin-multimineral supplements, and/or specific micronutrients required to treat a diagnosed deficiency (e.g., zinc, copper, vitamin B$_6$, vitamin

表 7.1 引起急性或慢性疾病住院患者蛋白质–能量营养不良和微量营养素缺乏的常见原因

由慢性或急性疾病引起的厌食，胃肠道症状（如恶心、呕吐、腹痛）或抑郁症和焦虑导致的自主进食减少
手术、诊断性或治疗性操作所需的饮食限制，以及这些操作后的胃肠功能障碍
由吸收不良（如乳糜泻、短肠综合征、炎症性肠病、囊性纤维化、腹泻），消化不良（如胰腺炎），呕吐，多尿（如糖尿病），伤口引流或肾脏替代治疗导致体内宏量营养素和微量营养素异常流失
能量消耗（热量需求）、蛋白质需求和微量营养素需求增加的时期（如重症疾病、炎症加剧）
反调节激素（如皮质醇、儿茶酚胺、胰高血糖素）的分解代谢作用，被激活的免疫细胞、内皮细胞及上皮细胞释放促炎性细胞因子 [如 IL（如 IL-1、IL-6、IL-8）和 TNF-α]，以及外周组织对促合成激素（胰岛素和 IGF- I ）抵抗
机械通气期间卧床休息、活动减少和化学性瘫痪（由蛋白质合成受损导致的骨骼肌萎缩）
应用可导致骨骼肌分解、胃肠道损伤或电解质及水溶性维生素流失的药物（如皮质类固醇、化疗药物、利尿剂、抗排斥方案）
社会经济贫困、缺乏照护者、在家中行动困难
住院期间能量、蛋白质和必需微量营养素（维生素、矿物质、微量元素）供应不足

降 ≥ 5% ～ 10% 的患者、体重 < 90% 的理想体重（IBW）的患者，以及 BMI < 18.5 kg/m^2 的患者，因为这些患者很可能存在营养不良。

在住院患者（特别是在 ICU 的患者）中，循环中的蛋白质（如白蛋白、前白蛋白）浓度通常很低，但由于缺乏特异性，不能用作评价蛋白质营养状况的生物标志物。由于肝脏合成减少和血液中蛋白质分解，在活动性炎症或感染期间、危重疾病状态及创伤性损伤后，血浆白蛋白和前白蛋白浓度通常会下降。其浓度受到非营养因素的显著影响，包括体液状态、毛细血管渗漏、肝脏合成减少和血液清除增加。在不考虑其他混杂因素的情况下，由于白蛋白的循环半衰期较长（18 ～ 21 天），即使给予患者充足的营养，其血液浓度仍然较低，且对营养补充的反应也较慢。前白蛋白的循环半衰期较短（数天），因此连续检测其血液浓度可作为评价临床状况稳定的门诊患者蛋白质情况的一般指标。

能量需求可通过使用标准公式来估算，如 Harris-Benedict 公式，该公式结合了患者的年龄、性别、体重和身高来确定基础能量消耗（BEE）。近期发布的欧洲和美国临床实践指南建议，大多数患者的充足能量目标估计为 20 ～ 25 kcal/（kg·d）（使用住院前最近一次的干体重），这大致相当于测量或估算的 BEE 乘以

1.0 ～ 1.3。正在进行的随机对照试验旨在更好地确定普通住院患者和 ICU 患者的能量需求指南。

通常情况下，给予 ICU 患者的能量较低（见下文）。床旁代谢车（间接量热计）通过测量呼出气体来确定氧气的消耗量和二氧化碳的产生量，可在大多数环境中提供准确的实际能量消耗数据，且非常有用。

基于过度喂养的已知并发症（见下文）和能量对临床结局影响的有限数据，一些学者主张给予 ICU 患者更低的能量 [相当于 15 ～ 20 kcal/（kg 干体重·d）]。对于临床状况稳定、营养不良且需要营养补充的非 ICU 患者，如果可避免再喂养综合征（见下文），通常能很好地耐受更高的能量 [高达 35 kcal/（kg·d）]。对于肥胖症患者（定义为体重较 IBW 高 20% ～ 25%），应根据以下公式，使用调整体重来计算能量和蛋白质需要量：

$$调整体重 =（当前体重 - IBW）× 0.25 + IBW$$

对非烧伤 ICU 患者的研究表明，超过 2.0 g/（kg·d）的蛋白质负荷可能无法被有效地用于蛋白质合成，而过量的蛋白质可能被氧化，导致氮质血症。对于大多数需要特殊喂养的分解代谢旺盛的患者，若肾功能正常，蛋白质的推荐摄入量为 1.5 g/（kg·d）。这约为健康成人膳食营养素供给量（RDA；0.8 g/kg）的 2 倍。应根据氮质血症（在没有透析治疗的情况下）及高胆红素血症的程度和速度，酌情下调蛋白质的用量。上述策略考虑了分解代谢旺盛患者相对难以有效利用外源性营养素，以及大多数蛋白质和瘦组织能在出院后数周到数月的康复期内得到补充的情况。充足的非蛋白质能量供应对于氨基酸被有效用于蛋白质合成而非用于氧化供能 [腺苷三磷酸（ATP）] 至关重要。对于大多数肝肾功能正常的成人，通常推荐的蛋白质 / 氨基酸每日摄入量为 1.2 ～ 1.5 g/kg（比 RDA 的 0.8 g/kg 高 50% ～ 100%）；而对于需要进行肾脏替代治疗或烧伤等特定住院患者，一些指南推荐给予更高剂量 [2.0 ～ 2.5 g/（kg·d）]。

营养支持

表 7.2 列出了可能需要专门应用口服 /EN 或 PN 支持的常见临床情况。在这些情况下，尽可能咨询多学科营养支持团队可减少并发症和降低医疗成本，并促进综合医院和社区医院对 EN 和 PN 的合理使用。

口服营养支持

口服营养补充包括提供营养均衡的普通饮食，并辅以完全型液体（或固体）营养产品、蛋白质补充剂（如可与饮料混合的水解乳清蛋白粉或酪蛋白粉）、高效复合维生素–复合矿物质补充剂和（或）治疗已确诊的营养素缺乏症所需的特定微量营养素（如锌、铜、

TABLE 7.2 Some Clinical Indications for Specialized Oral/Enteral or Parenteral Nutrition Support

Patient currently exhibits moderate to severe protein or protein-energy malnutrition or has evidence of specific deficiency of one or more essential micronutrients

Patient with involuntary body weight loss of 5-10% or more of their usual body weight in the previous few weeks or months, weighs less than 90% of ideal body weight, or has a BMI lower than 18.5 kg/m²

Dietary food intake in a hospital or outpatient setting likely to be <50% of needs for more than 5-10 days due to underlying illness

Patient with severe catabolic stress (e.g., ICU care, serious infection) and adequate nutrient intake unlikely for >3-5 days

After major gastrointestinal surgery or other major operation (e.g., hip replacement, partial organ resection)

Medical illness associated with prolonged (>5-10 days) GI dysfunction (diarrhea, nausea and vomiting, GI bleeding, severe ileus, partial obstruction) and/or short bowel syndrome, chronic or severe diarrhea, or other malabsorptive disorders

Clinical settings in which adequate oral food intake may be contraindicated or otherwise significantly decreased, such as respiratory or other acute or severe organ failure, dementia, dysphagia, chemotherapy or irradiation, inflammatory bowel disease, pancreatitis, high-output enterocutaneous fistula, alcoholism, drug addiction

Chronic obstructive lung disease, chronic infection, or other chronic inflammatory or catabolic disorders with documented poor nutrient intake and/or recent weight loss

BMI, Body mass index; *GI,* gastrointestinal; *ICU,* intensive care unit; *PN,* parenteral nutrition.

B_{12}, vitamin D). Special supplements designed for patients with chronic renal failure (featuring concentrated calories and low amounts of protein and electrolytes) are available, as are a variety of formulations designed for other specific disease categories (see later discussion). Several studies have shown that convalescence after stresses such as total hip replacement or gastrointestinal surgery is enhanced with the addition of one or two containers per day of complete liquid nutrient supplements. These provide calories, carbohydrate, high-quality protein, fat, and micronutrients; are lactose and gluten free; and may contain small peptides and medium-chain triglycerides to facilitate absorption of amino acid and fat, respectively. Some formulations also contain soluble fiber or prebiotics (e.g., fructo-oligosaccharides) designed to decrease diarrhea. It is probably prudent to place outpatients who exhibit or are at risk for undernutrition and can tolerate oral medications on a potent oral multivitamin-multimineral preparation, at least for several months.

Administration of Enteral Tube Feeding

Patients with conditions outlined in Table 7.2 may have a functional gastrointestinal tract and yet be unable to consume adequate diet orally due to medical or surgical conditions (e.g., mechanical ventilation, pancreatitis, dementia, dysphagia, trauma, or burns). Although PN is commonly administered in these settings, this practice is not evidence based; academic guidelines strongly suggest that oral nutritional supplements or enteral tube feedings should be used if specialized nutrition support is indicated in patients with a functional gastrointestinal tract ("if the gut works, use it"). EN is more physiologic, associated with less severe infectious, mechanical, and metabolic complications, and is less costly than PN. Although not evidence based, common contraindications to EN include paralytic ileus, bowel ischemia, and hemodynamic

instability requiring mid- to high-dose vasopressors, inability to gain access to the gastrointestinal (GI) tract, intestinal obstruction, intractable vomiting, severe diarrhea, and peritonitis.

These products can be used for oral nutrient supplementation as tolerated. When delivered in appropriate amounts, the liquid diets provide complete nutrition for most patients, although some ICU patients and patients with malabsorption or other conditions may have special needs (see later discussion).

The feedings can be delivered by conventional nasogastric tubes into the stomach or by small-bore nasogastric or nasojejunal tubes, percutaneous gastrostomy or jejunostomy tubes, or percutaneous gastrojejunostomy tubes (in which the gastric port may be used for suction and the jejunal port for feeding). Gastric feedings can be administered by either continuous or bolus feeds, whereas small bowel feeds must employ a continuous slow infusion using an infusion pump to avoid diarrhea. Tube feedings should be initiated at a slow rate (e.g., 10 to 20 mL/hr) for 8 to 24 hours and slowly advanced to the goal rate in 8- to 24-hour increments to deliver the calculated caloric and protein needs over the next 24 to 48 hours, depending on clinical tolerance and clinical conditions. Recent guidelines emphasize placing tube-fed patients in the semirecumbent position (e.g., increase head of bed), advancing feedings cautiously (with serial evaluations for diarrhea, nausea, emesis, abdominal distention, and significant gastric residuals), and using prokinetic agents and/or postpyloric feedings if gastric feedings are not well tolerated. Recent data suggest that higher volumes of gastric residuals (e.g., >250 mL) are usually well tolerated in patients being tube fed.

Primarily based on results of animal studies, EN is associated with improved gut barrier function, decreased infectious complications, less hypermetabolism, and decreased morbidity and mortality in catabolic models, compared with PN. Salutary clinical outcomes have been shown in randomized clinical trials in patients with pancreatitis receiving EN into the jejunum, compared with PN. The current Society for Critical Care Medicine (SCCM) and American Society for Parenteral and Enteral Nutrition (ASPEN) guidelines recommend starting early EN (within 24-48 hours) in ICU patients who cannot achieve adequate caloric needs (e.g., >60%) with oral diet and supplements alone, especially for patients with existing malnutrition. Many studies have shown that ICU patients actually receive only 60% to 75% of the amount of tube feeding ordered by physicians. This can occur because of tube feeding intolerance (e.g., high gastric residuals, emesis, diarrhea, tube dislodgement) or discontinuation of feeding for diagnostic tests or therapeutic interventions. Although supplemental PN (see later discussion) is commonly ordered in patients who are not able to achieve tube-feeding rates adequate for their needs, this practice remains controversial because of the limited number of good clinical trials. Rigorous studies are now in progress to address the efficacy of this approach, motivated by data suggesting that an increase in net caloric deficit (i.e., the difference between daily calorie requirements and daily actual calories delivered, summed over time) is associated with worse clinical outcomes in medical and surgical ICU patients.

Most outpatients and hospitalized ICU and non-ICU patients tolerate standard, inexpensive enteral formulas delivered via gastric or intestinal routes that provide between 1.0 and 1.5 kcal/mL. A large variety of enteral tube-feeding products are available for clinical use. Because EN products can be marketed without efficacy data from randomized, controlled clinical trials, there remains a clear need for such trials to determine optimal EN formulations for different clinical conditions.

表 7.2 需要专门应用口服 / 肠内营养或肠外营养支持的部分临床指征

患者当前表现出中重度蛋白质或蛋白质-能量营养不良，或有证据表明存在 1 种或多种必需微量营养素缺乏

患者在过去数周或数月内非自主体重下降 5% ～ 10% 或以上，体重＜ 90% 的理想体重，或 BMI ＜ 18.5 kg/m²

在医院或门诊环境中，由于基础疾病，患者膳食摄入量可能低于实际需要量的 50%，且持续超过 5 ～ 10 天

患者处于严重分解代谢应激状态（如 ICU 照护、严重感染），且难以获得充足的营养摄入超过 3 ～ 5 天

胃肠道或其他重大手术（如髋关节置换术、部分器官切除术）术后

长期（超过 5 ～ 10 天）胃肠道功能障碍（腹泻、恶心、呕吐、消化道出血、严重肠梗阻、部分梗阻）和（或）短肠综合征、慢性 / 严重腹泻或其他吸收不良性疾病

可能禁止或显著减少经口摄食的临床情况，如呼吸衰竭或其他急性或严重器官衰竭、痴呆、吞咽困难、化疗或放疗、炎症性肠病、胰腺炎、高流量肠瘘、酗酒和药物成瘾

患有慢性阻塞性肺疾病、慢性感染或其他慢性炎症或分解代谢性疾病，伴随营养摄入不足和（或）近期体重减轻

维生素 B_6、维生素 B_{12}、维生素 D）。目前已有针对慢性肾衰竭患者的特殊补充剂（其特点为能量密集且蛋白质及电解质含量低），以及为其他特定疾病设计的各种配方（见下文）。多项研究表明，在全髋关节置换术或胃肠手术等应激后，每天额外摄入 1 ～ 2 罐完全型液体全营养素补充剂可加速康复。这些补充剂可提供能量、碳水化合物、优质蛋白质、脂肪和微量营养素；不含乳糖和麸质；可能含有短肽和中链甘油三酯，能分别促进氨基酸和脂肪的吸收。有些旨在减少腹泻的配方中还含有可溶性纤维或益生元（如低聚果糖）。对于表现为营养不良或存在风险且能够耐受口服药物的门诊患者，给予口服高效复合维生素-复合矿物质制剂（持续使用数月）可能是明智的做法。

肠内管饲的实施

符合表 7.2 中所述情况的患者可能具有正常的胃肠道功能，但由于疾病或手术（如机械通气、胰腺炎、痴呆、吞咽困难、创伤或烧伤）而无法经口摄入充足的食物。尽管在这些情况下进行 PN 十分常见，但这种做法并非基于循证；学术指南强烈建议，如果患者的胃肠道功能正常，但需要特殊的营养支持，应使用口服营养补充剂或肠内管饲（"如果肠道能工作，就让它工作"）。与 PN 相比，EN 更符合生理学特点，感染、机械性并发症和代谢性并发症更少，成本也更低。虽然未被循证医学证实，但 EN 的常见禁忌证包括麻痹性肠梗阻、肠缺血、需要中高剂量血管活性药物治疗的血

流动力学不稳定、无法进入胃肠道通路、肠梗阻、难治性呕吐、严重腹泻和腹膜炎。

在患者能够耐受的情况下，这些膳食补充剂也可用于口服营养补充。当提供适当剂量时，这些流质饮食可为大多数患者提供全面的营养，尽管部分 ICU 患者、吸收不良或有其他情况的患者可能有特殊需求（见下文）。

液体管饲配方制剂可常规经鼻胃管送入胃内，也可经小口径鼻胃管或鼻空肠管、经皮胃造口或空肠造口管，或经皮胃空肠管（胃端口可能用于引流，空肠端口用于喂养）送入。胃内喂养可通过连续或间歇性喂养方式进行，但小肠喂养必须使用输注泵连续缓慢输注，以避免腹泻。管饲应从慢速开始（如 10 ～ 20 ml/h），持续 8 ～ 24 h，并在接下来的 24 ～ 48 h 根据患者的临床耐受性和临床状况，以 8 ～ 24 h 为节点缓慢增加至目标速度，以满足未来 24 ～ 48 h 的目标能量和蛋白质需求。近期指南强调将管饲患者置于半卧位（如抬高床头），谨慎增加喂养速度（对腹泻、恶心、呕吐、腹胀和有无大量胃残留物进行连续评估），若胃内喂养不耐受，则使用促动力剂和（或）幽门后喂养。近期数据表明，接受管饲的住院患者通常能很好地耐受较高的胃残留量（如＞ 250 ml）。

动物实验结果表明，与 PN 相比，EN 有助于改善肠道屏障功能、减少感染性并发症、减少高代谢状态，以及降低分解代谢模型动物的并发症发生率和死亡率。针对胰腺炎住院患者的随机临床试验显示，与 PN 相比，接受空肠 EN 有明显的临床获益。美国重症医学会（SCCM）和美国肠外肠内营养学会（ASPEN）指南建议，对于无法通过经口膳食摄入和补充剂而达到足够能量需求（如＞ 60%）的 ICU 患者，特别是已经存在营养不良的患者，应尽早开始 EN（24 ～ 48 h）。许多研究表明，ICU 患者实际上只获得医生开具的管饲剂量的 60% ～ 75%。这可能是由管饲不耐受（如胃残留量过多、呕吐、腹泻、导管脱落）或因诊断性检查或治疗干预而中断喂养所致。对于无法达到所需管饲速率的患者，虽然通常会开具补充性 PN（见下文），但由于缺乏高质量的临床试验，这种做法仍存在争议。目前正在进行严格的试验以评估这种方式的有效性，因为有数据表明，净能量不足（即随时间累积，每日能量需求与实际每日提供的能量之间的差异）的增加与内科和外科 ICU 患者的临床结局更差相关。

大多数门诊者及 ICU 和非 ICU 住院患者能够耐受经胃或肠道途径输送的价格低廉的标准 EN 制剂，其能量密度为 1.0 ～ 1.5 kcal/ml。临床上有多种类型的肠内管饲制剂可供选择。由于 EN 制剂可以在没有随机对照临床试验疗效数据的情况下上市销售，因此仍然迫切需要这样的试验，以确定不同临床状况下的最佳 EN 配方。

Complications of enteral feeding include diarrhea. Diarrhea is common in hospital patients receiving tube feedings but is typically caused by factors independent of the feeding, including administration of antibiotics, sorbitol-containing or hypertonic medications (e.g., acetaminophen elixir), and infections. Diarrhea caused by tube feeding itself does occur with rapid formula administration, in patients with underlying gut mucosal disease, and in those with severe hypoalbuminemia, which causes bowel wall edema. A fiber-containing enteral formula is sometimes useful to decrease diarrhea. Other complications of tube feeding include aspiration of tube feedings into the lung; mechanical problems with nasally placed feeding tubes, including discomfort, sinusitis, pharyngeal or esophageal mucosal erosion due to local tube trauma; and, with percutaneous feeding tubes, entrance site leakage, skin breakdown, cellulitis, and pain. Metabolic complications of tube feeding include fluid imbalances, hyperglycemia, electrolyte abnormalities, azotemia, and, occasionally, refeeding syndrome (discussed later). In general, if tube feedings are deemed to be required for more than 4 to 6 weeks, a percutaneous feeding tube should be placed.

In tube-fed patients who are receiving either subcutaneous or intravenous insulin to control hyperglycemia, significant hypoglycemia due to the continued actions of insulin may occur if tube feedings are discontinued inadvertently or for diagnostic or therapeutic tests. Hospitalized patients receiving tube feedings should have their blood glucose concentration monitored on a daily basis (or several times per day as indicated) and their blood electrolytes (including magnesium, potassium, and phosphorus) and renal function monitored several times each week (or daily in the ICU setting). Other blood chemistries should be determined at least weekly. This should be accompanied by close monitoring of intake and output records (including urine, stool, and drainage outputs) and gastrointestinal tolerance. When patients are able to consume oral food, tube feeding should be decreased and then discontinued (e.g., with daily calorie counts by a registered dietitian). For patients requiring home tube feeding, it is important to consult social service professionals to ensure appropriate care and follow-up.

EN administration must be individualized to each patient's specific needs. In order to determine the appropriate EN delivery method, GI tract integrity and functional capacity, presence and degree of malnutrition, underlying disease states, and patient tolerance must be assessed prior to and following the initiation of tube feeding. Gastrointestinal, mechanical, and metabolic complications, as well as pulmonary aspiration of feeds, can occur with enteral tube feeding. It is therefore essential to monitor enterally fed patients closely in order to identify complications.

A recent randomized study of 894 clinically similar, critically ill adults with medical or surgical issues at seven academic centers assigned patients to permissive enteral underfeeding (40-60% of calculated energy needs) versus standard EN (70-100% of calculated energy needs), with similar daily protein intake (approximately 60 g/day). During intervention, the permissive underfed group received 835 plus or minus 297 kcal/day versus 1299 plus or minus 467 kcal/day in the standard group; no difference in mortality or other clinical outcomes occurred.

Administration of Parenteral Nutrition

The basic principle in considering PN therapy is that the patient must be unable to achieve adequate nutrient intake via the enteral route. PN support includes administration of standard complete nutrient mixtures that contain dextrose, L-amino acids, lipid emulsion, electrolytes, vitamins, and minerals (in addition to certain medications as indicated, such as insulin or octreotide), given via a peripheral or central vein. Administration of complete PN therapy to patients with gastrointestinal tract dysfunction has become a standard of care in most hospitals and ICUs throughout the world, although use in individual institutions varies widely. PN is life-saving in patients with intestinal

failure (e.g., short bowel syndrome). Existing data indicate that PN benefits patients with preexisting moderate to severe malnutrition or critical illness by decreasing overall morbidity, and possibly mortality, compared with patients receiving inadequate EN or hydration (intravenous dextrose) therapy alone. A consensus is emerging, based on recent rigorous studies in critical illness, that PN should probably not be initiated until days 3 to 4 after ICU admission in patients who are unable to tolerate adequate EN.

Compared with PN, EN is less expensive, probably maintains intestinal mucosal structure and function to a greater extent, is safer in terms of mechanical and metabolic complications (see later discussion), and is associated with reduced rates of nosocomial infection. Therefore, the enteral route of feeding should be used and advanced whenever possible, and the amount of administered PN should be correspondingly reduced.

Generally recognized indications for PN include the following situations:

1. Patients with short bowel syndrome or other conditions causing intestinal failure (e.g., motility disorders, obstruction, severe ileus, severe inflammatory bowel disease), especially those with preexisting malnutrition.
2. Clinically stable patients in whom adequate enteral feeding (e.g., >50% of needs) is unlikely for 7 to 10 days because of an underlying illness.
3. Patients with severe catabolic stress requiring ICU care in whom adequate enteral nutrient intake is unlikely for more than 3 to 5 days.

There is no reason to withhold PN in hospitalized patients for any period of time if they exhibit preexisting moderate to severe malnutrition and are deemed to be unlikely to meet their needs by the oral or enteral route.

Generally accepted contraindications for PN include the following conditions:

1. If the GI tract is functional and access for enteral feeding is available.
2. If PN is thought to be required for 5 days or less.
3. If the patient cannot tolerate the extra intravenous fluid required for PN or has severe hyperglycemia or electrolyte abnormalities on the planned day of PN initiation.
4. If the patient has an uncontrolled bloodstream infection or severe hemodynamic instability.
5. If new placement of an intravenous line solely for PN poses undue risks based on clinical judgment.
6. On an individualized basis, if aggressive nutritional support is not desired by the competent patient or legally authorized representative, such as in premorbid patients or those with terminal illness.

PN can be delivered either as peripheral vein solutions or as central vein solutions through a percutaneous subclavian vein or internal jugular vein catheter for infusion into the superior vena cava (nontunneled in the hospital setting), through a subcutaneously tunneled central venous catheter (e.g., Hickman catheter) or central venous port (for chronic home PN therapy), or through a peripherally inserted central venous catheter (PICC). Although data are limited, it is clearly preferable to manage long-term central venous PN to be managed at home with the use of a tunneled central venous catheter rather than a PICC line because of the higher rate of local complications (e.g., phlebitis, catheter breakage) and possibly catheter-associated infections with PICC lines.

A comparison of typical fluid, macronutrient, and micronutrient content of peripheral and central vein PN solutions is shown in Table 7.3. Complete PN provides intravenous lipid emulsions (IVF) as a source of both energy and essential linoleic and linolenic fatty acids.

EN 的并发症包括腹泻。腹泻在接受管饲的住院患者中很常见，但通常由与喂养无关的因素引起，包括使用抗生素、含山梨醇的药物或高渗性药物（如对乙酰氨基酚口服液）和感染。管饲本身也会引起腹泻，尤其是在管饲速度过快、患有基础肠道黏膜疾病和严重低白蛋白血症（导致肠壁水肿）的患者中。含有纤维素的 EN 配方有时有助于减少腹泻。管饲的其他并发症包括将管饲物吸入肺部；经鼻置管相关机械问题，包括不适感、鼻窦炎、因局部置管创伤导致的咽部或食管黏膜糜烂；对于经皮饲管，可出现入口部位渗漏、皮肤破损、蜂窝织炎和疼痛。管饲的代谢性并发症包括液体失衡、高血糖、电解质紊乱、氮质血症，偶可出现再喂养综合征（见下文）。一般来说，如果认为管饲需要持续 4 ~ 6 周以上，则应放置经皮饲管。

对于正在接受皮下或静脉注射胰岛素以控制高血糖的管饲患者，如果不慎或因诊断或治疗性操作而中断管饲，由于胰岛素的持续作用，可能会发生严重低血糖。接受管饲的住院患者应每天（或根据需要每天数次）监测血糖浓度，每周监测（或在 ICU 中每天监测）数次电解质（包括镁、钾和磷）和肾功能。其他血液生化指标也应每周至少监测 1 次。这应与密切监测出入量（包括尿液、粪便和引流物）及胃肠道耐受性相结合。当患者能够经口进食时，应减少进而停止管饲（如由注册营养师进行每日能量计算）。对于需要家庭管饲的患者，咨询社会服务专业人员以确保适当的照护和后续随访非常重要。

EN 的实施必须针对每位患者的具体需求而个性化制订。为确定合适的 EN 给予方式，必须在管饲前后评估胃肠道的完整性和功能、营养不良状况和严重程度、基础疾病状况及患者耐受性。肠内管饲过程中可能会发生胃肠道、机械性和代谢性并发症，以及食物被误吸入肺部。因此，密切监测肠内管饲的患者以识别并发症至关重要。

近期，在一项纳入来自 7 个医疗中心的 894 名临床状况相似、患有内科或外科疾病的重症成人患者的随机试验中，患者被分配到允许性肠内低喂养组（给予计算的能量需求的 40% ~ 60%）与标准 EN 组（给予计算的能量需求的 70% ~ 100%），两组每日蛋白质摄入量相似（约 60 g/d）。在干预期间，允许性低喂养组患者每天接受（835±297）kcal 能量，而标准 EN 组患者每天接受（1299±467）kcal 能量；试验结果显示，两组患者的死亡率或其他临床结局无显著差异。

PN 的实施

考虑 PN 治疗的基本原则是患者无法通过肠内途径达到足够的营养摄入。PN 支持包括通过外周或中心静脉给予标准且完全的营养素混合物，其中包含葡萄糖、L- 氨基酸、脂肪乳、电解质、维生素、矿物质及某些指定的药物（如胰岛素或奥曲肽）。尽管不同医疗机构的使用情况差异很大，但对于胃肠功能障碍的患者，给予全肠外营养（TPN）治疗已成为全球大多数医院和 ICU 的医疗照护标准。对于肠功能衰竭（如短肠综合征）患者，PN 是挽救生命的治疗。现有数据表明，与仅接受不充分 EN 或水化（静脉输注葡萄糖）治疗的患者相比，PN 对中重度营养不良或危重症患者有益，可降低总并发症发生率，甚至可能降低死亡率。根据近期危重症医学领域的高质量研究，新的共识正在形成：对于不能耐受充分 EN 的 ICU 住院患者，PN 的启动可能不应晚于入住 ICU 后的 3 ~ 4 天。

与 PN 相比，EN 的成本更低，可能在更大限度上维持肠道黏膜的结构和功能，在机械性和代谢性并发症方面更安全（见下文），且与更低的院内感染率有关。因此，应尽可能使用 EN，并相应减少 PN 的用量。

一般认为，PN 的指征包括以下情况：

1. 患有短肠综合征或其他导致肠功能衰竭的情况（如胃肠动力障碍、梗阻、严重肠梗阻、严重炎症性肠病），特别是已经存在营养不良的患者。

2. 由于存在基础疾病，预计在 7 ~ 10 天无法获得足够的 EN 摄入（如达到 > 50% 的实际需求量）的临床状况稳定的患者。

3. 处于严重分解代谢应激且需要 ICU 照护的患者，并预计至少 3 ~ 5 天无法获得足够的 EN 摄入。

如果住院患者已经存在中重度营养不良，且被认为不太可能通过口服或 EN 满足自身需求，则没有理由在任何时间段内停用 PN。

一般而言，PN 的禁忌证包括以下情况：

1. 胃肠道功能正常且 EN 管路可用。

2. PN 所需时间 ≤ 5 天。

3. 患者不能耐受 PN 所需的额外静脉输注，或在计划开始 PN 的当天存在严重高血糖或电解质异常。

4. 患者存在未经控制的血流感染或严重血流动力学障碍。

5. 根据临床判断，专为 PN 放置的静脉导管可能带来不必要的风险。

6. 基于个体情况，有民事行为能力的患者本人或法定授权代理人不希望进行积极的营养支持，如发病前的患者或患有绝症的患者。

PN 可通过外周静脉溶液或中心静脉溶液的形式进行输送。后者可通过经皮锁骨下静脉或颈内静脉导管注入上腔静脉（在医院环境中为非隧道式），也可通过皮下隧道式中心静脉导管（如 Hickman 导管）或中心静脉输液港（用于长期家庭 PN 治疗），或通过经外周静脉穿刺的中心静脉导管（PICC）输注。尽管数据有限，但使用隧道式中心静脉导管（而非 PICC）来管理长期中心静脉 PN 显然是最优选择，因为 PICC 管路发生局部并发症（如静脉炎、导管断裂）的概率更高，且可能引发导管相关感染。

表 7.3 列出了外周静脉和中心静脉 PN 溶液典型的

In the United States, historically the only commercially available lipid emulsion was soybean oil (SO)-based; now, an intravenous soybean oil/olive oil emulsion, an intravenous soybean oil/medium-chain triglyceride mixture, a fish oil/medium-chain triglyceride/olive oil/soybean oil emulsion, and a fish oil–based emulsion have been approved for use in PN. The different formulations vary in the fatty acid content and dosing. The use of SO-based emulsions has been associated with elevated serum bilirubin levels, intestinal failure–associated liver disease, and cholestasis in some patients, particularly at chronic doses exceeding 1.0 g/kg/day. Recent reviews of fish oil–containing IVF lowered inflammatory markers, improved triglyceride levels and liver enzymes, and reduced infectious complications in ICU patients. When compared with SO-based IVF, olive oil–based IVF are a safe alternative but clinical and metabolic differences between these two IVF were not statistically significant.

The maximal recommended rate of fat emulsion infusion is approximately 1.0 g/kg/day but larger doses may be given for shorter term use in hospital settings and are well tolerated. Most patients are well able to clear triglyceride from plasma after intravenous administration of fat emulsion. It is important to monitor blood triglyceride levels at baseline and then approximately weekly and as indicated to assess clearance of intravenous fat; triglyceride levels should be maintained lower than 400 mg/dL to decrease the risk of pancreatitis or diminished pulmonary diffusion capacity in patients with severe chronic obstructive lung disease.

Central venous administration of PN allows higher concentrations of dextrose (3.4 kcal/g) and amino acids (4 kcal/g) to be delivered as hypertonic solutions; thus, lower amounts of fat emulsion are needed to reach caloric goals (see Table 7.3). Requirements for potassium, magnesium, and phosphorus are typically higher with central vein PN compared to peripheral vein PN. The higher concentrations of dextrose and amino acids allow most patients to achieve caloric and amino acid goals with only 1 to 1.5 L of PN per day. In central vein PN, initial orders typically provide 60% to 70% of non–amino acid calories as dextrose and 30% to 40% of non–amino acid calories as fat emulsion. These percentages are adjusted as indicated based on levels of blood glucose and triglyceride, respectively. Based on comprehensive data associating hyperglycemia with hospital morbidity and mortality, expert panels now recommend tight blood glucose control in ICU settings (between 80 and 130 to 150 mg/dL) and close blood glucose monitoring. Separate intravenous insulin infusions should usually be administered in the ICU when patients receiving central vein PN develop hyperglycemia.

Specific requirements for intravenous trace elements and vitamins have not been rigorously defined for patient subgroups, and in most stable patients, therapy is directed at meeting published recommended doses using standardized intravenous preparations to maintain blood levels in the normal range (see Table 7.3). Several studies have shown that a significant proportion of ICU patients have low levels of zinc, selenium, vitamin C, vitamin E, and vitamin D despite receiving specialized PN (or EN). Depletion of these essential nutrients may impair antioxidant capacity, immunity, wound healing, and other important body functions, and supplementation is recommended if serum concentrations are low. For example, zinc (and other micronutrients such as copper) should probably be increased in the PN of patients with burns, large wounds, significant gastrointestinal fluid losses, and other conditions if serum concentrations indicate low levels. Recent data suggest that thiamine depletion is not uncommon in patients receiving chronic diuretic therapy, renal replacement therapy, or in those with severe malabsorption.

The most common complication of peripheral vein PN is local phlebitis resulting from use of the catheter. In such cases, a small dose of hydrocortisone and heparin is typically added to the solution.

TABLE 7.3   Composition of Typical Parenteral Nutrition Solutions

Component[a]	Peripheral PN	Central PN
Volume (L/day)	2-3	1-1.5
Dextrose (%)	5	10-25
Amino acids (%)[b]	2.5-3.5	3-8
Lipid (%)[c]	3.5-5.0	2.5-5.0
Sodium (mEq/L)	50-150	50-150
Potassium (mEq/L)	20-35	30-50
Phosphorus (mmol/L)	5-10	10-30
Magnesium (mEq/L)	8-10	10-20
Calcium (mEq/L)	2.5-5	2.5-5
Trace elements[d]		
Vitamins[e]		

[a]Electrolytes in parenteral nutrition (PN) are adjusted as indicated to maintain serially measured serum levels within the normal range. The percentage of sodium and potassium salts as chloride is increased to correct metabolic alkalosis, and the percentage of salts as acetate is increased to correct metabolic acidosis. Regular insulin is added to PN as needed to achieve blood glucose goals (separate intravenous insulin infusions are commonly required with hyperglycemia in intensive care unit settings).

[b]Provides all essential amino acids and several nonessential amino acids. The dose of amino acids is adjusted downward or upward to goal as a function of the degree of azotemia or hyperbilirubinemia in patients with renal or hepatic failure, respectively.

[c]Lipid is given as soybean oil– or olive oil/soybean oil–based fat emulsion in the United States. Intravenous fish oil, olive oil, medium-chain triglycerides, and combinations of these are also now available for use in PN. Lipid is typically mixed with dextrose and amino acids in the same PN infusion bag ("all-in-one" solution).

[d]Trace elements added on a daily basis to peripheral vein and central vein PN are mixtures of chromium, copper, manganese, selenium, and zinc. (These elements can also be supplemented individually.)

[e]Vitamins added on a daily basis to peripheral vein and central vein PN are mixtures of vitamins A, B_1 (thiamine), B_2 (riboflavin), B_3 (niacinamide), B_6 (pyridoxine), B_{12}, C, D, and E, biotin, folate, and pantothenic acid. Vitamin K is added on an individual basis (e.g., for patients with cirrhosis). Specific vitamins can also be supplemented individually.

Alterations in blood electrolytes can be treated with adjustment of concentrations in the peripheral PN prescription. Hypertriglyceridemia typically responds well to lowering of the total PN lipid dose. Central vein PN is associated with a much higher rate of mechanical, metabolic, and infectious complications than peripheral vein PN. Mechanical complications include those related to insertion of the central venous catheter (e.g., pneumothorax, hemothorax, malposition of the catheter, thrombosis). Infectious complications include catheter-related bloodstream infections and non–catheter-related infections. The risk for these infections appears to be increased with use of non–subclavian vein central venous access (e.g., jugular vein, femoral vein) and multiple-use catheters with non-dedicated PN infusion ports used for additional purposes such as blood drawing or medication administration. Poorly controlled blood glucose levels (>140 to 180 mg/dL) are not uncommon in patients requiring central vein PN and are associated with an increased risk of nosocomial infection. Risk factors for hyperglycemia include poorly controlled blood glucose at PN initiation; use of high dextrose concentrations (>10%) in the initial few days of PN administration or too rapid an increase in total dextrose load; insufficient exogenous insulin administration; inadequate monitoring of blood glucose responses to central vein PN administration; and administration of corticosteroids and vasopressor agents such as

液体、宏量营养素和微量营养素含量的比较。TPN 提供静脉用脂肪乳剂（IVF）作为能量及必需亚油酸和亚麻酸的来源。在美国，历史上唯一市售的脂肪乳剂是以大豆油（SO）为基础的；目前，静脉用大豆油 / 橄榄油乳剂、大豆油 / 中链甘油三酯混合物、鱼油 / 中链甘油三酯 / 橄榄油 / 大豆油乳剂和鱼油基乳剂已被批准用于 PN。不同的配方在脂肪酸含量和剂量上有所不同。使用基于 SO 的乳剂与部分患者出现血清胆红素水平升高、肠功能衰竭相关肝病和胆汁淤积有关，特别是长期使用且剂量 ＞ 1.0 g/（kg·d）时。近期综述表明，含有鱼油的 IVF 可降低 ICU 患者的炎症标志物水平，改善甘油三酯和肝酶水平，并减少感染性并发症的发生。与基于 SO 的 IVF 相比，基于橄榄油的 IVF 是安全的替代方案，但这两种 IVF 在临床和代谢结局上无显著差异。

脂肪乳剂输注的最大推荐剂量约为 1.0 g/（kg·d），但在医院环境中短期使用可给予更大的剂量，且耐受性良好。大多数患者在接受静脉用脂肪乳剂输注后能够很好地清除血浆中的甘油三酯。重要的是，应定期监测甘油三酯水平（包括基线水平及之后约每周 1 次），并根据需要评估静脉脂肪的清除情况；甘油三酯水平应维持在 400 mg/dl 以下，以降低胰腺炎或严重慢性阻塞性肺疾病患者肺弥散功能下降的风险。

中心静脉 PN 允许更高浓度的葡萄糖（3.4 kcal/g）和氨基酸（4 kcal/g）作为高渗溶液输送；因此，需要较少的脂肪乳剂来达到能量目标（表 7.3）。与外周静脉 PN 相比，中心静脉 PN 对钾、镁和磷的需求量通常更高。高浓度葡萄糖和氨基酸可使大多数患者每天仅需 1 ～ 1.5 L PN 即可达到能量和氨基酸目标。在中心静脉 PN 中，初始处方中葡萄糖通常占非氨基酸能量的 60% ～ 70%，脂肪乳剂占 30% ～ 40%。可分别根据血糖和甘油三酯水平酌情调整上述百分比。基于高血糖与院内并发症发生率和死亡率的关联数据，目前专家小组推荐在 ICU 患者中严格控制血糖（80 ～ 150 mg/dl）并密切监测血糖。当接受中心静脉 PN 的患者出现高血糖时，通常应在 ICU 进行静脉胰岛素输注。

目前尚未严格制定不同亚群患者静脉微量元素和维生素的特定需求量，对于大多数病情稳定的患者，制订治疗方案的原则是使用标准化静脉制剂，以满足已公布的推荐剂量，从而维持正常的血液浓度（表 7.3）。多项研究表明，尽管接受了专门的 PN（或 EN），但仍有相当比例的 ICU 患者存在锌、硒、维生素 C、维生素 E 和维生素 D 水平低下。这些必需营养素的缺乏可能会损害机体的抗氧化能力、免疫力、伤口愈合能力及其他重要的身体功能，如果血清浓度较低，则建议补充。例如，在烧伤、大面积创伤、胃肠道液体大量流失及其他情况的患者中，如果血清锌浓度低下，则可能需要增加 PN 中锌及其他微量营养素（如铜）的含量。近期数据显示，在接受长期利尿剂治疗、肾脏替代治疗或患有严重

表 7.3　典型 PN 溶液的组成

组分 [a]	外周静脉 PN	中心静脉 PN
液体量（L/d）	2 ～ 3	1 ～ 1.5
葡萄糖（%）	5	10 ～ 25
氨基酸（%）[b]	2.5 ～ 3.5	3 ～ 8
脂肪（%）[c]	3.5 ～ 5.0	2.5 ～ 5.0
钠（mmol/L）	50 ～ 150	50 ～ 150
钾（mmol/L）	20 ～ 35	30 ～ 50
磷（mmol/L）	5 ～ 10	10 ～ 30
镁（mmol/L）	4 ～ 5	5 ～ 10
钙（mmol/L）	1.25 ～ 2.5	1.25 ～ 2.5
微量元素 [d]		
维生素 [e]		

[a] 根据需要来调整 PN 中的电解质含量，以保持连续检测的血清电解质水平处于正常范围内。增加氯化钠和氯化钾的占比可纠正代谢性碱中毒，增加醋酸盐占比可纠正代谢性酸中毒。根据需要在 PN 中添加常规胰岛素以实现血糖控制（在 ICU 中，通常需要单独静脉输注胰岛素来控制高血糖）。

[b] 提供所有必需氨基酸和多种非必需氨基酸。分别根据肾衰竭和肝衰竭住院患者氮质血症和高胆红素血症的程度，调整氨基酸的剂量以达到目标。

[c] 在美国，脂肪是通过以大豆油或橄榄油 / 大豆油为基础的脂肪乳剂给予。静脉注射鱼油、橄榄油、中链甘油三酯及其组合也可用于 PN。脂肪通常与葡萄糖和氨基酸混合在同一个 PN 输注袋中（"全合一"溶液）。

[d] 每日添加到外周静脉 PN 和中心静脉 PN 中的微量元素是铬、铜、锰、硒和锌的混合物（这些元素也可以单独补充）。

[e] 每日添加到外周静脉 PN 和中心静脉 PN 中的维生素是维生素 A、B_1（硫胺素）、B_2（核黄素）、B_3（烟酰胺）、B_6（吡哆醇）、B_{12}、C、D 和 E，以及生物素、叶酸和泛酸的混合物。根据个体情况添加维生素 K（如肝硬化患者）。也可单独补充特定维生素。

吸收不良的患者中，维生素 B_1 缺乏并不少见。

外周静脉 PN 最常见的并发症是导管所致的局部静脉炎。在这种情况下，通常需在溶液中加入少量氢化可的松和肝素。一旦血电解质浓度发生变化，可通过调整外周静脉 PN 处方中的电解质浓度来进行治疗。减少总 PN 中的脂肪剂量通常能有效改善高甘油三酯血症。与外周静脉 PN 相比，中心静脉 PN 的机械性并发症、代谢性并发症和感染性并发症的发生率显著升高。机械性并发症包括与置入中心静脉导管相关的并发症（如气胸、血胸、导管异位、血栓形成等）。感染性并发症包括与导管相关的血流感染和非导管相关的感染。使用非锁骨下静脉中心静脉通路（如颈内静脉、股静脉）和用于其他目的（如抽血和给药）的多用途导管似乎会增加感染的风险。在需要中心静脉 PN 的患者中，血糖控制不佳（＞ 140 ～ 180 mg/dl）并不少见，且与院内感染风险增加有关。高血糖的危险因素包括在开始 PN 时血糖控制不佳；在开始 PN 的最初数天使用高浓度葡萄糖（＞ 10%）或总葡萄糖负荷增加过快；外源性胰岛素剂量不足；给予中心静脉 PN 期间血糖监测不足；使用皮质类固醇和血管升压药，如去甲肾上

norepinephrine (which stimulate gluconeogenesis and cause insulin resistance).

Studies on nutrient utilization efficiency and metabolic complications in severely catabolic patients suggest that lower amounts of total energy and protein/amino acids should be administered than were routinely given in the past, particularly in unstable and ICU patients. High calorie, carbohydrate, amino acid, and fat loads ("hyperalimentation") are easily administered via central vein PN but can induce severe metabolic complications, including carbon dioxide overproduction, azotemia, hyperglycemia, electrolyte alterations, and hepatic steatosis and injury. Dextrose and lipid doses in PN should be advanced over several days after initiation, with close monitoring of the blood glucose concentration, electrolytes, triglycerides, organ function tests, intake and output measurements, and the clinical course.

Refeeding syndrome with central vein PN administration is relatively common in patients at risk, including those with preexisting malnutrition, electrolyte depletion, alcoholism, or prolonged periods of intravenous hydration therapy (e.g., 5% dextrose) without nutritional support, all of which are common in hospital patients. Refeeding syndrome is mediated by administration of excessive intravenous dextrose (>150 to 250 g, for example in 1 L of PN containing 15% to 25% dextrose). This, in turn, markedly stimulates insulin release, which rapidly lowers blood concentrations of potassium, magnesium, and especially phosphorus as a result of intracellular shifts and utilization in carbohydrate metabolic pathways. Administration of high doses of carbohydrate also consumes thiamine, which is required as a cofactor for carbohydrate metabolism and can precipitate symptoms of thiamine deficiency, especially in patients with poor thiamine nutriture at baseline. Hyperinsulinemia also tends to cause sodium and fluid retention at the level of the kidney. Together, fluid and sodium retention, the drop in electrolytes (which can cause arrhythmias), and hypermetabolism due to excessive calorie provision can result in heart failure, especially in patients with preexisting heart disease and cardiac muscle atrophy due to prolonged protein-energy malnutrition. Prevention of refeeding syndrome requires vigilance to identify patients at risk; use of initially low PN dextrose concentrations; empiric provision of higher doses of potassium, magnesium, and phosphorus based on current blood levels and renal function; and supplemental thiamine (100 mg/day for 3 to 5 days).

If home PN is indicated, the primary physician should consult with social service professionals to identify appropriate home care companies and nutrition support professionals to assess intravenous line access, metabolic status, and the home PN order and to arrange for follow-up care and monitoring of PN. It is important not to arrange for rapid discharge of hospitalized patients newly started on PN. Obtaining appropriate venous access and monitoring of fluid and electrolyte status over a 2- to 3-day period is an important aspect of care for most patients started on PN, and it is imperative for those with severe malnutrition and those at risk for refeeding syndrome.

For a deeper discussion on this topic, please see Chapters 203, ❖ "Protein-Energy Malnutrition," and 204, "Malnutrition: Assessment and Support," in *Goldman-Cecil Medicine*, 26th Edition.

SUGGESTED READINGS

Arabi VM, Aldawood AS, Haddad SH, et al: Permissive underfeeding or standard enteral feeding in critically ill adults, New Engl J Med 372:2398–2408, 2015.

Blaauw R, Osland E, Sriram K, et al: Parenteral provision of micronutrients to adult patients: an expert consensus paper, JPEN J Parenter Enteral Nutr 43(Suppl 1):S5–S23, 2019.

Boullata J, Carrera A, Harvey L, et al: ASPEN safe practices for enteral nutrition therapy, JPEN J Parenter Enteral Nutr 41:36–46, 2017.

Casaer MP, Mesotten D, Hermans G, et al: Early versus late parenteral nutrition in critically ill adults, N Engl J Med 365:506–517, 2011.

Doig GS, Simpson F, Sweetman EA, et al: Early PN Investigators of the ANZICS clinical trials group: early parenteral nutrition in critically ill patients with short-term relative contraindications to early enteral nutrition: a randomized controlled trial, J Am Med Assoc 309:2130–2138, 2013.

Harvey SE, Parrott F, Harrison DA, et al: Trial of the route of early nutritional support in critically ill adults, N Eng J Med 371:1673–1684, 2014.

Honeywell S, Zelig R, Radler DR: Impact of intravenous lipid emulsions containing fish oil on clinical outcomes in critically ill surgical patients: a literature review, JPEN J Parenter Enteral Nutr 26:112–122, 2019.

Manzanares W, Langlois PL, Hardy G: Intravenous lipid emulsions in the crucially ill: an update, Curr Opin Crit Care 22:308–315, 2016.

McClave SA, Taylor BE, Martindale RG, et al: Guidelines for the provision and assessment of nutrition support therapy in the adult critically ill patient: society of critical care medicine (SCCM) and American Society for Parenteral and Enteral Nutrition (A.S.P.E.N.), JPEN J Parenter Enteral Nutr 40(2):159–211, 2016.

Singer P, Blaser AR, Berger MM, et al: ESPEN guidelines on clinical nutrition in the intensive care unit, Clin Nutr 38:48–79, 2019.

Ziegler TR: Nutrition support in critical illness: bridging the evidence gap, N Engl J Med 365:562–564, 2011.

Ziegler TR: Parenteral nutrition in the critically ill patient, N Engl J Med 361:1088–1097, 2009.

腺素（刺激糖异生并导致胰岛素抵抗）。

针对严重分解代谢患者营养利用效率及代谢性并发症的研究表明，总能量和蛋白质/氨基酸的剂量应低于既往的常规给予量，特别是在病情不稳定和 ICU 的患者中。中心静脉 PN 易导致高能量、碳水化合物、氨基酸和脂肪负荷（"过度喂养"），进而可能导致严重的代谢性并发症，包括二氧化碳过度产生、氮质血症、高血糖、电解质紊乱、肝脂肪变性及肝损伤。PN 中的葡萄糖和脂质剂量应在开始治疗后的数天内逐渐增加，并密切监测血糖、电解质、甘油三酯、器官功能、出入量和临床病程。

在高危患者中，使用中心静脉 PN 出现再喂养综合征相对常见，这些患者包括已存在营养不良、电解质缺乏、酗酒或长时间静脉水化治疗（如 5% 葡萄糖）而未进行营养支持，上述情况在住院患者中均很常见。过量静脉给予葡萄糖（> 150 ～ 250 g，如 1 L PN 中含有 15% ～ 25% 葡萄糖）可介导再喂养综合征的发生。这又会显著刺激胰岛素的释放，由于电解质向细胞内转移和碳水化合物代谢过程中的利用增加，导致血钾、血镁、尤其是血磷水平降低。给予高剂量碳水化合物也会消耗维生素 B_1，后者是碳水化合物代谢所必需的辅因子，因此可能会诱发维生素 B_1 缺乏的症状，特别是在基线时就存在维生素 B_1 缺乏的患者中。高胰岛素血症易引起肾脏水平的水钠潴留。综上，水钠潴留、电解质水平下降（可导致心律失常）、过量供能所致的高代谢可能导致心力衰竭，特别是在已经患心脏病和由长期蛋白质-能量营养不良导致心肌萎缩的患者中。预防再喂养综合征需要谨慎识别高危者；起始 PN 给予低浓度葡萄糖；根据当前血电解质水平和肾功能状态经验性给予更高剂量的钾、镁和磷；补充维生素 B_1（100 mg/d，持续 3 ～ 5 天）。

如果需要家庭 PN，主治医生应与社会服务专业人员协商，确定合适的家庭照护机构和营养支持专业人员，以评估静脉通路、代谢状态和家庭 PN 医嘱，并安排后续的医疗照护和 PN 监测。重要的是，不要安排刚开始应用 PN 的住院患者迅速出院。对于大多数患者，用 2 ～ 3 天建立适当的静脉通路并监测液体和电解质情况是照护的重要方面，这对于严重营养不良和有再喂养综合征风险的患者尤为重要。

有关此专题的深入讨论，请参阅 *Goldman-Cecil* ❖ *Medicine* 第 26 版第 203 章"蛋白质-能量营养不良"和第 204 章"营养不良：评估和支持"。

推荐阅读

Arabi VM, Aldawood AS, Haddad SH, et al: Permissive underfeeding or standard enteral feeding in critically ill adults, New Engl J Med 372:2398–2408, 2015.

Blaauw R, Osland E, Sriram K, et al: Parenteral provision of micronutrients to adult patients: an expert consensus paper, JPEN J Parenter Enteral Nutr 43(Suppl 1):S5–S23, 2019.

Boullata J, Carrera A, Harvey L, et al: ASPEN safe practices for enteral nutrition therapy, JPEN J Parenter Enteral Nutr 41:36–46, 2017.

Casaer MP, Mesotten D, Hermans G, et al: Early versus late parenteral nutrition in critically ill adults, N Engl J Med 365:506–517, 2011.

Doig GS, Simpson F, Sweetman EA, et al: Early PN Investigators of the ANZICS clinical trials group: early parenteral nutrition in critically ill patients with short-term relative contraindications to early enteral nutrition: a randomized controlled trial, J Am Med Assoc 309:2130–2138, 2013.

Harvey SE, Parrott F, Harrison DA, et al: Trial of the route of early nutritional support in critically ill adults, N Eng J Med 371:1673–1684, 2014.

Honeywell S, Zelig R, Radler DR: Impact of intravenous lipid emulsions containing fish oil on clinical outcomes in critically ill surgical patients: a literature review, JPEN J Parenter Enteral Nutr 26:112–122, 2019.

Manzanares W, Langlois PL, Hardy G: Intravenous lipid emulsions in the crucially ill: an update, Curr Opin Crit Care 22:308–315, 2016.

McClave SA, Taylor BE, Martindale RG, et al: Guidelines for the provision and assessment of nutrition support therapy in the adult critically ill patient: society of critical care medicine (SCCM) and American Society for Parenteral and Enteral Nutrition (A.S.P.E.N.), JPEN J Parenter Enteral Nutr 40(2):159–211, 2016.

Singer P, Blaser AR, Berger MM, et al: ESPEN guidelines on clinical nutrition in the intensive care unit, Clin Nutr 38:48–79, 2019.

Ziegler TR: Nutrition support in critical illness: bridging the evidence gap, N Engl J Med 365:562–564, 2011.

Ziegler TR: Parenteral nutrition in the critically ill patient, N Engl J Med 361:1088–1097, 2009.

Disorders of Lipid Metabolism

Russell Bratman, Geetha Gopalakrishnan

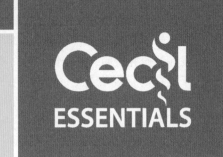

DEFINITION AND EPIDEMIOLOGY

Lipids such as free fatty acids (FFA), cholesterol, and triglycerides are hydrophobic molecules that bind proteins for transport. Nonesterified FFA travel as anions complexed to albumin. Esterified complex lipids are transported in lipoprotein particles. Lipoproteins have a hydrophobic core (cholesteryl esters and triglycerides) and an amphiphilic surface monolayer (phospholipids, unesterified cholesterol, and apolipoproteins). Ultracentrifugation separates lipoproteins into five classes based on their density (Table 8.1).

Proteins on the surface of lipoproteins (i.e., apolipoproteins) activate enzymes and receptors that guide lipid metabolism. Defects in the synthesis and catabolism of lipoproteins result in dyslipidemia. Prevalence of dyslipidemia in the United States is approximately 20% and varies with the population studied. An estimated 70% of individuals with premature coronary heart disease (CHD) have dyslipidemia. In clinical trials, treatment of dyslipidemia improved both CHD and all-cause mortality rates. Two classes of lipids, triglyceride and cholesterol, play a significant, yet modifiable, role in the pathogenesis of atherosclerosis and therefore are the focus of this chapter.

PATHOLOGY

In the intestinal lumen, dietary triglycerides and cholesterol esters are hydrolyzed by pancreatic lipase to produce glycerol, FFA, and free cholesterol. Bile acids aid in the formation of amphiphilic droplets known as micelles. Micelles enable the absorption of glycerol and FFA into the intestinal cell. The transport of free cholesterol is mediated by a cholesterol gradient that exists between the lumen and the intestinal cell. Within the cell, glycerol combines with three fatty acid chains to form triglycerides, and cholesterol is esterified to form cholesterol esters. Chylomicrons are formed from triglycerides (85% of chylomicron mass) and cholesterol esters assembled with surface lipoproteins. Chylomicrons enter the circulation and acquire more surface apolipoproteins such as apo C-II and apo E from high-density lipoprotein (HDL) particles (Fig. 8.1). Apo C-II activates lipoprotein lipase (LPL), which is located on the capillary endothelium. LPL hydrolyzes the core chylomicron triglycerides to release FFA. FFA functions as an energy source. Excess FFA are stored in adipose tissue or utilized in hepatic lipoprotein synthesis. The triglyceride-poor chylomicron remnant is then cleared from the circulation by hepatic LDL receptors. These receptors are activated by apo E located on the surface of chylomicrons.

Very-low-density lipoproteins (VLDL) are synthesized by the liver (see Fig. 8.1) using FFA and cholesterol obtained from the circulation or synthesized by the liver. Any condition that increases the flux of FFA to the liver, such as poorly controlled diabetes, will increase VLDL production. The liver assembles triglycerides (55% of VLDL mass), cholesterol (20%), and surface apolipoproteins to form VLDL particles. Apo C-II, the cofactor for LPL, hydrolyzes the triglyceride core of VLDL particles to generate VLDL remnant or intermediate-density lipoprotein (IDL). The IDL, depleted of triglycerides (25%), can be cleared from the circulation by apo E–mediated LDL receptors, or it can be hydrolyzed further to form low-density lipoproteins (LDL). LDL particles are triglyceride poor (5% of LDL mass) and consist mostly of cholesterol esters (60%) and apolipoproteins. Apo B100 on the surface of LDL binds LDL receptors and facilitates LDL clearance from the circulation. Internalized LDL-cholesterol is used to synthesize hormones, produce cell membranes, and store energy.

In the liver, LDL-cholesterol is used to synthesize bile acids (see Fig. 8.1), which are secreted into the intestinal lumen along with free cholesterol. Bile acids help transport fat. Approximately 50% of the cholesterol and 97% of the bile acid entering the lumen are reabsorbed back into the circulation. The reabsorbed cholesterol regulates cholesterol and LDL receptor synthesis.

Many cells in the body, including liver parenchymal cells, synthesize cholesterol (Fig. 8.2). Acetate is converted to 3-hydroxy-3-methylglutaryl–coenzyme A (HMG-CoA). HMG-CoA reductase converts HMG-CoA to mevalonic acid, which is then converted to cholesterol through a series of steps. HMG-CoA reductase catalyzes the rate-limiting step in the cholesterol synthesis pathway. Drugs that inhibit this enzyme decrease cholesterol biosynthesis and cellular cholesterol pools. The class of drugs that inhibit HMG-CoA inhibitors are often called "statins." Internalization of LDL particles into cells is regulated by negative feedback (see Fig. 8.2). A negative cholesterol balance increases the expression of LDL receptors and subsequent uptake of cholesterol from the circulation. A positive cell cholesterol balance suppresses LDL receptor expression and decreases uptake of LDL-cholesterol into cells. Circulating LDL then enters macrophages and other tissues via scavenger receptors. Because the scavenger receptors are not regulated, these cells accumulate excess intracellular cholesterol, resulting in the formation of foam cells and atheromatous plaques.

The anti-atherogenic effect of HDL is attributed to the removal of excess cholesterol from tissue sites and other lipoproteins. HDL is synthesized in the liver and intestine (see Fig. 8.1). Excess phospholipids, cholesterol, and apolipoproteins on remnant chylomicrons, VLDL, IDL, and LDL are transferred to HDL particles and thus increase HDL mass. Apo A-I, a surface lipoprotein on HDL particles, mobilizes cholesterol from intracellular pools and accepts cholesterol released during lipolysis of triglyceride-rich lipoproteins. It also activates lecithin-cholesterol acyltransferase (LCAT), an enzyme that esterifies cholesterol. These cholesterol esters move the hydrophilic HDL

脂代谢紊乱

梁思宇 译 阳洪波 潘慧 审校 宁光 通审

定义和流行病学

游离脂肪酸（FFA）、胆固醇和甘油三酯等脂质是疏水性分子，通过与蛋白质结合来进行转运。其中，非酯化的 FFA 以阴离子形式与白蛋白结合来进行转运。酯化的脂质复合物通过脂蛋白颗粒来进行转运。脂蛋白由疏水性的核心（胆固醇酯和甘油三酯）和两亲性的表面单层膜（磷脂、非酯化的胆固醇和载脂蛋白）组成。超速离心可根据其密度将脂蛋白分为 5 类（表 8.1）。

脂蛋白表面的蛋白质成分（即载脂蛋白）可激活引导脂代谢的酶和受体。脂蛋白合成和分解代谢过程中的缺陷可导致血脂异常。在美国，血脂异常的患病率约为 20%，不同人群的患病率存在差异。据估计，70% 的早发冠心病人群合并血脂异常。在临床试验中，治疗血脂异常可改善冠心病死亡率和全因死亡率。甘油三酯和胆固醇在动脉粥样硬化的发病机制中发挥着重要的作用，但两者也可作为调控的靶点，因此也是本章关注的重点。

病理学

在小肠腔中，食物中的甘油三酯和胆固醇酯被胰脂肪酶水解，产生甘油、FFA 和游离胆固醇。胆汁酸有助于使甘油和脂肪酸形成两亲性的脂滴（即微胶粒），进而被小肠细胞吸收。游离胆固醇的转运由肠腔和小肠细胞之间的胆固醇梯度介导。在细胞内，甘油与 3 条脂肪酸链结合形成甘油三酯，胆固醇酯化形成胆固醇酯。乳糜微粒由甘油三酯（占乳糜微粒质量的 85%）和胆固醇酯与表面脂蛋白组装而成。乳糜微粒进入循环后，从高密度脂蛋白（HDL）颗粒中获得更多的表面载脂蛋白，如载脂蛋白 C-Ⅱ 和载脂蛋白 E（图 8.1）。载脂蛋白 C-Ⅱ 可激活位于毛细血管内皮细胞上的脂蛋白脂肪酶（LPL）。LPL 可水解乳糜微粒核心中的甘油三酯，释放出 FFA。FFA 可提供能量。多余的 FFA 储存在脂肪组织中或用于肝脏脂蛋白合成。乳糜微粒表面的载脂蛋白 E 可激活肝脏低密度脂蛋白（LDL）受体，进而将含甘油三酯较少的残余乳糜微粒从血液循环中清除。

肝脏利用循环中或由肝脏合成的 FFA 和胆固醇合成极低密度脂蛋白（VLDL）（图 8.1）。任何增加肝脏中 FFA 的情况（如控制不佳的糖尿病）都会增加

VLDL 的生成。甘油三酯（占 VLDL 质量的 55%）、胆固醇（占 VLDL 质量的 20%）和表面载脂蛋白在肝脏中组装形成 VLDL 颗粒。载脂蛋白 C-Ⅱ 是 LPL 的辅因子，可水解 VLDL 颗粒的甘油三酯核心，产生 VLDL 残余物或中密度脂蛋白（IDL）。IDL 已去除 25% 的甘油三酯，可由载脂蛋白 E 介导被 LDL 受体从循环中清除，或被进一步水解形成 LDL。LDL 颗粒缺乏甘油三酯（占 LDL 质量的 5%），主要由胆固醇酯（占 60%）和载脂蛋白组成。LDL 表面的载脂蛋白 B100 可结合 LDL 受体，促进 LDL 从循环中清除。内化的 LDL 胆固醇可用于合成激素、形成细胞膜和储存能量。

在肝脏中，LDL 胆固醇用于合成胆汁酸（图 8.1），胆汁酸与游离胆固醇一起分泌至肠腔内。胆汁酸有助于脂肪转运。进入肠腔的约 50% 的胆固醇和 97% 的胆汁酸会被重吸收至循环中。被重吸收的胆固醇可调节胆固醇和 LDL 受体的合成。

人体的许多细胞（包括肝实质细胞）可合成胆固醇（图 8.2）。醋酸盐转化为 3- 羟基 -3- 甲戊二酸单酰辅酶 A（HMG-CoA）。HMG-CoA 还原酶可将 HMG-CoA 转化为甲羟戊酸，然后经过一系列步骤将其转化为胆固醇。HMG-CoA 还原酶的催化是胆固醇合成通路中的限速步骤。抑制该酶的药物会减少胆固醇的生物合成及细胞内储存的胆固醇。抑制 HMG-CoA 还原酶的药物通常被称为他汀类药物。LDL 颗粒在细胞内的内化受负反馈调节（图 8.2）。细胞内胆固醇减少会增加 LDL 受体的表达，继而从循环中摄取胆固醇。胆固醇增多则会抑制 LDL 受体的表达，并减少细胞对 LDL 胆固醇的摄取。循环中多余的 LDL 可通过清道夫受体进入巨噬细胞和其他组织。由于清道夫受体不受调节，这些细胞内会积聚过多的胆固醇，从而导致泡沫细胞和动脉粥样硬化斑块的形成。

HDL 能起到抗动脉粥样硬化作用是因为其能从组织和其他脂蛋白中清除多余的胆固醇。HDL 在肝脏和小肠中合成（图 8.1）。残余乳糜微粒、VLDL、IDL 和 LDL 上多余的磷脂、胆固醇和载脂蛋白可转移至 HDL 颗粒上，从而增加 HDL 的质量。HDL 颗粒表面有一种载脂蛋白，即载脂蛋白 A-Ⅰ，它能从细胞内池中动员胆固醇，并接受富含甘油三酯的脂蛋白在脂肪分解过程中释放的胆固醇。载脂蛋白 A-Ⅰ 还能激活卵磷脂胆固醇酰基转移酶（LCAT），LCAT 是一种能酯化胆固醇的酶。

TABLE 8.1   Properties of Lipoproteins

Lipoprotein Class	Density (g/mL)	Origin	Apolipoproteins	Lipid
Chylomicrons	<0.95	Intestine	B48, C-II, E	TG (85%), cholesterol (10%)
VLDL	<1.006	Liver	B100, C-II, E	TG (55%), cholesterol (20%)
IDL	1.006–1.019	VLDL catabolism	B100, E	TG (25%), cholesterol (35%)
LDL	1.019–1.063	IDL catabolism	B100	TG (5%), cholesterol (60%)
HDL	1.063–1.25	Liver, intestine	A-I, E	TG (5%), cholesterol (20%)

HDL, High-density lipoprotein; *IDL,* intermediate-density lipoprotein; *LDL,* low-density lipoprotein; *TG,* triglyceride; *VLDL,* very-low-density lipoprotein.

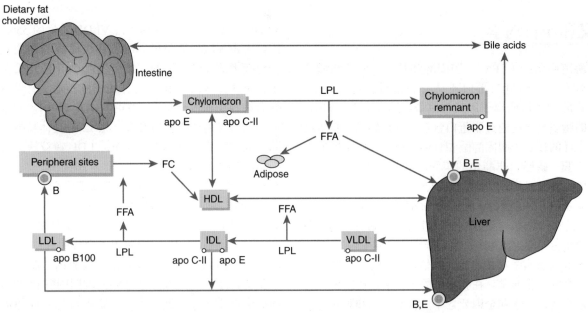

Fig. 8.1 Normal metabolism of plasma lipoproteins (see text for details). *apo,* Apolipoprotein; *B,E,* membrane receptor for lipoproteins containing apo B and apo E (synonymous with the LDL receptor); *FC,* free (unesterified) cholesterol; *FFA,* free (unesterified) fatty acids; *HDL,* high-density lipoprotein; *IDL,* intermediate-density lipoprotein; *LDL,* low-density lipoprotein; *LPL,* lipoprotein lipase; *VLDL,* very-low-density lipoprotein.

surface to the hydrophobic HDL core. Cholesterol ester transfer protein (CETP) transfers core HDL cholesterol esters to other lipoproteins such as VLDL. These lipoproteins deliver cholesterol to peripheral sites for hormone and cell membrane synthesis.

Defects in the production or removal of lipoproteins results in dyslipidemia. Both genetic and acquired conditions have been implicated in the pathogenesis of lipid disorders (Tables 8.2 and 8.3). These are discussed later in the chapter.

CLINICAL PRESENTATION

Dyslipidemia plays a significant role in the development of atherosclerosis. Increased incidence of CHD with high LDL- and low HDL-cholesterol is well documented. Excess LDL can result in the formation of cholesterol plaques that deposit in arteries (atheroma), skin and tendon (xanthomas), eyelids (xanthelasma), and iris (corneal arcus). The impact of triglycerides on vascular disease is less clear. Metabolic disorders such as diabetes and obesity are often associated with vascular disease and hypertriglyceridemia. The atherogenic impact of other elements associated with metabolic disorders is difficult to separate from the effect of hypertriglyceridemia. However, in several population-based studies, abnormal triglyceride levels correlated with

increased risk for CHD. Marked hypertriglyceridemia (>1000 mg/dL) is associated with the chylomicronemia syndrome, characterized by pancreatitis and xanthomas.

DIAGNOSIS

Dyslipidemia is defined by a total cholesterol, triglyceride, or LDL level greater than the 90th percentile or an HDL level lower than the 10th percentile for the general population. Because chylomicrons are present in plasma for up to 10 hours after a meal, fasting total cholesterol, triglyceride, and lipoprotein assessments are required for diagnosis. It is advisable to confirm dyslipidemia with two separate determinations.

Total cholesterol, triglyceride, and HDL levels can be measured directly. VLDL and LDL levels usually are calculated. If the triglyceride concentration is lower than 400 mg/dL, then VLDL is calculated by dividing the triglyceride level by 5. LDL-cholesterol is estimated by subtracting VLDL and HDL from the total cholesterol. This is known as the Friedewald equation. LDL cholesterol calculated utilizing this equation is used to set therapeutic targets in most clinical trials and treatment guidelines. However, calculated LDL cholesterol becomes progressively inaccurate with increasing triglyceride levels and should not be estimated if triglyceride levels are greater the 400 mg/dL. In

表 8.1 脂蛋白的特征

脂蛋白类型	密度（g/ml）	来源	载脂蛋白	脂质
乳糜微粒	< 0.95	小肠	B48、C-Ⅱ、E	TG（85%）、胆固醇（10%）
VLDL	< 1.006	肝脏	B100、C-Ⅱ、E	TG（55%）、胆固醇（20%）
IDL	1.006 ~ 1.019	VLDL 分解代谢	B100、E	TG（25%）、胆固醇（35%）
LDL	1.019 ~ 1.063	IDL 分解代谢	B100	TG（5%）、胆固醇（60%）
HDL	1.063 ~ 1.25	肝脏、小肠	A-Ⅰ、E	TG（5%）、胆固醇（20%）

HDL，高密度脂蛋白；IDL，中密度脂蛋白；LDL，低密度脂蛋白；TG，甘油三酯；VLDL，极低密度脂蛋白。

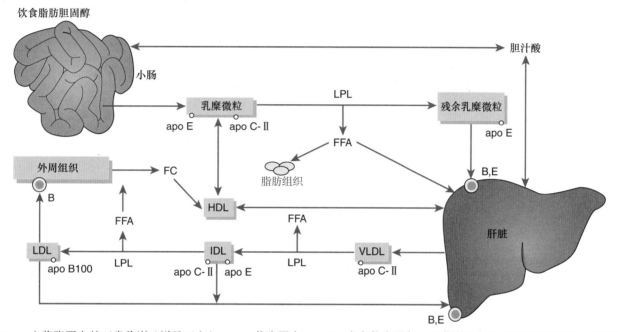

图 8.1 血浆脂蛋白的正常代谢（详见正文）。apo，载脂蛋白；B,E，含有载脂蛋白 B 和载脂蛋白 E 的脂蛋白膜受体（等同于 LDL 受体）；FC，游离（非酯化）胆固醇；FFA，游离（非酯化）脂肪酸；HDL，高密度脂蛋白；IDL，中密度脂蛋白；LDL，低密度脂蛋白；LPL，脂蛋白脂肪酶；VLDL，极低密度脂蛋白

这些胆固醇酯可从亲水性的 HDL 表面转移到疏水性的 HDL 核心。胆固醇酯转移蛋白（CETP）可将 HDL 的胆固醇酯转移至其他脂蛋白（如 VLDL）。这些脂蛋白会将胆固醇输送到外周组织，用于合成激素和细胞膜。

脂蛋白的生成或清除缺陷可导致血脂异常。血脂异常的发病机制与多种遗传性和获得性疾病相关（表 8.2 和表 8.3）。这些将在下文详细讨论。

临床表现

血脂异常在动脉粥样硬化的发展中发挥重要作用。越来越多的研究证实，高 LDL 胆固醇和低 HDL 胆固醇水平与冠心病发病风险增加相关。过多的 LDL 会导致胆固醇斑块形成，这些斑块会沉积在动脉壁（即粥样硬化斑块）、皮肤和肌腱（即黄色瘤）、眼睑（即眼睑黄斑瘤）及虹膜中（即角膜环）。甘油三酯对血管疾病的影响尚不清楚。糖尿病和肥胖症等代谢性疾病通常与血管疾病和高甘油三酯血症有关。与代谢性疾病相关的其他因素对动脉粥样硬化的影响很难与高甘油三酯血症的影响区分开来。然而，在多项基于人群

的研究中，甘油三酯水平异常与冠心病风险增加相关。明显的高甘油三酯血症（> 1000 mg/dl）与乳糜微粒血症综合征相关，其特征为胰腺炎和黄色瘤。

诊断

血脂异常是指总胆固醇、甘油三酯或 LDL 水平高于普通人群的第 90 百分位数，或 HDL 水平低于普通人群的第 10 百分位数。由于餐后 10 h 内血浆中仍存在乳糜微粒，因此诊断血脂异常需要依据空腹总胆固醇、甘油三酯和脂蛋白检测值。建议通过两次单独的测定来确认血脂异常。

总胆固醇、甘油三酯和 HDL 水平可直接检测。VLDL 和 LDL 水平通常经计算得出。若甘油三酯 < 400 mg/dl，则 VLDL ＝甘油三酯水平 ÷5。估算的 LDL 胆固醇＝总胆固醇－VLDL－HDL。这就是著名的 Friedewald 公式。大多数临床试验和指南中的 LDL 胆固醇治疗目标都是利用该公式计算得出。然而，计算得出的 LDL 胆固醇在甘油三酯水平升高的情况下不准确。若甘油三酯 > 400 mg/dl，则不能用公式计算 VLDL 和 LDL 水平。在这种情况下，

LDL Cholesterol Uptake from Circulation

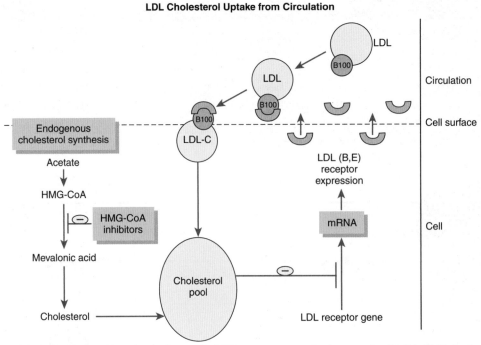

Fig. 8.2 Regulation of low-density lipoprotein (LDL) receptor expression (see text for details). *B100,* Apolipoprotein B100; *B,E,* membrane receptor for lipoproteins containing apo B and apo E (synonymous with the LDL receptor); *HMG-CoA,* 3-hydroxy-3-methylglutaryl–coenzyme A; *LDL-C,* LDL-cholesterol; *mRNA,* messenger RNA.

TABLE 8.2	**Genetic Disorders of Lipid Metabolism**	
Disorder	**Genetic Defect**	**Dyslipidemia**
Familial hypercholesterolemia	Mutation in the gene that encodes LDL receptor	Elevated TC and LDL
	Gain of function mutation in *PCSK9* gene	
	Mutation in the apolipoprotein B100 gene	
Elevated plasma Lp(a)	Increased binding of LDL to apolipoprotein(a)	Elevated Lp(a)
Polygenic hypercholesterolemia	Increased binding of apo E4–containing lipoprotein to LDL receptor resulting in downregulation of the LDL receptor	Elevated TC and LDL
Familial combined hyperlipoproteinemia	Polygenic disorder associated with increased hepatic VLDL production, resulting in increased LDL and decreased HDL production; some individuals have a mutation in the LPL gene that affects expression and function of LPL	Elevated TC, LDL, and TG Low HDL
Familial dysbetalipoproteinemia	Lower affinity of apo E2 for LDL receptor	Elevated TG, TC, and LDL
Lipoprotein lipase deficiency	Mutation in the *LPL* gene	Elevated TG
Apolipoprotein C-II deficiency	Decrease in activation of LPL due to a deficiency of apo CII	Elevated TG
Familial hypertriglyceridemia	Overproduction of hepatic VLDL and increased catabolism of HDL	Elevated TG Low HDL

HDL, High-density lipoprotein; *LDL,* low-density lipoprotein; *TC,* total cholesterol; *TG,* triglyceride; *VLDL,* very-low-density lipoprotein.

that case, assays are available to directly measure the concentration of LDL cholesterol. Furthermore, the lipoprotein abnormality associated with triglyceride levels greater than 400 mg/dL can be identified by inspecting the serum. When the triglyceride level exceeds 350 mg/dL, the serum is cloudy. After refrigeration, a white surface layer depicts excess chylomicrons, whereas a dispersed, opaque infranatant reflects a VLDL dysfunction.

In general, universal screening is recommended starting at 35 years of age for men and at 45 years of age for women. There is a paucity of data supporting long-term benefits from universal screening of younger individuals. Most guidelines suggest selective screening

of children who have a family history of lipoprotein abnormality or premature vascular disease. Baseline lipid levels are also recommended in adults with CHD, risk factors for CHD, or CHD equivalent (i.e., symptomatic carotid artery disease, peripheral arterial disease, abdominal aortic aneurysm, or diabetes). CHD risk factors include hypertension, diabetes mellitus, cigarette smoking, and family history of premature CHD (i.e., affected male first-degree relative <55 years or female first-degree relative <65 years of age). Either a fasting or a nonfasting total cholesterol and HDL measurement can be the initial screen. Treatment initiation is based on 10-year and lifetime risk of atherosclerotic cardiovascular disease (ASCVD) (Table 8.4).

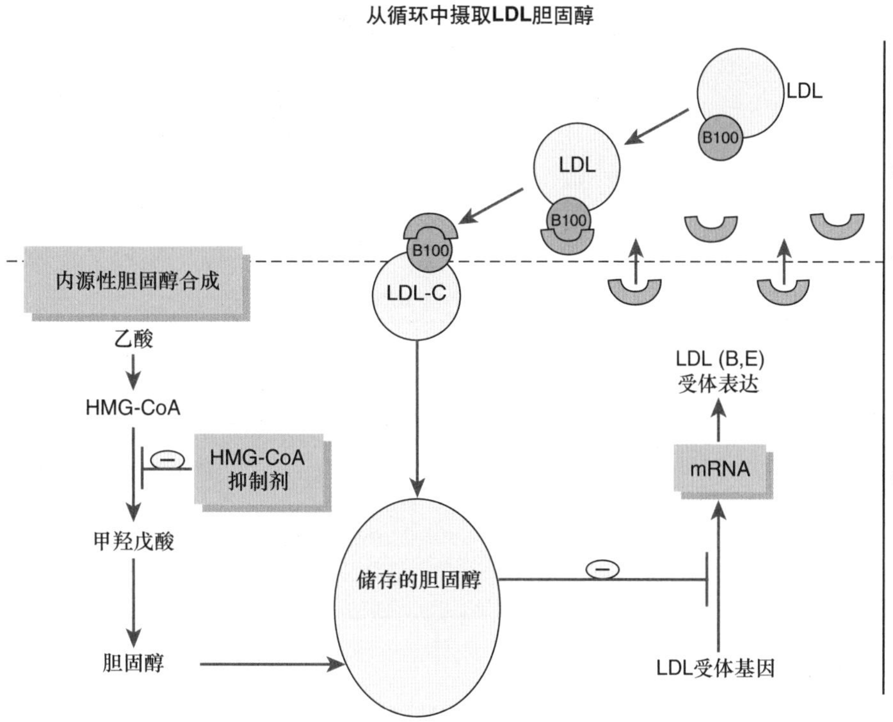

从循环中摄取LDL胆固醇

图 8.2　低密度脂蛋白（LDL）受体表达的调控（详见正文）。B100，载脂蛋白 B100；B,E，含载脂蛋白 B 和载脂蛋白 E 的脂蛋白膜受体（等同于 LDL 受体）；HMG-CoA，3- 羟基 -3- 甲戊二酸单酰辅酶 A；LDL-C，LDL 胆固醇；mRNA，信使 RNA

表8.2　**遗传性脂代谢紊乱**		
疾病	基因缺陷	血脂异常
家族性高胆固醇血症	编码 LDL 受体的基因突变 *PCSK9* 基因功能获得突变 载脂蛋白 B100 基因突变	TC 和 LDL 水平升高
高脂蛋白（a）血症	LDL 与载脂蛋白（a）的结合增加	脂蛋白（a）水平升高
多基因性高胆固醇血症	含有载脂蛋白 E4 的脂蛋白与 LDL 受体结合增加，导致 LDL 受体下调	TC 和 LDL 水平升高
家族性混合性高脂蛋白血症	与肝脏 VLDL 生成增加相关的多基因疾病，导致 LDL 生成增加、HDL 生成减少；部分患者存在 *LPL* 基因突变，影响 LPL 的表达和功能	TC、LDL 和 TG 水平升高 HDL 水平降低
家族性异常 β 脂蛋白血症	载脂蛋白 E2 与 LDL 受体的亲和力降低	TG、TC 和 LDL 水平升高
脂蛋白脂肪酶缺乏症	*LPL* 基因突变	TG 水平升高
载脂蛋白 C-Ⅱ 缺乏症	载脂蛋白 C-Ⅱ 缺乏导致 LPL 活性降低	TG 水平升高
家族性高甘油三酯血症	肝脏 VLDL 过量生成，HDL 分解代谢增加	TG 水平升高 HDL 水平降低

HDL，高密度脂蛋白；LDL，低密度脂蛋白；TC，总胆固醇；TG，甘油三酯；VLDL，极低密度脂蛋白。

需要直接检测 LDL 胆固醇水平。此外，检查血液标本可发现伴随甘油三酯＞ 400 mg/dl 的脂蛋白异常。当甘油三酯＞ 350 mg/dl 时，血清会变得浑浊。血液标本冷藏后出现白色表面层则表示乳糜微粒过多，出现分散的不透明浑浊底层则反映了 VLDL 异常。

一般来说，推荐男性从 35 岁、女性从 45 岁开始筛查血脂异常。对更年轻的人群筛查血脂异常是否有长期获益，尚缺乏证据支持。大多数指南建议对有脂蛋白异常或早发血管疾病家族史的儿童进行选择性筛

查。对于患有冠心病、具有冠心病危险因素或患有冠心病等危疾病（即有症状的颈动脉疾病、外周动脉疾病、腹主动脉瘤或糖尿病）的成人，建议检测基线血脂水平。冠心病危险因素包括高血压、糖尿病、吸烟和早发冠心病家族史（男性一级亲属发病年龄＜ 55 岁或女性一级亲属发病年龄＜ 65 岁）。空腹或非空腹总胆固醇和 HDL 可作为初始筛查。启动治疗的依据是动脉粥样硬化性心血管疾病（ASCVD）的 10 年风险和终身风险（表 8.4）。未达到治疗阈值的个体应每 3 ～ 5

TABLE 8.3	Mechanisms of Secondary Hyperlipidemia	
Clinical	**Elevated Lipoprotein**	**Mechanism**
Diabetes	Chylomicron, VLDL, LDL	Increase in VLDL production and decrease in VLDL/LDL clearance
Obesity	Chylomicron, VLDL, LDL	Increase in VLDL production and decrease in VLDL/LDL clearance
Lipodystrophy	VLDL	Increase in VLDL production
Hypothyroidism	LDL, VLDL	Decrease in LDL/LDL clearance
Estrogen	VLDL	Increase in VLDL production
Glucocorticoids	VLDL, LDL	Increase in VLDL production and conversion to LDL
Alcohol	VLDL	Increase in VLDL production
Nephrotic syndrome	VLDL, LDL	Increase in VLDL production and conversion to LDL

LDL, Low-density lipoprotein; *VLDL,* very-low-density lipoprotein.

TABLE 8.4	Cardiovascular Risk Prevention		
	Primary Prevention (Age 40–75 Years)		**Secondary Prevention**
Risk assessment	LDL 70–190 or 10-year risk of ASCVD 7.5–20% or diabetes	LDL >190 or 10-year risk of ASCVD >20% or diabetes with risk factors	Known ASCVD
Statin dosing	Moderate intensity statin	High intensity statin	High intensity statin to lower LDL-C >50%
LDL target	<100	<100	<50–70

TABLE 8.5	Recommendations for Nutritional Intake	
Nutrient	**Recommended Intake**	
Total fat	25–35% of total calories	
Saturated	<7%	
Polyunsaturated	<10%	
Monounsaturated	<20%	
Carbohydrates	50–60% of total calories	
Protein	15% of total calories	
Cholesterol	<200 mg/day	
Fiber	20–30 g/day	

Individuals who do not meet the threshold for treatment should be screened every 3 to 5 years.

TREATMENT

Treatment of elevated total and LDL-cholesterol can slow the development and progression of CHD. Meta-analysis of primary and secondary prevention trials indicates that CHD mortality decreases by approximately 15% for every 10% reduction in serum cholesterol. LDL-cholesterol treatment strategies are based on risk indicators. There is strong evidence that dietary modifications can reduce LDL-cholesterol and triglyceride levels (Table 8.5). However, evidence that lifestyle-induced lipid modifications improve cardiovascular outcomes is limited. Ample evidence supports statin use in primary and secondary prevention of CHD (see Table 8.4 and Table 8.6). Treatment effects of statins can be assessed after 1 to 2 months. Additional agents can be considered if target goals are not achieved with maximal drug dosing (Table 8.7).

A fasting lipid panel is required to diagnose hypertriglyceridemia. Triglyceride levels higher than 200 mg/dL are classified as abnormal. Borderline triglyceride levels range from 150 to 200 mg/dL, and normal values are lower than 150 mg/dL. A diet and exercise program is recommended for all individuals with abnormal triglyceride levels. However, pharmacologic treatments to reduce triglyceride levels may be considered if fasting levels are higher than 200 mg/dL, especially if the individual is at risk for CHD or pancreatitis (see Table 8.7). Fibrates, fish oil, and nicotinic acid should be considered if the triglyceride level is higher than 500 mg/dL. However, for levels lower than 500 mg/dL, statins are first-line therapy.

Low HDL concentrations (<40 mg/dL) can also increase the risk for CHD. In the Framingham Heart Study, every decrease in HDL of 5 mg/dL increased the risk for myocardial infarction. Both lifestyle modifications (e.g., diet low in saturated fat, exercise) and pharmacologic therapy (e.g., nicotinic acid, fibrate) can improve HDL levels. However, target goals and treatment recommendations have not been established due to a lack of evidence.

Lifestyle Modification

Lifestyle modification should be the initial step in the management of hyperlipidemia (see Table 8.5). Restricting the dietary intake of fat lowers total cholesterol by approximately 15% and LDL cholesterol by 25%. Low-fat diets that limit saturated fat content promote LDL receptor expression and increase the uptake of LDL-cholesterol from the circulation. By contrast, saturated fat downregulates hepatic LDL receptors and increases circulating LDL. Because unsaturated fats (polyunsaturated and monounsaturated) generally do not have this effect, they are the preferred form of fat intake. However, polyunsaturated fats containing fatty acids with a *trans* rather than *cis* double bond configuration (*trans*-fatty acids) increase plasma cholesterol levels similarly to saturated fat.

Limiting the intake of saturated and *trans*-unsaturated fatty acids requires appropriate calorie substitutions. Increasing carbohydrate content to achieve this goal can increase the hepatic synthesis of triglyceride. Dietary substitution with soluble fibers (e.g., oat bran) has been recommended, because these fibers have a limited effect on triglyceride levels. They also bind bile acids in the gut and thereby decrease cholesterol levels. Other polyunsaturated fats, such as omega-3 fatty acids, are cardioprotective. They are abundant in fatty fish, flaxseed oil, canola oil, and nuts. They reduce VLDL production, inhibit platelet

表 8.3 继发性高脂血症的机制

临床	升高的脂蛋白	机制
糖尿病	乳糜微粒、VLDL、LDL	VLDL 生成增加，VLDL/LDL 清除减少
肥胖症	乳糜微粒、VLDL、LDL	VLDL 生成增加，VLDL/LDL 清除减少
脂肪营养不良	VLDL	VLDL 生成增加
甲状腺功能减退症	LDL、VLDL	LDL/LDL 清除减少
雌激素	VLDL	VLDL 生成增加
糖皮质激素	VLDL、LDL	VLDL 生成增加，VLDL 向 LDL 转化增加
酒精	VLDL	VLDL 生成增加
肾病综合征	VLDL、LDL	VLDL 生成增加，VLDL 向 LDL 转化增加

LDL，低密度脂蛋白；VLDL，极低密度脂蛋白。

表 8.4 心血管疾病的预防

	一级预防（40～75 岁）		二级预防
风险评估	LDL 70～190 mg/dl 或 ASCVD 10 年风险 7.5%～20% 或糖尿病	LDL > 190 mg/dl 或 ASCVD 10 年风险 > 20% 或糖尿病且有危险因素	患有 ASCVD
他汀类药物剂量	中等强度他汀类药物	高强度他汀类药物	高强度他汀类药物，LDL-C 水平降低 > 50%
LDL 目标	< 100 mg/dl	100 mg/dl	< 50～70 mg/dl

表 8.5 营养摄入的建议

营养素	推荐摄入量
总脂肪	占总热量的 25%～35%
饱和脂肪	< 7%
多不饱和脂肪	< 10%
单不饱和脂肪	< 20%
碳水化合物	占总热量的 50%～60%
蛋白质	占总热量的 15%
胆固醇	< 200 mg/d
膳食纤维	20%～30 g/d

年接受 1 次筛查。

治疗

治疗高总胆固醇和高 LDL 胆固醇水平可延缓冠心病的发生和发展。对一级和二级预防试验的荟萃分析表明，血清胆固醇每降低 10%，冠心病的死亡率降低约 15%。LDL 胆固醇治疗策略基于风险指标。已有明确证据表明，调整饮食可降低 LDL 胆固醇和甘油三酯水平（表 8.5）。然而，有关调整生活方式后血脂异常的改善是否能改善心血管结局的证据尚有限。大量证据支持他汀类药物用于冠心病的一级和二级预防（表 8.4 和表 8.6）。他汀类药物的疗效可在服药后 1～2 个月进行评估。如果应用最大剂量的他汀类药物仍不能使血脂达标，则可考虑加用其他药物（表 8.7）。

诊断高甘油三酯血症需要进行空腹检查。甘油三酯 > 200 mg/dl 被定义为异常，临界甘油三酯范围为 150～200 mg/dl，< 150 mg/dl 为正常。建议所有甘油三酯水平异常的患者均应调整饮食，并进行运动干预。然而，若空腹甘油三酯 > 200 mg/dl，尤其是对于有冠心病或胰腺炎风险的人群，建议药物治疗（表 8.7）。若甘油三酯 > 500 mg/dl，则应考虑使用贝特类药物、鱼油和烟酸。若甘油三酯 < 500 mg/dl，他汀类药物为一线治疗药物。

HDL 水平过低（< 40 mg/dl）也会增加冠心病风险。在弗明翰心脏研究（Framingham Heart Study）中，HDL 每降低 5 mg/dl 均会增加心肌梗死的风险。生活方式调整（如低饱和脂肪酸饮食、运动）和药物治疗（如烟酸、贝特类药物）均可提高 HDL 水平。然而，由于缺乏足够证据，治疗目标和推荐治疗尚不明确。

生活方式调整

生活方式调整是高脂血症治疗中的首要步骤（表 8.5）。限制饮食中的脂肪摄入可使总胆固醇降低约 15%，LDL 胆固醇降低 25%。限制饱和脂肪含量的低脂饮食会促进 LDL 受体表达，并增加对循环中 LDL 胆固醇的摄取。相反，饱和脂肪会下调肝脏中 LDL 受体的表达，并升高循环中的 LDL 水平。由于不饱和脂肪（多不饱和脂肪和单不饱和脂肪）通常不会产生上述影响，因此不饱和脂肪是更优的脂肪摄入形式。然而，具有反式（而非顺式）双键结构的脂肪酸（即反式脂肪酸）可产生类似饱和脂肪的作用，摄入含反式脂肪酸的多不饱和脂肪会升高胆固醇水平。

限制饱和脂肪酸和反式不饱和脂肪酸的摄入需要适当的热量替代补充。为实现这一目标，如果增加碳水化合物含量，则会增加肝脏合成甘油三酯。建议用可溶性纤维（如燕麦麸）饮食替代，因为这些纤维对甘油三酯水平的影响很小。它们还能与肠道中的胆汁酸结合，从而降低胆固醇水平。其他多不饱和脂肪（如 ω-3 脂肪酸）具有心脏保护作用。这些多不饱和脂肪酸在多脂鱼、亚麻籽油、菜籽油和坚果中的含量较多。它们可减

TABLE 8.6 Statins

High-Intensity Statins: Lowers LDL-C by >50%	Moderate-Intensity Statins: Lowers LDL-C 30–50%	Low-Intensity Statins: Lowers LDL-C by 30%
Atorvastatin 40–80 mg Rosuvastatin 20–40 mg	Atorvastatin 10–20 mg Rosuvastatin 5–10 mg Simvastatin 20–40 mg Pravastatin 40–80 mg Lovastatin 40 mg Fluvastatin 80 mg Pitavastatin 2–4 mg	Simvastatin 10 mg Pravastatin 10–20 mg Lovastatin 20 mg Fluvastatin 20–40 mg Pitavastatin 1 mg

TABLE 8.7 Drugs Commonly Used for the Treatment of Hyperlipidemia

Drug Class	LDL (% Change)	HDL (% Change)	Triglycerides (% Change)	Side Effects
HMG-CoA inhibitors	↓ 20–60	↑ 5–10	↓ 10–30	Liver toxicity, myositis, rhabdomyolysis; enhanced warfarin effect
Cholesterol absorption inhibitors	↓ 17	No effect	↓ 7–8	Abnormal liver enzymes in combination with an HMG-CoA inhibitor, myalgia, hepatitis, rhabdomyolysis, pancreatitis, potential increase in cancer risk and cancer death
PCSK-9 inhibitor	↓ 38–72	↑ 4–9	↓ 2–23	Injection site reaction, hypersensitivity, drug neutralizing antibody
Bempedoic acid	↓ 15–19	No change	No change	Hyperuricemia, tendon rupture, and may potentiate statin-related myopathy
Bile acid sequestrants	↓ 15–30	Slight increase	No effect	Nausea, bloating, cramping, abnormal liver function; interferes with absorption of other drugs such as warfarin and thyroxine
Fibric acid	↓ 6–20	↑ 5–20	↓ 41–53	Nausea, cramping, myalgias, liver toxicity, enhanced warfarin effect
Nicotinic acid	↓ 10–25	↑ 15–35	↓ 25–30	Hepatotoxicity, hyperuricemia, hyperglycemia, flushing, pruritus, nausea, vomiting, diarrhea
Omega-3 fatty acids	Variable	↑ 5–9	↓ 23–45	Eructation, taste perversion, dyspepsia

HMG-CoA, Hydroxymethylglutaryl–coenzyme A reductase.

aggregation, and decrease CHD. Even two servings per week of fatty fish such as salmon can be beneficial.

Dietary restriction of fat (<10%) is essential for the treatment of marked hypertriglyceridemia. Other factors such as carbohydrate and alcohol intake can also increase the synthesis of triglyceride. Restriction of alcohol intake to one or two servings per week and adherence to a low-fat, high-fiber diet will improve hypertriglyceridemia.

Exercise has been shown to increase LPL activity. Even a single exercise session can reduce triglycerides and increase HDL. The impact of exercise on LDL is less clear. With low- to moderate-intensity exercise regimens, clearance of VLDL particles increases LDL production. However, this effect is not seen with high-intensity exercise programs. A decrease in LDL-cholesterol occurs with high-intensity exercise, and this effect is independent of weight loss.

Pharmacotherapy

In addition to diet and exercise modifications, pharmacologic agents are prescribed to reduce cardiovascular risk and to achieve therapeutic goals. The ASCVD Risk algorithm is used to calculate a 10-year risk of heart disease or stroke. This algorithm calculates risk by evaluating the following factors: history of ASCVD, LDL-cholesterol levels, age, current diagnosis of diabetes, gender, race, total cholesterol, HDL-cholesterol levels, medication controlled hypertension, and smoking history. History of the following conditions is considered as known

ASCVD: acute coronary syndrome, myocardial infarction, stable angina, coronary revascularization, stroke, transient ischemic attack, or peripheral arterial disease. Cardiovascular risk profile determines therapeutic plan including drug dosing and LDL targets in individuals 40 to 75 years of age (see Tables 8.4 and 8.6). High-risk patients may require additional agents to achieve target goals. Likely benefit of each agent needs to be balanced against potential adverse effects when determining drug therapy (see Table 8.7). In individuals younger than 40 years or with 10-year risk below 7.5%, lifestyle modification is recommended unless risk enhancers such as family history of premature ASCVD, LDL-cholesterol greater than 160 mg/dL, chronic kidney disease, and metabolic syndrome, are noted.

HMG-CoA reductase is the rate-limiting enzyme involved in cholesterol biosynthesis. Inhibition of this enzyme decreases intracellular cholesterol pools and subsequently increases uptake of LDL cholesterol from the circulation. HMG-CoA reductase inhibitors (e.g., atorvastatin and rosuvastatin) increase cholesterol utilization, decrease VLDL synthesis, and increase HDL synthesis. As a result, lower LDL and triglyceride levels and higher HDL levels are observed with treatment. Meta-analysis of primary and secondary CHD prevention trials found reductions in all-cause and cardiovascular mortality rates with statin therapy. These agents limit progression and may even cause regression of coronary atherosclerosis. Therefore, they represent first-line therapy in the management of abnormal LDL-cholesterol levels and

表 8.6　他汀类药物

高强度他汀类药物：使 LDL 胆固醇水平降低 > 50%	中等强度他汀类药物：使 LDL 胆固醇水平降低 30%～50%	低强度他汀类药物：使 LDL 胆固醇水平降低 < 30%
阿托伐他汀 40～80 mg 瑞舒伐他汀 20～40 mg	阿托伐他汀 10～20 mg 瑞舒伐他汀 5～10 mg 辛伐他汀 20～40 mg 普伐他汀 40～80 mg 洛伐他汀 40 mg 氟伐他汀 80 mg 匹伐他汀 2～4 mg	辛伐他汀 10 mg 普伐他汀 10～20 mg 洛伐他汀 20 mg 氟伐他汀 20～40 mg 匹伐他汀 1 mg

表 8.7　高脂血症的常用治疗药物

药物种类	LDL 改变（%）	HDL 改变（%）	甘油三酯改变（%）	副作用
HMG-CoA 抑制剂	↓ 20～60	↑ 5～10	↓ 10～30	肝毒性、肌炎、横纹肌溶解；增强华法林的作用
胆固醇吸收抑制剂	↓ 17	无作用	↓ 7～8	与 HMG-CoA 抑制剂合用导致肝酶异常；肌痛、肝炎、横纹肌溶解、胰腺炎，可能增加癌症风险和癌症相关死亡
PCSK-9 抑制剂	↓ 38～72	↑ 4～9	↓ 2～23	注射部位反应、过敏、药物中和抗体
贝派地酸	↓ 15～19	不改变	不改变	高尿酸血症、肌腱断裂，可能加重他汀类药物相关肌病
胆汁酸螯合剂	↓ 15～30	轻微增加	无作用	恶心、腹胀、腹部痉挛痛、肝功能异常；干扰其他药物（如华法林和甲状腺）的吸收
贝特类药物	↓ 6～20	↑ 5～20	↓ 41～53	恶心、腹部痉挛痛、肌痛、肝毒性、增强华法林的作用
烟酸	↓ 10～25	↑ 15～35	↓ 25～30	肝毒性、高尿酸血症、高血糖、皮肤潮红、瘙痒、恶心、呕吐、腹泻
ω-3 脂肪酸	不确定	↑ 5～9	↓ 23～45	嗳气、味觉异常、消化不良

HMG-CoA，3- 羟基 -3- 甲戊二酸单酰辅酶 A。

少 VLDL 产生、抑制血小板聚集和降低冠心病风险。即使每周食用 2 次多脂鱼（如三文鱼等）也有获益。

限制脂肪（< 10%）的饮食对于治疗显著的高甘油三酯血症至关重要。碳水化合物和酒精摄入等其他因素也会增加甘油三酯的合成。限制饮酒至每周 1～2 次，并坚持低脂、高纤维饮食，有助于改善高甘油三酯血症。

大量证据表明，运动可增加 LPL 的活性。即使单次运动也可降低甘油三酯水平、升高 HDL 水平。运动对 LDL 的影响尚不清楚。中低强度运动可清除 VLDL 颗粒，增加 LDL 产生。但是，高强度运动会降低 LDL 胆固醇水平，而这种效果与体重减轻无关。

药物治疗

除调整饮食和运动外，还可应用药物降低心血管风险并达到治疗目标。ASCVD 风险评估被用于计算心脏病和脑卒中的 10 年风险。该算法通过评估以下因素来计算风险：ASCVD 病史、LDL 胆固醇水平、年龄、糖尿病病史、性别、种族、总胆固醇水平、HDL 胆固醇水平、药物控制的高血压、吸烟史。以下情况被视为已患 ASCVD：急性冠脉综合征、心肌梗死、稳定型心绞痛、冠状动脉血运重建、卒中、短暂性脑缺血发作、外周动脉疾病。心血管风险评估结果决定后续治疗的药物剂量和 40～75 岁人群的 LDL 目标值（表 8.4 和表 8.6）。高风险患者可能需要额外加用药物来达到治疗目标。在确定药物治疗时，需要平衡每种药物可能带来的获益和潜在的不良反应（表 8.7）。对于年龄 < 40 岁或 ASCVD 10 年风险 < 7.5% 的患者，建议先调整生活方式，除非存在早发 ASCVD 家族史、LDL 胆固醇 > 160 mg/dl、慢性肾脏病和代谢综合征等增加 ASCVD 风险的因素。

HMG-CoA 还原酶是胆固醇合成的限速酶。抑制该酶可减少细胞内储存的胆固醇，从而增加循环中 LDL 胆固醇的摄取。HMG-CoA 还原酶抑制剂（如阿托伐他汀和瑞舒伐他汀）可升高胆固醇利用率，减少 VLDL 合成，增加 HDL 合成。因此，治疗后可观察到 LDL 和甘油三酯水平降低、HDL 水平升高。对冠心病一级和二级预防试验的荟萃分析显示，他汀类药物可降低全因死亡率和心血管死亡率。这些药物可限制其至逆转冠状动脉粥样硬化的进展。因此，他汀类药物是治疗 LDL 胆固醇水平异常和预防心血管疾病的一线治疗。肝酶升高和肌肉损伤是潜在的剂量相关并发症。单独使用他汀类药物可能会发生肌炎，与烟酸或贝特类药物联用时风险更高。

for prevention of cardiovascular outcomes. Elevated liver enzymes and muscle toxicity are potential dose-related complications. Myositis can occur with statins alone, but the risk is higher when statins are used in combination with nicotinic acid or fibric acid derivatives.

Ezetimibe is a Niemann-Pick C1 Like 1 (NPC1L1) inhibitor. NPC1L1 is a protein that aids in the transport of cholesterol across the intestinal brush border. Ezetimibe inhibits this enzyme, decreasing cholesterol absorption and thus increasing cholesterol utilization and decreasing LDL-cholesterol levels. Ezetimibe may be used as a single agent or in combination with an HMG-CoA reductase inhibitor to lower LDL-cholesterol levels. In combination with a statin, this agent may reduce cardiovascular events in high-risk individuals.

Proprotein convertase subtilisin kexin type 9 (PCSK9) inhibitors represent an exciting new frontier in LDL-cholesterol reduction. PCSK9 is a protease whose function is the degradation of LDL receptors. Inhibition of this protease leads to increased LDL receptor survival, which in turn leads to the reduction of circulating LDL-cholesterol. The two approved agents, evolocumab and alirocumab, are both monoclonal antibodies against PCSK9 that are administered by subcutaneous injection every 2 to 4 weeks. They are indicated in patients with LDL greater than 190 mg/dL or ASCVD judged to be high risk who have not achieved desired LDL reduction on statin and ezetimibe. Cost of these therapies is significant and may be a limiting factor. Antisense therapy (injectable oligonucleotides to prevent mRNA translation) against PCSK9 mRNA is an area of active investigation.

Bempedoic acid inhibits adenosine triphosphate citrate lyase, an enzyme in the cholesterol biosynthesis pathway. This enzyme is upstream of 3-hydroxy-3methylglutarly-CoA reductase, the target of statin drugs. Bempedoic acid alone or in combination with other agents lowers LDL-cholesterol and is recommended for individuals intolerant to statins, unable to achieve target goals, and in circumstances where PCSK-9 inhibitors are not an option.

Drugs that interfere with the absorption of cholesterol from the intestinal lumen increase cholesterol utilization and decrease circulating levels of cholesterol. Bile acid sequestrants (e.g., cholestyramine, colestipol, and colesevelam) bind bile acids in the intestinal lumen and increase fecal excretion. Subsequently, more LDL-cholesterol is used by the liver to synthesis bile acids. The decrease in cellular cholesterol pools upregulates LDL receptors and decreases the amount of LDL-cholesterol in the circulation. Mild increases in HDL-cholesterol are also seen with this agent as a result of increased intestinal HDL formation. Treatment is associated with a reduction in the incidence of CHD. Bile acid sequestrants may be used alone for mild lipid dysfunction or in combination with another lipid-lowering agent such as an HMG-CoA reductase inhibitor. Abnormal liver function and gastrointestinal symptoms (e.g., nausea, bloating, cramping) are common side effects that limit the use of bile acid sequestrants. They can also interfere with the absorption of other drugs such as warfarin and thyroxine.

Fibric acid derivatives such as gemfibrozil and fenofibrate increase FFA oxidation in muscle and liver. The reduced lipogenesis in the liver decreases VLDL and subsequent LDL production. Fibric acid derivatives also enhance LPL activity and HDL synthesis. As a result, treatment is usually associated with not only lower triglyceride and LDL levels, but also higher HDL levels. Reduced cardiovascular events have been demonstrated in a subset of individuals with high triglyceride (>200 mg/dL) and low HDL (<40 mg/dL) levels, but improvements in cardiovascular or all-cause mortality otherwise have not been confirmed with these agents. Liver toxicity and myositis are potential side effects of fibric acid derivatives, and they also interfere with the metabolism of warfarin, leading to a need for its dose adjustment.

Nicotinic acid has an antilipolytic effect and therefore decreases the influx of FFA to the liver. As a result, hepatic VLDL synthesis and LDL production are reduced. Nicotinic acid also decreases HDL catabolism. Lower triglyceride and LDL levels and higher HDL levels are observed with treatment. In addition, nicotinic acid stimulates tissue plasminogen activator and prevents thrombosis. It also reduces lipoprotein(a), or Lp(a), which is an independent risk factor for developing vascular disease (discussed later). The cardioprotective effect of nicotinic acid may be linked to its effect on Lp(a) and HDL. Side effects include hepatotoxicity, hyperuricemia, hyperglycemia, and flushing.

Omega-3 fatty acids reduce VLDL production and subsequently lower triglyceride levels (by 35%). They also modestly increase HDL (3%) and LDL (5%). The impact on lipids can occur over months to years and requires treatment doses as high as 3 to 4 g of fish oil per day. Omega-3 fatty acids constitute 30% of fish oil supplements and 85% of prescribed pharmacologic preparations (i.e., Lovaza and Vascepa). In clinical trials, both Lovaza and Vascepa 4 g/day lowered triglyceride levels by 45%. Fish oil supplements seem to be a reasonable, cost-effective means to reduce triglyceride levels; side effects include eructation, taste perversion, and dyspepsia. A large clinical trial recently demonstrated that Vascepa may reduce the incidence of cardiovascular events in patients with cardiovascular disease, well-controlled LDL, and modest triglyceride elevations.

Other agents to consider are neomycin, lomitapide, and mipomersen. These agents can be considered in the management of patients with refractory LDL elevations. Neomycin complexes with bile acid and lowers LDL levels. It also inhibits production of apolipoprotein(a) in the liver and lowers Lp(a). It is recommended as adjuvant therapy for patients with familial hypercholesterolemia and Lp(a) excess. Important side effects include nephrotoxicity and ototoxicity. Lomitapide inhibits microsomal triglyceride transfer protein in the liver and decreases apo B. Significant reductions in LDL (up to 50%) are seen with treatment. Liver toxicity is a serious adverse event associated with this agent. Mipomersen is another agent approved for use in homozygous familial hypercholesterolemia. It binds apo B messenger RNA and inhibits apo B production. Apo B is a structural component of VLDL, IDL, and LDL. Treatment reduces LDL by up to 50%. Side effects include flu-like symptoms, injection site reactions, elevations in liver enzymes, and liver toxicity. The side effect profile and expense associated with both lomitapide and mipomersen limit the use of these agents to individuals with homozygous familial hypercholesterolemia.

LIPID DISORDERS

A number of specific disorders of overproduction or impaired removal of lipoproteins result in dyslipidemia (see Tables 8.2 and 8.3). These disorders are often familial, but secondary causes also need to be considered. Comorbid conditions (diabetes, hypothyroidism), medications (estrogen, glucocorticoids, β-adrenergic receptor blockers), and lifestyle factors (diet, alcohol) can increase the production and clearance of lipoproteins. Addressing these factors can often normalize lipid levels. If abnormalities persist, evaluation of genetic factors and treatment with pharmacologic therapy may need to be considered.

Familial Hypercholesterolemia

Familial hypercholesterolemia (FH) is an autosomal dominant disorder that alters LDL receptor synthesis and function. It is caused by mutations in one of three genes that decrease the clearance of LDL particles and increase circulating LDL levels. Gene mutations that result in FH exhibit an additive effect with more severe clinical presentations noted in individuals with homozygous or compound heterozygous mutations. A defect in the LDL (apo B/E) receptor gene is the most

依折麦布是尼曼-皮克 C1 型类似蛋白 1（NPC1L1）抑制剂。NPC1L1 是一种协助胆固醇穿过小肠刷状缘边界运输的蛋白质。依折麦布可抑制 NPC1L1，减少胆固醇吸收，从而提升胆固醇利用率，降低 LDL 胆固醇水平。依折麦布可单独使用或与 HMG-CoA 还原酶抑制剂联用，以降低 LDL 胆固醇水平。与他汀类药物联用时，可减少高风险人群的心血管事件。

前蛋白转化酶枯草杆菌蛋白酶 kexin 9 型（PCSK9）抑制剂是降低 LDL 胆固醇水平的前沿治疗。PCSK9 是一种可降解 LDL 受体的蛋白酶。抑制 PCSK9 可提高 LDL 受体水平，进而减少循环中的 LDL 胆固醇。依洛尤单抗和阿利西尤单抗是已获批的针对 PCSK9 的单克隆抗体，每 2 ~ 4 周皮下注射 1 次。这两种药物适用于 LDL > 190 mg/dl 或 ASCVD 高风险、使用他汀类药物和依折麦布未达到 LDL 治疗目标的患者。PCSK9 抑制剂的费用较高，可能限制其应用。此外，目前备受关注的研究热点还有针对 PCSK9 mRNA 的反义治疗（通过注射寡核苷酸阻止 mRNA 翻译）。

贝派地酸能抑制腺苷三磷酸柠檬酸裂解酶。该酶在胆固醇生物合成通路中位于 HMG-CoA 还原酶（他汀类药物的靶点）的上游。贝派地酸可单独使用或与其他药物联合使用以降低 LDL 胆固醇水平，建议不耐受他汀类药物、无法达到治疗目标及无法选择 PCSK-9 抑制剂的患者考虑使用贝派地酸。

干扰肠腔吸收胆固醇的药物会提升胆固醇的利用率，降低循环中的胆固醇水平。胆汁酸螯合剂（如考来烯胺、考来替泊和考来维仑）可在肠腔内结合胆汁酸，并增加粪便中胆汁酸的排泄。因此，更多的 LDL 胆固醇会被肝脏用于合成胆汁酸。细胞胆固醇池的减少可上调 LDL 受体的表达，并减少循环中的 LDL 胆固醇。胆汁酸螯合剂还可增加肠内 HDL 形成，从而使 HDL 胆固醇水平轻度升高。胆汁酸螯合剂可降低冠心病的发病风险。这类药物可单药用于治疗轻度血脂异常，或与 HMG-CoA 还原酶抑制剂等其他降脂药物联用。肝功能异常和胃肠道症状（如恶心、腹胀、腹部疼挛痛）是胆汁酸螯合剂的常见副作用，可能限制其使用。这些药物还可能干扰其他药物的吸收（如华法林和甲状腺素）。

吉非罗齐和非诺贝特等贝特类药物可增加肌肉和肝脏中的 FFA 氧化。肝脏脂肪生成减少会降低 VLDL 产生，进而减少 LDL 的产生。贝特类药物还可增强 LPL 活性和 HDL 合成。因此，这类药物不仅能降低甘油三酯和 LDL 水平，还能提高 HDL 水平。在高甘油三酯（> 200 mg/dl）和低 HDL（< 40 mg/dl）水平人群中，使用贝特类药物可减少心血管事件，但在心血管死亡率或全因死亡率方面的改善尚未得到证实。肝毒性和肌炎是贝特类药物的潜在副作用，它们还会干扰华法林的代谢，导致需要调整华法林剂量。

烟酸具有抗脂肪分解作用，因此可减少 FFA 进入肝脏，导致肝脏 VLDL 合成和 LDL 产生均减少。烟酸还能减少 HDL 分解代谢。治疗后可观察到甘油三酯和 LDL 水平降低，HDL 水平升高。此外，烟酸可刺激组织纤溶酶原激活物，并预防血栓形成。烟酸还能降低脂蛋白（a）[Lp（a）] 水平，其是血管疾病的独立危险因素（见下文）。烟酸的心脏保护作用可能与其对 Lp（a）和 HDL 的影响有关。副作用包括肝毒性、高尿酸血症、高血糖和潮红。

ω-3 脂肪酸可减少 VLDL 的产生，降低甘油三酯水平（35%），适度升高 HDL（3%）和 LDL（5%）水平。每日使用 3 ~ 4 g 鱼油对血脂的影响可持续数月至数年。ω-3 脂肪酸在鱼油补充剂中占 30%，在处方药（如 Lovaza 和 Vascepa）中占 85%。在临床试验中，服用 4 g/d Lovaza 和 Vascepa 使甘油三酯水平降低 45%。鱼油补充剂似乎是降低甘油三酯水平的经济有效的方法；副作用包括嗳气、味觉异常和消化不良。近期一项大型临床试验表明，对于患心血管疾病、LDL 水平控制良好、甘油三酯水平轻度升高的患者，Vascepa 可降低心血管事件的发生率。

其他药物包括新霉素、洛美他派和米泊美生。这些药物可用于管理难治性 LDL 升高的患者。新霉素可与胆汁酸结合，从而降低 LDL 水平。它还能抑制肝脏中载脂蛋白（a）的生成而减少 Lp（a）。推荐将新霉素作为家族性高胆固醇血症（FH）和 Lp（a）水平过高的辅助治疗。主要副作用包括肾毒性和耳毒性。洛美他派可抑制肝脏中的微粒体甘油三酯转移蛋白，降低载脂蛋白 B 水平，并显著降低 LDL 水平（高达 50%）。洛美他派的严重不良反应是肝毒性。米泊美生已获批用于治疗纯合型 FH。它能与载脂蛋白 B 信使 RNA 结合，抑制其生成。载脂蛋白 B 是 VLDL、IDL 和 LDL 的结构性组分，米泊美生治疗可使 LDL 水平降低 50%。副作用包括流感样症状、注射部位反应、肝酶水平升高和肝毒性。洛美他派和米泊美生的副作用及高费用使其在纯合型 FH 人群中的应用受限。

脂代谢紊乱

许多引起脂蛋白生成过多或清除障碍的特定疾病可导致血脂异常（表 8.2 和表 8.3）。这些疾病通常为家族性，但也需考虑是否存在继发性因素。合并症（如糖尿病、甲状腺功能减退症），药物（如雌激素、糖皮质激素、β 受体阻滞剂）和生活方式（如饮食、饮酒）均会增加脂蛋白的生成和清除。解决这些因素通常可使血脂水平恢复正常。如果血脂异常持续存在，可能需要考虑评估遗传性病因并进行药物治疗。

家族性高胆固醇血症

FH 是一种常染色体显性遗传病，其特点为 LDL 受体的合成和功能改变。FH 由 3 个基因之一发生突变所致，这些基因突变会减少 LDL 颗粒的清除并升高循环中的 LDL 水平。导致 FH 的基因突变具有叠加效应，纯合突变或多个杂合突变个体的临床表现更重。LDL（载脂蛋白 B, E）受体基因缺陷是导致 FH 的最常见原因。受体缺陷可根据受体活性分为受体缺失（活性 < 2%）和受体缺

common cause of FH. Receptor defects are classified based on receptor activity: receptor-negative (<2% activity) and receptor-defective (2% to 25% activity). Defects in the PCSK9 and apolipoprotein B gene are less common. PCSK9 is a serine protease produced by the liver. It binds the LDL receptor leading to internalization and eventual destruction of the LDL receptor. Gain of function mutation in the PCSK9 gene results in decreased LDL receptor expression, decreased LDL catabolism, and increased LDL-cholesterol. Mutation in the apolipoprotein B gene results in impaired binding of LDL particles to the LDL receptors. Apo B100 protein defect has a milder presentation than LDL (apo B/E) receptor defect. This is because apo E–mediated clearance of remnant particles is still functional.

The homozygous form of the LDL receptor mutation is rare. Affected individuals present early in life with elevated levels of total cholesterol (600 to 1000 mg/dL) and LDL-cholesterol (550 to 950 mg/dL). Triglyceride and HDL-cholesterol levels are normal. These patients develop CHD, aortic stenosis due to atherosclerosis of the aortic root, and tendon xanthomas (often in the Achilles tendon). If the condition remains untreated, patients with homozygous familial hypercholesterolemia typically die of myocardial infarction before 20 years of age. The heterozygous form of FH affects 1 in every 500 individuals. Partial receptor defect results in cells that display half the normal number of fully functional LDL receptors. These individuals have lower concentrations of total cholesterol (>300 to 600 mg/dL) and LDL-cholesterol (250 to 500 mg/dL) than do those with the homozygous form. Premature CHD and tendon xanthomas are characteristic clinical findings.

Although the diagnosis of familial hypercholesterolemia can be established by genetic testing, the diagnosis is usually made based on clinical features. Elevated total cholesterol (>300 mg/dL) and LDL-cholesterol (>250 mg/dL) in an individual with a personal or family history of premature CHD and tendon xanthomas identifies patients at risk for familial hypercholesterolemia. Treatment requires a low-fat (<20% of total calories), low-cholesterol (<100 mg/day) diet in combination with drug therapy. Usually, patients with familial hypercholesterolemia require multiple agents including high-intensity statin, ezetimibe, and/or PCSK9 inhibitors to lower cholesterol levels to the target range. For patients who are unable to achieve target goals, additional intervention with liver transplantation to provide functional receptors, ileal bypass surgery to decrease gastrointestinal absorption of bile acids, LDL apheresis to remove excess LDL, and novel therapies with lomitapide and mipomersen may be considered.

Elevated Plasma Lipoprotein(a)

Lp(a) is a specialized form of LDL that is assembled extracellularly from apolipoprotein(a) and LDL. Lp(a), when present at elevated levels, interferes with fibrinolysis by competing with plasminogen. This leads to decreased thrombolysis and increased clot formation. Lp(a) also binds macrophages, promoting foam cell formation and atherosclerotic plaques. Screening should be considered in individuals who have a family or personal history of premature CHD without dyslipidemia and in those for whom cholesterol-lowering therapy has failed. The diagnosis can be made by documenting Lp(a) levels higher than 30 mg/dL in a patient with premature CHD. The primary goal of therapy is to lower LDL levels with agents such as statins, ezetimibe, and PCSK-9 inhibitors. Niacin can also reduce Lp(a); however, the effectiveness of this strategy in ASCVD prevention remains unproven.

Polygenic Hypercholesterolemia

Hypercholesterolemia in a population is mostly due to small influences of many different genes. The exact nature of these genetic defects is poorly defined, but apo E may play a role in the pathogenesis. Apo

E4 on chylomicrons and VLDL remnants has a high affinity for the LDL receptor. Elevated binding of apo E4–containing lipoproteins to LDL receptors may downregulate LDL receptor synthesis and increase circulating LDL levels. Environmental factors such as diet can influence production of chylomicrons and VLDL, resulting in downregulation of the LDL receptor in conditions with high apo E4. This leads to an increased propensity for CHD, and treatment with LDL-lowering agents is recommended based on risk factors (see Table 8.7).

Familial Combined Hyperlipoproteinemia

Familial combined hyperlipoproteinemia (FCHL) is a polygenic disorder that affects 1% to 2% of the population. Factors such as diet, glucose intolerance, and medications can influence the phenotypic presentation. In FCHL, the liver synthesizes excess VLDL. VLDL is hydrolyzed by LPL to produce LDL. Mutations in the *LPL* gene affecting its expression or function can decrease the efficiency of VLDL catabolism. Dysfunction of LPL is observed in one third of patients with FCHL. Diminished LPL activity increases circulating VLDL-triglyceride; furthermore, fewer VLDL remnant particles are available for HDL synthesis. Therefore, FCHL needs to be considered in all patients whose total cholesterol level is greater than 250 mg/dL, triglycerides greater than 175 mg/dL, or HDL-cholesterol less than 35 mg/dL.

There are no definitive diagnostic tests, but family screening can help confirm the diagnosis. The phenotype of FCHL is variable, with individuals displaying high LDL-cholesterol, high VLDL-triglyceride, or both based on the genetic defect and environmental factors. Patients also typically have high apo B (>120 mg/dL) and a low ratio of LDL-cholesterol to apo B100 (<1.2). They accumulate small dense LDL particles, which are thought to be atherogenic and contribute to premature CHD. Xanthomas or xanthelasmas are not a feature of this disorder. Affected individuals require a low-fat, low-cholesterol diet plus multiple lipid-lowering drugs to achieve target goals. Statins are recommended to lower LDL-cholesterol and to reduce the risk of cardiovascular disease and mortality. Addition of ezetimibe, fibric acid derivatives, niacin, and omega-3 fatty acid are often considered to achieve LDL-cholesterol and triglyceride target goals. However, these agents have not been shown to decrease cardiovascular events or improve overall survival.

Familial Dysbetalipoproteinemia

Apo E on the surface of lipoprotein particles binds LDL receptors and facilitates clearance of remnant particles from the circulation. The apo E2 allele has a lower affinity for LDL receptors than apo E3 or apo E4. In individuals who are homozygous for apo E2, LPL hydrolyzes the triglyceride core and the resulting cholesterol-rich chylomicrons. VLDL and IDL remnant particles accumulate in the circulation. Expression of this phenotype usually requires a precipitating condition that increases lipoprotein production (e.g., diabetes, alcohol consumption) or decreases clearance (e.g., hypothyroidism). In addition to the more common autosomal recessive mutation of apo E described previously, several apo E mutations have been described that result in an autosomal dominant phenotype manifesting in childhood. Premature CHD, peripheral vascular disease, and xanthomas involving the palmar crease are characteristic clinical features. Individuals with familial dysbetalipoproteinemia have elevated levels of total cholesterol (300 to 400 mg/dL) and triglycerides (300 to 400 mg/dL). Definitive diagnosis requires genetic testing to identify apo E2 homozygosity or mutation. Treatment of coexisting conditions such as diabetes and hypothyroidism can normalize lipid levels in apo E2 homozygotes. If target levels are not achieved, dietary therapy and lipid-lowering drugs such as fibric acid derivatives and HMG-CoA reductase inhibitors should also be considered.

陷（活性为 2% ～ 25%）。PCSK9 和载脂蛋白 B 基因缺陷较少见。PCSK9 是由肝脏生成的丝氨酸蛋白酶。PCSK9 可与 LDL 受体结合，导致 LDL 受体内化并被降解。PCSK9 基因的功能获得突变会导致 LDL 受体表达降低、LDL 分解代谢减少、LDL 胆固醇增加。载脂蛋白 B 基因突变会导致 LDL 颗粒与 LDL 受体结合受损。与 LDL 受体缺陷相比，载脂蛋白 B100 缺陷的临床表现较轻，这是因为载脂蛋白 E 仍可介导清除残余的 LDL 颗粒。

LDL 受体的纯合突变很罕见。纯合突变患者在生命早期出现总胆固醇（600 ～ 1000 mg/dl）和 LDL 胆固醇（550 ～ 950 mg/dl）水平升高，而甘油三酯和 HDL 胆固醇水平正常。这些患者易患冠心病、主动脉根部动脉粥样硬化导致主动脉狭窄，以及肌腱黄色瘤（常见于跟腱）。若不及时治疗，纯合型 FH 患者通常在 20 岁前死于心肌梗死。杂合型 FH 的患病率为 1/500，LDL 受体部分缺陷会导致细胞中仅有 1/2 的 LDL 受体功能正常。这些患者的总胆固醇（> 300 ～ 600 mg/dl）和 LDL 胆固醇（250 ～ 500 mg/dl）水平低于纯合型患者。早发冠心病和肌腱黄色瘤是其特征性临床表现。

虽然 FH 可通过基因检测确诊，但诊断通常基于临床表现。在有早发冠心病和肌腱黄色瘤史或家族史的患者中，总胆固醇（> 300 mg/dl）和 LDL 胆固醇（> 250 mg/dl）水平升高提示有 FH 风险。治疗包括低脂肪（<总热量的 20%）低胆固醇（< 100 mg/d）饮食联合药物治疗。FH 患者通常需多种药物治疗［包括高强度他汀类药物、依折麦布和（或）PCSK9 抑制剂］才能将胆固醇水平降至目标范围。对于无法达标的患者，可考虑肝移植（提供功能性受体）、回肠旁路手术（减少胃肠道吸收胆汁酸）、LDL 分离（清除过量的 LDL），以及洛美他派和米泊美生等新治疗。

高脂蛋白（a）血症

Lp（a）是一种特殊形式的 LDL，由载脂蛋白（a）和 LDL 在细胞外组装而成。当 Lp（a）水平升高时，可与纤溶酶原竞争，干扰纤维蛋白溶解，导致血栓溶解减少，血栓形成增加。Lp（a）可与巨噬细胞结合，促进泡沫细胞及动脉粥样硬化斑块的形成。对于有早发冠心病史或家族史但无血脂异常的人群及降胆固醇治疗未达标的人群，应考虑筛查高脂蛋白（a）血症。诊断依据为 Lp（a）> 30 mg/dl 且有早发冠心病。主要治疗目标是使用他汀类药物、依折麦布和 PCSK-9 抑制剂等药物来降低 LDL 水平。烟酸能降低 Lp（a）水平，但其预防 ASCVD 的有效性尚未被证实。

多基因性高胆固醇血症

多数高胆固醇血症由多种基因的共同作用所致。这些基因缺陷的确切作用尚不清楚，但载脂蛋白 E 可能在发病机制中发挥作用。乳糜微粒和 VLDL 残余物上的载脂蛋白 E4 与 LDL 受体具有强亲和力。含载脂蛋白 E4 的脂蛋白与 LDL 受体结合增加可下调 LDL 受体的合成，增加循环 LDL。饮食等环境因素可影响乳糜微粒和 VLDL 的产生，导致载脂蛋白 E4 水平升高、LDL 受体下调。这会导致冠心病的发病风险增加，建议根据危险因素应用降低 LDL 的药物治疗（表 8.7）。

家族性混合性高脂蛋白血症

家族性混合性高脂蛋白血症（FCHL）是多基因疾病，发病率为 1% ～ 2%。饮食、糖耐量异常和药物等因素可影响其表型。在 FCHL 中，肝脏合成过量的 VLDL，VLDL 被 LPL 水解产生 LDL。*LPL* 基因突变会影响其表达或功能，从而降低 VLDL 分解代谢的效率。1/3 的 FCHL 患者存在 LPL 功能异常。LPL 活性降低会增加循环中的 VLDL- 甘油三酯，使可用于 HDL 合成的 VLDL 残余物颗粒减少。因此，总胆固醇 > 250 mg/dl、甘油三酯 > 175 mg/dl 或 HDL 胆固醇 < 35 mg/dl 的患者均应考虑 FCHL。

目前 FCHL 缺乏确诊性检查，但家庭史筛查可帮助诊断。FCHL 有多种表型，根据遗传缺陷和环境因素，患者可表现出高 LDL 胆固醇和（或）高 VLDL- 甘油三酯。患者通常合并载脂蛋白 B 水平升高（> 120 mg/dl）和 LDL/ 载脂蛋白 B100 比值降低（< 1.2）。患者体内会积聚小而密的 LDL 颗粒，这些颗粒会导致动脉粥样硬化，进而引发早发冠心病。黄色瘤和眼睑黄斑瘤不是 FCHL 的临床特点。FCHL 患者需要低脂肪低胆固醇饮食，并联合多种降脂药物以达到血脂控制目标。建议使用他汀类药物降低 LDL 胆固醇，以减少心血管疾病和死亡风险。通常还需联合依折麦布、贝特类药物、烟酸和 ω-3 脂肪酸，以达到 LDL 胆固醇和甘油三酯的目标值。然而，这些药物未被证明能减少心血管事件或提高总生存率。

家族性异常 β 脂蛋白血症

脂蛋白颗粒表面的载脂蛋白 E 可结合 LDL 受体，促进残余颗粒从血液循环中清除。载脂蛋白 E2 等位基因型对 LDL 受体的亲和力低于载脂蛋白 E3 或 E4。在纯合型载脂蛋白 E2 基因突变的患者中，LPL 水解甘油三酯核心及其产生的富含胆固醇的乳糜微粒。VLDL 和 IDL 残余颗粒会在血液循环中累积。通常在脂蛋白生成增加（如糖尿病、饮酒）或清除减少（如甲状腺功能减退症）等诱因存在时才会出现表型。除了较常见的常染色体隐性遗传的载脂蛋白 E 突变，还有多种常染色体显性遗传的载脂蛋白 E 突变，后者在儿童期即可出现表型。早发冠心病、周围血管疾病和累及掌皱襞的黄色瘤是其特征性临床表现。家族性异常 β 脂蛋白血症患者的总胆固醇（300 ～ 400 mg/dl）和甘油三酯（300 ～ 400 mg/dl）水平升高。确诊需要进行基因检测确定是否存在载脂蛋白 E2 的纯合型或杂合型突变。治疗糖尿病和甲状腺功能减退症等合并症可使纯合型载脂蛋白 E2 患者的血脂水平恢复正常。如果未达到治疗目标，应考虑调整饮食和联合降脂药物，如贝特类药物和 HMG-CoA 还原酶抑制剂。

Familial Chylomicronemia

Mutations in the *LPL* gene resulting in deficiency of LPL synthesis or function lead to increased circulating chylomicron and VLDL particles and severe hypertriglyceridemia. Homozygous LPL deficiency is rare. It manifests in childhood with triglyceride levels higher than 1000 mg/dL. Heterozygous LPL deficiency occurs in 2% to 4% of the population and usually requires a precipitating factor, such as uncontrolled diabetes or estrogen therapy, to manifest the phenotype. These individuals have moderate hypertriglyceridemia (250 to 750 mg/dL) that can increase to levels greater than 1000 mg/dL with secondary factors. This can result in the chylomicronemia syndrome, which is characterized by marked hypertriglyceridemia (>1000 to 2000 mg/dL), pancreatitis, eruptive xanthomas, lipemia retinalis, and hepatosplenomegaly. Visual inspection demonstrates lipemic plasma. After refrigeration for 12 hours, a creamy top layer (increased chylomicrons) or turbid plasma infranatant (increased VLDL), or both, can be demonstrated. Documentation of diminished LPL activity confirms the diagnosis. A diet low in fat (<10% of total calories or 20 to 25 g/day) is the primary treatment. Secondary factors such as uncontrolled diabetes and alcohol use should be addressed, and VLDL-lowering agents (e.g., fibric acid derivatives, niacin) may be needed to prevent severe hypertriglyceridemia.

Apolipoprotein C-II Deficiency

Apo C-II is an activating cofactor for LPL. Deficiency of apo C-II is a rare autosomal recessive disorder that leads to increased chylomicrons and VLDL particles in the circulation, resulting in severe hypertriglyceridemia. Clinical manifestations are similar to those of LPL deficiency, including hypertriglyceridemia (>1000 mg/dL) and symptoms of pancreatitis, eruptive xanthomas, lipemia retinalis, and hepatosplenomegaly. Treatment recommendations include appropriate management of secondary factors such as diabetes and hypothyroidism, dietary fat restriction (<10% of calories), and drug therapy (e.g., fibric acid derivatives). For severe hypertriglyceridemia, plasma transfusion (with apo C-II) can be considered.

Familial Hypertriglyceridemia

Familial hypertriglyceridemia is an autosomal dominant disorder that is characterized by overproduction of hepatic VLDL. The exact defect or mutation is unknown. Secondary factors that increase VLDL, such as diabetes, alcohol ingestion, and estrogen therapy, appear to exacerbate this condition. Low HDL associated with familial hypertriglyceridemia is related to increased catabolism. Individuals with this condition have hypertriglyceridemia (200 to 500 mg/dL) and low HDL-cholesterol (<35 mg/dL) at presentation. This diagnosis is considered in individuals who have a family and personal history of hypertriglyceridemia, CHD, and normal LDL levels. Cloudy infranatant after overnight refrigeration of plasma identifies a disorder of VLDL metabolism. Treatment starts with management of secondary factors that may exacerbate the condition. Dietary fat restriction (<10% of calories) and drug therapy with fish oil, niacin, and fibric acid derivatives should be initiated if target goals are not achieved.

For a deeper discussion on this topic, please see Chapter 195, ❖ "Disorders of Lipid Metabolism," in *Goldman-Cecil Medicine*, 26th Edition.

SUGGESTED READINGS

Eckel RH, Jakicic JM, Ard JD, et al: 2013 AHA/ACC guideline on lifestyle management to reduce cardiovascular risk, Circulation 129:S76–S99, 2014.

Grundy SM, Stone NJ, Bailey AL, et al: 2018 AHA/ACC multisociety guideline on the management of blood cholesterol, J Am Coll Cardiol 73:e285, 2019.

Jellinger PS, Handelsman Y, Rosenblit PD, et al: American association of clinical endocrinologist and American College of Endocrinology guidelines for the management of dyslipidemia and prevention of cardiovascular disease, Endocr Pract 23:1–87, 2017.

U.S. Preventive Services Task Force: Statin use for the primary prevention of cardiovascular disease in adults: Preventive medication: U.S. Preventive Services Task Force recommendation statement, 2016, Available at: https://www.uspreventiveservicestaskforce.org/Page/Document/RecommendationStatementFinal/statin-use-in-adults-preventive-medication1. Accessed June 2020.

家族性乳糜微粒血症

LPL 基因突变会引起 LPL 合成或功能障碍，导致循环乳糜微粒和 VLDL 颗粒增加，以及严重高甘油三酯血症。纯合型 LPL 缺乏症非常罕见，在儿童期即会出现高甘油三酯血症（> 1000 mg/dl）。杂合型 LPL 缺乏症的发病率为 2% ~ 4%，通常需要诱因才会出现表型，如未控制的糖尿病或雌激素治疗。这些杂合型患者可有中度高甘油三酯血症（250 ~ 750 mg/dl），若合并继发因素，甘油三酯水平也可升高至 1000 mg/dl 以上。这可能导致乳糜微粒血症综合征，其特征是明显的高甘油三酯血症（> 1000 ~ 2000 mg/dl）、胰腺炎、发疹性黄色瘤、视网膜脂血症和肝脾大。肉眼观察可见乳糜血。血液标本冷藏 12 h 后可观察到乳白色表层（乳糜微粒增加）和（或）浑浊的血浆底层（VLDL 增加）。有 LPL 活性降低的证据可确诊。低脂饮食（脂肪＜总热量的 10%，或＜ 20 ~ 25 g/d）是主要的治疗方法。应控制继发因素（如未控制的糖尿病、酗酒），还可能需要使用降低 VLDL 的药物（如贝特类药物、烟酸）来预防严重的高甘油三酯血症。

载脂蛋白 C-Ⅱ 缺乏症

载脂蛋白 C-Ⅱ 是 LPL 的活化辅因子。载脂蛋白 C-Ⅱ 缺乏症是一种罕见的常染色体隐性遗传病，可导致循环中乳糜微粒和 VLDL 颗粒增多，进而导致严重的高甘油三酯血症。临床表现类似于 LPL 缺乏症，包括高甘油三酯血症（> 1000 mg/dl）、胰腺炎、出疹性黄色瘤、视网膜脂血症和肝脾大等。推荐治疗包括控制继发因素（如糖尿病和甲状腺功能减退症）、限制饮食中的脂肪摄入（＜总热量的 10%）和药物治疗（如贝特类药物）。对于严重的高甘油三酯血症，可考虑输注含有载脂蛋白 C-Ⅱ 的血浆。

家族性高甘油三酯血症

家族性高甘油三酯血症是一种常染色体显性遗传病，其特征是肝脏 VLDL 生成过多。相关基因缺陷 / 突变尚不明确。糖尿病、饮酒和雌激素治疗等增加 VLDL 的继发因素可加重该病。家族性高甘油三酯血症导致的低 HDL 水平与分解代谢增加有关。患者可表现为高甘油三酯血症（200 ~ 500 mg/dl）和低 HDL 胆固醇水平（< 35 mg/dl）。有高甘油三酯血症病史及家族史、有冠心病但 LDL 水平正常的患者，应考虑诊断该病。血浆过夜冷藏后出现浑浊的底层物质可考虑 VLDL 代谢紊乱。初始治疗为控制可能加重病情的继发因素。如果血脂不能达标，则应开始限制饮食中的脂肪摄入（＜总热量的 10%），并使用鱼油、烟酸和贝特类药物等进行治疗。

有关此专题的深入讨论，请参阅 *Goldman-Cecil* ❖ *Medicine* 第 26 版第 195 章 "脂代谢紊乱"。

推荐阅读

Eckel RH, Jakicic JM, Ard JD, et al: 2013 AHA/ACC guideline on lifestyle management to reduce cardiovascular risk, Circulation 129:S76–S99, 2014.

Grundy SM, Stone NJ, Bailey AL, et al: 2018 AHA/ACC multisociety guideline on the management of blood cholesterol, J Am Coll Cardiol 73:e285, 2019.

Jellinger PS, Handelsman Y, Rosenblit PD, et al: American association of clinical endocrinologist and American College of Endocrinology guidelines for the management of dyslipidemia and prevention of cardiovascular disease, Endocr Pract 23:1–87, 2017.

U.S. Preventive Services Task Force: Statin use for the primary prevention of cardiovascular disease in adults: Preventive medication: U.S. Preventive Services Task Force recommendation statement, 2016, Available at: https://www.uspreventiveservicestaskforce.org/Page/Document/RecommendationStatementFinal/statin-use-in-adults-preventive-medication1. Accessed June 2020.

SECTION II

Women's Health

女性健康

Women's Health Topics

Vidya Gopinath, Yael Tarshish, Kelly McGarry

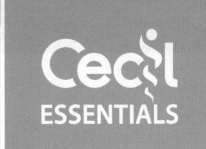

INTRODUCTION

The field of women's health grew out of the recognition that certain medical conditions are unique to women. Sex- and gender-specific differences exist in disease manifestation and management. Sex differences are defined as variations between males and females due to the specific composition and expression of their chromosomes. Gender differences are derived from sociocultural origins. For instance, women are disproportionately affected by poverty, intimate partner violence (IPV), unstable housing, substance use disorders, lack of transportation, lack of insurance, and the necessity of finding child care, all of which pose barriers to care and thereby influence their health. Variations in health outcomes between men and women are related to a complex interplay among lifestyle, environmental, behavioral, molecular, and cellular differences.

Women's health as a specialty focuses on conditions unique to women, diseases that disproportionately affect women, present differently or are managed in ways that are specific to women. Diagnoses unique to women include polycystic ovarian syndrome, menstrual irregularities, and endometriosis. Conditions that disproportionately affect women include breast cancer, osteoporosis, lupus, hypothyroidism, and urinary incontinence. Women have an increased susceptibility for developing certain conditions. For example, a woman who smokes the same number of cigarettes as a man is 20% to 70% more likely to develop lung cancer. Women are also more susceptible to alcohol-induced liver disease. Among individuals who consume 28 to 41 alcoholic beverages per week, the relative risk of alcohol-induced cirrhosis is 17.0 in women and 7.0 in men. During unprotected intercourse, women are 10 times more likely to contract human immunodeficiency virus (HIV) than men. The field of women's health has become more robust and includes practitioners from a multitude of disciplines: obstetrician-gynecologists, general internists, subspecialty internists, family medicine, emergency medicine, radiologists, and surgeons. Pharmacokinetics and pharmacodynamics of numerous drugs have sex-specific differences that are being discovered and require further study. The National Institutes of Health has made significant progress in the inclusion of women in clinical trials; they were historically excluded for numerous reasons including concerns about hormonal fluctuations affecting the data and teratogenic effects in women who were or could become pregnant. In 1977, the US Food and Drug Administration (FDA) recommended excluding women with "childbearing potential" from phase 1 and early phase 2 clinical studies. There is now growing recognition of the need for research studies to fully analyze sex-specific differences and include individuals of both sexes.

The seeds of this disparity in research and representation stem in part from the fact that women have been underrepresented in the field of medicine. In 1849, Elizabeth Blackwell earned the first medical degree granted to an American woman, but the advancement of female physicians has been gradual. In 1950, only 6% of practicing physicians were female. Currently, female physicians make up 36% of the workforce. In 2017, for the first time, the number of women enrolling in US medical schools exceeded the number of men, with females representing 50.7% of the 21,338 new enrollees, compared with 49.8% in 2016. Given these statistics, women will have an expanding impact on shaping the profession and the world of health care.

In this chapter, we focus on medical issues unique to women and highlight what is known about sex and gender differences in common diseases. Although "females" and "women" are often used interchangeably, we recognize that biological sex and gender are not synonymous. We aim to be inclusive of sexual minorities and recognize that some topics may be relevant only to biological females or women who choose to have sexual relationships with males. For more detailed discussions of specific topics, please refer to the appropriate chapters in this edition of *Cecil Essentials of Medicine* and the 26th edition of *Goldman-Cecil Medicine*.

THE MENSTRUAL CYCLE

The menstrual cycle is a complex hormonal process resulting in the release of a single oocyte, an immature ovum or egg. The menstrual cycle consists of two phases, the follicular phase and the luteal phase. The follicular phase begins with the first day of menses. Several follicles grow until a single dominant follicle is selected. Meanwhile, the uterine endometrium gradually thickens. The follicular phase ends the day prior to the luteal hormone (LH) surge that marks the first day of the luteal phase. The LH surge initiates the release of the follicle from the ovary to travel down the fallopian tube to the uterine cavity. The luteal phase ends when either the oocyte becomes fertilized and implants in the endometrium or without fertilization, when levels of estradiol and progesterone decline. Without high levels of estradiol or progesterone, endometrial blood supply decreases, which then leads to sloughing of the endometrial lining and thus marks the onset of menses. The physiologic changes that define the menstrual cycle, including variations in hormones, the uterine lining, and morning basal body temperature, are graphically represented in Fig. 9.1 . The average adult menstrual cycle is 28 to 35 days. Variability in length of cycle is common during adolescence; between ages 20 to 40 years old, women tend to have consistent cycle lengths.

Menstrual disorders are common and categorized as amenorrhea or abnormal uterine bleeding. Amenorrhea is defined as the lack of menses in a sexually mature female. It is further delineated as primary

女性健康

段佳丽 郑清月 译 陈蓉 审校 朱兰 通审

引言

女性健康领域的发展源于人们认识到某些医学问题是女性所特有的。疾病的临床表现和诊疗方式存在着生理性别（sex）和社会性别（gender）的差异。生理性别差异（sex differences）来自男性（male）与女性（female）染色体的组成和表达的不同，而社会性别差异（gender differences）则是源自社会文化。例如，贫困、亲密伴侣间暴力（IPV）、住房不稳定、物质使用障碍、交通不便、缺乏保险及需要为孩子寻找看护等因素对女性的影响更为严重，这些情况对女性的医疗保健构成更多障碍，继而影响女性健康。男性和女性健康结局的差异与生活方式、环境、行为、分子和细胞层面的差异之间的复杂相互作用有关。

女性健康专业重点关注女性特有的、对女性影响更严重、临床表现或治疗方式具有女性特异性的疾病。女性特有的疾病包括多囊卵巢综合征、月经失调和子宫内膜异位症。对女性影响更严重的疾病包括乳腺癌、骨质疏松症、系统性红斑狼疮、甲状腺功能减退症和尿失禁。女性较男性对某些疾病更易感。例如，在吸烟量相同的情况下，女性比男性患肺癌的风险高20%～70%。女性也更易罹患酒精性肝病，同样是每周饮用28～41杯酒精饮料，女性患酒精性肝硬化的相对风险为17.0，而男性为7.0。女性在无保护性行为中感染HIV的风险是男性的10倍。女性健康领域不断发展健全，涉及妇产科医生、全科内科医生、专科内科医生、家庭医生、急诊科医生、放射科医生和外科医生等多学科医护工作者。许多药物的药代动力学和药效学存在性别差异，这些差异正在逐渐被发现并需要进一步深入研究。美国国立卫生研究院（NIH）在将女性纳入临床试验方面取得了重大进展。历史上女性受试者曾因多种原因被排除在外，如研究者担心女性的激素波动会影响研究数据、药物可能对已经妊娠或可能妊娠的女性产生致畸作用。1977年，美国食品药品监督管理局（FDA）建议Ⅰ期和早期Ⅱ期临床试验将"有生育潜能"的女性排除在外。现在，人们越来越认识到深入分析生理性别差异的需要，并应当在临床研究中同时纳入男性和女性受试者。

对女性研究不足的部分原因是女性在医疗领域中的占比较小。1849年，Elizabeth Blackwell成为第一位获得医学学位的美国女性，但此后女医生数量的增长较为缓慢。到1950年，仅有6%的执业医生是女性。目前，女医生的占比约为36%。2017年，美国医学院入学的21 338名新生中女性占比为50.7%，女性新生占比首次超过男性，这一比例在2016年为49.8%。根据以上数据，女性将对医生这一职业及医疗保健领域产生越来越大的影响。

本章重点关注女性特有的健康问题，并强调常见疾病中已知的生理性别和社会性别差异。尽管"female"（生理性别）和"women"（社会性别）这两个词经常被混用，但生理性别和社会性别并非同义词。我们旨在包含性少数群体，并认为某些主题仅与生理性别为女性的群体或选择与男性发生性关系的社会性别为女性的群体相关。有关此主题的深入讨论，请参阅本书和*Goldman-Cecil Medicine*第26版中的相应章节。

月经周期

月经周期中复杂的激素变化使得单个卵母细胞（未成熟的卵细胞）释放。月经周期包括卵泡期和黄体期。卵泡期始于月经第1天。在此期间，数个卵泡持续生长直至单个优势卵泡被选择；同时，子宫内膜逐渐增厚。卵泡期结束于黄体生成素（LH）激增的前一天，LH激增标志着黄体期的第1天。LH激增促使卵泡从卵巢排出，沿着输卵管进入子宫腔。当卵母细胞受精形成受精卵并植入子宫内膜，或未受精且雌二醇和孕酮水平下降时，黄体期结束。当缺乏高水平的雌二醇或孕酮时，子宫内膜血供减少，导致子宫内膜脱落，标志着月经的开始。图9.1形象地展示了月经周期中的各种生理学变化，包括激素水平、子宫内膜和晨起基础体温。成年女性的月经周期平均为28～35天。青春期时月经周期常不稳定；20～40岁女性的月经周期通常较为规律。

月经失调较为常见，可分为闭经和异常子宫出血。闭经是指性发育成熟的女性无月经来潮的现象，可进

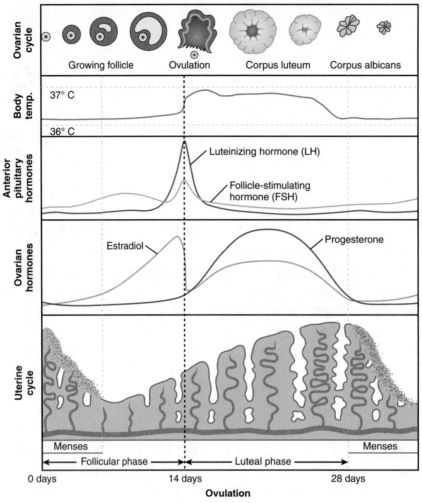

Ovarian cycle

Growing follicle   Ovulation   Corpus luteum   Corpus albicans

Body temp.

37° C

36° C

Anterior pituitary hormones

Luteinizing hormone (LH)

Follicle-stimulating hormone (FSH)

Ovarian hormones

Estradiol   Progesterone

Uterine cycle

Menses   Menses

Follicular phase   Luteal phase

0 days   14 days   28 days

Ovulation

Fig. 9.1 The physiologic changes that define the menstrual cycle.

or secondary amenorrhea. These abnormalities may indicate problems related to the reproductive system or may be an early sign of an important underlying systemic illness. A pregnancy test must always be done to exclude pregnancy in cases of amenorrhea along with a thorough history and physical exam.

Primary Amenorrhea

Primary amenorrhea is most often caused by genetic or anatomic abnormalities. It is defined as the lack of menarche by age 15 or 16 despite normal sexual development or the lack of menarche by age 13 or 14 in the absence of sexual development. Breast development, the presence of a uterus, and levels of LH, follicle-stimulating hormone (FSH), thyroid-stimulating hormone (TSH), and prolactin are important factors in determining the cause of primary amenorrhea. Work-up may include karyotyping and pelvic or brain imaging. The most common cause of primary amenorrhea is gonadal dysgenesis, which is found in Turner syndrome. The second most common cause is müllerian agenesis, a congenital malformation resulting in lack of uterine development and vaginal hypoplasia. If the uterus is present, an outflow tract obstruction such as an imperforate hymen or a transverse vaginal septum may be identified. FSH and LH levels can differentiate between functional hypothalamic amenorrhea and primary ovarian insufficiency.

Secondary Amenorrhea

Secondary amenorrhea is the absence of menses for 3 months in women with regular menses or 6 months in women with irregular menses outside of the setting of pregnancy or lactation. Oligomenorrhea occurs when menses are irregular or infrequent, with a cycle length usually greater than 35 to 40 days or fewer than nine menstrual cycles in 12 months, and it is often associated with chronic anovulation or oligo-ovulation. The most common cause of secondary amenorrhea is pregnancy. Lactation causes amenorrhea for up to 6 months in women who are exclusively breast-feeding. Prolonged amenorrhea can follow cessation of some hormonal contraceptives, especially depot medroxyprogesterone acetate (DMPA). Menopause should be suspected in a woman older than 45 years of age.

Amenorrhea and oligomenorrhea may be caused by pathologic changes at any point in the endometrial-ovarian-pituitary-hypothalamic axis. The differential diagnosis for other causes of secondary amenorrhea is broad. Most cases are associated with polycystic ovary syndrome (PCOS), hypothalamic amenorrhea, hyperprolactinemia or primary ovarian insufficiency.

PCOS and hyperandrogenism are associated with hirsutism, acne, and history of irregular menses. Hypothalamic amenorrhea can be functionally caused by stress, change in weight, diet or exercise or an eating disorder. Headaches and visual field deficits are concerning for hypothalamic-pituitary disease; galactorrhea indicates

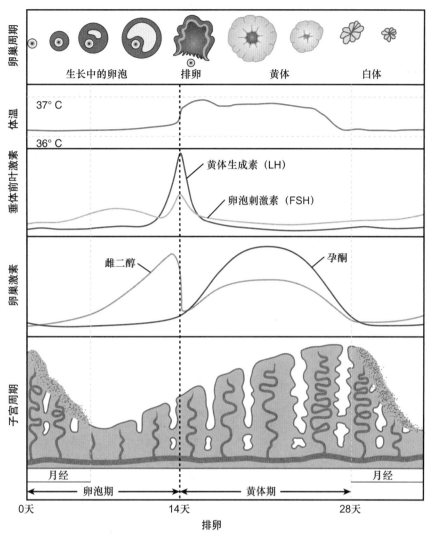

图 9.1　月经周期的生理学变化

一步分为原发性闭经和继发性闭经。这些异常提示可能存在生殖系统疾病，也可能是潜在全身疾病的早期征象。出现闭经时，必须进行妊娠试验以除外妊娠的可能性，并进行全面的病史采集和体格检查。

原发性闭经

原发性闭经最常见的病因是遗传或解剖异常。原发性闭经的定义是有第二性征发育但 15 岁或 16 岁时无月经来潮，或无第二性征发育且 13 岁或 14 岁时无月经来潮。乳房有无发育、子宫是否存在，以及 LH、FSH、促甲状腺激素（TSH）和催乳素的水平是鉴别原发性闭经病因的重要依据。相关检查还包括染色体核型分析、盆腔影像学检查和头颅影像学检查。原发性闭经最常见的病因是特纳综合征的性腺发育不全。第二大病因是米勒管发育不全，这是一种表现为子宫缺失、阴道发育不全的先天性畸形。若患者有子宫，则可能发现流出道梗阻，如处女膜闭锁或阴道横隔。FSH和 LH 水平有助于鉴别功能性下丘脑性闭经和原发性卵巢功能不全。

继发性闭经

继发性闭经是指在排除妊娠或哺乳的情况下，既往月经规律的女性 3 个月无月经来潮，或既往月经不规律的女性 6 个月无月经来潮。月经稀发是指月经周期不规律或月经次数较少，通常月经周期超过 35 ～ 40 天或 12 个月内月经来潮＜ 9 次，多与慢性无排卵或稀发排卵有关。继发性闭经最常见的原因是妊娠。哺乳可导致纯母乳喂养的女性闭经长达 6 个月。停用某些激素避孕药，尤其是长效醋酸甲羟孕酮（DMPA）后，可能会出现长时间闭经。45 岁以上女性出现闭经应考虑绝经可能。

子宫内膜-卵巢-垂体-下丘脑轴中任何环节的病理学改变均可能导致闭经和月经稀发。继发性闭经的鉴别诊断范围很广。多数病例与多囊卵巢综合征（PCOS）、下丘脑性闭经、高催乳素血症或原发性卵巢功能不全相关。

PCOS 和高雄激素血症与多毛症、痤疮和月经不规律病史有关。下丘脑性闭经可能由压力、体重 / 饮食 / 运动变化或进食障碍引起。头痛和视野缺损提示下丘脑-垂体疾病；溢乳提示高催乳素血症。卵巢功能不全的证据包括雌激素缺乏症状，如潮热、阴道干燥和性

hyperprolactinemia. Evidence of ovarian insufficiency includes symptoms of estrogen deficiency such as hot flashes, vaginal dryness, and decreased libido. Initial labs include FSH, TSH, prolactin, and possibly total testosterone. Pituitary MRI, progestin withdrawal test, and hysteroscopy may be a part of the work-up if initial tests are unrevealing.

Abnormal Uterine Bleeding

Abnormal uterine bleeding (AUB) affects approximately one third of women at some point in their life. Terms such as menorrhagia and metrorrhagia were updated in 2011 by the International Federation of Gynecology and Obstetrics. Instead they recommend use of the terms heavy menstrual bleeding (HMB), which is defined as ovulatory bleeding for more than 8 days or interfering with quality of life, and abnormal uterine bleeding with ovulatory dysfunction (AUB-O), which is defined as irregular bleeding.

In the PALM-COEIN classification, the etiology of HMB and AUB-O is divided into structural and nonstructural causes. The four main structural causes are *p*olyp, *a*denomyosis, *l*eiomyoma, and *m*alignancy or hyperplasia. The five nonstructural causes are *c*oagulopathy, *o*vulatory dysfunction, *e*ndometrial, *i*atrogenic, and *n*ot yet classified.

Key elements of the history include details about bleeding, including the onset, duration, pattern, and quantity of bleeding. This history and information about breast tenderness and cramping prior to onset of bleeding can establish evidence of ovulatory cycles. The evaluation should also confirm the source of bleeding as uterine and not gastrointestinal, urinary, or vulvar. Pregnancy must be ruled out in all patients including those who are using contraception or deny being sexually active.

Evaluation includes a pelvic exam with a vaginal speculum and bimanual exam to characterize the uterus. Pap smear and cervical cultures should be obtained to assess for cervical disease or infection. Laboratory testing should include a complete blood count (CBC), thyroid studies, and serum ferritin. It may also include coagulation studies because a significant fraction (5% to 32%) of women with heavy menstrual bleeding have an underlying bleeding disorder.

Endometrial sampling should be performed for women age 45 or older and for women younger than 45 years of age who are at risk for endometrial hyperplasia or endometrial cancer (i.e., women with obesity or a history of chronic anovulation, failed medical therapy or persistent symptoms). For women with suspected structural abnormalities, a transvaginal ultrasound study should be pursued.

Management of abnormal bleeding depends on the underlying pathology identified and the degree of anemia caused by the bleeding. Hemodynamically unstable women may require uterine curettage or intravenous estrogen. For hemodynamically stable women, control of bleeding is usually achieved through a combination of estrogen and progestin preparations, usually in the form of oral contraceptive pills. In women with a contraindication to estrogen, levonorgestrel-releasing intrauterine devices (IUDs) and high-dose oral progestins can be used. Irregular bleeding often continues with hormonal management but declines over time. Nonsteroidal anti-inflammatory drugs (NSAIDs) can be used by women who do not require contraception, because NSAIDs have been shown to decrease bleeding. Standard iron supplementation is recommended for patients with resultant anemia or iron deficiency. Surgical options include less-invasive treatments like endometrial ablation and uterine artery embolization as well as definitive therapy with hysterectomy. These are usually reserved for women who have failed other treatments, decline long-term medical therapy, and do not desire future pregnancy.

CONTRACEPTION

Approximately 62% of reproductive-age women in the United States are using some form of contraception and 99% of women who have ever been sexually active with men have used a form of contraception in their lifetime. However, nearly half of pregnancies in the United States are unintended. When helping patients choose a contraceptive method, several important variables should be considered. Patient preference and likelihood of adherence to a given method are important components to consider in selecting a mode of contraception. Efficacy depends on appropriate use. Patients' past experiences with different forms of contraception and personal preferences help to predict how well they will adhere to current regimens. Observational studies have demonstrated patient-provider relationships are important in family planning care.

Obtaining a thorough personal and family medical history is important to determine what methods are appropriate for a patient. Certain medical issues can make a choice too risky for one patient but provide a health benefit for another. For example, oral contraceptives that increase the risk of thrombosis are contraindicated for a patient with a strong family history of venous thrombosis, but they could correct anemia in a patient with menorrhagia. The patient's sexual history and assessment of the risk for sexually transmitted infections (STIs) play a role in contraceptive choice and education about the use of barrier methods.

Methods of Contraception

Barrier methods include the diaphragm, cervical cap, male condom, and female condom. These methods do not disrupt fertility beyond their moment of use. The diaphragm and cervical cap need to be fitted by a medical professional and therefore require a prescription. With each sexual encounter spermicide must be applied and the device needs to be left in 6 to 8 hours after intercourse to be efficacious. The male condom can be purchased over the counter and is among the most cost-effective options. It has the added benefit of reducing the transmission of STIs. Prevention of conception and STI transmission depends on correct and consistent use: the male condom must be used during the entire sexual act. The female condom is also over the counter and protects against transmission of STIs, though there are less data on decreased STI transmission compared to male condoms.

Combination hormonal contraceptives are the most common form of hormonal birth control. They typically contain a low dose of estrogen (≤35 µg) and one of several progestins. Delivery methods include pills, patches, and intravaginal rings. These methods carry similar contraindications and have the same contraceptive mechanism: prevention of ovulation. Combined oral contraceptives (COCs) are classified as either monophasic, which release a constant hormone dose throughout the menstrual cycle, or multiphasic, which contain variable levels of hormones to be taken over the course of the month. Monophasic COCs are preferred because they have been more extensively studied, may be associated with improved mood variability compared to multiphasic formulations in susceptible women, and are simpler to use. No clear benefit has been demonstrated for multiphasic COCs. Continuous or extended cycle COCs allow for less frequent withdrawal bleeding and more control over timing of withdrawal bleeding, though this can be associated with more unpredictable bleeding. After cessation of combination hormonal contraceptives, menses typically return in 1 month. Fertility and menses are expected in all women within 90 days of stopping the medication.

The transdermal patch is applied weekly for 3 weeks per month followed by a week without the patch in order to allow for withdrawal bleeding. The patch is applied to a different site on the body each time. It delivers a higher average dose of estrogen but lower peak doses. One key difference between COCs and the patch is that the latter bypasses hepatic first pass metabolism; thus, the patch has fewer drug interactions and requires lower peak hormonal doses in order to be effective

欲减退。初始实验室检验包括 FSH、TSH、催乳素及总睾酮水平。若上述检查未发现异常，后续检查可包括垂体 MRI、孕激素撤退试验和宫腔镜检查。

异常子宫出血

约 1/3 的女性在一生中的某个阶段会出现异常子宫出血（AUB）。国际妇产科联盟于 2011 年更新了"menorrhagia（月经过多）""metrorrhagia（子宫不规则出血）"等术语，建议改用"heavy menstrual bleeding（HMB；月经过多）"和"abnormal uterine bleeding with ovulatory dysfunction（AUB-O；排卵障碍性异常子宫出血）"这两个术语。前者的定义为月经出血超过 8 天或影响生活质量，后者的定义为不规则出血。

PALM-COEIN 分类系统将 AUB 的病因分为结构性原因和非结构性原因两大类。4 种结构性原因包括子宫内膜息肉、子宫腺肌病、子宫平滑肌瘤、子宫内膜恶变或不典型增生。5 种非结构性原因包括凝血功能障碍、排卵障碍、子宫内膜局部异常、医源性和尚未分类的其他病因。

病史采集的要点为出血的细节，包括如何起病、出血持续时间、出血模式和出血量。出血情况结合出血前有无乳房触痛或绞痛有助于确定患者的排卵周期。此外，还应确认出血的来源是子宫，而不是胃肠道、泌尿道或外阴。所有患者均需排除妊娠可能，包括正在使用避孕药及否认有性生活的患者。

可采用阴道窥器和双合诊检查对患者进行妇科查体，以了解子宫情况。应通过巴氏染色涂片和宫颈分泌物培养评估有无宫颈病变或感染。实验室检查应涵盖全血细胞计数、甲状腺功能和血清铁蛋白水平。考虑到相当比例（5%～32%）表现为月经过多的女性患有潜在的出血性疾病，还应检查患者的凝血功能。

对于 45 岁以上女性，或 45 岁以下但有子宫内膜增生或子宫内膜癌风险的女性（如肥胖症、慢性无排卵史、药物治疗失败或症状持续存在），应进行子宫内膜活检。对于怀疑有结构异常的女性，应进行经阴道超声检查。

AUB 的治疗取决于病因和出血所致贫血的严重程度。血流动力学不稳定的女性可能需要刮宫或静脉注射雌激素。对于血流动力学稳定的女性，通常联合使用雌孕激素来控制出血，常用口服避孕药。对于有雌激素使用禁忌证的女性，可使用释放左炔诺孕酮的宫内节育器和口服大剂量孕激素。不规则出血通常在激素治疗后仍持续出现，但会随着时间的推移而减少。非甾体抗炎药（NSAID）已被证明能够减少出血，可用于没有避孕需求的女性。对于因出血导致贫血或缺铁的患者，建议服用标准铁补充剂。手术治疗方式包括微创治疗（如子宫内膜切除术和子宫动脉栓塞术）和根治性治疗（如子宫切除术）。手术治疗通常仅用于其他治疗无效、拒绝长期药物治疗且没有生育需求的女性。

避孕

在美国，约 62% 的育龄期女性正在使用某种方式进行避孕，99% 与男性发生过性行为的女性在其一生中使用过某种形式的避孕措施。然而，美国近 1/2 的妊娠是意外妊娠。在选择避孕方式时，患者偏好和使用依从性是需要考虑的重要因素。避孕的效果取决于使用方式是否正确。患者既往使用不同避孕方式的经验和个人偏好有助于预测她们能否很好地遵守当前方案。观察性研究表明，患者与医护人员的关系在计划生育服务中十分重要。

获取患者全面的个人史和家族史对于确定哪些方法适合该患者非常重要。某些健康问题会使特定避孕方式对某一患者来说风险过大，但对另一患者来说却有益。例如，口服避孕药会增加血栓形成的风险，因此有静脉血栓家族史的患者禁用口服避孕药；但对于月经过多的患者，口服避孕药可纠正贫血。患者的性生活史和性传播疾病感染风险评估在避孕方式的选择和屏障避孕法的宣教中发挥重要作用。

避孕方式

屏障避孕法包括阴道隔膜、宫颈帽、男用避孕套和女用避孕套。使用这些方法后不会影响生育能力。阴道隔膜和宫颈帽需要由医护人员放置，因此需要开具处方。每次性交时均必须使用杀精剂，且该装置需在性交后 6～8 h 放置才有效。男用避孕套可以在柜台购买，是最经济实惠的选择之一。男用避孕套还有助于减少性传播疾病。避孕和预防性传播疾病需要正确使用男用避孕套，并在性行为过程中全程使用。女用避孕套也是非处方药，并可预防性传播疾病传播，但与男用避孕套相比，其减少性传播疾病传播的相关数据较少。

复方激素避孕药是最常用的激素避孕方式。它们通常含有小剂量雌激素（≤ 35 μg）和几种孕激素中的一种。给药途径包括药片、贴剂和阴道避孕环。这些方法的禁忌证类似，避孕的机制也类似：抑制排卵。复方口服避孕药（COC）分为单相片和多相片。单相片在整个月经周期释放的激素剂量恒定，而多相片在月经周期不同时期释放的激素剂量不同。由于相关研究较多、可能比多相片更有助于改善敏感女性的情绪波动，且使用更为简便，因此目前首选单相片。多相片尚未被证实有明确优势。持续或长期使用 COC 可降低撤退性出血的频率，并更好地控制撤退性出血发生的时间，但这可能与更不可预测的出血有关。停用 COC 后，患者通常会在 1 个月内恢复月经来潮。所有女性在停药后 90 天内都有望恢复生育能力和月经来潮。

复方激素避孕药经皮贴剂需要每周使用 1 次，连用 3 周，然后停用 1 周，以出现撤退性出血。每次需将贴剂贴在身体的不同部位。贴剂可提供更高的雌激素平均剂量，但峰值剂量较低。COC 和贴剂的一个主要区别是后者避开了肝脏首过代谢；因此，与 COC 相比，贴剂的药物相互作用较少，起效所需的峰值激素剂量更低。由于外源性激素在 3 天内就会降至很低的

as compared to COCs. Return to fertility can occur immediately after patch discontinuation because exogenous hormones reach very low levels within 3 days.

The ring is inserted vaginally and left in place for 3 weeks and then removed for 1 week to allow for withdrawal bleeding. Extended ring regimens are possible whereby a new ring is inserted the same day as the prior one is removed. This can be done every 3 weeks for up to a year to delay withdrawal bleeding, though it is associated with spotting. The patch and the ring are reasonable options for patients concerned with taking a daily medication.

Contraindications to combination hormonal contraception are related to the estrogen component. Contraindications include a personal history of a thromboembolic event or known thrombogenic mutation, cerebrovascular accident (CVA), coronary artery disease (CAD), uncontrolled hypertension, migraine with aura, smoking after age 35, breast cancer, estrogen-dependent neoplasms, undiagnosed abnormal vaginal bleeding, liver tumors, and pregnancy. There is no evidence that COCs cause weight gain. Upon initiation, some patients report breast tenderness, nausea, and bloating. Most symptoms go away quickly with continued use. Irregular bleeding typically resolves within 3 months. If COCs are started more than 5 days since onset of menses, back-up contraception is recommended for 7 days.

Potential noncontraceptive benefits of combination oral contraceptives include regulation of menstrual flow and improvement in ovarian cyst recurrence, endometriosis, chronic pelvic pain, acne, polycystic ovarian syndrome, hyperandrogenism, and mittelschmerz (i.e., midcycle pain). Long-term use of combination oral contraceptives has been associated with a reduced lifetime risk of endometrial and ovarian cancers. Bone density is higher in perimenopausal women who used COCs compared to women who did not.

Progesterone-only contraceptives are an option for women intolerant of estrogen or at increased risk for thromboembolic events. They can be taken continuously without a hormone-free interval. Contraindications include active CAD, breast cancer, hepatic tumor, and phlebitis. They are slightly less efficacious than the combination pills, and women may experience breakthrough bleeding. They have a short duration of action and half-life so they must be taken at the same time each day. Back-up contraception is required if a dose is taken more than 3 hours late. Upon cessation, the return of fertility is rapid. Compared to COCs, ovulation is not consistently suppressed.

DMPA is a progesterone-only injection administered every 12 weeks. Major side effects include irregular bleeding (which resolves over time) and amenorrhea (50% at 1 year). Weight gain, hair changes, and acne are possible side effects. The FDA issued a black box warning that DMPA may decrease bone density, especially in adolescents and perimenopausal women. This possible association between DMPA use and fracture risk remains controversial without definitive data; however, a retrospective cohort study found no significant fracture risk difference. Return to fertility can be delayed and is dependent on body weight: women with lower body weights conceive sooner after discontinuation as compared to women with higher body weight. If conception is desired within 1 to 2 years of initiating a contraceptive method, DMPA is not recommended.

The IUD can be a great option for women who do not desire pregnancy in the next 5 to 10 years. Worldwide, it is the most widely used method of reversible contraception. Two types of IUDs are available in the United States, and both are as effective as sterilization. The copper IUD can be left in 10 years. There are four progesterone-emitting IUDs available in the United States and they can be left in from 3 to 5 years depending on the formulation. The copper IUD can be associated with heavier menstrual bleeding and cramps. The progesterone IUD may initially have breakthrough bleeding, but almost one half of users become amenorrheic. Return of fertility is rapid after removal of IUD.

The progesterone contraceptive subdermal implant was originally marketed as Implanon and is now Nexplanon. Unlike Implanon, Nexplanon is radiopaque. It is a 40-mm progesterone rod that is implanted under the skin of the upper arm and is highly effective for 3 years. It can be placed in outpatient offices and is helpful in reducing dysmenorrhea, but it is associated with irregular menses.

Postcoital emergency contraception (EC) can be achieved with one or several hormonal options or with placement of a copper IUD. EC is not considered an abortifacient. It functions to either disrupt ovulation or prevent fertilization. The copper IUD is the most effective option and can be used within 5 days of unprotected intercourse. Hormonal oral contraceptives can be used in a specifically formulated EC dose (Plan B) or off-label with a regimen of COCs. The recommendation is for use of Plan B within 72 hours of unprotected intercourse. It is available without a prescription. Efficacy of hormonal contraception decreases with increasing body mass index (BMI) above 25 kg/m². The only absolute contraindication to EC is pregnancy.

INFERTILITY

According to the Centers for Disease Control (CDC), 12% of US women have trouble conceiving. However, infertility is a unique medical condition in that it involves a couple rather than an individual. Infertility is a failure to conceive after 1 year of regular intercourse without contraception in women under age 35 or 6 months in women 35 years and older. The term fecundability is the probability of achieving pregnancy in one menstrual cycle. Impaired fecundity describes women who have difficulty getting pregnant or carrying a pregnancy to term. It is unclear if the prevalence of infertility has changed or if the heightened awareness of infertility is due to the combination of factors such as deferment of pregnancy to later in life, technological advances, and increase in awareness of infertility. Causes of infertility are likely varied among different demographic and socioeconomic groups.

Infertility may be caused by female factors, male factors or both. Approximately 20% to 30% of couples experience unexplained infertility. History should focus on menstrual and contraceptive history, surgeries, sexual dysfunction, medications, and family history of early menopause or reproductive issues. The physical exam should include a thyroid, breast and pelvic exam. The most common female cause is a problem involving ovulation (20% to 35%), followed by tubal disease (20% to 25%) and uterine factors (5% to 15%). Ovulatory dysfunction can be evaluated from patient report, but up to one third of women with normal menses are anovulatory; therefore, objective measures can be used to confirm ovulation with progesterone and LH levels, evaluation of cervical mucus and basal body temperature. Testing also typically includes TSH, FSH, and prolactin levels in women with irregular menses. Initial male evaluation includes semen analysis and a reproductive history. Further testing is performed by reproductive specialists and may include evaluation of ovarian reserve through a transvaginal ultrasound and hysterosalpingography to visualize the uterus and fallopian tubes and ensure tubal patency. The diagnosis of infertility is associated with significant stress for most couples and a provider's awareness can help to mitigate its effects.

PREGNANCY COMPLICATIONS AND RISK OF FUTURE DISEASES

During pregnancy, a woman is typically primarily cared for by her obstetrics provider. However, women with complex medical conditions or pregnancy complications may require a maternal fetal

水平，因此停用贴剂后可立刻恢复生育能力。

阴道避孕环需在阴道中放置 3 周，然后取出 1 周，以出现撤退性出血。也可在取出前一个环的同一天放入 1 个新环，以延长阴道避孕环的疗程。这种方式可每 3 周进行 1 次，最多持续 1 年，从而延迟撤退性出血，但可能发生阴道点滴出血。如果患者对每日服药有顾虑，贴剂和阴道避孕环是合理的选择。

复方激素避孕的禁忌证与其中的雌激素成分有关，包括既往血栓栓塞事件或有已知的致血栓形成突变、脑血管意外、冠状动脉疾病、未控制的高血压、偏头痛先兆、35 岁后吸烟、乳腺癌、雌激素依赖性肿瘤、未确诊的异常阴道出血、肝脏肿瘤和妊娠。尚无证据表明 COC 会导致体重增加。开始使用 COC 时，部分患者会出现乳房触痛、恶心和腹胀。大多数症状在继续服药的过程中很快消失。不规则出血通常在 3 个月内消退。如果在月经来潮后 5 天以上才开始使用 COC，建议初始的 7 天同时使用其他避孕方式。

COC 的潜在非避孕获益包括调节月经量、减少卵巢囊肿复发、改善子宫内膜异位症、慢性盆腔疼痛、痤疮、多囊卵巢综合征、高雄激素血症和经间期疼痛（即月经中期疼痛）。长期使用 COC 与降低子宫内膜癌和卵巢癌的终身风险有关。与未使用过 COC 的女性相比，使用过 COC 的女性在围绝经期的骨密度更高。

对于雌激素不耐受或血栓栓塞风险较高的女性，可考虑使用仅含孕激素的避孕药。这些药物可以连续服用，无需停药间隔。禁忌证包括冠状动脉疾病活动期、乳腺癌、肝脏肿瘤和静脉炎。它们的疗效略弱于复方避孕药，患者可能会出现突破性出血。仅含孕激素的避孕药的药效持续时间和半衰期较短，因此必须在每天的同一时间服用。如果服药时间延迟 3 h 以上，需要使用备用避孕方式。停药后，生育能力可迅速恢复。与 COC 相比，使用这类药物后排卵不会持续受抑制。

长效醋酸甲羟孕酮（DMPA）是一种仅含孕激素的注射剂，每 12 周注射 1 次。主要副作用包括不规则出血（随着时间的推移而消退）和闭经（1 年时的发生率约为 50%）。体重增加、毛发变化和痤疮也是可能的副作用。FDA 曾发布过黑框警告，提示 DMPA 可能降低骨密度，特别是在青春期和围绝经期女性中。由于没有确凿的数据，DMPA 的使用与骨折风险的关联仍存在争议；一项回顾性队列研究显示，骨折风险并没有显著差异。患者生育能力恢复的时间受体重影响：体重较轻的女性在停药后更快实现妊娠。如果在启动避孕的 1 ~ 2 年有生育需求，则不建议使用 DMPA。

对于未来 5 ~ 10 年没有生育需求的女性，宫内节育器（IUD）是一个很好的选择。它是全球使用最广泛的可逆性避孕方法。美国有两类 IUD：含铜 IUD 和释放孕激素的 IUD（译者注：IUD 中均为合成孕激素，而非天然孕激素，原文 progesterone 一词有误），两类 IUD 的有效性均与绝育相当。含铜 IUD 可放置 10 年。美国有 4 种释放孕激素的 IUD，根据配方的不同可放置 3 ~ 5 年不等。

含铜 IUD 可能与月经过多和腹部痉挛痛有关。释放孕激素的 IUD 在置入初期可能出现突破性出血，但几乎 1/2 的使用者会出现闭经。取出 IUD 后，生育能力可迅速恢复。

孕激素皮下埋植剂包括最初上市的依托孕烯植入剂和现有的 Nexplanon，后者不透射线。孕激素皮下埋植剂是一根 40 mm 长的含有孕激素的小棒，被植入上臂皮下后有效期可达 3 年。放置皮下埋植剂的操作可在门诊进行，放置后有助于减轻痛经，但与月经不规律相关。

性交后的紧急避孕（EC）方式包括激素（使用 1 种或多种）和放置含铜 IUD。EC 不被视作堕胎药，其作用机制是干扰排卵或阻止受精。含铜 IUD 是最有效的方式，可在无保护性交后 5 天内使用。激素口服避孕药可使用特殊的 EC 剂量（计划 B），或采取超说明书用药的 COC 方案。建议在无保护性交后 72 h 内使用计划 B，无需处方即可获得。体重指数（BMI）> 25 kg/m^2 者，激素避孕的有效性会降低。EC 的唯一绝对禁忌证是妊娠。

不孕症

根据美国疾病预防控制中心（CDC）的数据，12% 的美国女性难以受孕。然而，不孕症是一种独特的疾病，它涉及夫妇双方，而不是单一个体。不孕症是指 < 35 岁的女性未避孕且规律性交 1 年仍未受孕，或 ≥ 35 岁的女性未避孕且规律性交 6 个月仍未受孕。生育能力是指在 1 个月经周期内妊娠的概率。生育能力受损是指难以妊娠或无法足月妊娠的女性。目前尚不明确不孕症的患病率是否发生了变化，也不清楚大众对不孕症的认知是否因妊娠年龄推迟和技术进步等因素的共同作用而提高。不孕症的病因在具有不同人口学特征和社会经济地位的人群中可能有所不同。

不孕症的病因包括女方因素、男方因素或男女双方因素。20% ~ 30% 的夫妇面临不明原因的不孕症。病史采集应关注月经情况、避孕史、手术史、性功能障碍、用药情况、早绝经或生育问题的家族史。体格检查应包括甲状腺、乳房和盆腔检查。不孕症最常见的女方原因是排卵问题（20% ~ 35%），其次是输卵管疾病（20% ~ 25%）和子宫因素（5% ~ 15%）。排卵功能障碍可根据患者的描述进行评估，但多达 1/3 的月经正常的女性其实并未排卵。因此，可通过客观指标来确认有无排卵，如孕激素和 LH 水平、宫颈黏液评估和基础体温测定。针对月经失调女性的实验室检查通常还包括 TSH、FSH 和催乳素水平。针对男方的初步评估包括精液分析和生育史采集。进一步的检查应由生殖医学专家进行，可能包括经阴道超声（评估卵巢功能储备）、子宫输卵管造影（观察子宫和输卵管并确保输卵管通畅）。不孕症的诊断会给多数夫妇带来巨大的心理压力，医生知晓这一点有助于减小诊断带来的负面影响。

妊娠并发症及未来疾病风险

孕妇通常由产科医生照护，但患有复杂疾病或出

medicine (MFM) specialist or an obstetric medicine specialist to participate in their care. MFM is a specialty in obstetrics and gynecology that manages high-risk pregnancies as well as unexpected complications in pregnancy such as a trauma to the mother, early labor, and bleeding. Obstetric medicine is a specialty of internal medicine that manages medical problems in pregnancy such as hypertension, kidney disease, thyroid disease, diabetes mellitus, and heart disease.

Pregnancy can be associated with exacerbations of chronic illnesses, unmasking a new illness or predicting future disease. An understanding of the long-term consequences of certain complications in pregnancy can smooth the transition back to primary care.

Gestational diabetes affects 4% to 8% of pregnancies in the United States. All pregnant women receiving routine obstetric care are screened for gestational diabetes. Women with a history of gestational diabetes are at increased risk for diabetes later in life. They should be screened 6 to 12 weeks postpartum with an oral glucose tolerance test and diagnosed with nonpregnancy diagnostic criteria for diabetes. They should have lifelong screening at least every 3 years.

Women whose pregnancies were complicated by a gestational hypertensive disorder, such as preeclampsia or gestational hypertension, are at increased risk for subsequent essential hypertension. A history of preeclampsia is associated with twice the risk of heart disease and stroke and four times the risk of hypertension. Currently, there are no additional screening or preventive interventions recommended for these women.

MENOPAUSE

Menopause is defined as the absence of a menstrual period for 12 consecutive months or the cessation of the menstrual cycle due to oophorectomy. The average age at menopause in the United States is 51 years, with a range of 40 to 58 years. Natural menopause prior to the age of 40 is considered premature ovarian failure. Menopause after the age of 55 is considered late menopause. The life expectancy of women in the United States is almost 80 years; therefore, many women spend at least one third of their lifetime in the postmenopausal period. Although symptoms such as hot flashes and vaginal dryness may develop during menopause, the process itself is a normal part of aging for women.

Transition From Perimenopause to Menopause

The transition to menopause can be erratic and prolonged over a 5- to 10-year period. It is characterized by ovarian and endocrine changes that ultimately result in the depletion of primordial oocyte stores and the cessation of ovarian estrogen production. An accelerated loss of follicles begins at about 37 years of age and is correlated with a small increase in FSH and a decrease in inhibin levels. As the FSH concentration increases, the follicular phase of the cycle decreases. One of the earliest clinical signs of the menopausal transition is shortening of the menstrual cycle from a mean length of 30 days in the early reproductive years to 25 days in the early menopausal transition.

Later in the menopausal transition, the few remaining follicles respond poorly to FSH, and anovulation may occur. Menstrual cycles may become erratic with prolonged periods of oligomenorrhea. Ovulation may still occur, and women in this time period are advised to continue effective contraception until 12 months of amenorrhea have occurred. Ultimately, when ovarian follicles are depleted, the ovary no longer secretes estradiol but continues to secrete androgens due to continued stimulation by LH.

Perimenopausal Symptoms

Menstrual irregularities are experienced by almost 75% of women and are usually the first change noticed by women entering the menopausal transition. Although changes in the menstrual flow are expected and

most women can be reassured, clinicians need to be aware of bleeding patterns that may represent underlying pathology and require evaluation.

Sleep disturbances in perimenopausal women are a well-documented phenomenon. Hot flashes can disturb sleep patterns and interfere with sleep quality, resulting in fatigue, irritability, and difficulty concentrating. Vaginal dryness and dyspareunia are common symptoms that can interfere with sexual function and increase the risk of urinary tract infections. Another genitourinary symptom that increases with age is urinary incontinence, which affects approximately 25% of postmenopausal women. The etiology is multifactorial. The endothelium of the bladder and urethra become more fragile and less elastic; urethral tone decreases with age. Uterine prolapse, cystoceles, rectoceles, and increasing BMI all increase the risk of urinary incontinence.

Change in mood is a common complaint during the menopausal transition, but a causative link between hormonal fluctuations and mood disturbances has not been established. Women who experience significant depression around menopause are more likely to have experienced depression earlier in their lives, particularly at times of hormonal change (e.g., postpartum depression, premenstrual dysphoric disorder [PMDD]). Mood issues during the perimenopausal transition should be approached in the same manner as at other ages.

In addition to mood symptoms, many women in perimenopause complain of difficulties with concentration and memory. A large multisite, multiethnic cohort study, the Study of Women's Health Across the Nation (SWAN), demonstrated that women had a small, transient decline in cognitive abilities during perimenopause. However, anxiety and depression also had independent negative effects on cognition. Most epidemiologic studies do not demonstrate an increased risk of depression or a decline in cognitive skills during the menopausal transition.

Hot flashes or vasomotor symptoms are the hallmark symptom of menopause. In the United States, up to 75% of women who experience a natural menopause and 90% of women who experience surgical menopause have vasomotor symptoms. Hot flashes may occur a few times per year or several times each day; 10% to 15% of women have hot flashes that are very frequent or severe. For most women, vasomotor symptoms are self-limited, lasting on average 1 to 2 years; however, up to 25% of women may have symptoms for longer than 5 years.

The exact cause of a hot flash is not understood, although it is related to a disturbance of hypothalamic thermoregulation. A hot flash consists of a sudden onset of a warm sensation over the face and upper body that ranges from mild to markedly uncomfortable. This may be accompanied by significant perspiration and typically lasts 2 to 4 minutes. It can be followed by chills. There are racial and ethnic differences in reported hot flashes, with African American women experiencing higher rates compared with white women and Hispanic and Asian women experiencing lower rates. Frequency of hot flashes is also affected by smoking, obesity, and stress.

In the 1950s, the use of estrogen to relieve hot flashes became widespread. In 1975, a study published in the *New England Journal of Medicine* showed that women who used estrogen for more than 7 years had a 14-fold increase in uterine cancer. Subsequent research determined that the increased risk of endometrial hyperplasia and uterine cancer is reduced to essentially zero when concurrent low-dose progestin is continued for 12 to 13 days per month. Women on estrogen with an intact uterus must use progestin therapy to prevent endometrial hyperplasia and cancer.

Menopausal hormone therapy (MHT) is the use of estrogen or combined estrogen and progestin for women with an intact uterus. MHT remains the most effective treatment of menopausal vasomotor symptoms. It is also FDA approved for the treatment of urogenital

现妊娠并发症的孕妇可能需要母胎医学（MFM）专家或产科内科学专家参与诊疗。MFM 是妇产科的一个亚专业，负责处理高危妊娠和妊娠期意外并发症，如母亲外伤、早产和出血。产科内科学是内科的一个亚专业，负责处理妊娠期的内科问题，如高血压、肾病、甲状腺疾病、糖尿病和心脏病。

妊娠可能与慢性疾病恶化、新发疾病显露或预测未来疾病有关。了解特定妊娠并发症的长期结局有助于患者平稳过渡至初级医疗保健机构。

在美国，4%～8% 的妊娠女性会出现妊娠期糖尿病。所有接受产检的孕妇均应进行妊娠期糖尿病筛查。有妊娠期糖尿病病史的女性后续患糖尿病的风险增加，因此应在产后 6～12 周接受口服葡萄糖耐量试验筛查，并根据非妊娠糖尿病诊断标准进行诊断。此后，应至少每 3 年进行 1 次筛查，并持续终身。

患有妊娠期高血压相关疾病（如先兆子痫或妊娠期高血压）的孕妇后续患原发性高血压的风险增加。有先兆子痫病史的女性患心脏病和卒中的风险是无病史女性的两倍，患高血压的风险是无病史女性的 4 倍。目前，尚无针对这些患者进行额外筛查或预防干预的建议。

绝经

绝经是指连续 12 个月无月经来潮或由于卵巢切除术导致月经周期停止。美国女性绝经的平均年龄是 51 岁，范围为 40～58 岁。40 岁之前自然绝经被认为是卵巢早衰。55 岁之后绝经被认为是绝经晚。美国女性的预期寿命接近 80 岁；因此，许多女性一生中至少有 1/3 的时间处于绝经后期。虽然绝经过程中可能会出现潮热和阴道干燥等症状，但绝经本身是女性衰老的正常阶段。

围绝经期过渡到绝经

绝经过渡期长度不稳定，持续时间可达 5～10 年。其特征是卵巢和内分泌功能改变，最终导致原始卵母细胞储备耗竭，卵巢停止产生雌激素。约从 37 岁开始，卵泡丢失加速，与 FSH 水平的小幅升高和抑制素水平的下降有关。随着 FSH 浓度升高，月经周期的卵泡期缩短，月经周期从育龄期的平均 30 天缩短到绝经过渡期早期的 25 天，这是绝经过渡期最早的临床标志之一。

在绝经过渡期后期，残余的少量卵泡对 FSH 反应不佳，可能会出现无排卵。月经周期可能变得不稳定，月经稀发的时间延长。由于仍有可能发生排卵，故建议此时期的女性继续采取有效的避孕措施，直至停经 12 个月。最终，当卵泡耗尽时，卵巢不再分泌雌激素，但由于 LH 的持续作用，卵巢会继续分泌雄激素。

围绝经期症状

近 75% 的围绝经期女性会经历月经失调，这通常是女性进入绝经过渡期时最早注意到的变化。虽然月经量的变化在预料之中，多数女性可以对此感到放心，但临床医生应考虑出血模式可能提示存在潜在疾病，需要进一步评估。

围绝经期女性的睡眠障碍是一种常见现象。潮热会扰乱睡眠模式，影响睡眠质量，导致疲劳、易怒和注意力难以集中。阴道干燥和性交困难是常见症状，会影响性功能并增加尿路感染的风险。另一种随年龄增长而增加的泌尿生殖道症状是尿失禁，可见于约 25% 的绝经后女性。尿失禁由多因素所致：膀胱和尿道的上皮（译者注：原文 endothelium 应为 epithelium）变得更脆弱，弹性降低；尿道张力随年龄增长而降低；子宫脱垂、膀胱膨出、直肠膨出和 BMI 升高均会增加尿失禁的风险。

情绪变化是绝经过渡期的常见症状，但激素波动和情绪变化之间的因果关系尚未确立。围绝经期表现出严重抑郁症状的患者更可能是有抑郁症病史的患者，特别是既往在激素变化时期出现过抑郁症［如产后抑郁、经前焦虑症（PMDD）］的患者。围绝经期情绪问题的处理方式与其他年龄段人群相同。

除了情绪症状外，许多围绝经期女性还会表现出注意力难以集中和记忆力减退。一项大型多中心、多种族队列研究（SWAN 试验）表明，女性的认知功能在围绝经期会出现短暂小幅下降。然而，焦虑和抑郁症状也会对认知功能产生独立的负面影响。大多数流行病学研究并未发现围绝经期女性抑郁症风险增加或认知功能下降。

潮热或血管舒缩症状是绝经的标志性症状。在美国，高达 75% 的自然绝经女性和 90% 的手术绝经女性会出现血管舒缩症状。潮热可能每年发生数次或每天发生数次；10%～15% 女性的潮热发作非常频繁或非常严重。对于大多数女性，血管舒缩症状具有自限性，平均持续 1～2 年；然而，25% 女性的症状可能持续超过 5 年。

尽管潮热被认为与下丘脑体温调节紊乱有关，但其确切病因尚不清楚。潮热是指面部和上半身突然出现热感，程度可从轻微到非常不适，可能伴有大量出汗，通常持续 2～4 min，随后可能发冷。潮热存在种族差异，非裔美国女性的潮热发生率高于美国白人女性，而西班牙裔和亚洲裔女性的潮热发生率较低。吸烟、肥胖症和压力也会影响潮热发生的频率。

20 世纪 50 年代，雌激素被广泛用于缓解潮热症状。1975 年，《新英格兰医学杂志》发表的一项研究表明，使用雌激素超过 7 年的女性患子宫内膜癌的概率增加了 14 倍。后续研究发现，当每月同时使用低剂量孕激素 12～13 天时，子宫内膜增生和子宫癌症的风险基本不会增加。子宫完整的患者在使用雌激素时必须同时使用孕激素治疗，以预防子宫内膜增生和子宫癌症。

绝经激素治疗（MHT）是指对子宫完整的女性使用雌激素或雌孕激素联合治疗。MHT 仍然是治疗绝经期血管舒缩症状最有效的治疗。FDA 还批准其用于治疗泌尿生殖道萎缩和预防骨质疏松症。有证据表明，超低剂量的雌激素足以防止骨质流失。虽然 FDA 尚未

atrophy and the prevention of osteoporosis. Evidence suggests that ultra-low-dose estrogen is sufficient to prevent bone loss. Although not FDA approved for treatment of osteoporosis, there is some research supporting its use in preventing fractures and increasing bone density.

Early epidemiologic studies demonstrated a decrease in coronary heart disease (CHD) events in women on MHT. However, the opposite conclusion was found in dedicated randomized trials. One large study demonstrated an overall null effect but an increased number of CHD events in the first year of treatment. Another large randomized controlled trial to evaluate MHT was stopped early because there was more harm than benefit with the treatment intervention. Therefore, menopausal hormone therapy is not recommended for primary prevention of CHD or chronic disease.

Postmenopausal Therapy
Hormone Therapy

Estrogen and estrogen-progestin therapy are appropriate and the most effective treatment for moderate to severe vasomotor symptoms. If hormone therapy is initiated, the lowest dose needed to treat the symptoms should be used and usually for short-term use. Women with a uterus require progesterone and estrogen. Combination MHT is recommended for 3 to 5 years total if initiated and limited by the increased risk of breast cancer. Estrogen-only therapy has a more favorable risk profile and can be used for 7 years in women without a uterus. Oral contraceptives can be used for management of menopausal symptoms for women who require contraception until age 51. The estrogen dose in oral contraceptives is 4 to 7 times higher than in MHT, and thus the use of COCs confers an unnecessary risk to postmenopausal women. One recommendation on determining ability to transition from oral contraception to MHT is to check FSH levels at age 50 to evaluate for menopause. Estrogen administration can be oral, transdermal, or topical. There are some minor differences in their risk profile. For example, transdermal estrogen is associated with decreases in blood pressure compared to oral administration. When administered transdermally, estrogen bypasses liver metabolism resulting in decreased angiotensin production thereby lowering blood pressure. MHT needs to be tapered when stopping because abrupt cessation could cause a recurrence of symptoms.

For women who have primarily vaginal symptoms such as vaginal dryness or urogenital atrophy, referred to as "genitourinary symptoms of menopause," estrogen can be used transvaginally. Transvaginal estrogen can be high dose, in which case it has the risk profile of systemic oral or transdermal MHT. Low-dose transvaginal estrogen does not require progesterone in women who have a uterus and does not confer the same risks as systemic estrogen. For example, the low-dose estrogen ring releases 7.5 mcg of estradiol daily compared to the high dose ring that releases 50 to 100 mcg daily and is considered systemic estrogen.

Nonhormonal Therapies

During the 1990s, newer antidepressants that affect serotonin and/or norepinephrine (SSRIs and SNRIs) were observed to improve hot flashes. Randomized controlled trials studying the effects of SSRIs and SNRIs on vasomotor symptoms have demonstrated varied efficacy, but a large meta-analysis and systemic review found all SSRIs were more effective than placebo; escitalopram was found to be the most effective. However, the only FDA-approved nonhormonal treatment for hot flashes is paroxetine.

Gabapentin and pregabalin have also been demonstrated to decrease intensity and frequency of hot flashes. One study found the efficacy of gabapentin to be comparable to SSRIs. Clonidine is another nonhormonal option but is considered second line because it

is typically poorly tolerated due to dizziness and dry mouth. In practice, the SSRIs/SNRIs and gabapentin/pregabalin are commonly used off-label given demonstrated efficacy.

Complementary Therapy

As many as 75% of menopausal women have used some form of alternative or complementary treatment to relieve menopausal symptoms. Behavioral options such as dressing in layers, regular exercise, stress reduction techniques, and avoidance of known triggers are safe and may be helpful for many women. Cognitive behavioral therapy has also been demonstrated to be modestly effective. Some of the more common herbal remedies for menopausal symptoms include isoflavones and phytoestrogens (e.g., soy, chickpeas, red clover) and black cohosh. None of these therapies has been shown to decrease hot flashes beyond placebo.

BREAST PAIN, DISCHARGE, AND MASSES

Breast pain, masses, and nipple discharge are common symptoms that providers face when taking care of female patients. Women who present with breast symptoms often fear that any abnormality indicates the presence of malignancy. Although it is essential to keep breast cancer on the differential diagnosis throughout the clinical evaluation, most breast-related complaints are not manifestations of cancer. For example, in recent studies, breast pain was a presenting symptom in close to 6% of women who had breast cancer, whereas 70% of women report breast pain over the course of their lifetime.

Mastalgia

Breast pain can originate from the breast tissue itself, which is termed "true mastalgia," or appear as referred pain from the chest wall. Chest wall pain is often isolated to the medial or lateral side of the breast. Intercostal nerves originating from T3 to T5 innervate the breast and nipple. Any irritation along their course can lead to pain experienced in the breast. Causes of nerve irritation include cervical and thoracic spondylosis, lung disease, and gallstones.

True mastalgia is often classified as cyclical or non-cyclical pain. Etiologies of non-cyclical pain include trauma, mastitis, superficial thrombophlebitis, cysts or tumors. Cyclical breast pain is the most common type of breast pain and is hormone dependent. The onset of pain occurs during the weeks before menstruation, and the start of menstruation marks resolution. A unifying etiology of cyclical breast pain remains unclear. Studies demonstrate that progesterone, prolactin, ratio of fatty acids, and type of estrogen receptors may play a role. The presence of breast pain in women on hormone replacement therapy suggests that hormones have a causative impact; however, hormone manipulation rather than concentration of estrogen appears to influence the occurrence of pain. Amount of caffeine intake has not been shown to have any impact on developing mastalgia, despite popular belief.

Evaluation of mastalgia often consists of age-appropriate breast cancer screening. Focal pain and pain that is progressively worsening may warrant further imaging. Unfortunately, obtaining a history of symptoms that follow a cyclical versus non-cyclical pattern has not proven to help differentiate between etiologies of pain.

Research shows that most women presenting with mastalgia respond well to reassurance. Adjustments in type of brassiere or additional breast support during the night can improve pain levels. Treatments with proven effectiveness for cyclical pain include danazol, tamoxifen, progestogen, and progesterone, as well as non-hormone–based therapies including selective serotonin reuptake inhibitors and the fruit extract agnus castus. Use of therapies such as danazol and

批准其用于骨质疏松症的治疗，但一些研究结果支持其用于预防骨折和增加骨密度。

早期流行病学研究表明，使用 MHT 的女性的冠心病事件减少，但随机对照试验得到了相反的结论。一项大型研究表明，治疗 1 年时患者的冠心病事件增加，但未达到统计学显著差异。另一项评估 MHT 的大型随机对照试验因干预结果弊大于利而提前终止。因此，不推荐为了预防冠心病或慢性疾病而使用 MHT。

绝经后治疗

激素治疗

雌激素和雌孕激素治疗是中重度血管舒缩症状最恰当且最有效的治疗方法。如果开始激素治疗，应使用最低有效剂量，并通常短期使用。有子宫的女性需同时使用雌激素和孕激素。受乳腺癌风险增加的限制，建议雌孕激素联合治疗的总时间不超过 3 ～ 5 年。仅含雌激素的治疗风险更低，无子宫的女性可使用 7 年（译者注：参照《国际绝经学会 2016 版指南》《北美绝经协会 2022 年激素治疗立场声明》和《中国绝经管理与绝经激素治疗指南 2023 版》，MHT 的使用期限无特殊限制，长期使用应规范随访）。对于 51 岁前有避孕需求的女性，可使用口服避孕药来缓解绝经症状。口服避孕药中雌激素的剂量比 MHT 高 4 ～ 7 倍，因此口服避孕药会给绝经后女性带来不必要的风险。建议在 50 岁时检测 FSH 水平评估绝经状态，以判断能否从口服避孕药过渡到 MHT。雌激素给药方式包括口服、经皮或局部给药。不同给药方式的风险略有差异。例如，与口服相比，经皮给药与血压下降相关。这是由于经皮给药的雌激素会避开肝脏代谢，导致血管紧张素生成减少，从而降低血压。MHT 应逐渐停药，突然停药可能会导致症状复发。

对于以阴道症状为主的女性，可以经阴道使用雌激素。阴道症状又被称为绝经泌尿生殖症状，包括阴道干涩和泌尿生殖道萎缩等。经阴道使用大剂量雌激素时，其风险情况与 MHT 全身给药或经皮给药相似。对于有子宫的女性，经阴道使用低剂量雌激素不会带来全身应用雌激素的风险，无须同时使用孕激素。例如，低剂量雌激素环每天释放 7.5 μg 雌二醇，而高剂量雌激素环每天释放 50 ～ 100 μg 雌二醇，后者等同于全身应用雌激素的剂量。

非激素治疗

在 20 世纪 90 年代，研究发现影响 5- 羟色胺和（或）去甲肾上腺素的抗抑郁药可以改善潮热症状，如选择性 5- 羟色胺再摄取抑制剂（SSRI）和 5- 羟色胺去甲肾上腺素再摄取抑制剂（SNRI）。随机对照试验表明，SSRI 和 SNRI 对血管舒缩症状的疗效不同，但大型荟萃分析和系统综述显示，所有 SSRI 均比安慰剂更有效，其中艾司西酞普兰最有效。但是，帕罗西汀是唯一经 FDA 批准用于治疗潮热的非激素类药物。

加巴喷丁和普瑞巴林也被证实可降低潮热的程度和频率。一项研究发现，加巴喷丁的疗效与 SSRI 相当。可乐定是另一种非激素类药物，但患者常因其头晕和口干的副作用而耐受不良，故被认为是二线选择。由于 SSRI/SNRI 和加巴喷丁 / 普瑞巴林已被证明有效，故在临床实践中经常超说明书用药。

其他治疗

多达 75% 的绝经女性使用某种形式的其他治疗来缓解绝经症状。多穿衣物、规律运动、缓解压力、避免已知诱因等行为干预措施是安全的，且对于许多女性是有效的。认知行为疗法也被证明有一定效果。一些常用于缓解绝经症状的草药，包括异黄酮类、植物雌激素类（如大豆、鹰嘴豆、红三叶草）和黑升麻，均未被证实能比安慰剂更有效地减轻潮热。

乳房疼痛、乳头溢液和肿物

乳房疼痛、乳头溢液和肿物是女性常见的症状。出现乳房症状的女性常担心患有乳腺癌。虽然乳腺癌是临床评估过程中必不可少的鉴别诊断，但大多数乳房相关主诉不是癌症的临床表现。例如，近期研究表明，只有约 6% 的乳腺癌女性患者表现为乳房疼痛，而 70% 的女性在一生中出现过乳房疼痛。

乳房疼痛

乳房疼痛可能源自乳房本身，即真性乳房疼痛，也可能是来自胸壁的牵涉痛。胸壁疼痛通常局限于乳房的内侧或外侧。起源于 T3 ～ T5 的肋间神经支配乳房和乳头。在神经走行区域的任何刺激均可导致乳房疼痛的感觉。神经刺激的原因包括颈椎病、胸椎病、肺部疾病和胆石症。

真性乳房疼痛通常被分为周期性疼痛和非周期性疼痛。非周期性疼痛的原因包括创伤、乳腺炎、浅表血栓性静脉炎、囊肿或肿瘤。周期性乳房疼痛是最常见的类型，且呈激素依赖性，从月经来潮前数周开始，在月经来潮时缓解。其潜在病因仍不明确。研究发现，孕激素、催乳素、脂肪酸比例和雌激素受体类型可能在发病机制中发挥作用。接受 MHT 的女性出现乳房疼痛提示激素与乳房疼痛存在因果关系；但是，影响疼痛发生的似乎是激素控制，而不是雌激素浓度。虽然人们普遍认为咖啡因摄入会对乳房疼痛产生影响，但事实并非如此。

乳房疼痛的评估通常包括适合年龄的乳腺癌筛查。局部疼痛和疼痛进行性加重提示需要进一步行影像学检查。遗憾的是，周期性疼痛或非周期性疼痛的症状史不能帮助鉴别疼痛的病因。

研究表明，大多数表现出乳房疼痛的女性对安抚的反应良好。调整胸罩类型或在夜间增加乳房支撑可缓解疼痛。经证实的对周期性乳房疼痛有效的治疗包括达那唑、他莫昔芬、孕激素和黄体酮，以及非激素治疗（如 SSRI

tamoxifen are limited by side effects of the medications. NSAIDS and steroid injections have been effective in managing chest wall pain.

Nipple Discharge

Based on history and examination, nipple discharge can be classified into three categories to guide evaluation and management. If the discharge is serous, sanguineous, or serosanguineous, spontaneously occurring, unilateral, originating from a single duct, and found to be reproducible on examination, then a mammogram and ultrasound are recommended for women over 30. An ultrasound is recommended as initial evaluation for women under 30. If the discharge is milky and bilateral, then a pregnancy test followed by a work-up for galactorrhea should be initiated. Work-up includes measuring TSH and prolactin levels. In women over 40, if the discharge is nonspontaneous, originates from multiple ducts, and cannot be characterized as serous, sanguineous, or serosanguineous, a diagnostic mammography plus ultrasonography is recommended. For women younger than 40, observation and education around avoiding nipple manipulation is appropriate. In summary, nipple discharge suggestive of malignancy occurs without provocation, is persistent, unilateral, presents in an older patient, is of serous, sanguineous, or serosanguineous quality or is associated with a mass or lump.

Breast Masses

There are four categories of breast masses: abscesses, benign masses, benign tumors, and cancer. Benign masses are further subdivided into categories of nonproliferative (i.e., cyst), proliferative without atypia (i.e., fibroadenoma), and atypical hyperplasia, which guide further evaluation and predict risk of becoming malignant. Cancerous masses are typically painless, occur in older women, and do not vary by menstrual cycle. Although breast cancers have characteristically been described as hard and immobile with irregular borders, no self or clinical examination finding reliably distinguishes between a benign and cancerous mass.

For women over 30, any palpable mass requires a diagnostic mammogram. Further diagnostic evaluation depends on a combination of radiographic qualities (i.e., solid vs. fluid filled) classified according to the Breast Imaging Reporting Data System (BI-RADS) and level of clinical suspicion. For example, if a mass gets a BI-RADS classification of 1, then an ultrasound is recommended. If it gets a BI-RADS classification of 4, then a tissue biopsy follows. For masses rated as BI-RADS 1 to 3, ultrasound findings in combination with clinical suspicion guide further evaluation versus observation. For women under 30, if clinical suspicion for malignancy is low, then a mass can be observed for several menstrual cycles. If clinical suspicion is high, then an ultrasound is the first line of imaging. BI-RADS from the ultrasound reading guides additional testing. If biopsies prove negative for malignancy or imaging determines that the mass is a cyst, masses are surgically removed and cysts aspirated only if the patient is symptomatic.

Breast Cancer Screening

Breast cancer is the most common type of cancer in women. Despite significant prevalence, it has a high survival rate of close to 90% at 5 years, which is attributed to early detection and effective treatment. Individuals are considered high risk for breast cancer if they have a personal history of breast cancer, a previous diagnosis of a high-risk breast lesion, a genetic mutation associated with risk for developing breast cancer, or if they have received radiation therapy to the chest. Although other risk factors such as early menarche, late menopausal onset, oral contraceptive or menopausal hormone therapy, increased breast density on mammography, and family member with a history of breast cancer have been identified, they do not change an individual's

categorization as average or high risk according to most guidelines. Screening consists of a mammogram for average-risk patients and an MRI in addition to mammography for high-risk patients. Different medical societies and international health organizations offer different guidelines regarding the appropriate age to begin screening for breast cancer in average risk women. These guidelines shift based on the results of risk-benefit models and the current data available. Current recommendations from US Preventive Services Task Force (USPSTF) are for screening average-risk women at age 50 and continuing every 2 years until age 75 years. Shared decision making around starting screening between age 40 and 49 should take place between the patient and provider. The American College of Obstetrics and Gynecology, in contrast, recommends that screening should start at age 40. Harms from screening mammography include false-positive results that could lead to overdiagnosis and overtreatment. Self-exams and breast exams as part of a routine physical for the purpose of screening are no longer recommended by most medical societies.

CERVICAL CANCER SCREENING

Cervical cancer screening is an important example of success in preventative medicine over the second half of the last century: mortality rates decreased by 50% between 1975 and 2008. In women found to have cervical cancer, 50% percent of them had not undergone screening in the preceding 3 to 5 years. The success of screening rests on the fact that cervical cancer progresses slowly.

Infections with high-risk strains of HPV (16 and 18) are responsible for approximately 70% of cervical cancer cases. Peak incidence of HPV infection occurs among women younger than 25 years of age, but most of these infections are transient. Approximately 10% of women remain HPV positive 5 years after infection. Current guidelines recommend Papanicolaou (Pap) tests with cytology starting at age 21 to be repeated every 3 years if normal. At age 30, both cytology and HPV co-testing can be sent and if both are negative, then testing can be spaced to every 5 years until age 65. A Pap test obtains cervical cells that are analyzed for the presence of abnormal cells to identify squamous intraepithelial lesions (SIL). SIL identified in the cytological report mandates a cervical biopsy via colposcopy. Biopsy results are graded in terms of cervical intraepithelial lesion (CIN) 1, 2 or 3. Depending on grade, they are treated and then monitored for possible progression into cancer according to a different algorithm of surveillance than normal screening. In addition, recommendations for screening differ for women who have had diethylstilbestrol (DES) exposure in utero or for women who are immunocompromised. The CDC recommends vaccination for HPV starting at age 11 and 12 (see *CDC Vaccines and Preventable Diseases* for full recommendations).

OSTEOPOROSIS

Eighty percent of the ten million Americans with osteoporosis are women. The risk of osteoporosis increases with age. Estrogen is protective of bones and many women experience significant bone density loss in the 5 to 7 years after menopause. Approximately one in two women over the age of 50 will experience a bone fracture due to osteoporosis. These fractures are associated with significant morbidity and mortality both directly and indirectly related to the fracture, including acute myocardial infarction, pulmonary embolus, loss of independence, decreased quality of life, and multiple hospitalizations. Twenty-one percent to 30% of patients with a hip fracture die within 1 year.

The USPSTF recommends screening for osteoporosis in average risk white women age 65 and older with bone density evaluation. The most common method of bone density evaluation is dual-energy

和穗花牡荆果实提取物）。达那唑和他莫昔芬的使用受其副作用的限制。NSAID 和类固醇注射对控制胸壁疼痛有效。

乳头溢液

根据病史和检查，可将乳头溢液分为 3 类，从而指导评估和治疗。若溢液为浆液性、血性或浆液血性，自发溢出，单侧溢液，来自单一乳腺导管，且检查时反复出现，则 30 岁以上女性建议行乳腺 X 线摄影和超声检查；30 岁以下女性建议行超声检查作为初步评估。若溢液呈乳白色且为双侧，则应先进行妊娠试验，再进行溢乳检查，包括检测 TSH 和催乳素水平。对于 40 岁以上女性，若溢液非自发溢出，来自多个乳腺导管，且不是浆液性、血性或浆液血性，则建议进行诊断性乳腺 X 线摄影和超声检查；40 岁以下的女性应观察并宣教避免刺激乳头的相关内容。总之，提示恶性肿瘤的乳头溢液的特点包括无诱因、持续性、单侧；乳头溢液呈浆液性、血性或浆液血性；患者年龄较大；伴有肿物或包块。

乳腺肿物

乳腺肿物分为 4 类：脓肿、良性肿物、良性肿瘤和癌症。良性肿物可进一步分为非增生性肿物（即囊肿）、无不典型增生的增生性肿物（即纤维腺瘤）和不典型增生，可用于指导进一步评估并预测恶变的风险。癌性肿物通常呈无痛性，多见于年龄较大的女性，且不随月经周期而变化。虽然乳腺癌的特征是质硬、活动性差且边界不规则，但没有任何自我检查或临床检查结果能可靠地区分良性肿物和癌性肿物。

对于 30 岁以上的女性，任何可触及的肿物都需要进行诊断性乳腺 X 线摄影。进一步的诊断评估取决于基于乳腺影像学报告数据系统（BI-RADS）分类的影像学性质（即实性 vs. 液性）和临床怀疑程度。例如，若肿物为 BI-RADS 1 类，则建议进行超声检查；若为 BI-RADS 4 类，则应进行组织活检。对于 BI-RADS 1 ~ 3 类的肿物，超声检查结果结合临床可指导进一步评估或观察。对于 30 岁以下的女性，若临床怀疑恶性的可能性较低，则可观察数个月经周期。若临床高度怀疑，则超声检查是一线影像学检查。基于超声的 BI-RADS 可指导进一步检查。若活检证明无恶性肿瘤或影像学检查确定肿物为囊肿，则应手术切除肿物，只有在患者出现症状时才抽吸囊肿。

乳腺癌筛查

乳腺癌是女性最常见的癌症类型。尽管患病率高，但得益于早期发现和有效治疗，其 5 年生存率很高（接近 90%）。若有乳腺癌病史、曾被诊断为高危乳腺病变、有乳腺癌相关基因突变或曾接受胸部放疗，则被视为乳腺癌高危人群。其他危险因素包括初潮早、绝经晚、使用口服避孕药或绝经激素治疗史、乳腺 X 线摄影显示乳房密度增加、乳腺癌家族史等，但根据大多数指南，这些因素并不会改变个体的风险分类（一般风险或高风险）。一般风险患者的筛查选择乳腺 X 线摄影，高风险患者在此基础上还需进行 MRI。各专业学会和国际卫生组织针对一般风险的女性开始乳腺癌筛查的年龄给出了不同的建议。这些指南的变化是基于风险-效益模型的结果和现有数据。美国预防服务工作组（USPSTF）目前的建议是，一般风险的女性在 50 岁时开始筛查，之后每 2 年筛查 1 次，直到 75 岁。关于是否在 40 ~ 49 岁开始筛查，应由患者和医务人员共同决策。美国妇产科学会（ACOG）则建议应从 40 岁开始筛查。乳腺 X 线摄影筛查的危害是可能产生假阳性结果，这可能导致过度诊断和过度治疗。大多数学会不再推荐以筛查为目的的自我检查和常规体检进行乳房检查。

宫颈癌筛查

宫颈癌筛查是 20 世纪后半叶预防医学的一个重要的成功案例，它使得 1975—2008 年宫颈癌死亡率下降了 50%。在宫颈癌患者中，50% 在之前的 3 ~ 5 年没有接受过筛查。宫颈癌进展缓慢是筛查成功的基础。

约 70% 的宫颈癌病例是由感染高危型人乳头状瘤病毒（HPV）（16 型和 18 型）所致。HPV 感染的高峰期为 25 岁以前，但大多数感染呈一过性。约 10% 的女性在感染 5 年后 HPV 仍阳性。目前的指南建议从 21 岁开始进行巴氏染色涂片细胞学检查，若检查结果正常，则每 3 年复查 1 次。在 30 岁时，可进行细胞学和 HPV 联合检测，若均为阴性，则可间隔 5 年检测 1 次，直到 65 岁。巴氏染色涂片检查可分析获取的宫颈细胞中是否有异常细胞，以确定是否存在鳞状上皮内病变（SIL）。细胞学检查报告 SIL 需要进一步行阴道镜下宫颈活检。活检结果分为宫颈上皮内病变（CIN）1 级、2 级和 3 级。患者应基于分级接受相应治疗，然后根据与常规筛查不同的监测流程，对可能进展成癌症的情况进行监测。此外，对于既往宫内暴露己烯雌酚（DES）或免疫功能低下的女性，筛查建议有所不同。CDC 建议从 11 岁或 12 岁开始接种 HPV 疫苗（完整建议参见 *CDC Vaccines and Preventable Diseases*）。

骨质疏松症

在 1000 万患有骨质疏松症的美国人中，女性占 80%。骨质疏松症的风险随年龄的增长而增加。雌激素对骨骼具有保护作用，许多女性在绝经后 5 ~ 7 年会出现骨密度明显下降。约 1/2 的 50 岁以上女性会因骨质疏松症而骨折。这些骨折直接或间接地与严重并发症发生率和死亡率升高相关，包括急性心肌梗死、肺栓塞、丧失自理能力、生活质量下降和多次住院。21% ~ 30% 的髋部骨折患者会在 1 年内死亡。

USPSTF 建议对 ≥ 65 岁的一般风险白人女性进行骨密度检查，以筛查骨质疏松症。最常见的骨密度检查方

x-ray absorptiometry (DXA) of the hip and lumbar spine. Several risk assessment tools exist to evaluate a woman's risk of osteoporosis. The most commonly used is the FRAX tool. Risk factors for osteoporosis include a family history of hip fracture, smoking, long-term steroid use, and low body weight. Women younger than age 65 with at least one risk factor should have their osteoporosis risk assessed and then have bone density evaluation if their risk equals that of a 65-year-old white woman without risk factors. The recommendation is based on the risk of osteoporosis in white women because they have been historically the population studied. Ethnic background affects risk and management of osteoporosis, and racial minorities are diagnosed and treated less frequently. Women found to have osteoporosis who are treated have a moderate reduction in osteoporotic fracture. Treatment options include bisphosphonates, estrogen, and raloxifene. Individuals with osteopenia and osteoporosis are recommended to have adequate calcium and vitamin D intake through diet and/or supplements.

INTIMATE PARTNER VIOLENCE

IPV is a preventable public health problem that affects 1 in 4 American women during their lifetime. Nearly half of female homicide victims in the United States are killed by a current or former male intimate partner. IPV is any behavior that causes physical, sexual or psychological harm by a current or former intimate partner or spouse. There are numerous health consequences beyond the direct effects of IPV such as depression, anxiety disorders, chronic pain, and posttraumatic stress disorder (PTSD). Even when historical or physical examination clues are evident, IPV often remains undiagnosed by providers.

The USPSTF recommends that clinicians screen for IPV in women of childbearing age and refer women who screen positive to support services. The strongest evidence supporting screening is in women who are pregnant or postpartum, but the recommendation is to screen all women of childbearing age. There are several screening instruments to detect IPV. When screening for and discussing IPV, the clinician must be nonjudgmental, compassionate, and ensure confidentiality. Clinicians should normalize the screening interview with an explanation of IPV as an important health issue.

Identified risk factors for IPV victimization include younger age, female sex, lower SES, and a family history or personal history of violence. Suspicion for IPV should increase when there is a history of frequent emergency room visits, delay in seeking treatment, an inconsistent explanation of injuries, missed appointments, repeated abortions, late initiation of prenatal care or medication noncompliance. If a patient appears with an inappropriate affect, overly attentive or verbally abusive partner, apparent social isolation, and reluctance to undress or difficulty with examination of genitals or rectum, providers should further evaluate for IPV. Patients who are experiencing IPV present with a diverse range of complaints that include somatic and psychological symptoms as well as sexually transmitted infections. Women who screen positive for IPV should be evaluated for their risk of immediate harm. They should be provided with information about safety planning and a list of local and national resources.

OBESITY, METABOLIC SYNDROME, AND POLYCYSTIC OVARY SYNDROME

Obesity/Metabolic Syndrome

Rates of obesity (BMI >30) have increased in recent decades, yielding a rate of 40% in US adults in 2016. Overall, obesity appears to affect men and women equally, although the distribution by income varies by sex. Women in the lowest socioeconomic group have the highest rates of obesity. Men in the highest and lowest socioeconomic groups had a higher rate of obesity compared to the middle-income group. Obesity increases the risk for many diseases. In women, central obesity (waist-hip ratio >0.9) predicts the risk of CAD. The risk of many cancers (e.g., endometrial cancer, breast cancer, kidney cancer, ovarian cancer) is increased for obese individuals. Obesity has specific implications for women during pregnancy, increasing the risk of numerous pregnancy-related complications, including gestational diabetes mellitus, fetal macrosomia, hypertension, shoulder dystocia, and cesarean delivery, and contributes to postpartum complications such as thrombosis and infection. Obesity is also associated with irregular menses and higher rates of anovulation.

The risk of cardiovascular disease related to the metabolic syndrome appears to have a stronger correlation in women. There are several definitions of the metabolic syndrome. The most commonly used defines metabolic syndrome as the presence of three or more of five risk factors that increase the chance of developing heart disease or stroke: central obesity, elevated triglyceride levels, low levels of high-density lipoprotein (HDL) cholesterol, hypertension, and impaired fasting glucose values. Women with the metabolic syndrome should be monitored and counseled about their increased risk of cardiovascular events and overt diabetes mellitus.

Polycystic Ovary Syndrome

PCOS is a complex endocrine disorder without a known etiology that affects approximately 5% to 10% of women worldwide. The key diagnostic criteria are androgen excess, ovulatory dysfunction and/or polycystic ovaries. The most commonly used diagnostic criteria is the Rotterdam 2003 criteria which requires two out of three of the above criteria. Risk factors for PCOS include first-degree relatives with PCOS, diabetes mellitus, obesity, and certain ethnic groups such as Mexican Americans. Reproductive and metabolic effects include anovulation, infertility, acne, hirsutism, obesity, nonalcoholic fatty liver disease, and metabolic syndrome. Increased insulin resistance is a significant consequence of the syndrome, increasing the risk of type 2 diabetes, particularly in obese women. Therefore, women with a diagnosis of PCOS require screening for diabetes.

Management of PCOS is primarily symptom based. For women who are overweight or obese, lifestyle modifications are recommended. COCs are the first line in PCOS to regulate menses and decrease hyperandrogenism in women not attempting to conceive. After COCs, second-line treatment for hyperandrogenism is an antiandrogen such as spironolactone or finasteride. Insulin sensitivity can be increased with metformin and thiazolidinediones. Metformin also regulates menses. These medications are contraindicated during pregnancy, and an effective form of contraception is required because these medications are teratogenic. Women with PCOS often struggle to conceive. Ovulation-inducing medications such as clomiphene citrate or letrozole are frequently required. Women with PCOS are at increased risk for endometrial and ovarian cancers. COCs decrease risk for endometrial hyperplasia and may decrease risk of endometrial cancer.

FIBROMYALGIA

The prevalence of fibromyalgia ranges from 2% to 8% depending on the diagnostic criteria used. Historically, the diagnosis of fibromyalgia has been significantly more common in women. Original diagnostic criteria involved the quantity of tender points present on exam. Either women were likely to report more tender points or the symptom manifestation between women and men differed, which led to a disproportionate number of women with the condition as compared to

法是髋关节和腰椎双能 X 射线吸收法（DXA）。多种风险评估工具可用于评估女性患骨质疏松症的风险，其中最常用的是 FRAX 工具。骨质疏松症的危险因素包括髋部骨折家族史、吸烟、长期使用类固醇和体重过轻。< 65 岁且至少有 1 个危险因素的女性应进行骨质疏松症风险评估；若其风险与无危险因素的 65 岁白人女性相同，则应进行骨密度检查。该建议是基于白人女性的骨质疏松症风险，因为白人女性在既往研究中是主要的研究对象。种族背景会影响骨质疏松症的风险和管理，少数种族群体的诊断和治疗频率较低。接受治疗后，女性患者的骨质疏松性骨折发生率会适度降低。治疗方法包括双膦酸盐、雌激素和雷洛昔芬。建议骨量减少和骨质疏松症患者通过饮食和（或）补充剂摄入足够的钙和维生素 D。

亲密伴侣间暴力

　　亲密伴侣间暴力（IPV）是一个可预防的公共卫生问题，每 4 名美国女性中就有 1 名在其一生中受到 IPV 的影响。在美国，近 1/2 的女性凶杀案受害者是被现任或前任男性亲密伴侣杀害。IPV 是指现任或前任亲密伴侣或配偶造成躯体、性或心理伤害的任何行为。除了直接影响外，IPV 还有许多健康后果，如抑郁症、焦虑症、慢性疼痛和创伤后应激障碍（PTSD）。即使在病史或体格检查有明显线索的情况下，IPV 也通常没有被诊断。

　　USPSTF 建议临床医生对育龄期女性进行 IPV 筛查，并将筛查结果呈阳性的女性转诊至支持服务机构。目前最有力的证据支持对孕妇或产后女性进行筛查，但建议对所有育龄期女性进行筛查。多种筛查工具可用于识别 IPV。在筛查和讨论 IPV 时，临床医生必须不作评判、富有同情心并确保保密，应通过解释 IPV 是一个重要的健康问题使筛查访谈正常化。

　　已明确的 IPV 受害危险因素包括年龄较小、女性、社会经济地位较低、家族或个人暴力史。若患者有频繁的急诊就诊史、延迟就诊、对受伤的解释前后不一、错过就诊时间、反复人工流产、产检开始较晚或不遵医嘱用药，则应增加对 IPV 的怀疑。若患者表现出不适当的情绪、伴侣过分殷勤或存在语言暴力、明显的社会隔离、抗拒脱衣、检查生殖器或直肠困难，医务人员应进一步评估是否存在 IPV。遭受 IPV 的患者可能有多种主诉，包括躯体和心理症状及性传播感染。对于 IPV 筛查呈阳性的女性，应评估是否有受到直接伤害的风险。应向她们提供有关安全规划的信息及当地和国家资源清单。

肥胖症、代谢综合征与多囊卵巢综合征

肥胖症 / 代谢综合征

　　近几十年来，肥胖症（BMI > 30 kg/m^2）发病率不断上升，2016 年美国成人的肥胖症发病率为 40%。总体而言，肥胖症对男性和女性的影响相同，但收入对肥胖症的影响因性别而异。社会经济地位最低的女性的肥胖症发病率最高。与中等收入群体相比，社会经济地位最高和最低的男性的肥胖症发病率更高。肥胖症可增加许多疾病的风险。在女性中，向心性肥胖（腰臀比 > 0.9）可预测罹患冠状动脉疾病的风险。肥胖症患者中多种癌症（如子宫内膜癌、乳腺癌、肾癌、卵巢癌）的风险也会增加。肥胖症对妊娠期女性有特殊影响，会增加许多妊娠相关并发症的风险，包括妊娠期糖尿病、巨大儿、高血压、肩难产和剖宫产，并导致血栓形成和感染等产后并发症。肥胖症还与月经失调和无排卵率较高有关。

　　心血管疾病风险与代谢综合征在女性中似乎有更强的相关性。代谢综合征有多种定义，最常用的定义是以下 5 个增加患心脏病或卒中概率的危险因素中存在 ≥ 3 个：向心性肥胖、甘油三酯水平升高、高密度脂蛋白胆固醇水平降低、高血压和空腹血糖受损。患代谢综合征的女性应接受监测，并针对其心血管事件和显性糖尿病的风险增加而进行咨询。

多囊卵巢综合征

　　多囊卵巢综合征（PCOS）是一种复杂的内分泌失调症，病因不明，全球有 5% ～ 10% 的女性患病。主要诊断标准是雄激素过多、排卵功能障碍和（或）卵巢多囊。最常用的诊断标准是 2003 年鹿特丹标准，该标准要求满足上述 3 项标准中的 2 项。PCOS 的危险因素包括一级亲属患有 PCOS、糖尿病、肥胖症和特定种族人群（如墨西哥裔美国人）。PCOS 对生殖和代谢功能的影响包括无排卵、不孕症、痤疮、多毛、肥胖症、非酒精性脂肪性肝病和代谢综合征。胰岛素抵抗增加是该综合征的一个重要后果，会增加 2 型糖尿病的风险，尤其是在肥胖症患者中。因此，被诊断为 PCOS 的女性需要进行糖尿病筛查。

　　PCOS 的治疗主要为对症治疗。对于超重或肥胖症女性，建议调整生活方式。COC 是 PCOS 的一线治疗，可调节月经，降低无妊娠需求女性的高雄激素水平。高雄激素血症的二线治疗方法是螺内酯或非那雄胺等抗雄激素药物。二甲双胍和噻唑烷二酮类药物可提高胰岛素敏感性，二甲双胍还能调节月经。这些药物有致畸作用，故妊娠期间禁用，使用时需采取有效的避孕措施。PCOS 女性通常很难受孕，常需使用枸橼酸氯米芬或来曲唑等促排卵药物。PCOS 患者子宫内膜癌和卵巢癌的风险增加。使用 COC 可降低子宫内膜增生的风险，并可能降低子宫内膜癌的风险。

纤维肌痛

　　纤维肌痛的患病率为 2% ～ 8%，具体取决于所使用的诊断标准。历史上，纤维肌痛在女性中更常见。最初的诊断标准涉及检查时压痛点的数量。由于女性报告的压痛点更多或女性和男性的症状表现不同，

men. With the change in diagnostic criteria, however, the disease has a smaller female to male ratio at 2:1. Since 2011, diagnosis has been determined by a symptom survey. Because of the vague set of symptoms and lack of laboratory findings, it has been a complicated and controversial diagnosis that continues to evolve.

Fibromyalgia is characterized by persistent pain, sleep disturbance, and fatigue lasting more than 3 months. The pain state is thought to be driven by how the central nervous system interprets peripheral nociceptive input. The central nervous system magnifies a given signal based on the levels of neurotransmitters, which then intensifies the pain response. The centralized pain phenomenon can be associated with other chronic pain states that have similar pathophysiology involving a specific organ system, such as chronic headaches, dysmenorrhea, irritable bowel syndrome, interstitial cystitis, or endometriosis. In addition, 10% to 30% of rheumatologic conditions are thought to have fibromyalgia as an associated diagnosis. The etiology is likely multifactorial, involving the influence of the environment, infection, and genetic predisposition.

Physical exam without any findings other than diffuse tenderness to palpation is characteristic. Treatment recommendations involve an integrated approach including both pharmacologic and nonpharmacologic modalities. Studies show that gabapentinoids, serotonin norepinephrine reuptake inhibitors, and gamma-hydroxybutyrate have efficacy in addressing symptoms of fibromyalgia. Choice of medication should be driven by predominant symptom, but multiple agents from different classes can be used for a synergistic effect. General patient-centered education, exercise, cognitive behavioral therapy, as well as some complementary and alternative medicine therapies such as tai chi, yoga, acupuncture, and trigger point injections, have been shown to be effective in increasing functionality. Setting expectations around the fact that fibromyalgia is a chronic disease that needs to be managed is an important part of the clinical care of these patients.

INTERSTITIAL CYSTITIS/HYPERSENSITIVE BLADDER

Interstitial cystitis, bladder pain syndrome, hypersensitive bladder, or painful bladder syndrome is a diagnosis that has evolved, changed names, and included different criteria for diagnosis over time. Based on literature from the Society for Urodynamics and Female Urology (SUFU), which was adapted by the American Urological Association, the current definition of interstitial cystitis is: "an unpleasant sensation (pain, pressure, discomfort) perceived to be related to the urinary bladder, associated with lower urinary tract symptoms of more than 6 weeks' duration, in the absence of infection or other identifiable causes." Interstitial cystitis disproportionately affects women, with studies reporting ratios ranging from 2:1 to 8:1. It most often presents in the fourth decade of life. Quality-of-life scores demonstrate a significant negative impact on functioning. Diagnosis involves ruling out infection or other physiologic causes of symptoms. No lab test aids in the diagnosis of the disease; however, antinuclear antibodies are often present and can confound the diagnosis. Based on symptoms and risk factors different imaging modalities may be employed.

The exact etiology remains unknown. Possibilities include epithelial dysfunction, neurogenic inflammation on the level of the urothelium, and mast cell activation leading to a heightened pain response. Theories involving central amplification of a pain signal, similar to the pathophysiology used to explain pain in fibromyalgia, have been applied to interstitial cystitis. Hunner lesion interstitial cystitis is defined by the presence of well-circumscribed reddened mucosal areas with small vessels radiating towards a central scar visualized on cystoscopy. This form of the disease most often occurs in older patients and presents

with more severe symptoms and fewer associated other chronic pain conditions. Treatment involves an elimination diet geared towards decreasing foods with high acid and potassium content. Fulguration and electrocautery can be performed by a urologist.

Patients without identifiable lesions are more likely to have dyspareunia, vulvodynia, and bowel symptoms in addition to having more comorbid conditions. Guidelines for treatment involve starting with conservative options and progressing to more aggressive measures only in the case that initial treatments fail. Treatment often begins with diet modifications. Other nonpharmacologic approaches include pelvic floor physical therapy, cognitive behavioral therapy, and complementary therapy such as acupuncture and massage. Tricyclic antidepressants and antihistamines have led to a decrease in symptoms and an increase in functional status. Intravesical injections of BOTOX and combinations of dimethyl sulfoxide, heparin, or lidocaine, as well as nerve blocks and neuromodulators have been shown to be effective.

HUMAN IMMUNODEFICIENCY VIRUS INFECTION

HIV demands special attention in women's health care due to both epidemiologic and pathophysiologic factors. In the United States, only 7% of people with known HIV infections were women when the epidemic began; however, women now account for 25% of the population of people living with HIV, with women representing 20% of new infections in 2017. There is a higher incidence in rates of infection in African American women, which points to an inequality in education regarding HIV transmission and access to care. Heterosexual sexual encounters cause most HIV infections in women. Unprotected vaginal sex is a much higher risk for women than for men, and unprotected anal sex carries higher risk than unprotected vaginal sex.

The virus itself has a different physiologic impact on women: women typically have lower viral loads than men despite the same level of CD4 counts. Yet the rates of disease progression and opportunistic infections are similar for men and women. Awareness of gynecologic infections as initial manifestations of HIV/AIDS is important when treating women. Counseling for women of childbearing age around risk for vertical transmission and infection through breast milk are important considerations.

Although antiretroviral therapy and follow-up monitoring are similar for men and women with HIV/AIDS, general primary care for women with HIV requires special considerations. Risk for cervical abnormalities and cervical cancer is related to the degree of immunosuppression, age, and co-infection with high-risk HPV genotypes (16, 18, 52, and 58). Women with HIV infection are more likely to progress more rapidly to cervical cancer. The CDC recommends two cervical cytology screens at 6-month intervals in the first year after an HIV diagnosis and then annually. If there are three normal screens, then testing can be every 3 years. For more detail see the HIV opportunistic infection guidelines at *CDC.gov*. Vulvar and perianal intraepithelial neoplasia are more common in women with HIV than HIV-seronegative women, therefore any lesions present need careful evaluation.

EATING DISORDERS

Eating disorders are disturbances to a person's eating behaviors that result in significant health or psychosocial impairment. They often involve having a distorted body image. Common eating disorders include binge eating disorder, bulimia nervosa, and anorexia nervosa. Median age of onset is between 18 and 21 years old. The lifetime prevalence of binge eating disorder, bulimia nervosa, and anorexia nervosa are 2.8%, 1.0%, and 0.6%, respectively. Rates of eating disorders are

女性患者人数与男性不成比例。但是，随着诊断标准的改变，该病的女性和男性比例缩小为 2∶1。自 2011 年起，诊断依据改为症状调查。由于症状模糊且缺乏实验室检查结果，该病的诊断复杂且存在争议，并仍在不断变化。

纤维肌痛的特点是持续疼痛、睡眠障碍和疲劳，持续时间超过 3 个月。疼痛状态被认为是由中枢神经系统如何解释外周痛觉输入所驱动的。中枢神经系统会根据神经递质水平放大特定的信号，从而加剧疼痛反应。中枢性疼痛现象可能与其他慢性疼痛状态有关，这些慢性疼痛状态具有类似的病理生理学特征，但涉及特定器官系统，如慢性头痛、腹泻、肠易激综合征、间质性膀胱炎或子宫内膜异位症。此外，10% ～ 30% 的风湿病被认为与纤维肌痛有关。纤维肌痛的病因可能是多因素的，涉及环境、感染和遗传易感性。

纤维肌痛的特征是体格检查除弥漫性触痛外无任何其他发现。推荐采用包括药物治疗和非药物治疗的综合治疗。研究表明，加巴喷丁类药物、SNRI 和 γ- 羟基丁酸盐对缓解纤维肌痛症状有效。应根据主要症状选择药物，但也可使用不同类别的多种药物以产生协同效应。以患者为中心的教育、运动、认知行为疗法，以及辅助治疗和替代医学治疗（如太极拳、瑜伽、针灸和扳机点注射）已被证明能有效增强功能。让患者认识到纤维肌痛是一种需要控制的慢性疾病并建立合理预期，是临床治疗纤维肌痛的重要一环。

间质性膀胱炎 / 高敏感性膀胱

间质性膀胱炎、膀胱疼痛综合征、高敏感性膀胱或疼痛性膀胱综合征是指同一种疾病，其命名和诊断标准随着时间推移而不断发展和变化。根据改编自美国泌尿外科协会的尿动力学和女性泌尿外科学会（SUFU）的文献，目前间质性膀胱炎的定义是：与膀胱有关的不适感（疼痛、压迫、不适），伴有持续 6 周以上的下尿路症状，且无感染或其他可确定的病因。间质性膀胱炎多见于女性，研究报告的女性和男性发病比例为（2 ～ 8）∶1，31 ～ 40 岁的患病率最高。生活质量评分显示，该病对功能有显著的负面影响。诊断需要排除感染或其他引起症状的生理学原因。没有任何实验室检查有助于该病的诊断；但是，该病患者的抗核抗体常为阳性，可能会混淆诊断。根据患者的症状和危险因素，可能会采用不同的影像学检查来辅助诊断。

间质性膀胱炎的确切病因尚不清楚。可能的病因包括上皮细胞功能障碍、尿路上皮神经源性炎症、肥大细胞激活导致疼痛反应增强。间质性膀胱炎的病理生理学解释与纤维肌痛的疼痛类似，涉及疼痛信号的中枢性放大。洪纳病变（Hunner lesion）间质性膀胱炎的定义是：在膀胱镜检查中可见界限清晰的发红的黏膜区伴有向中央瘢痕放射的小血管。这种类型多见于

年龄较大的患者，症状更为严重，且较少伴有其他慢性疼痛。治疗方法包括减少食用酸和钾含量高的食物。可由泌尿科医生进行电灼术。

未发现明显病变的患者更有可能伴有性生活障碍、外阴疼痛和肠道症状，并可能有更多的合并症。治疗指南建议先进行保守治疗，只有在初始治疗失败的情况下才采取更积极的措施。治疗通常从调整饮食开始。其他非药物治疗包括盆底物理治疗、认知行为疗法，以及针灸和按摩等辅助治疗。三环类抗抑郁药和抗组胺药可减轻症状，改善功能状态。膀胱内注射 A 型肉毒毒素和组合药物（二甲基亚砜＋肝素或利多卡因），以及神经阻滞剂和神经调节剂已被证明有效。

人类免疫缺陷病毒感染

由于流行病学和病理生理学两方面的因素，女性医疗保健需特别关注 HIV。在美国，艾滋病（AIDS）刚开始流行时，仅有 7% 的已知 HIV 感染者是女性；但现在，女性占 HIV 感染者总数的 25%；2017 年，新发感染者中女性占 20%。非裔美国女性的感染率更高，这表明在 HIV 传播途径的教育和保健获取方面存在不平等。异性性行为是女性感染 HIV 的主要原因，女性在无保护的阴道性行为中的感染风险远高于男性，无保护的肛交风险高于无保护的阴道性行为。

病毒本身对女性的生理学影响不同：尽管 CD4 细胞计数水平相近，但女性的病毒载量通常低于男性。然而，男性和女性的疾病进展率和机会性感染率相似。在治疗女性患者时，认识到妇科感染是 HIV/AIDS 的初期表现非常重要。围绕垂直传播和经母乳感染的风险为育龄期女性提供咨询十分重要。

虽然男性和女性的抗逆转录病毒治疗和随访监测相似，但女性 HIV 感染者的一般初级保健需要特殊注意。宫颈异常和宫颈癌的风险与免疫抑制程度、年龄及合并感染高危 HPV 基因型（16 型、18 型、52 型和 58 型）有关。感染 HIV 的女性更可能迅速进展为宫颈癌。CDC 建议，在确诊感染 HIV 后的第 1 年，每隔 6 个月进行 1 次宫颈细胞学筛查，之后每年筛查 1 次。若 3 次筛查结果正常，则可以每 3 年检测 1 次。详情请参阅 CDC.gov 网站上的 HIV 机会性感染指南。相比于 HIV 血清阴性的女性，外阴和肛周上皮内瘤变在 HIV 感染女性中更常见，因此任何病变均需仔细评估。

进食障碍

进食障碍是指个体的进食行为受到干扰，从而导致严重的健康或心理障碍，通常涉及体象变形。常见的进食障碍包括暴食、神经性贪食和神经性厌食。中位发病年龄为 18 ～ 21 岁。暴食、神经性贪食和神经性厌食的终身患病率分别为 2.8%、1.0% 和 0.6%。进食障碍的发

increasing, and white females tend to be disproportionately affected. According to the National Institute of Mental Health, the prevalence of eating disorders ranges between 2 to 5 times higher in women than in men. In contrast, some studies based on clinical practice have found a 20- to 30-fold higher prevalence in women. There is a high comorbidity with other mental disorders, primarily anxiety disorders. Physicians who care for adolescents should monitor weight and BMI and screen for alterations in body image and behaviors that suggest disordered eating. A number of screening instruments are available. Somatic symptoms are common and include dyspnea, chest pain, headache, and gastrointestinal problems. Self-induced vomiting is associated with erosion of dental enamel, parotid gland swelling, scarring or calluses on the dorsum of the hand, and esophageal complications such as Mallory-Weiss syndrome. Individuals with eating disorders should be evaluated for severe medical complications that require hospitalization. Unstable vital signs, moderate to severe refeeding syndrome and dehydration are indications for hospitalization for medical stabilization. Long-term treatment of anorexia may require inpatient hospitalization if there is minimal response to outpatient treatment or weight remains under 70% to 75% of ideal body weight. Management of eating disorders often requires a multidisciplinary approach with a primary care physician, psychologist, and nutritionist. Treatment for binge eating disorder is typically CBT. Treatment for bulimia includes a combination of pharmacotherapy, of which fluoxetine is first line, and psychotherapy. Treatment for anorexia is nutritional rehab and psychotherapy. If individuals fail to respond to outpatient treatment, they may require inpatient treatment for closer monitoring and more intensive treatment.

CARDIOVASCULAR DISEASE

CAD remains the leading cause of death for both women and men; however, significant sex and gender differences in the epidemiology, pathophysiology, and clinical manifestations of cardiovascular disease exist. Women with ischemic heart disease are more likely than men to experience atypical symptoms, such as fatigue, abdominal pain, indigestion, nausea and vomiting, and shortness of breath. These non-classic symptoms may partially explain why women tend to seek health care later than men. Even when women seek health care, they have a longer time to diagnosis and a longer time to medical intervention than men. Women are also more likely to have sudden cardiac death at presentation. They are less likely to receive proven effective therapies, such as β-blockers, aspirin, thrombolytics, and statins, and they are less often referred for invasive testing and coronary artery bypass grafting (CABG). Women are also more likely to die after a myocardial infarction and CABG compared with men. Inequalities are at play in the management of heart disease along racial lines: African American women are offered reperfusion therapy and coronary angiography at lower rates, and in-hospital mortality rates are higher compared with those of white women.

Women who present with acute coronary syndrome more frequently have coronary arteries absent of thrombus, but with distal emboli. This points to pathophysiologic differences in ischemic heart disease based on sex. Vasoreactivity and endothelial dysfunction are more common in women, which is demonstrated in the phenomenon of spontaneous coronary artery dissection, an underdiagnosed cause of acute coronary syndromes (ACS) seen in women between the ages of 45 and 60 and associated with pregnancy and the postpartum period. Takotsubo syndrome (stress cardiomyopathy) represents an estimated 8% of ACS cases in women, whereas it is the cause of less than 1% of ACS cases in men. Women with ischemic heart disease tend to present with ACS an average of 7 to 10 years later than men. The predominance

of disease in women post menopause suggests the protective role of higher estrogen states. Estrogen enhances HDL cholesterol and influences atherosclerotic plaque progression and regression. Estrogen may also be beneficial due to its vasodilatory, anti-inflammatory, and antioxidative properties.

Much of the evidence used to guide the treatment of coronary disease in women is based on trials that predominantly enrolled men. The studied treatments and interventions may not induce the same benefit and may even cause harm. For example, due to the tendency for women to have smaller arteries and fewer lesions, initial noninvasive tests have a higher likelihood of producing false-positive results that lead to invasive testing for evaluation of obstructive CAD.

PRECONCEPTION COUNSELING AND PRE-PREGNANCY CARE

Preconception counseling involves a combination of taking a thorough social, family, and medical history to assess potential risks to the mother and potential fetus and offering guidance around maintaining a healthy lifestyle, nutritional supplementation, and avoidance of potential toxins. The first step of a visit involves assessing desire of the patient to become pregnant, discussing what factors are influencing her decision, and offering contraception if pregnancy is not wanted. Women with a personal or family history of genetic disorders may benefit from formal genetic counseling. During a preconception visit, blood work is assessed and immunizations can be administered.

All prescribed and over-the-counter medications and herbal supplements need review to identify potential teratogens. Medications not considered necessary for the well-being of the mother should be stopped. This is not always possible or indicated for women treated for chronic medical conditions where the risk in stopping the medication outweighs the potential harm to the fetus. All women planning pregnancy or capable of becoming pregnant should be advised to take a daily multivitamin with folic acid (400 μg) to reduce the risks of neural tube defects and other congenital anomalies, including cardiovascular defects, urinary defects, and cleft lip.

Medical conditions known to increase the risk of adverse pregnancy outcomes for women and their offspring include obesity, diabetes, thyroid disease, seizure disorders, hypertension, rheumatoid arthritis, chronic renal disease, thrombophilias, asthma, and cardiovascular disease. Preconception care of these conditions can improve pregnancy outcomes. Patients usually are referred to high-risk pregnancy care for evaluation. Addressing obesity prior to pregnancy is important because although higher BMIs lead to adverse outcomes for both the woman and baby, weight loss should not occur during pregnancy.

Approximately 1% of pregnancies in the United States are complicated by pregestational diabetes. Gestational diabetes (GDM) occurs in approximately 7% of pregnancies. GDM has a high recurrence rate (30% to 80%) in subsequent pregnancies and a significantly increased risk for future development of type 2 diabetes. In women with pregestational diabetes and GDM, adequate control of diabetes reduces the risk of congenital malformations. Goal for HbA_{1C} prior to conception is less than 6.5%.

Hyperthyroidism and overt hypothyroidism occur in approximately 0.2% and 2.5% of all pregnancies, respectively. Adequate treatment of thyroid illness improves pregnancy outcomes. Approximately 70% to 80% of women with rheumatoid arthritis experience remission of disease during pregnancy, although the remaining women have active or worsening disease in pregnancy. Women with systemic lupus erythematosus (SLE) often experience exacerbations in pregnancy. SLE increases the risk of adverse fetal outcomes, including spontaneous abortion, fetal growth restriction, and preterm birth. Maternal

病率呈上升趋势，白人女性患者的比例最高。根据美国国家心理健康研究所的数据，女性进食障碍的患病率是男性的 2 ～ 5 倍。相比之下，一些基于临床实践的研究显示，女性的患病率比男性高出 20 ～ 30 倍。进食障碍常合并其他精神疾病（主要是焦虑症）。为青少年提供医疗保健的医生应监测其体重和 BMI，当出现提示进食障碍的体象和行为改变时，应注意筛查。目前有多种筛查工具可供使用。进食障碍的躯体症状很常见，包括呼吸困难、胸痛、头痛和胃肠道症状。催吐与牙釉质侵蚀、腮腺肿胀、手背瘢痕或胼胝、食管并发症［如马洛里-魏斯综合征（Mallory-Weiss 综合征）］有关。进食障碍患者应进行评估，以确定是否存在需要住院治疗的严重并发症。生命体征不稳定、中重度再喂养综合征和脱水是住院治疗的指征。若厌食患者对门诊治疗反应甚微或体重持续低于理想体重的 70% ～ 75%，则可能需要住院接受长期治疗。进食障碍的治疗通常需要初级保健医生、心理学家和营养学家的多学科合作。暴食的治疗通常采用认知行为疗法。贪食的治疗包括药物治疗（氟西汀是一线药物）和心理治疗。厌食的治疗包括营养康复和心理治疗。患者对门诊治疗无反应时，可能需要住院接受更严密的监测和进一步治疗。

心血管疾病

冠状动脉疾病仍是男性和女性的主要死亡原因；然而，心血管疾病在流行病学、病理生理学和临床表现方面存在显著的性别差异。女性缺血性心脏病患者比男性更易表现为非典型症状，如疲劳、腹痛、消化不良、恶心、呕吐和气短。症状不典型是女性就医通常晚于男性的部分原因。即使就医，女性获得诊断和医疗干预的时间也晚于男性。女性更可能在发病时出现心源性猝死。她们使用已被证实有效的药物（β 受体阻滞剂、阿司匹林、溶栓药和他汀类药物等）的可能性更小，且更少被转诊至接受侵入性检查和冠状动脉旁路移植术（CABG）。与男性相比，女性在心肌梗死和 CABG 后死亡的可能性也更大。在心脏病的治疗中，种族之间也存在不平等：非裔美国女性接受再灌注治疗和冠状动脉造影的比例低于白人女性，院内死亡率高于白人女性。

急性冠脉综合征（ACS）女性患者的冠状动脉中通常没有血栓，但有远端栓子。这说明缺血性心脏病的病理生理学存在性别差异。血管反应性和内皮功能障碍在女性中更常见，表现为自发性冠状动脉夹层现象，这是 45 ～ 60 岁女性 ACS 诊断不足的原因，并与妊娠和产后有关。据估计，在女性 ACS 病例中，Takotsubo 综合征（应激性心肌病）占 8%，而在男性 ACS 病例中，Takotsubo 综合征的占比不足 1%。患有缺血性心脏病的女性通常比男性平均晚 7 ～ 10 年出现 ACS。女性主要在绝经后发病，这表明较高的雌激素水平具有保护作用。雌激素可使高密度脂蛋白胆固醇水平升高，影响动脉粥样硬化斑块的进展和消退。雌激素的扩张血管、抗炎和抗氧化特性也可能对人体有益。

指导女性冠心病治疗的大部分证据是基于以男性受试者为主的试验。其所验证的治疗和干预措施在女性中可能不会带来同样的益处，甚至可能造成伤害。例如，由于女性的动脉较小、病变较少，最初的非侵入性检查产生假阳性结果的可能性较大，导致进行侵入性检查以评估阻塞性冠状动脉疾病。

孕前咨询和孕前保健

孕前咨询包括全面了解家族史和个人史，以评估母亲和胎儿的潜在风险，并提供保持健康生活方式、补充营养和避免潜在有毒物质等方面的指导。接诊的第一步包括评估患者生育意愿，讨论影响其决定的因素，并在患者无生育计划的情况下提供避孕指导。有遗传病个人史或家族史的女性可能会受益于正规的遗传咨询。在孕前就诊时，应进行血液检查及免疫接种。

需要对所有处方药、非处方药和草药补充剂进行审查，以发现潜在的致畸剂。对母亲健康没有必要的药物，应停止使用。这并不总是可行或适用的，对于部分接受慢性疾病治疗的女性，停药的风险大于对胎儿的潜在伤害。应建议所有备孕或可能妊娠的女性每天服用含叶酸（400 μg）的多种维生素，以降低胎儿神经管缺陷和其他先天性畸形的风险，包括心血管缺陷、泌尿系统缺陷和唇裂。

已知会增加不良妊娠结局（母亲及其后代）风险的疾病包括肥胖症、糖尿病、甲状腺疾病、癫痫发作、高血压、类风湿关节炎、慢性肾脏病、血栓性疾病、哮喘和心血管疾病。对这些疾病进行孕前保健可改善妊娠结局。患者通常会被转诊到高危妊娠诊疗机构进行评估。在妊娠前解决肥胖症问题非常重要，因为虽然较高的 BMI 会对孕妇和胎儿造成不良后果，但不应在妊娠期间减肥。

在美国，约 1% 的妊娠女性合并妊娠前糖尿病。约 7% 的妊娠女性会发生妊娠期糖尿病（GDM）。GDM 在后续妊娠中的复发率很高（30% ～ 80%），且未来发展为 2 型糖尿病的风险也会显著增加。对于妊娠前糖尿病和 GDM，充分控制糖尿病可降低先天性畸形的风险。孕前 HbA1c 的目标值为 < 6.5%。

甲状腺功能亢进症和显性甲状腺功能减退症分别约占所有妊娠女性的 0.2% 和 2.5%。对甲状腺疾病的充分治疗可改善妊娠结局。70% ～ 80% 的类风湿关节炎女性患者的病情可在妊娠期得到缓解，但其他病情会在妊娠期活动或加重。系统性红斑狼疮（SLE）通常会在妊娠期加重。SLE 会增加胎儿不良结局的风险，包括自然流产、胎儿生长受限和早产。孕产妇死亡与肺动脉高压［尤其

mortality is associated with conditions such as pulmonary hypertension (especially Eisenmenger's syndrome), congenital heart disease with hypoxia and poor functional class, and arrhythmias.

Assessing for substance use and providing support around abstinence from tobacco, alcohol, and other illicit substances is important in addressing fertility concerns, for the general well-being of the woman, and for the development of the fetus. Routine laboratory evaluation includes rubella titer, varicella titer (in women with a negative history of varicella), hepatitis B surface antigen, and a complete blood count to assess for hemoglobinopathy. Women should receive screening for HIV, chlamydia, and syphilis.

Immunity to measles, mumps, rubella, tetanus, diphtheria, poliomyelitis, and varicella should be ensured through vaccination. Women should receive influenza vaccine in pregnancy due to the increased risk of complications from influenza infection. Ideally, women should receive all indicated vaccinations at least 1 month before conception. Live vaccines (e.g., rubella) should not be given during pregnancy.

PERINATAL DEPRESSION

Depression during pregnancy and in the postpartum period is a significant and common occurrence for childbearing women. Although more efforts to understand the cause, impact, and adequate management are emerging, stigma and underdiagnosis have led to missed opportunities to provide women with appropriate care. Defining and categorizing the specific type of depression particular to this period varies, thereby making it more challenging to study, recognize, and treat. Perinatal depression as delineated by ACOG is defined as major or minor episodes of depression that occur during pregnancy or within the first 12 months after delivery. The DSM-V, however, defines postpartum depression (PPD) as the onset of depressive symptoms within the first 4 weeks of delivery. Studies show that 33% of women with PPD had symptoms during pregnancy, whereas 27% had symptoms pre-pregnancy. In 2016, USPSTF issued a recommendation for routine depression screening in the general adult population and specifically including pregnant and postpartum women, which highlights perinatal depression as a condition worthy of attention but at the same time does not clearly delineate it from other types of depression.

Changes in sleep, appetite, and libido directly caused by responsibilities associated with caring for a newborn may complicate evaluation of postpartum depression based on symptomatology. Postpartum, 50% of women experience a change in mood, called "postpartum blues," marked by intensified emotions that are transient, lasting for the first few weeks after birth. Postpartum blues can develop into PPD. Anxiety or obsessions regarding the health and safety of the baby are common in the postpartum period; the degree to which these thoughts and feelings lead to a debilitating state varies and thereby drives the diagnosis of the psychological condition of PPD. Studies of PPD have found that 20% of women with this diagnosis have suicidal thoughts. Risk factors for PPD include depression and anxiety during pregnancy, traumatic birth experience, previous history of depression, and complications in the health of the infant.

Pathophysiology is multifactorial, likely including genetic, hormonal, immune, and social influences. Although changes in hormones have been assumed to be at the center of PPD, studies have failed to demonstrate a clear association between reproductive levels in women with PPD. Management should be driven by severity of symptoms. First steps involve providing support around self-care and psychosocial needs, which includes encouraging exercise and sleep. In moderate cases, cognitive behavioral therapy and the addition of an SSRI is recommended. In severe cases, additional classes of antidepressants are added, if a switch in SSRI does not yield improvement. ECT

is recommended when suicidality and/or psychosis are present. The FDA has recently approved a treatment for severe postpartum depression that consists of an intravenous formulation of allopregnanolone, a steroid that works on GABA receptors. However, applicability only to women with severe symptoms and cost limit current use of this medication.

SEXUAL DYSFUNCTION

Sexual dysfunction is a term that describes a range of sexual health–related concerns that cause personal distress. The etiology is often multifactorial with psychological, sociocultural, biologic, and physiologic components. It is experienced by approximately 40% of women in the United States. Women around menopause, between the ages of 45 and 65, are most commonly affected. It is often underdiagnosed and undertreated. Numerous medical conditions can impact sexual function due to changes in desire, arousal, orgasm or the presence of pain. Aging itself is associated with decreased libido and sexual responsiveness. The decline in estrogen during menopause causes thinning of the vaginal epithelium, decreased vaginal elasticity, and decreased lubrication. Medications are also implicated in sexual dysfunction, most commonly SSRIs. Evaluation includes a thorough medical and sexual history and the physical exam should also include testing for STIs. Management depends on the etiology but is frequently multifactorial. Some treatment options include pelvic physical therapy, psychotherapy or sex therapy, and mindfulness-based interventions. Pharmacologic options are limited but there are two recently FDA-approved medications. Flibanserin is a daily oral medication approved for premenopausal women with low sexual desire; however, its use is limited by a black box warning, an interaction with alcohol, and significant nausea and dizziness. Bremelanotide, a subcutaneous injection administered as needed prior to sexual activity, was approved in June 2019 for premenopausal women with low sexual desire. Hormone therapies such as systemic estrogen and testosterone have been used off label. Systemic estrogen was not found to improve sexual dysfunction in postmenopausal women in the Women's Health Initiative. Testosterone has been found to improve sexual dysfunction in peri- and postmenopausal women in most studies. Testosterone is metabolized to estrogen, thus its use can be associated with abnormal uterine bleeding and breast symptoms.

PELVIC PAIN

Pelvic pain is characterized as acute or chronic, and both types are commonly encountered in primary care practice. Acute pelvic pain usually manifests over hours to days and may be gynecologic, gastrointestinal, or urologic in origin. Life-threatening conditions, including ruptured ectopic pregnancy and appendicitis, need to be ruled out. Gynecologic causes include complications of pregnancy, acute pelvic infection, and ovarian pathology, including cyst and torsion.

Chronic pelvic pain (CPP) is lower abdominal pain of at least 6 months' duration, and it is severe enough to cause functional impairment or require treatment. Approximately 10% of ambulatory gynecologic referrals are for CPP. The history obtained for evaluation of CPP should include characteristics of the pain; a thorough review of systems; prior medical, surgical, gynecologic, and obstetric history; and a thorough psychiatric and social history, including episodes of domestic violence as a child or an adult and periods of substance abuse.

The most common conditions associated with CPP are endometriosis, chronic pelvic inflammatory disease, interstitial cystitis, irritable bowel syndrome, pelvic floor myalgia, myofascial pain, and neuralgia.

是艾森门格综合征（Eisenmenger 综合征）]、先天性心脏病伴缺氧和心功能不全，以及心律失常等疾病有关。

评估物质使用障碍情况，并在戒烟、戒酒和戒断其他非法药物等方面提供支持，对于解决生育问题、女性整体福祉和胎儿发育至关重要。常规实验室检查包括检测风疹病毒、水痘病毒（未患过水痘的女性）、乙型肝炎表面抗原、全血细胞计数（含血红蛋白），以及 HIV、衣原体和梅毒筛查。

孕前应接种疫苗，以确保对麻疹、流行性腮腺炎、风疹、破伤风、白喉、脊髓灰质炎和水痘有免疫力。由于感染流行性感冒病毒会增加并发症的风险，女性在妊娠期应接种流感疫苗。理想情况下，女性应在受孕前至少 1 个月接种所有指定的疫苗。妊娠期不应接种活疫苗（如风疹疫苗）。

围产期抑郁症

妊娠期抑郁症和产后抑郁症（PPD）是育龄期女性的常见病和多发病。尽管人们正在努力了解抑郁症的病因、影响和治疗方法，但病耻感和诊断不足导致错失了为女性提供恰当治疗的机会。对这一时期特有的抑郁症类型的定义和分类各不相同，使得研究、识别和治疗更具挑战性。根据 ACOG 的定义，围产期抑郁症是指在妊娠期或产后 12 个月内发生的严重或轻微的抑郁发作。然而，《精神障碍诊断与统计手册》第 5 版（DSM-V）将 PPD 定义为产后 4 周内出现的抑郁症状。研究表明，33% 的 PPD 女性在妊娠期出现症状，而 27% 的女性在妊娠前就有症状。2016 年 USPSTF 发布了一项关于在普通成年人群中进行常规抑郁症筛查的建议，并特别将孕妇和产妇纳入其中。该建议将围产期抑郁症作为一种值得关注的疾病，但并未将其与抑郁症其他类型明确区分开。

与照顾新生儿相关的责任直接导致了睡眠、食欲和性欲的变化，这可能会使根据症状学对 PPD 的评估变得复杂。50% 的女性在产后会出现情绪变化，被称为产后忧郁，其特征是产后最初数周内的短暂情绪激化。产后忧郁可发展为 PPD。对婴儿健康和安全的焦虑或强迫症在产后很常见；这些想法和感觉可引起不同程度的衰弱状态，导致了 PPD 这一心理疾病的诊断。针对 PPD 的研究显示，诊断 PPD 的产妇中 20% 有自杀的想法。PPD 的危险因素包括妊娠期抑郁症和焦虑症、创伤性分娩经历、既往抑郁症病史及婴儿健康并发症。

PPD 的病理生理学机制是多因素的，可能包括遗传、激素、免疫和社会影响。虽然激素变化一直被认为是 PPD 的核心，但研究未能证明生殖激素水平与 PPD 之间存在明确关系。应根据症状的严重程度采取相应的治疗措施。第一步是围绕自我护理和心理需求提供支持，包括鼓励运动和睡眠。对于中度 PPD，建议采用认知行为疗法并使用 1 种 SSRI。对于重度 PPD，若更换 SSRI 不能改善病情，则应增加抗抑郁药的种类。当出现

自杀和（或）精神病时，建议使用电休克疗法（ECT）。FDA 近期批准静脉注射异丙孕酮（一种作用于 GABA 受体的类固醇）用于治疗重度 PPD。然而，该治疗仅适用于症状严重的女性，且价格昂贵，这限制了其应用。

性功能障碍

性功能障碍这一术语包含了一系列给个体带来困扰的性健康相关问题。其病因通常是多因素的，包括心理、社会文化、生物和生理因素。在美国，约 40% 的女性经历过性功能障碍，围绝经期女性（45 ~ 65 岁）最常见。性功能障碍通常诊断不足、治疗不及时。许多疾病会因改变性欲、性唤起、性高潮或疼痛而影响性功能。衰老本身也与性欲和性反应能力下降有关。绝经时雌激素水平下降会导致阴道上皮变薄、阴道弹性下降和润滑度降低。药物也与性功能障碍有关，最常见的是 SSRI。性功能障碍的评估包括全面的病史和性生活史，体格检查应包括性传播疾病感染（STI）检测。治疗方法取决于病因，但通常是综合治疗。治疗方案包括盆腔物理治疗、心理治疗或性治疗、正念干预。药物治疗的选择有限，但近期有两种药物获得了 FDA 批准。氟班色林是一种口服药物，获批用于治疗绝经前女性的性欲低下；但由于与酒精的相互作用、引起明显的恶心和头晕等，其使用受到黑框警告的限制。布美诺肽是一种在性活动前按需使用的皮下注射药物，于 2019 年 6 月获批用于治疗绝经前女性的性欲低下。激素治疗（如全身使用雌激素和睾酮）已被超说明书使用。在女性健康倡议（Women's Health Initiative）中，全身使用雌激素并不能改善绝经后女性的性功能障碍。大多数研究发现，睾酮可改善围绝经期和绝经后女性的性功能障碍。睾酮会代谢为雌激素，因此使用睾酮可能与异常子宫出血和乳房症状有关。

盆腔疼痛

盆腔疼痛分为急性和慢性，两种类型在初级保健实践中均很常见。急性盆腔疼痛通常持续数小时至数天，可能由妇科疾病、胃肠道疾病或泌尿系统疾病引起。需要排除危及生命的疾病，包括异位妊娠破裂和阑尾炎。妇科原因包括妊娠并发症、急性盆腔感染和卵巢病变（包括囊肿和扭转）。

慢性盆腔疼痛（CPP）是指持续至少 6 个月的下腹部疼痛，其严重程度足以导致功能障碍或需要治疗。妇科门诊中约 10% 是因 CPP 转诊。评估 CPP 时需获取的病史包括疼痛的特征；全面系统回顾既往内科、外科、妇科和产科病史；全面的精神病史和社会史（包括儿童或成人时期的家庭暴力事件和药物滥用）。

与 CPP 相关的最常见疾病包括子宫内膜异位症、慢性盆腔炎、间质性膀胱炎、肠易激综合征、盆底肌痛、肌筋膜痛和神经痛。

Interstitial cystitis or painful bladder syndrome is a clinical diagnosis consisting of pain, pressure, or discomfort related to the bladder and associated with lower urinary tract symptoms lasting more than 6 weeks and occurring in the absence of infection or other identifiable causes. Mental health issues, including substance abuse, somatization, depression, and physical or sexual abuse, can also cause CPP and are important to identify so that women need not undergo unnecessary testing and interventions.

Physical examination should assess for focal areas of pain, scars, hernias, or masses in the abdomen, and a pelvic examination should be performed. After the most likely diagnosis has been identified, an empirical, targeted treatment may be instituted and followed for efficacy. Further work-up should be considered if the patient does not respond or symptoms change. If empirical therapy and a thorough investigation do not yield a diagnosis, laparoscopy may be considered to identify pelvic pathology.

Any identified peripheral etiology to CPP should be treated; however, CPP of unclear etiology is common and does not have definitive treatment. Depending on the underlying cause, management strategies may include heat therapy (for musculoskeletal pain), counseling and psychiatric referral, gastrointestinal referral, medications (e.g., gabapentin for neuropathic pain, NSAIDs, hormonal contraceptives), hysterectomy, and nerve transection procedures. Multidisciplinary approaches, including medications and interventions that address dietary and psychosocial factors, may be superior to medical treatment alone.

GENDER AND FEMALE SEXUAL MINORITIES

The health care needs of female sexual and gender minorities have significant overlap with the general population but require specific attention and sensitivity given significant barriers to care and differences in both sexual health concerns and certain medical issues. Females who have sex with females come from diverse racial, ethnic, and socioeconomic backgrounds and may choose to identify as lesbian, gay, or bisexual or transgender. Gender minorities, such as individuals who identify as transgender or genderqueer, identify and/or express a different gender than the gender traditionally associated with their assigned sex at birth. Gender and sexual minorities are significantly more likely than heterosexual women to experience implicit and explicit discrimination during health care visits. Many providers do not take a sexual history or inquire about sexual orientation. Health care providers may inadvertently assume heterosexuality and communicate heterosexist attitudes, making it more difficult for patients to disclose their sexual orientation. A lack of cultural competency means that providers do not understand appropriate terminology around gender identity and sexual orientation, which can create further challenges in provider-patient relationships.

Rates of STIs between females who have sex with females are not well studied; however, the assumption that there is lower risk for STIs through female-female sex as compared to heterosexual intercourse is not based in adequate research. Female-female sex allows for transmission of infection through vaginal fluids, menstrual blood, mucosal contact, and via sex toys. Dental dams, condoms, or latex sheet provide a barrier for transmission of bacterial and viral infections. Using condoms on sex toys and cleaning sex toys between use can decrease the spread of infection. Lubrication can also decrease infection transmission by preventing breakdown and bleeding of mucosal areas. Rates of bacterial vaginosis are higher in females who have sex with females, which has suggested transmissibility of bacterial vaginosis and that it should be classified as an STI.

Sexual minorities should receive the same age-appropriate preventative health care and cancer screenings as heterosexual women. For transgender individuals, the decision as to whether to screen for breast cancer or cervical cancer should be based on current anatomy and risk as opposed to gender identity of the individual. Recognition that the individual's relationship to the organ in need of cancer screening may be dysphoric for the individual should inform how screenings are introduced and discussed during a clinic visit.

Sexual and gender minority stress as a result of prejudice and systemic discrimination has direct and indirect impacts on the health of individuals. Recent studies comparing the health and health risk factors between individuals who identified as lesbian, gay or bisexual (LGB) and heterosexual individuals demonstrate LGB persons have higher rates of psychological distress, heavy alcohol and tobacco use, obesity, cardiovascular disease, type 2 diabetes, and breast and gynecological cancers compared to heterosexual women. These differences are not explained by any innate biological differences between heterosexuals/cisgendered individuals and sexual/gender minorities but are felt to be heavily influenced by minority stress and decreased access of medical care. Lifetime rates of intimate personal violence are higher for lesbian, bisexual, and transgender peoples. Although the differences in health outcomes for sexual and gender minorities do not change screening recommendations, provider awareness is important in meeting the physical and emotional health needs of all patients.

SUGGESTED READINGS

American College of Obstetricians and Gynecologists' Committee on Practice Bulletins—Gynecology: Practice bulletin No. 164: diagnosis and management of benign breast disorders, Obstet Gynecol 127(6):e141–e156, 2016.

Bots SH, Peters SAE, Woodward M: Sex differences in coronary heart disease and stroke mortality: a global assessment of the effect of ageing between 1980 and 2010, BMJ Glob Health 2(2):e000298, 2017.

Clayton AH, Margarita Valladares Juarez E: Female sexual dysfunction, Med Clin 103(4):681–698, 2019.

Eriksen EF, Díez-Pérez A, Boonen S: Update on long-term treatment with bisphosphonates for postmenopausal osteoporosis: a systematic review, Bone 58(January):126–135, 2014.

Guy J, Peters MG: Liver disease in women: the influence of gender on epidemiology, natural history, and patient outcomes, Gastroenterol Hepatol 9(10):633–639, 2013.

Han E, Nguyen L, Sirls L, Peters K: Current best practice management of interstitial cystitis/bladder pain syndrome, Ther Adv Urol 10(7):197–211, 2018.

Iddon J, Dixon JM: Mastalgia, BMJ 347(December):f3288, 2013.

Infertility Workup for the Women's Health Specialist—ACOG. n.d. https://www.acog.org/Clinical-Guidance-and-Publications/Committee-Opinions/Committee-on-Gynecologic-Practice/Infertility-Workup-for-the-Womens-Health-Specialist?IsMobileSet=false. Accessed July 3, 2019.

Kaunitz AM: Abnormal uterine bleeding in reproductive-age women, J Am Med Assoc, 2019, https://doi.org/10.1001/jama.2019.5248.

Kodner C: Common questions about the diagnosis and management of fibromyalgia, Am Fam Physician 91(7):472–478, 2015.

Mehler PS: Diagnosis and care of patients with anorexia nervosa in primary care settings, Ann Intern Med 134(11):1048–1059, 2001.

Millett ERC, Peters SAE, Woodward M: Sex differences in risk factors for myocardial infarction: cohort study of UK biobank participants, BMJ 363(November):k4247, 2018.

Nonhormonal Management of Menopause-Associated Vasomotor Symptoms: 2015 Position Statement of the North American Menopause Society. 2015. Menopause 22 (11): 1155-1172; quiz 1173-1174.

Stewart DE, Vigod SN: Postpartum depression: pathophysiology, treatment, and emerging therapeutics, Annu Rev Med 70(January):183–196, 2019.

间质性膀胱炎或疼痛性膀胱综合征包括与膀胱有关的疼痛、压迫或不适，伴有持续 6 周以上的下尿路症状，且没有感染或其他可识别的原因。精神卫生问题（包括物质滥用、躯体化、抑郁症、躯体虐待或性虐待）也可能导致 CPP，因此必须加以识别，以避免女性接受不必要的检查和干预。

体格检查应评估腹部是否有局部疼痛区域、瘢痕、疝气或肿块，并进行盆腔检查。在确定最有可能的诊断后，应有针对性地采取经验性治疗并跟踪疗效。若治疗无效或症状发生变化，则应考虑进一步检查。若经验性治疗和全面检查均无法确诊，可考虑进行腹腔镜检查以确定盆腔病变。

任何已确定的 CPP 病因均应给予治疗；但是，病因不明的 CPP 很常见，且没有明确的治疗方法。根据潜在病因，治疗策略可能包括热疗（用于肌肉骨骼疼痛），心理咨询和精神科转诊，消化科转诊，药物治疗[如加巴喷丁（用于治疗神经性疼痛）、NSAID、激素避孕药]，子宫切除术和神经横断术。多学科治疗（包括药物治疗及针对饮食和心理社会因素的干预措施）可能优于单纯药物治疗。

性少数群体和女性性少数群体

女性性少数群体和性少数群体的医疗保健需求与普通人群有很大的重叠，但由于这些群体在获得医疗保健方面存在障碍，以及性健康问题和某些医疗问题的差异，因此需要给予特别关注。与女性发生性关系的女性来自不同的种族、民族和社会经济背景，她们可能认同自己是女同性恋、男同性恋、双性恋或跨性别者。性少数群体（如跨性别者或性别酷儿）所认同和（或）表达的性别与其出生时的传统性别不同。与异性恋女性相比，性少数群体在就医过程中遭受隐性和显性歧视的可能性明显增大。许多医务人员不会询问性生活史或性取向。医务人员可能会无意识地假定患者是异性恋，并传达异性恋主义的态度，从而使患者更难透露自己的性取向。缺乏文化竞争力意味着医务人员不了解有关性别认同和性取向的适当术语，这可能会给医患关系带来更多挑战。

女女性行为的 STI 率尚未得到充分研究；但是，与异性性交相比，女女性行为的 STI 风险更低，这一假设并非基于充分的研究。女女性行为可通过阴道分泌物、经血、黏膜接触和性玩具而传播感染。口腔保护膜、避孕套或乳胶片可阻隔细菌和病毒感染的传播。在性玩具上使用安全套并在两次使用之间清洁性玩具可减少感染传播。润滑剂可防止黏膜破裂和出血，从而减少感染传播。细菌性阴道病在与女性发生性关系的女性中发病率较高，这表明细菌性阴道病具有传播性，应将其归类为 STI。

性少数群体应与异性恋女性一样接受适龄的预防保健和癌症筛查。对于跨性别者，是否进行乳腺癌或宫颈癌筛查应基于当前的解剖学结构和风险，而不是个体的性别认同。医生应认识到个体与需要癌症筛查的器官之间的关系可能会使其感到不适，并在就诊时介绍和讨论筛查的方式。

偏见和歧视造成的性别 / 性少数群体压力会对个体健康产生直接和间接的影响。近期研究比较了被认定为女同性恋者、男同性恋者或双性恋者（LGB）和异性恋者之间的健康和健康危险因素，结果表明，与异性恋女性相比，LGB 人群的心理困扰、重度饮酒和吸烟、肥胖症、心血管疾病、2 型糖尿病、乳腺癌和妇科癌症发病率更高。异性恋 / 顺性别者与性别 / 性少数群体之间的先天生理学区别无法解释这些差异，但性少数群体的压力和医疗保健服务的减少被认为对这些差异产生了重大影响。女同性恋、双性恋和跨性别者在一生中遭受亲密伴侣间暴力的比例更高。虽然性别 / 性少数群体在健康结局方面的差异不会改变筛查建议，但医务人员的认识对于满足所有患者的躯体和情感健康需求非常重要。

推荐阅读

American College of Obstetricians and Gynecologists' Committee on Practice Bulletins—Gynecology: Practice bulletin No. 164: diagnosis and management of benign breast disorders, Obstet Gynecol 127(6):e141–e156, 2016.

Bots SH, Peters SAE, Woodward M: Sex differences in coronary heart disease and stroke mortality: a global assessment of the effect of ageing between 1980 and 2010, BMJ Glob Health 2(2):e000298, 2017.

Clayton AH, Margarita Valladares Juarez E: Female sexual dysfunction, Med Clin 103(4):681–698, 2019.

Eriksen EF, Díez-Pérez A, Boonen S: Update on long-term treatment with bisphosphonates for postmenopausal osteoporosis: a systematic review, Bone 58(January):126–135, 2014.

Guy J, Peters MG: Liver disease in women: the influence of gender on epidemiology, natural history, and patient outcomes, Gastroenterol Hepatol 9(10):633–639, 2013.

Han E, Nguyen L, Sirls L, Peters K: Current best practice management of interstitial cystitis/bladder pain syndrome, Ther Adv Urol 10(7):197–211, 2018.

Iddon J, Dixon JM: Mastalgia, BMJ 347(December):f3288, 2013.

Infertility Workup for the Women's Health Specialist—ACOG. n.d. https://www.acog.org/Clinical-Guidance-and-Publications/Committee-Opinions/Committee-on-Gynecologic-Practice/Infertility-Workup-for-the-Womens-Health-Specialist?IsMobileSet=false. Accessed July 3, 2019.

Kaunitz AM: Abnormal uterine bleeding in reproductive-age women, J Am Med Assoc, 2019, https://doi.org/10.1001/jama.2019.5248.

Kodner C: Common questions about the diagnosis and management of fibromyalgia, Am Fam Physician 91(7):472–478, 2015.

Mehler PS: Diagnosis and care of patients with anorexia nervosa in primary care settings, Ann Intern Med 134(11):1048–1059, 2001.

Millett ERC, Peters SAE, Woodward M: Sex differences in risk factors for myocardial infarction: cohort study of UK biobank participants, BMJ 363(November):k4247, 2018.

Nonhormonal Management of Menopause-Associated Vasomotor Symptoms: 2015 Position Statement of the North American Menopause Society. 2015. Menopause 22 (11): 1155-1172; quiz 1173-1174.

Stewart DE, Vigod SN: Postpartum depression: pathophysiology, treatment, and emerging therapeutics, Annu Rev Med 70(January):183–196, 2019.

Men's Health

男性健康

Men's Health Topics

Niels V. Johnsen, Douglas F. Milam, Joseph A. Smith, Jr.

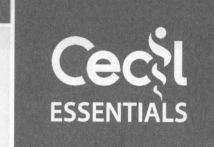

INTRODUCTION

Men's health has grown into a subspecialty field that includes primary care physicians, urologists, and endocrinologists, among others. Men's health needs and concerns are becoming more evident and often require the expertise of those with dedicated interest in men's health topics. This chapter aims to address benign disorders that are unique to men because they specifically involve the male genitalia and reproductive system. Male genitourinary malignancies and infertility are addressed in Chapters 4.

TESTOSTERONE DEFICIENCY

Definition and Epidemiology

The prescribing and use of testosterone in the United States has risen dramatically in the past decade. However, many men continue to fail to receive treatment when appropriate due to lack of provider knowledge or unsupported clinical concerns, while others continue to receive testosterone despite the lack of a clear clinical indication. Furthermore, escalations in direct-to-consumer marketing and the rise of well-publicized centers dedicated solely to the management of men's health issues have further increased patient interest in and desire to receive testosterone therapy.

Previously referred to by a number of different terms, *testosterone deficiency* is the preferred terminology adopted by the American Urological Association (AUA) to describe the condition of low serum testosterone in men in conjunction with signs or symptoms associated with low serum testosterone levels. The true prevalence of testosterone deficiency is not known. Estimates range between 2% and 77% of the US male population. This wide variability in estimates stems from inconsistencies both in definitions of testosterone deficiency applied within the literature, as well as variabilities in the assays and cut-off values used to determine low serum testosterone levels.

Testosterone deficiency does not refer to a low serum testosterone level alone, but by definition requires additional clinical signs or symptoms associated with low serum testosterone. Previous recommendations have attempted to quantify a required number of associated symptoms or signs for diagnosis of testosterone deficiency in a patient with a low total serum testosterone; however, the current AUA guidelines simply state that patients must have at least one sign or symptom in addition to low serum testosterone levels for diagnosis. These include symptoms such as fatigue, depression, erectile dysfunction, cognitive dysfunction, decreased libido, and decreased endurance; as well as signs such as loss of body hair, weight gain, or loss of lean muscle mass. Unfortunately, while some signs and symptoms are more suggestive of testosterone deficiency, many are nonspecific and can often be manifestations of other illnesses or disease states (Table 10.1). Thus, it is vital that clinicians have a thorough understanding of testosterone deficiency in order to ensure patients are both offered appropriate care when indicated and not offered care when not indicated.

Pathophysiology

Testosterone is produced primarily by the testicles as a result of stimulation by luteinizing hormone (LH) secreted from the anterior pituitary gland, which in turn is stimulated by the hypothalamus. This hypothalamic-pituitary-gonadal (HPG) axis can often be disrupted by aging, with multiple studies showing that the prevalence of testosterone deficiency increases significantly with advancing age. Disruptions in the HPG axis can occur at multiple points and lead to differing classifications of testosterone deficiency. *Primary hypogonadism* is a condition due to testicular failure, in which the testicles fail to produce adequate amounts of testosterone (and sperm) despite adequate stimulation by LH from the anterior pituitary. *Secondary hypogonadism*, on the other hand, is a low serum testosterone level as a result of failure of the pituitary to secrete sufficient amounts of LH. In this state, the Leydig cells of the testicle are not adequately stimulated and thus do not produce testosterone. *Secondary hypogonadism* can be the result of disease processes such as pituitary tumors, hemochromatosis, or obstructive sleep apnea.

As the predominant androgen in men, testosterone circulates within the bloodstream in four distinct forms. Approximately 44% of testosterone is tightly bound to sex hormone-binding globulin (SHBG) and represents the non-bioavailable component of serum testosterone. However, 50% is loosely bound to albumin, 4% loosely bound to corticotropin-binding globulin, and 2% freely circulating within the blood stream, representing the bioavailable form of testosterone. The 2% of circulating testosterone that it is not bound to serum proteins, however, is the most biochemically active form of testosterone and referred to as free testosterone (FT).

Laboratory tests of total testosterone (TT) measure both the bound and unbound forms of testosterone. In patients with either borderline-low serum TT levels or in patients with low-normal TT levels with significant associated signs or symptoms, measurement of FT may be helpful in making a clinical diagnosis. Increased levels of SHBG in the serum can decrease the level of FT, as more testosterone becomes bound to SHBG. The level of SHBG may increase with smoking, excessive coffee consumption, age, and disease processes such as hepatitis and hyperthyroidism. Therefore, increased levels of SHBG can contribute to testosterone deficiency. Conversely, while obesity may

男性健康

朱军 译 吴寒 林浩成 审校 姜辉 通审

引言

男性健康已经发展成为一个包括初级保健医生、泌尿外科医生和内分泌科医生等在内的亚专科领域。男性对健康的需求及关注度日益凸显，通常需要专注于男性健康问题的专科医生提供专业知识。本章旨在讨论涉及男性生殖器和生殖系统的良性疾病。男性泌尿生殖系统恶性肿瘤和不育症见第4章。

睾酮缺乏症

定义和流行病学

在过去十年间，美国的睾酮处方量及用量急剧上升。然而，由于医护人员的知识不足或缺乏依据，许多男性仍然未能在适当的时机接受治疗，而部分男性在没有明确临床指征的情况下仍持续接受睾酮治疗。此外，直接面向消费者的营销升级和专门治疗男性健康问题的知名中心的兴起，进一步增加了患者对接受睾酮治疗的兴趣和意愿。

睾酮缺乏症既往有多种术语命名，美国泌尿外科协会（AUA）推荐将"睾酮缺乏症"作为首选术语，用于描述男性血清睾酮水平低下并伴有相应症状或体征的情况。睾酮缺乏症的实际患病率尚不明确，美国男性的患病率估计为2%～77%。如此大的差异主要是因为文献中对睾酮缺乏症的定义不一致，以及实验室检测睾酮水平的方法和诊断睾酮缺乏症采用的临界值存在差异。

睾酮缺乏症并不单纯指血清睾酮水平低下，根据定义，还需伴随低血清睾酮相关的临床症状或体征。以往的建议试图量化血清总睾酮水平低的患者被诊断为睾酮缺乏症所需的相关症状或体征。然而，目前的AUA指南规定，除了低血清睾酮水平外，患者至少有1种症状或体征即可诊断。这些症状包括疲劳、抑郁、勃起功能障碍、认知功能障碍、性欲减退和耐力下降等；体征方面包括体毛减少、体重增加或肌肉量减少等。遗憾的是，虽然某些体征和症状对于睾酮缺乏症具有较好的提示作用，但许多是非特异性的，往往也

是其他疾病或疾病状态的表现（表10.1）。因此，临床医生必须对睾酮缺乏症有透彻的理解，以确保在患者具备相应指征时为其提供合理的治疗，并在无指征时避免不必要的干预。

病理生理学

睾酮主要由睾丸在黄体生成素（LH）的刺激下产生，而LH由垂体前叶分泌，这一过程受下丘脑的调控。衰老通常会影响下丘脑-垂体-性腺（HPG）轴，多项研究表明，随着年龄的增长，睾酮缺乏症的患病率显著升高。HPG轴功能异常可以发生在多个环节，并导致不同类型的睾酮缺乏症。原发性性腺功能减退症由睾丸功能衰竭导致，尽管有足够的LH刺激，睾丸仍无法产生足够的睾酮（和精子）。继发性性腺功能减退症是由于垂体未能分泌足够的LH而导致血清睾酮水平降低。在这种状态下，睾丸间质细胞（Leydig细胞）未受到充分刺激，因此不能产生睾酮。继发性性腺功能减退症可由垂体肿瘤、血色病或阻塞性睡眠呼吸暂停等疾病引起。

作为男性体内主要的雄激素，睾酮在血液中以4种形式循环。约44%的睾酮与性激素结合球蛋白（SHBG）紧密结合，这是血清睾酮中非生物可利用的成分。另有50%的睾酮松散地结合于白蛋白，4%的睾酮松散地结合于促肾上腺皮质激素结合球蛋白，其余2%的睾酮则在血液中自由循环，为睾酮的生物可利用形式。其中，2%未与血清蛋白质结合的循环睾酮是睾酮中最具生化活性的形式，被称为游离睾酮（FT）。

总睾酮（TT）的实验室检测包括结合和未结合形式的睾酮。对于血清TT水平低于临界值或TT水平偏低但伴有明显相关体征或症状的患者，检测FT可能有助于临床诊断。血清SHBG水平升高会使FT水平降低，因为更多的睾酮会与SHBG结合。吸烟、过量饮用咖啡、年龄增长及疾病（肝炎和甲状腺功能亢进症等）可使SHBG水平升高。因此，SHBG水平升高可导致睾酮缺乏症。相反，尽管肥胖症可能会降低SHBG水平，但其也可通过脂肪细胞中睾酮向雌激素的外周转化而导致睾酮缺乏症。此外，过度运动、药物滥用、

TABLE 10.1   Signs and Symptoms of Testosterone Deficiency

Specific Signs and Symptoms	Less Specific Signs and Symptoms
Reduced sexual desire (libido) and activity	Decreased energy and self-confidence
Decreased spontaneous erections	Feeling sad, depressed mood
Breast discomfort, gynecomastia	Poor concentration and memory
Less axillary and pubic hair and less shaving	Sleep disturbance and sleepiness
Very small or shrinking testes	Mild anemia (normochromic, normocytic)
Infertility and low sperm count	Reduced muscle bulk and strength
Height loss and low bone mineral density	Increased body fat and body mass index
Hot flashes and sweats	Diminished physical or work performance

decrease levels of SHBG, it too can contribute to testosterone deficiency through the peripheral conversion of testosterone into estrogen within adipose cells. Lastly, conditions such as extreme exercise, recreational drug use, nutritional deficiency, stress, use of certain medications, and acute illness can transiently lower serum testosterone.

Clinical Presentation

Low testosterone levels can affect a patient's general, sexual, physical, and psychological health. In Table 10.1, these symptoms are grouped according to their specific relation to testosterone deficiency. Various studies have categorized and used the symptoms of testosterone deficiency in different ways. For example, one clinical trial looking at the incidence of testosterone deficiency defined the syndrome as the presence of 3 of 12 clinical symptoms combined with a low serum FT or TT level, whereas, in a similar trial, patients were considered to be testosterone deficient if they had a low TT and exhibited three specific sexual symptoms. Current guidelines state that clinicians should use these different symptomologies as a means to determine the appropriateness and potential benefit of checking a patient's serum testosterone level, while also noting that decreased libido is the most common presenting symptom.

Diagnosis

For several reasons, the diagnosis of testosterone deficiency is not straightforward. By the very simplest of definitions, diagnosis requires a low serum testosterone level on at least two separate occasions in conjunction with at least one clinical symptom. Most clinical guidelines suggest measuring an early morning TT in any adult man who has symptoms associated with testosterone deficiency and, if low, repeating a subsequent early morning test using the same assay to confirm low testosterone. An early morning blood draw is recommended given the diurnal variation in serum testosterone levels. According to the AUA, a serum TT level of less than 300 ng/dL serves as the appropriate threshold value for identifying testosterone deficiency. However, it should be noted that there is significant variability between different testosterone assays that may alter the range of normal for each particular test, so providers should be sure to evaluate their assay-specific ranges when making determinations for therapy. In highly symptomatic patients with borderline or normal TT, FT should be assessed; however, FT tests are not recommended initially due to higher variability, increased time, and increased costs. In addition, screening of asymptomatic men for low testosterone is not medically necessary or appropriate.

In men with borderline testosterone levels, repeat measurement of a morning testosterone level is warranted because there may be significant day-to-day and diurnal variability. Ideally, levels should be checked within 4 hours of waking (usually between 7 and 11 AM), when testosterone levels are highest. It is not necessary to fast before a testosterone laboratory test; however, in a study from 2013, there was a 25% reduction in TT levels in healthy men 60 minutes after an oral glucose tolerance test. Strength training may also transiently decrease serum testosterone levels in healthy men (but typically not outside the normal range).

Testosterone levels should not be checked during acute or subacute illness. However, physicians should have a lower threshold to check the testosterone level in patients with chronic illnesses that are known to cause a symptomatically lower testosterone concentration, such as diabetes mellitus, chronic obstructive lung disease, inflammatory arthritic disease, renal disease, human immunodeficiency virus (HIV)-related disease, obesity, metabolic syndrome, and hemochromatosis. In fact, some have argued that patients who have a pituitary mass, HIV-associated weight loss, unexplained anemia, chronic narcotic use, or chronic steroid use should have their testosterone level checked regardless of symptoms.

In patients with a confirmed low TT in the presence of symptoms, LH levels should be checked to determine the etiology of testosterone deficiency and to rule out secondary hypogonadism. Testosterone-deficient patients with a low LH likely have a defect at the level of the hypothalamus or pituitary (hypogonadotropic hypogonadism), whereas those with elevated LH levels have a primary testicular defect (hypergonadotropic hypogonadism). There are a number of conditions that may cause hypogonadotropic hypogonadism, including Kallmann syndrome, pituitary tumors, infiltrative pituitary disorders such as hemochromatosis or sarcoidosis, hyperprolactinemia, and prior head trauma. Patients with this disorder warrant further investigation to determine the source of the testosterone deficiency, such as serum prolactin measurements or possible endocrine evaluation. Hypergonadotropic hypogonadism, on the other hand, may be the result of prior infection or trauma to the testes, autoimmune damage, or possibly Klinefelter's syndrome, which would prompt karyotyping for diagnosis.

Men over the age of 40 being considered for testosterone replacement should have their prostate-specific antigen (PSA) level measured and a digital rectal examination (DRE) performed to assess the prostate. If either is abnormal, referral to a urologist should be considered. Table 10.2 provides helpful guidelines for evaluating possible testosterone deficiency. For patients with documented testosterone deficiency who are interested in future fertility, reproductive medicine evaluation should be performed because testosterone therapy markedly decreases sperm production. Return of normal spermatogenesis takes a variable amount of time, if at all.

Treatment

Testosterone therapy is recommended for men with confirmed testosterone deficiency on two separate tests who also have associated signs or symptoms of deficiency, or in the select cases mentioned above. The primary purpose of testosterone therapy is to provide symptom

表 10.1　睾酮缺乏症的体征和症状	
特异性体征和症状	非特异性体征和症状
性欲减退和性行为减少	精力和自信下降
自发性勃起减少	心情悲伤、心境低落
乳房不适、男性乳房发育	注意力和记忆力差
腋毛和阴毛减少，剃须次数减少	睡眠障碍和嗜睡
睾丸非常小或睾丸萎缩	轻度贫血（正细胞正色素性贫血）
不育症和精子计数降低	肌肉量减少、肌力减弱
身高下降和骨密度降低	体脂增多、体重指数增大
潮热、出汗	体能或工作表现下降

营养缺乏、压力、某些药物和急性疾病等也可能短暂地降低血清睾酮水平。

临床表现

低睾酮水平可能影响患者的一般健康、性健康、生理健康和心理健康。在表 10.1 中，根据这些症状与睾酮缺乏症的具体关系对其进行了分类。多项研究对睾酮缺乏症的症状进行了不同的分类和运用。例如，一项研究睾酮缺乏症发生率的临床试验将其定义为出现 12 种临床症状中的 3 种，并伴有低血清 FT 或 TT 水平；而在另一项类似的试验中，如果患者具有低 TT 水平并存在 3 种特异性的性相关症状，则可诊断睾酮缺乏症。目前的指南建议临床医生利用这些症状来决定是否需要检测血清睾酮水平及其可能的获益，同时应注意性欲减退是患者最常见的症状。

诊断

由于多种原因，睾酮缺乏症的诊断并不简单。根据最简单的定义，诊断需要至少 2 次不同时间点的血清睾酮水平降低，且伴有至少 1 种临床症状。大多数临床指南建议，对于有睾酮缺乏症相关症状的成年男性，均应在晨间检测血清 TT 水平。如果 TT 水平低，应择期使用相同的检测方法复查晨间 TT 水平以确认低血清睾酮水平。建议在早晨进行抽血检测是因为血清睾酮水平存在昼夜变化。根据 AUA 的建议，血清 TT 水平 < 300 ng/dl 是诊断睾酮缺乏症的合理阈值。然而，应该注意的是，不同的血清睾酮检测方法之间存在显著差异，这可能导致每种特定方法测得的血清睾酮正常值范围存在差异。因此，医生应在决定治疗时评估其检测方法的特定正常值范围。对于症状明显的患者，如果 TT 水平处于临界值或正常值范围内，应进一步检测 FT；值得注意的是，由于 FT 检测的变异性更高、耗时更长、成本更高，故不推荐将 FT 作为初始筛查项目。此外，对无症状的男性进行睾酮检测在医学上是没有必要且不合理的。

对于睾酮水平处于临界值的男性，建议复查晨间睾酮水平，因为睾酮水平可能存在显著的日间和昼夜变化。理想情况下，检测应在清醒后 4 h 内完成（通常在 07:00 至 11:00），此时睾酮水平最高。在检测睾酮水平前无须禁食；然而，2013 年的一项研究显示，健康男性在进行口服葡萄糖耐量试验后 60 min，TT 水平下降了 25%。力量训练也可能短暂降低健康男性的血清睾酮水平（但通常不会低于正常值范围）。

在急性或亚急性疾病期间不应进行睾酮水平检测。但是，对于患有已知能够导致症状性低睾酮的慢性疾病患者，如糖尿病、慢性阻塞性肺疾病、炎症性关节病、肾病、HIV 相关疾病、肥胖症、代谢综合征和血色病等，医生应相应放宽睾酮检测的标准。事实上，有些学者认为，对于患有垂体瘤、HIV 相关性体重减轻、原因不明的贫血、长期使用麻醉剂或类固醇的患者，无论其是否有症状，均应检测睾酮水平。

对于已确认低 TT 水平且存在相关症状的患者，应进一步检查血清 LH 水平，以明确睾酮缺乏症的病因，并排除继发性性腺功能减退症。LH 水平降低的睾酮缺乏症患者可能存在下丘脑或垂体功能缺陷（低促性腺激素性性腺功能减退症），而 LH 水平升高的患者则可能存在原发性睾丸功能缺陷（高促性腺激素性性腺功能减退症）。多种情况可能导致低促性腺激素性性腺功能减退症，包括 Kallmann 综合征、垂体肿瘤、浸润性垂体疾病（如血色病或结节病）、高催乳素血症和既往头部创伤等。对于这类患者，需行进一步检查明确睾酮缺乏症的病因，如血清催乳素检测或内分泌评估。此外，既往睾丸感染或损伤、自身免疫损伤或 Klinefelter 综合征（需进行染色体核型分析以确诊）等均可能导致高促性腺激素性性腺功能减退症。

对于考虑进行睾酮替代治疗的 40 岁以上男性，应进行前列腺特异性抗原（PSA）检测和直肠指检（DRE），以评估前列腺的情况。如果其中任何一项发现异常，应考虑转诊至泌尿外科。表 10.2 列出了评估睾酮缺乏症的相关指南意见。对于将来有生育计划的睾酮缺乏症患者，应进行生殖医学评估，因为睾酮替代治疗会显著减少精子生成。治疗后恢复正常精子发生所需的时间长短不一，有时甚至无法恢复。

治疗

对于 2 次检测确认睾酮缺乏症并伴有相关症状或体征的男性，或前文所述的特定病例，建议进行睾酮治疗。睾酮治疗的主要目的是通过将患者的睾酮水平

TABLE 10.2 **Testosterone Deficiency Diagnosis Do's and Don'ts**

Do check total testosterone (TT) in every symptomatic adult male >40 yr

Do confirm low testosterone results with a second test

Do check in the morning

Do have a lower threshold to check testosterone in patients with certain chronic illnesses

Do consider measuring prolactin and LH level in patients with low testosterone

Do check hematocrit and PSA levels prior to initiating testosterone therapy

Don't check the testosterone level during acute or subacute illness

Don't start with measurement of free testosterone

Don't monitor testosterone treatment with measurements of free testosterone

Don't consider testosterone therapy in a patient trying to father a child

LH, Luteinizing hormone; *PSA,* prostate-specific antigen.

---

relief by returning patients to normal physiologic levels of testosterone. This, in turn, may improve symptoms such as erectile dysfunction, decreased libido, anemia, depressive mood, or low bone mineral density. However, the data are not as clear as to the benefits of testosterone therapy in improving cognitive function, fatigue, or metabolic syndrome measures. Patients should also be counseled that although the data on the cardiovascular risks or benefits of testosterone therapy are currently inconclusive, low testosterone is a known risk factor for cardiovascular disease. Clinicians should also obtain a baseline hematocrit, because polycythemia (hematocrit >52%) is known to occur significantly more frequently in men on testosterone therapy. This is especially true for men receiving intramuscular testosterone injections and those with hormone pellet implants. Polycythemia can often be addressed with dose adjustment, but it will occasionally require phlebotomy or hematology consultation.

There are numerous testosterone replacement formulations. In the United States, the most commonly used forms are testosterone enanthate or cypionate by intramuscular (IM) injection, transdermal testosterone patches, testosterone gels, and implantable timed-release pellets. The goal of therapy should be to achieve a serum TT level in the middle tertile of the reference range for the assay being used. Because of the frequency of significant skin irritation with the testosterone patch, many practitioners prefer one of the other modalities, usually based on patient preference. There is also the risk of transference with gel applications, particularly worrisome for those who come in contact with pregnant women or young children. For specifics on dosing and formulations, the AUA Guideline on Evaluation and Management of Testosterone Deficiency provides a comprehensive table with recommendations. In general though, daily gel applications mimic diurnal variation with early morning application, produce middle tertile testosterone levels, and have a relatively low rate of polycythemia. Intramuscular injection (often biweekly) does not produce diurnal variation, causes very high testosterone levels initially that often fall to subtherapeutic levels before the next injection, and is more likely to produce polycythemia than gel preparations. Pellets do not mimic diurnal variation, often produce polycythemia, but have the advantage of dosage intervals as long as 6 months.

Side Effects of Testosterone Therapy

Testosterone therapy causes decreased sperm production and usually decreased testicular volume, and it may cause acne, oily skin, and breast tenderness. Testosterone replacement is not a treatment for infertility and has, in fact, been investigated as a method of male contraception.

Patients who are interested in fathering children should not take testosterone and those with a desire for future fertility should be informed that the return of normal spermatogenesis after cessation of testosterone is variable. If necessary, human chorionic gonadotropin (HCG), selective estrogen receptor modulators (SERM), aromatase inhibitors, or a combination thereof may be administered for testosterone-deficient men wishing to preserve fertility.

In addition, as previously discussed, testosterone can increase hematocrit levels and cause life-threatening polycythemia. Generally, patients experience a rise over the first 6 months of treatment, with a plateau thereafter. If the hematocrit becomes significantly elevated, testosterone replacement should be suspended and only resumed at a modified dose after levels have normalized. Occasionally, patients require phlebotomy to avoid or treat dangerous polycythemia.

Testosterone therapy may worsen obstructive sleep apnea and congestive heart failure; therefore, patients in whom these conditions are untreated should not be started on testosterone therapy. Present data suggest that testosterone therapy does not worsen levels of high-density lipoproteins and there is no definitive evidence linking testosterone therapy to an increased risk of venothrombotic events.

Testosterone Therapy and the Prostate

It has previously been advocated that testosterone therapy should be avoided in men with a history of prostate cancer, given the known association of testosterone with prostate cancer pathophysiology. Although this topic remains controversial, a number of providers now treat patients with confirmed testosterone deficiency and a history of prostate cancer in select cases. The current AUA guidelines state that there is inadequate evidence to quantify the risk-benefit ratio of testosterone therapy in men with a history of prostate cancer. However, in patients with a history of prostatectomy with low-risk pathology, current studies show no increased risk of cancer recurrence with testosterone therapy. Similar results have been seen in low-risk prostate cancer patients treated with radiation. Patients with a history of high-risk cancer treated by radiation, however, have experienced increased rises in post-treatment PSA values and should be cautioned about the risks with testosterone therapy. These patients, as well as those with active or recurrent prostate cancer, who desire testosterone therapy should be referred to centers with experience and expertise in this clinical scenario.

Monitoring Testosterone Treatment

Patients on testosterone therapy should have regular laboratory testing to confirm that appropriate serum testosterone levels are being achieved. As stated previously, therapy should be targeted to achieving the middle tertile of normal on the particular testosterone assay being used. In general, patients using gels or patches, as well as intranasal formulations, should have levels checked within 4 weeks of initiation of treatment, and then every 6 to 12 months once on steady dosing. For patients on short-acting injectable formulations, it is generally recommended to check testosterone levels after four cycles and then every 6 to 12 months. For patients who achieve target testosterone levels for 3 to 6 months but still do not feel that their inciting symptoms have improved, testosterone therapy should likely be discontinued in all but select cases (for example, patients with prior documented bone mineral density loss).

ERECTILE DYSFUNCTION

Erectile dysfunction (ED) is defined as the inability to achieve and/or maintain an erection sufficient for satisfactory sexual performance and is known to affect some 150 million men worldwide. According to

表 10.2　睾酮缺乏症诊断的注意事项
年龄＞ 40 岁且有症状的男性均应检测 TT 水平
需进行 2 次检测以确认睾酮水平低
在晨间进行睾酮检测
对于患有某些慢性疾病的患者，应放宽睾酮检测的适应证
低睾酮水平患者应检测催乳素和 LH 水平
开始睾酮治疗前应检测血细胞比容和 PSA 水平
不建议在急性或亚急性疾病期间检测睾酮水平
不建议初始直接检测游离睾酮水平
不建议通过游离睾酮水平来监测睾酮治疗
不建议对拟生育的患者进行睾酮治疗

LH，黄体生成素；PSA，前列腺特异性抗原；TT，总睾酮。

恢复到正常生理水平以缓解症状。这种治疗可能改善勃起功能障碍、性欲减退、贫血、心境低落或骨密度降低等症状。然而，关于睾酮治疗在改善认知功能、疲劳或代谢综合征等方面的益处，尚无明确的数据支持。医生应告知患者，尽管目前关于睾酮治疗的心血管风险或获益尚无定论，但睾酮水平低是心血管疾病的已知危险因素。临床医生还应获取患者的基线血细胞比容数值，因为在接受睾酮治疗的男性中，尤其是接受睾酮肌内注射和植入睾酮药丸的患者，红细胞增多症（血细胞比容＞ 52%）的发生率显著升高。红细胞增多症通常可以通过调整剂量来解决，少数情况需要进行静脉切开术或血液科会诊。

目前有许多睾酮替代制剂。在美国，最常用的剂型是肌内注射用庚酸睾酮或环戊丙酸睾酮、睾酮透皮贴剂、睾酮凝胶及植入型定时释放睾酮药丸。治疗目标是使 TT 水平达到所使用检测方法参考值范围的中间三分位区间。由于睾酮透皮贴剂常会引起严重的皮肤刺激，许多医生更倾向于根据患者偏好选择其他剂型。使用凝胶时存在接触风险，特别是需要与孕妇或幼儿接触的患者。关于剂量和剂型的具体信息，AUA 发布的睾酮缺乏症评估和治疗指南中提供了综合建议。一般来说，每天早晨使用凝胶可模拟昼夜节律变化，达到中间三分位的睾酮水平，且红细胞增多症的发生率相对较低。肌内注射睾酮（通常每 2 周 1 次）并不能模拟睾酮的昼夜节律变化，最初会导致睾酮水平非常高，在下一次注射前通常会降至治疗水平以下，并且比凝胶制剂更可能导致红细胞增多症。药丸同样不能模拟睾酮水平的昼夜节律变化，常引起红细胞增多症，但具有用药间隔长达 6 个月的优势。

睾酮治疗的副作用

睾酮治疗会抑制生精，且通常会使睾丸体积缩小，并可能引起痤疮、皮肤油腻和乳房触痛。睾酮替代治疗并不是不育症的治疗方法，事实上，它已被研究作为一种男性避孕的手段。有生育需求的患者不应进行睾酮治疗，应告知已接受睾酮治疗且有生育需求的患者，停用睾酮后睾丸的精子发生功能恢复所需的时间

并不固定。必要情况下，对于希望保留生育能力的睾酮缺乏症患者，可以考虑使用人绒毛膜促性腺激素（HCG）、选择性雌激素受体调节剂（SERM）、芳香化酶抑制剂或联合用药进行治疗。

此外，如前所述，睾酮可增加血细胞比容水平并引起危及生命的红细胞增多症。一般来说，患者在治疗的前 6 个月会出现血细胞比容升高，随后达到稳定水平。如果血细胞比容水平显著升高，应暂停睾酮替代治疗，待血细胞比容水平恢复正常后，调整睾酮剂量恢复治疗。少数患者需行静脉切开术，以避免或治疗凶险的红细胞增多症。

睾酮治疗可能会加剧阻塞性睡眠呼吸暂停和充血性心力衰竭；因此，存在这些情况且未经治疗的患者不应进行睾酮治疗。目前的数据表明，睾酮治疗不会降低高密度脂蛋白水平，也没有确凿证据表明睾酮治疗会增加静脉血栓栓塞事件的风险。

睾酮治疗与前列腺

鉴于睾酮与前列腺癌病理生理学之间的关联，既往一直主张有前列腺癌病史的男性应避免接受睾酮治疗。尽管这一问题仍有争议，但现在许多医生也对确诊睾酮缺乏症且有前列腺癌病史的特定患者进行睾酮治疗。AUA 指南指出，目前缺乏足够的证据来量化有前列腺癌病史的男性接受睾酮治疗的风险获益比。然而，现有研究表明，在前列腺切除术后病理证实低风险的患者中，睾酮治疗并未增加其癌症复发的风险。在曾接受放疗的低风险前列腺癌患者中也观察到了类似结果。但是，对于曾接受放疗的高风险前列腺癌患者，接受睾酮治疗后 PSA 水平升高的风险增加，因此应充分告知此类患者睾酮治疗的风险。对于这类患者和有活动性或复发性前列腺癌并希望进行睾酮治疗的患者，应转诊至具备相应治疗经验和专业知识的中心进行治疗评估。

睾酮治疗的监测

接受睾酮治疗的患者应定期进行实验室检查，以确定血清睾酮是否达到合适水平。如前所述，治疗目标是达到所用检测方法参考值范围的中间三分位区间。一般来说，使用凝胶、贴剂和鼻内制剂的患者应在开始治疗后的 4 周内检测血清睾酮水平，然后在用药剂量稳定后每 6 ～ 12 个月检测 1 次。对于使用短效注射制剂的患者，通常建议在治疗 4 个周期后检测睾酮水平，然后每 6 ～ 12 个月检测 1 次。对于在 3 ～ 6 个月达到目标睾酮水平但仍未感觉初始症状有所改善的患者，除特定情况（如既往存在骨密度降低）外，应考虑停止睾酮治疗。

勃起功能障碍

勃起功能障碍（ED）的定义为男性无法达到和（或）维持足够的勃起以完成满意的性生活，估计全球

the Massachusetts Male Aging Study, 52% of men older than 40 years of age are afflicted with some degree of ED, with the prevalence of ED tripling between the ages 40 and 70 years. By age 70 years, 15% of men will experience complete ED. While age and physical health are the most important predictors of the onset of ED, smoking remains one of the most important modifiable lifestyle factors impacting one's risk for ED.

Recently, many clinics that specifically treat ED and men's sexual health have opened across America, designed to meet a growing need for treatment of this condition. However, these clinics often charge out-of-pocket fees for treatments and medications that primary care physicians can provide and that are often covered by insurance. Therefore, it is more important than ever for primary care physicians to have a thorough understanding of this disease process and its management in order to provide appropriate and medically supervised care.

Mechanism of Erection

Afferent signals capable of initiating erection can originate within the brain, as with psychogenic stimulation, or as a result of peripheral tactile stimulation. While there is no discreet center for psychogenic erections, the temporal lobe appears to be important in this process. The pelvic plexus receives input from both the sympathetic and the parasympathetic nervous system and propagates these signals into the cavernous nerves of the penis. Sympathetic fibers involved originate in the thoracolumbar spinal cord, while parasympathetic fibers originate in the second through fourth sacral spinal cord segments (S2 through S4). Afferent somatic sensory signals are carried from the penis through the pudendal nerve to the S2 through S4 nerve roots. This information is then routed both to autonomic centers of the brain and to the spinal cord. Parasympathetic innervation is largely involved in achieving an erection (tumescence), whereas sympathetic, adrenergic innervation plays a vital role in the process of ending an erection (detumescence).

Sexual stimulation and the resultant propagation of efferent signaling through the pelvic plexus causes the release of nitric oxide (NO) by the cavernous nerves into the neuromuscular junction at the level of the smooth muscle of the corpora cavernosa of the penis (Fig. 10.1). NO subsequently activates guanylyl cyclase, which converts guanosine triphosphate (GTP) into cyclic guanosine monophosphate (cGMP). Protein kinase G is activated by cGMP and in turn activates several proteins that cause a decrease in the intracellular concentration of calcium ions (Ca^{2+}). Decreased Ca^{2+} concentration in the smooth muscle results in muscular relaxation, cavernosal artery dilation, increased blood flow, and subsequent tumescence. With the resultant cavernosal expansion from increased blood flow, venous sinuses that usually drain the penis are compressed and venous outflow from the penis is reduced, allowing for a persistent increased pressure within the penis and maintenance of the erection. At the end of erection, sympathetic nerves release norepinephrine, which ultimately results in smooth muscle contraction and detumescence. Similarly, phosphodiesterase type 5 (PDE5) works within the smooth muscle cells of the cavernosal tissue to degrade cGMP, ending the propagation of the signaling cascade for erection.

Causes of Erectile Dysfunction

Although often multifactorial in etiology, ED can be generally classified into two types: psychogenic ED and organic ED. Psychogenic ED was once thought to be the most common type of ED; however, advances in understanding of the mechanics and neurophysiology of erectile function have identified other more common causes. As a result, psychogenic ED is now thought to account for fewer than 15% of patients seen by ED specialists. Patients with psychogenic ED have otherwise intact vascular and neural physiology and are often able to

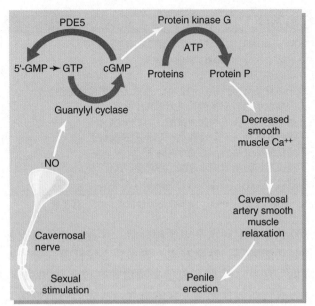

Fig. 10.1 Sexual stimulation causes the release of nitric oxide (NO) by the cavernous nerve into the neuromuscular junction. *ATP*, Adenosine triphosphate; *cGMP*, cyclic guanosine monophosphate; *GMP*, guanosine monophosphate; *GTP*, guanosine triphosphate; *PDE5*, phosphodiesterase type 5.

achieve erections either nocturnally or with self-stimulation, but continue to have difficulties with ED. This is most often related to issues such as depression, stress, anxiety or other psychiatric illness.

Organic ED represents the majority of ED seen clinically and can be classified as vasculogenic, neurogenic, endocrinologic or a combination thereof. For many patients, atherosclerotic arterial disease results in poor vascular inflow, impacting the ability to achieve an erection. Recent estimates suggest that atherosclerosis alone accounts for up to 60% of ED cases seen in men over the age of 60. Furthermore, a diagnosis of ED has been strongly associated with future cardiovascular disease in US men.

Cardiovascular Disease

In the United States, atherosclerotic vascular disease, hyperlipidemia, smoking, and hypertension are frequent causes of ED. These relationships are not surprising, as erection is achieved by a combination of relaxation of arteriolar smooth muscle and increased venous resistance of channels penetrating the wall of the corpora cavernosa. Cardiovascular disease may decrease erectile ability by decreasing blood flow to the penile arteries, mechanical obstruction of the vascular lumen, or, more commonly, due to the resultant endothelial dysfunction. Endothelial dysfunction is the most common cause of ED, in which there is an interruption of the neural control mechanism of vascular smooth muscle function due to a decreased ability of endothelial cells to release NO, leading to decreased blood flow and pressure in the corpora cavernosa. Given this close relationship between ED and cardiovascular disease, men presenting with ED should undergo appropriate cardiovascular risk factor evaluation and management. Men presenting with new onset ED in their forties are particularly at risk with an approximately 15 times increased risk of a myocardial event.

The principal blood vessels supplying the corpora cavernosa are the cavernosal arteries, which are terminal branches of the internal pudendal artery. Diseases of large and small arteries may decrease corporal blood pressure and lead to decreased penile lengthening and

约有 1.5 亿男性患有 ED。根据美国马萨诸塞州男性老龄化研究，52% 的 40 岁以上男性患有不同程度的 ED，且 ED 的患病率在 40 ～ 70 岁增加了 2 倍。到 70 岁，15% 的男性会彻底丧失勃起功能。虽然年龄和身体健康状况是 ED 发病最重要的预测因素，但吸烟仍然是影响 ED 发病风险的最重要且可调整的生活方式因素之一。

近年来，美国各地开设了许多专门治疗 ED 和男性性健康的诊所，以满足日益增长的治疗需求。然而，这些诊所采用的治疗和药物通常为自费，而这些是初级保健医生可以提供的，且这些治疗和药物通常在医疗保险覆盖范围内。因此，初级保健医生更应深入了解 ED 的病程及其管理，以便提供适当且规范的诊疗。

阴茎勃起的机制

勃起的传入信号可能源自大脑的心因性刺激或外周的触觉刺激。虽然没有明确的心因性勃起中枢，但颞叶在这个过程中似乎很重要。盆腔神经丛接收来自交感神经和副交感神经系统的信号，并传递至阴茎的海绵体神经。交感神经纤维起源于胸腰段脊髓，副交感神经纤维则起源于第 2 ～ 4 骶髓节段（S2 ～ S4）。传入的躯体感觉信号通过阴部神经从阴茎传至 S2 ～ S4 神经根。这些信号随后被传至大脑的自主神经中枢和脊髓。副交感神经主要参与实现勃起（胀大期），而交感神经和肾上腺素能神经则在结束勃起（消退期）中发挥重要作用。

性刺激及其产生的通过盆腔神经丛传递的传出信号促使海绵体神经向阴茎海绵体平滑肌水平的神经肌肉接头释放一氧化氮（NO）（图 10.1）。NO 激活鸟苷酸环化酶（GC），将鸟苷三磷酸（GTP）转化为环磷酸鸟苷（cGMP）。cGMP 可激活蛋白激酶 G（GPKG），进而激活多种蛋白质，导致细胞内钙离子（Ca^{2+}）浓度下降。平滑肌中 Ca^{2+} 浓度降低会引起平滑肌松弛，海绵体动脉扩张，血流增加，随后阴茎胀大。随着血流增加导致海绵体扩张，通常负责阴茎回流的静脉窦被挤压，阴茎的静脉回流减少，从而使阴茎内的压力持续增加并维持勃起。勃起结束时，交感神经释放去甲肾上腺素，最终导致平滑肌收缩和勃起消退。此外，5 型磷酸二酯酶（PDE5）在海绵体组织的平滑肌细胞内降解 cGMP，终止勃起信号的级联传播。

ED 的病因

虽然 ED 的病因通常涉及多因素，但一般可将 ED 分为两类：心因性 ED 和器质性 ED。心因性 ED 曾被视为最常见的类型；然而，随着对勃起功能的机制和神经生理学的深入研究，人们发现了其他更常见的原因。因此，目前认为在接受专科治疗的患者中，心因性 ED 的比例低于 15%。心因性 ED 患者的血管和神经生理学

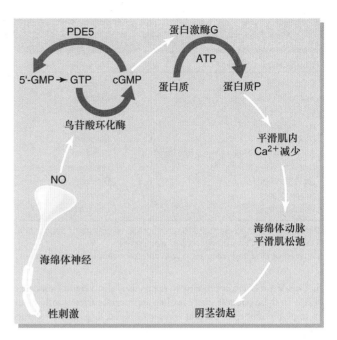

图 10.1　性刺激引起海绵体神经向神经肌肉接头释放一氧化氮（NO）。ATP，腺苷三磷酸；cGMP，环磷酸鸟苷；GMP，鸟苷一磷酸；GTP，鸟苷三磷酸；PDE5，5 型磷酸二酯酶

功能正常，通常在夜间或自我刺激时能够勃起，但仍有勃起困难的问题，这通常与抑郁、压力、焦虑或其他精神疾病相关。

临床上观察到的绝大多数患者为器质性 ED，其可分为血管源性、神经源性、内分泌性或混合型。对许多患者来说，动脉粥样硬化引起的血流不足影响了勃起功能。近期研究表明，仅动脉粥样硬化就占 60 岁以上男性 ED 病因的 60%。此外，在美国男性中，ED 与未来心血管疾病的风险密切相关。

心血管疾病

在美国，动脉粥样硬化、高脂血症、吸烟和高血压是 ED 的常见病因。这些因素导致 ED 并不令人意外，因为勃起依赖于小动脉平滑肌的松弛和阴茎海绵体静脉阻力的增加。心血管疾病可能通过减少阴茎动脉的血流、引起血管腔机械性阻塞或血管内皮功能障碍（更常见）来降低勃起功能。血管内皮功能障碍是导致 ED 的最主要原因，由于内皮细胞释放 NO 的能力下降，血管平滑肌功能的神经控制机制中断，导致海绵体内的血流减少和压力降低。鉴于 ED 与心血管疾病之间的密切联系，表现出 ED 症状的男性应接受适当的心血管危险因素评估及管理。特别是 40 岁以上首次出现 ED 症状的男性，其心肌事件的风险增加约 15 倍。

阴茎海绵体的主要供血动脉是海绵体动脉，它是阴部内动脉的终末分支。大动脉和小动脉疾病可能降低海绵体的血压，导致阴茎长度和硬度下降。此外，阴茎的静脉闭塞性疾病也是导致 ED 的重要原因。在这

TABLE 10.3   Frequency of Decreased Erectile Rigidity and Ejaculatory Dysfunction by Medication Class

Medication Class	Decreased Erectile Rigidity	Ejaculatory Dysfunction
β-Adrenergic antagonists	Common	Less common
Sympatholytics	Expected	Common
α1-Agonists	Uncommon	Uncommon
α2-Agonists	Common	Less common
α1-Antagonists	Uncommon	Less common[a]
Angiotensin-converting enzyme inhibitors	Uncommon	Uncommon
Diuretics	Less common	Uncommon
Antidepressants	Common[b]	Uncommon[c]
Antipsychotics	Common	Common
Anticholinergics	Less common	Uncommon

[a]Patients are able to ejaculate, but retrograde ejaculation is seen in 5% to 30%.
[b]Uncommon with serotonin reuptake inhibitors.
[c]Delayed or inhibited ejaculation with serotonin reuptake inhibitors.

rigidity. Veno-occlusive disease in the penis is also a significant cause of ED. In these patients, there is often appropriate arterial inflow but an impaired ability to prevent leakage of blood through the venous system out of the penis. As such, these patients often experience normal initial rigidity but quickly lose their erection before ejaculation occurs.

Neurogenic Erectile Dysfunction

Because the nervous system plays an integral role in the physiology of erection, any disease process that affects the brain, the spinal cord, or the peripheral nerves can cause ED. For example, dementia, Parkinson's disease, and stroke are diseases of the brain associated with ED. Patients with spinal cord injury commonly have ED. Because of an intact spinal reflex pathway, most patients with spinal cord injury respond to tactile sensation, but they usually require medical therapy to maintain the erection through intercourse. Iatrogenic injury to nerves during surgery (e.g., prostatectomy, rectal surgery) is also a common cause of neurogenic ED. Neurogenic ED due to decreases in penile tactile sensation can occur with increasing age.

Endocrine Disorders

Testosterone plays a permissive role in erectile function, and many endocrine disorders can directly or indirectly decrease plasma free or bound testosterone. However, while testosterone deficiency is an uncommon primary cause of ED as erectile ability is only partially androgen dependent, the current AUA guidelines do recommend checking a morning serum testosterone in men with ED to confirm that they are not testosterone deficient. Patients with testosterone deficiency typically have decreased or absent libido in addition to loss of erectile rigidity. If testosterone deficiency is confirmed on two separate morning testosterone tests, testosterone therapy should be offered. If erectile rigidity fails to improve with 3 to 6 months of testosterone therapy, testosterone supplementation should be discontinued. Testosterone therapy is not indicated for patients with normal circulating testosterone levels and ED.

The most common endocrine disorder affecting erectile ability is diabetes mellitus. In addition to causing atherosclerosis and microvascular disease, diabetes affects both the autonomic and the somatic nervous systems, including loss of function of long autonomic nerves. The loss of function of these long cholinergic neurons results in interruptions of the efferent arm of the erectile reflex arc. Diabetes also appears to produce dysfunction of the neuromuscular junction at the level of arterial smooth muscle in the penile corpora

cavernosa. Studies have indicated markedly decreased acetylcholine and NO concentrations in the trabeculae of the corpora cavernosa in diabetic patients. These findings probably represent a combination of neural loss and neuromuscular junction dysfunction. Other endocrine disorders, such as hypothyroidism, hyperthyroidism, and adrenal dysfunction, can also cause ED. Because of the uncommon occurrence of thyroid and adrenal disorders in patients presenting for treatment of ED, testing of those axes is not a part of the routine work-up of ED.

Medication-Induced Erectile Dysfunction

Many commonly prescribed medications can cause or contribute to decreased erectile function. Table 10.3 lists the major classes of medications implicated in ED and suggests how commonly these medications interfere with erectile function. Changing medications may restore erectile function in some patients. However, proceeding directly to treatment of ED is usually a better option in all but the most straightforward cases.

Medical and Surgical Therapies

Since the introduction of sildenafil in 1998, the Process of Care Model for the evaluation and treatment of ED has been adopted. This model targets the primary care provider as the initial source of care for patients with ED. Currently available therapies for ED include oral PDE5 inhibitors, intraurethral alprostadil, intracavernosal vasoactive injection therapy, vacuum constriction devices, and penile prosthesis implantation. Although a stepwise treatment approach starting with oral agents and progressing to more invasive therapeutic interventions has generally been advocated, many men's health specialists now advocate assessing each patient individually and ensuring that all options are discussed (Fig. 10.2). All patients who are candidates for oral medications should generally try these prior to more invasive procedures given their relative high success and low risk profile; however, all patients are not required to proceed incrementally up the chain of treatment measures, as long as they are fully informed of the available options. Informed patient decision making is critical to successful progression through the Process of Care pathway. Patient referral is primarily based on the need or desire for specialized diagnostic testing and management. Most importantly, all men with comorbidities known to negatively affect erectile function should be counseled that lifestyle modifications such as improved diet and physical activity may have a significant positive impact on their erectile function.

表 10.3　不同药物类别导致勃起硬度降低和射精功能障碍的发生频率

药物类别	勃起硬度降低	射精功能障碍
β 受体阻滞剂	常见	较少见
交感神经阻滞剂	可预见	常见
α₁ 受体激动剂	不常见	不常见
α₂ 受体激动剂	常见	较少见
α₁ 受体阻滞剂	不常见	较少见 [a]
血管紧张素转换酶抑制剂	不常见	不常见
利尿剂	较少见	不常见
抗抑郁药	常见 [b]	不常见 [c]
抗精神病药	常见	常见
抗胆碱药	较少见	不常见

[a] 患者能够射精，但有 5%～30% 的患者出现逆行射精。
[b] 使用选择性 5- 羟色胺再摄取抑制剂的患者不常见。
[c] 选择性 5- 羟色胺再摄取抑制剂可能导致射精延迟或受抑制。

类疾病中，患者的动脉血流通常正常，但阻止血液通过静脉系统流出阴茎的能力受损。因此，这些患者虽然在性活动初期可能表现出正常的勃起硬度，但通常在射精前很快失去勃起。

神经源性 ED

由于神经系统在勃起的生理过程中发挥核心作用，任何影响大脑、脊髓或周围神经的疾病都可能导致 ED。例如，痴呆、帕金森病和卒中都是与 ED 相关的脑疾病。脊髓损伤患者通常会出现 ED。由于保留完整的脊髓反射通路，多数患者对触觉刺激有反应，但通常需要药物治疗才能在性交过程中维持勃起。手术（如前列腺切除术、直肠手术）导致的医源性神经损伤也是神经源性 ED 的常见原因。随着年龄的增长，阴茎触觉减弱也会导致神经源性 ED。

内分泌疾病

睾酮在勃起功能中发挥重要作用，许多内分泌疾病可以直接或间接降低血浆中游离或结合睾酮的水平。尽管睾酮缺乏症并非 ED 的主要病因（因为勃起功能仅部分依赖于雄激素），但当前的 AUA 指南仍建议对 ED 患者进行晨间血清睾酮检测，以确认是否存在睾酮缺乏症。睾酮缺乏症患者通常会出现性欲减退或缺失，以及勃起硬度下降。如果 2 次单独的晨间睾酮检测确诊睾酮缺乏症，应考虑进行睾酮治疗。如果经过 3～6 个月的睾酮治疗后勃起硬度仍未改善，应考虑停止睾酮治疗。对于睾酮水平正常的 ED 患者，不建议进行睾酮治疗。

糖尿病是影响勃起功能最常见的内分泌疾病。除了导致动脉粥样硬化和微血管疾病外，糖尿病还会影响自主神经和躯体神经系统，包括导致长自主神经功能丧失。这种长胆碱能神经元功能的丧失会导致勃起反射弧传出中断。糖尿病还可能导致阴茎海绵体动脉平滑肌水平的神经肌肉接头功能障碍。研究表明，糖尿病患者海绵体小梁中的乙酰胆碱和 NO 浓度显著降低，这可能是神经损伤和神经肌肉接头功能障碍的共同结果。其他内分泌疾病（如甲状腺功能减退症、甲状腺功能亢进症和肾上腺功能障碍）也可导致 ED。由于甲状腺疾病和肾上腺疾病在接受 ED 治疗的患者中并不常见，因此其相关检查未纳入 ED 的常规检查中。

药物引起的 ED

很多常用的处方药可能导致或加重 ED。表 10.3 列举了与 ED 相关的主要药物类别，并总结了这些药物干扰勃起功能的可能性。更换药物可能使部分患者的勃起功能恢复。然而，除了明确由药物导致的 ED 外，直接治疗 ED 通常是更合适的选择。

药物和外科治疗

自 1998 年西地那非上市以来，ED 的评估和治疗即采用"综合诊疗流程模型"。该模型将初级保健医生作为 ED 患者的初始诊疗提供者。目前可用的 ED 治疗方法包括：口服 PDE5 抑制剂、前列地尔尿道内给药、海绵体内注射血管活性药、真空收缩装置及阴茎假体植入术。虽然普遍主张采用循序渐进的治疗方法，先从口服药物开始，然后逐步过渡到更具侵入性的治疗手段，但许多男性健康专科医生推荐对每位患者进行个体化评估，并确保对所有治疗选择进行讨论（图 10.2）。所有适合口服药物的患者通常均应在尝试更具侵入性的方法前试用药物治疗，因为口服药物的治疗成功率相对较高且风险较低；然而，只要患者充分了解可用的治疗选择，则并非所有患者都需要严格按照固定的治疗流程逐步进行。知情决策对于有效推进诊疗流程至关重要。患者转诊主要基于对专业诊断和治疗的需求或意愿。最重要的是，所有患有已知对勃起功能有负面影响的合并症的患者均应被告知，通过改善饮食和增加体力活动等生活方式的调整，可能显著改善勃起功能。

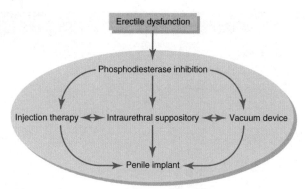

Fig. 10.2 A logical treatment algorithm for erectile dysfunction.

Oral Phosphodiesterase Type 5 Inhibitors

Current medical therapy is based on inhibition of PDE5, which degrades cGMP to inactive 5′-GMP, as shown in Fig. 10.1. Sildenafil, vardenafil, avanafil, and tadalafil all competitively inhibit PDE5 breakdown of cGMP. Use of a PDE5 inhibitor results in improved erectile rigidity even in patients with decreased NO or cGMP synthesis. However, not all patients respond to PDE5 inhibition. Adequate sexual stimulation and intact neural and vascular pathways are necessary to produce an adequate amount of NO and cGMP to increase deep penile artery blood flow. PDE5 inhibitors have been shown to be effective in men with vasculogenic, psychogenic, neurogenic, and mixed cases of ED. The overall response rate to PDE5 inhibitors is 70%.

Unless contraindicated, PDE5 inhibition should be considered first-line therapy for most men. The combination of PDE5 inhibitors and α-adrenergic receptor blockers (often used in men with lower urinary tract symptoms related to an enlarged prostate) can result in transient hypotension; however, in general it is safe to use selective α-blockers such as tamsulosin and alfluzosin with any PDE5 inhibitor, particularly once a patient is already established on therapy with the α-blocker. However, PDE5 inhibitors should not be used concurrently with nitrate medications due to the significant risk of a large (>25 mm Hg) synergistic drop in blood pressure. Periodic follow-up is necessary to determine therapeutic efficacy, assess for side effects related to PDE5 inhibition, and evaluate any changes in health status. Commonly reported side effects include headaches and flushing, while some patients have reported changes in vision due to unintended inhibition of PDE6 in the retina.

Alprostadil Intraurethral Drug Therapy

In patients for whom PDE5 inhibition is unsuccessful, one potential second-line medical treatment is intraurethral administration of prostaglandin E₁ (alprostadil). Alprostadil pellets are inserted directly into the urethra with the use of a pellet applicator and then diffuse into the surrounding tissue, initiating a second messenger cascade involving cAMP and inducing erection. This method of delivery assumes substantial venous communications between the corpus spongiosum surrounding the urethra and the corpus cavernosum and is effective in many patients who fail oral PDE5 inhibitor medications. A number of patients experience difficulty initiating this type of treatment due to discomfort or concerns in using the applicator, so it may be beneficial to administer the first dose in an office setting. To lubricate the urethra, patients should void prior to insertion of the pellet.

Up to one third of patients have normal, transient burning penile pain, and this should be discussed with the patient before treatment. Dizziness and presyncope are uncommon complications. Intraurethral alprostadil results in rapid onset erection after administration and has a minimal risk of priapism. It can be used with increased efficacy in combination with PDE5 inhibitors. Transient burning pain in the sexual partner can occur and is caused by leakage of the medication from the urethra into the vagina. This method of achieving erection is also contraindicated in men having intercourse with a pregnant female, due to the above risks of transference. This can be managed by wearing a condom.

Intracavernosal Injection Therapy

Pharmacologic injection therapy involves the injection of vasodilator agents into the corpora cavernosa to produce erection by stimulating dilation of the corporal artery smooth muscle. More than 90% of patients with ED respond to this type of therapy. Commonly used agents, either alone or in combination, include alprostadil, papaverine, and phentolamine. As monotherapy, alprostadil is most commonly used. Of the three, only alprostadil has been evaluated in rigorous clinical trials and has specific marketing approval from the US Food and Drug Administration for the treatment of ED. Phentolamine is often used to potentiate the action of papaverine and can be used in combination with both alprostadil and papaverine. These vasoactive drugs can be formulated with different combinations of medications and concentrations to achieve increased efficacy and decreased side effects. *Bimix* and *trimix* are terms often used to refer to a combination of two or three of these medications, respectively.

The most common side effects of this type of treatment are bruising and penile pain (50%). Penile pain is more common in young patients and is usually worse with alprostadil. Therefore, a combination using lower-dose alprostadil or formulations of papaverine and phentolamine alone might be beneficial in younger patients. Other, more serious risks of injection therapy include priapism and corporal scarring. Priapism has been reported to occur in 1% to 4% of patients but is more commonly reported in patients with neurogenic ED, especially young men with spinal cord injury. Significant acquired penile curvature due to corporal scarring (Peyronie's disease) is seen uncommonly and usually follows several years of injection therapy. Penile curvature appears to be less common with the use of alprostadil than with papaverine. The most common problem with pharmacologic injection therapy, however, is continuation of treatment, as up to 50% to 60% of patients stop using the technique within 1 year due to poor tolerance and satisfaction.

As with intraurethral alprostadil, initial treatment should be performed under the supervision of a physician. The medication can be injected using a self-contained medication-syringe kit or a 29-gauge (5/8-inch) insulin syringe with medication drawn from a refrigerated vial. It is advisable to start with a small test dose and slowly titrate the dosage for desired effect over several weeks. The patient should not use the medication more than once in a 24-hour period and should be instructed to seek medical care promptly for prolonged erections lasting longer than 4 hours. Typically, administration of the test dose should be carried out in the morning, and the patient should be expected to stay in close proximity to the medical office to monitor for priapism. Should a patient develop priapism, it usually resolves without sequelae after intracavernosal injection of phenylephrine in a setting where blood pressure and heart rate can be continuously monitored. Formal guidelines for the treatment of priapism are available on the website of the AUA.

Vacuum Constriction Devices

Vacuum constriction devices enclose the penis in a plastic tube with an airtight seal at the penile base. Air is pumped out of the cylinder, creating a vacuum and pulling blood into the corporal bodies, leading to penile erection. A constriction band is then slid from the cylinder to the base of the penis to constrict venous outflow and maintain the erection. Simultaneous use of a vacuum device and a PDE5 inhibitor is safe

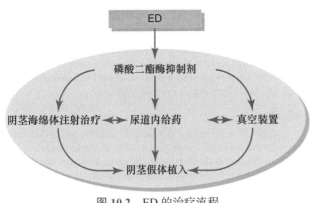

图 10.2　ED 的治疗流程

口服 PDE5 抑制剂

目前的药物治疗是基于对 PDE5 的抑制作用，如图 10.1 所示，PDE5 可将 cGMP 降解为无活性的 5′-GMP。西地那非、伐地那非、阿伐那非及他达拉非等药物能竞争性抑制 PDE5 对 cGMP 的降解。即使在 NO 或 cGMP 合成减少的患者中，使用 PDE5 抑制剂也能改善勃起硬度。然而，并非所有患者都对 PDE5 抑制剂有良好的反应。为了产生足够的 NO 和 cGMP 以增加阴茎深动脉的血流，仍需充分的性刺激及完整的神经和血管通路。研究表明，PDE5 抑制剂可有效治疗血管源性、心因性、神经源性及混合型 ED，其总体有效率约为 70%。

对于大多数男性患者，除非有禁忌证，PDE5 抑制剂应被视为一线治疗。PDE5 抑制剂与 α 受体阻滞剂（通常用于治疗由前列腺增生引起的下尿路症状）联合使用时，可能会引起短暂的低血压；但是，通常情况下，选择性 α 受体阻滞剂（如坦索罗辛和阿夫唑嗪）与 PDE5 抑制剂联合使用是安全的，特别是患者已稳定使用 α 受体阻滞剂时。然而，PDE5 抑制剂不应与硝酸盐类药物同时使用，因为血压大幅下降（> 25 mmHg）的风险会显著增加。在治疗过程中，需要定期进行随访以评估治疗效果，监测 PDE5 抑制剂相关的副作用，并评估健康状况的变化。常见副作用包括头痛和面部潮红，部分患者报告出现视力变化，这是由于 PDE5 抑制剂对视网膜中的 PDE6 产生预期外的抑制作用。

前列地尔尿道内给药

对于 PDE5 抑制剂治疗无效的患者，二线药物治疗的选择之一是前列腺素 E$_1$（前列地尔）尿道内给药。前列地尔药丸可使用药丸施药器直接置入尿道，然后扩散到周围组织，启动 cAMP 相关的第二信使级联反应，从而诱发勃起。这种给药方法是基于尿道周围的海绵体和阴茎海绵体之间有大量的静脉交通，对许多口服 PDE5 抑制剂无效的患者有效。使用施药器可能引起不适或担忧，因此首次使用最好在医疗机构进行。为了润滑尿道，患者应在置入药丸前排尿。

治疗过程中，多达 1/3 的患者可能会经历短暂的阴茎灼痛，应在治疗前与患者充分沟通。头晕和晕厥是不常见的并发症。前列地尔尿道内给药后能迅速诱发

勃起，且阴茎异常勃起的风险极低。此外，前列地尔可与 PDE5 抑制剂联合使用，以增强治疗效果。药物渗漏至性伴侣的阴道内可导致性伴侣出现短暂阴道灼痛，因此该治疗不适用于与妊娠期女性性交的男性，但上述风险可通过使用避孕套来有效规避。

海绵体内注射治疗

药物注射治疗是指将血管扩张剂注射到阴茎海绵体中，通过刺激海绵体动脉平滑肌的松弛来诱导勃起。超过 90% 的 ED 患者对该治疗有反应。常用药物包括前列地尔、罂粟碱和酚妥拉明，这些药物可单独使用或联合使用。单药治疗时，最常用前列地尔。在这 3 种药物中，前列地尔是唯一经过严格临床试验验证并获得 FDA 批准用于治疗 ED 的药物。酚妥拉明通常用于增强罂粟碱的效果，并可与前列地尔和罂粟碱组合使用。这些血管活性药物可以按不同的药物组合和浓度配置，以提高疗效并减少副作用。Bimix 和 trimix 通常分别指以上 2 种或 3 种药物的组合。

此类治疗最常见的副作用包括瘀伤和阴茎疼痛（50%）。年轻患者中阴茎疼痛更为常见，特别是在使用前列地尔时。因此，年轻患者使用低剂量前列地尔或仅使用罂粟碱和酚妥拉明的配方可能更合适。注射治疗的其他严重风险包括异常勃起和阴茎海绵体瘢痕。异常勃起可见于 1% ～ 4% 的患者，在年轻的神经源性 ED 患者中较常见，尤其是有脊髓损伤的年轻男性。阴茎海绵体瘢痕引起的显著阴茎弯曲（阴茎硬结症）较少见，通常发生在多年注射治疗后，使用前列地尔时阴茎弯曲的发生率似乎低于使用罂粟碱时。然而，药物注射治疗最常见的问题是治疗的持续性，由于耐受性差和满意度低，多达 50% ～ 60% 的患者会在 1 年内停止治疗。

与前列地尔尿道内给药类似，初次治疗应在医生的监督下进行。可以使用自装药物注射器套装，或 29 号针规（5/8 英寸针长）的胰岛素注射器从冷藏瓶中抽取药物进行注射。建议从低试验剂量开始，并在数周内缓慢调整剂量以达到期望的效果。患者 24 h 内最多用药 1 次，医生需告知患者，如果勃起持续超过 4 h，应立即就诊。通常情况下，试验剂量应在早晨给药，且患者应留在医疗机构附近，以便监测阴茎异常勃起。如果发生阴茎异常勃起，在持续监测血压和心率的情况下行海绵体内注射去氧肾上腺素通常可缓解且不会导致后遗症。关于阴茎异常勃起治疗的官方指南可查阅 AUA 网站。

真空收缩装置

真空收缩装置是将阴茎置于可密封的塑料管内，管底紧贴阴茎根部，通过抽出空气在管道内形成真空，从而将血液抽入海绵体使阴茎勃起。随后，约束环从管道中滑至阴茎根部，以限制静脉回流并维持勃起。真空收缩装置与 PDE5 抑制剂同时使用是安全的，且研

and has been shown to improve erectile rigidity and patient satisfaction with the vacuum device. Some of the common side effects that affect patient satisfaction with these devices are coldness, numbness, and bruising of the penis, as well as the cumbersome nature of the process.

Penile Prosthesis

A penile prosthesis is an either semirigid or inflatable device that is implanted into the penis in the operating room under general anesthesia. These devices allow for men to achieve rigid erections suitable for penetration and sexual function. In contemporary series, most patients prefer the inflatable devices over semirigid options because of the more natural erection when inflated and a fully flaccid penis when deflated. Although implantation of a penile prosthesis is more invasive than the other techniques, this device is the most effective long-term option for impotence treatment, with nearly 90% of patients and partners satisfied with the result.

Important interval improvements have been made in the design of implantable penile prostheses to make them more durable and resistant to infection. Improvements in the connections between tubing and corporal cylinders have cut the mechanical failure rate to less than 5% in 5 years. Components now also have special coatings that either contain antibiotics or absorb antibiotics applied topically at the time of implantation in order to decrease the risk of infection.

PEYRONIE'S DISEASE

Peyronie's disease (PD) is an acquired condition of the penis that involves fibrosis of the tunica albuginea, resulting in contracture and ultimately penile curvature and/or deformity. It may affect up to 6% of men in the United States. This disease can be quite debilitating to men for both psychological as well as functional reasons. Other than embarrassment related to the appearance of their penises, many men experience depression, relationship difficulties, and diminished quality of life, not to mention pain and difficulty in sexual activity, both for themselves and for their partners. There have been a number of significant advances over the past decade in the management of PD, progressing from a purely surgical disease process to one that now is often amenable to minimally invasive injection therapies.

Pathophysiology

PD is the result of fibrosis in the tunica albuginea of the penis and is believed to be secondary to repetitive microvascular trauma and buckling events over time. While some individuals will present with a clear history of a significant prior penile injury, most recall no inciting event. The natural history of PD itself is variable as well. Most men report a gradual worsening of curvature with associated penile pain for a number of months prior to presentation to a physician. For men who remain untreated for PD after presentation to a physician, approximately 12% will note improvement in their curvature over the ensuing year, while the remainder will either remain stable or worsen with time.

PD is defined temporally by *active* and *stable* phases of disease. The active phase is generally characterized by changes in the degree of curvature with time, as well as other degrees of penile modeling changes such as development of an "hourglass" appearance or induration. The prime characteristic of the active phase of disease, however, is the presence of pain, particularly with erection. The stable phase of disease is defined by at least 3 months of stable, unchanged curvature and/or other deformity. Pain with manipulation should be absent once a patient has reached the stable phase of the disease.

Differential Diagnosis

Acquired penile curvature due to PD may be difficult to differentiate from congenital penile curvature in some individuals, especially those who become sexually active later in life. Patients with congenital curvature generally have lifelong ventral curvature and no palpable fibrotic plaque consistent with PD. Acute penile trauma may cause pain and/or induration that may be confused for the active phase of PD. Rarely, patients with acute penile fractures may develop PD later in life due to inappropriate collagen deposition following injury.

Evaluation

The most common presenting symptom for patients with PD is dorsal curvature (the penis curves up towards the abdomen) with a palpable fibrotic plaque on the dorsum of the penis. However, there is tremendous variation in the degree and extent of curvature that patients may develop, with many patients having ventral, lateral, or multiplanar, compound curvatures. Furthermore, many patients develop the previously mentioned "hourglass" appearance due to circumferential constriction of the tunica albuginea by fibrosis within the corpora cavernosa. PD has been shown to occur simultaneously in patients with Dupuytren contracture of the hands or Ledderhose disease of the plantar fascia, so patients should be appropriately evaluated for these diseases as well. While some patients will occasionally present with photographs of their erect penis for evaluation, providers should be comfortable inducing a pharmacologic erection to evaluate the degree, extent, and location of curvature in the office. Concomitant penile duplex ultrasonography may be useful to evaluate the vascular integrity of the penis, as well as for possible calcifications of the fibrotic plaque, but this is best performed by individuals specifically trained in this technique.

Measurements of penile length and specific notation on the location and size of the plaque are useful in determining treatment strategies. A thorough sexual history is similarly vital in the initial evaluation. The degree or extent of ED must be ascertained, as PD commonly coexists with ED and the presence of ED impacts potential treatment options. Treatment of penile curvature due to Peyronie's disease will not improve decreased penile rigidity. Similarly, a thorough history of the duration and stability of curvature, as well as the presence of pain with erections and/or intercourse, should be obtained in order to determine if a patient is in the active and stable phase of disease.

Treatment
Active Phase

Active phase disease represents an ongoing physiologic process in which collagen deposition is incomplete and variable. Many attempts have been made in the past to alter this process through the use of medications; however, no proven therapies have been found to be efficacious, other than simple nonsteroidal anti-inflammatory drugs (NSAIDs) for the pain associated with active disease. Surgical treatments for PD are not indicated during the active phase of the disease. Although a number of proposed oral therapies have been previously advocated with hopes of preventing or reversing curvature, there is currently insufficient evidence for their use. The most commonly used oral medication, vitamin E, has had a number of both observational and randomized control trials performed, all of which have failed to demonstrate efficacy in reducing curvature, pain or progression. The primary aim for management of patients in the active phase of disease is symptom control with NSAIDs.

Stable Phase

For patients in the stable phase of PD, in whom curvature has been stable for at least 3 months and there is no significant pain with erections, treatment is geared towards improving sexual function and quality of life. There is no urgent medical indication for intervening on PD in the absence of patient bother. Treatment decisions are based on patient

究证实其能提高勃起硬度和患者对真空装置的满意度。影响患者对这些装置的满意度的常见原因包括阴茎冰凉感、麻木、瘀伤及使用过程繁琐。

阴茎假体

阴茎假体是一种半硬性或可膨胀装置，通常在全身麻醉下植入阴茎。假体能够使男性达到适合性交的勃起硬度。在现代产品中，大多数患者更倾向于选择可膨胀假体而非半硬性假体，因为可膨胀假体在充气时阴茎勃起更为自然，放气后阴茎可完全松弛。尽管阴茎假体植入术比其他方法更具侵入性，但它是治疗阳痿最有效的长期方案，近 90% 的患者及其伴侣对手术结果感到满意。

植入式阴茎假体在设计上取得的重要技术改进使其更耐用、抗感染性能更强。管道和阴茎海绵体假体之间连接的改进使 5 年内机械故障率降低至 5% 以下。现有的组件具有特殊涂层，这些涂层含有抗生素或在植入时可吸收的局部应用抗生素，以减少感染风险。

阴茎硬结症

阴茎硬结症（PD）是一种获得性阴茎白膜纤维化病变，可导致白膜收缩并最终引起阴茎弯曲和（或）畸形。美国约 6% 的成年男性受此病影响。这种疾病可在心理和功能方面对男性造成严重困扰。除了使患者因阴茎外观改变而感到尴尬外，许多 PD 患者还可能经历抑郁症、人际关系障碍及生活质量下降等问题，以及在性生活中所感受到的疼痛和困难，这些问题不仅影响患者自身，也影响他们的伴侣。在过去十年中，PD 的治疗取得了显著进展，从主要依靠外科手术治疗发展到现在通常可以通过微创注射治疗有效处理。

病理生理学

PD 由阴茎白膜纤维化造成，继发于长期反复的微血管损伤和导致阴茎弯曲的事件。尽管一些患者有明确的阴茎创伤史，但大多数患者并不记得有明显的诱因。PD 的自然病程因人而异，大部分男性主诉在就诊前几个月阴茎弯曲逐渐加重，并伴有疼痛。对于就诊后未接受治疗的 PD 患者，约 12% 的患者在接下来的 1 年内阴茎弯曲有所改善，其他患者病情稳定或随时间逐渐恶化。

PD 的病程可分为活动期和稳定期。活动期的一般特征是阴茎弯曲度改变及其他阴茎形态改变（如"沙漏"样外观或硬结）。然而，活动期的主要特征是疼痛，特别是在勃起时。稳定期是指疾病在至少 3 个月内无进一步变化，弯曲和（或）其他畸形保持稳定。一旦进入稳定期，触诊阴茎应不再出现疼痛。

鉴别诊断

在某些患者中，由 PD 引起的获得性阴茎弯曲可能难以与先天性阴茎弯曲进行鉴别，特别是对于那些开始性生活较晚的患者。先天性阴茎弯曲的患者通常自出生以来就存在阴茎向腹侧弯曲，并且无法触及与 PD 相一致的纤维性斑块。急性阴茎创伤可能导致疼痛和（或）硬结形成，这可能会被误诊为 PD 活动期。在极少数情况下，急性阴茎折断患者由于创伤后胶原蛋白沉积不当，可能会在后续发展成 PD。

评估

在 PD 患者中，最常见的症状是阴茎背侧弯曲（阴茎向腹部弯曲）伴有阴茎背侧可触及纤维性斑块。然而，患者的弯曲程度和类型可能有很大差异，许多患者可能出现腹侧弯曲、侧面弯曲或多平面复合弯曲。此外，许多患者由于海绵体内纤维化导致白膜环向收缩而出现"沙漏"样外观。手部掌腱膜挛缩或足底筋膜 Ledderhose 病患者可合并 PD，因此这些疾病也应得到适当评估。虽然一些患者可能会提供阴茎勃起的照片以供评估，但医生也应通过药物诱导勃起，以精确评估弯曲的角度、程度和具体位置。此外，阴茎多普勒超声检查有助于评估阴茎的血管完整性及纤维性斑块的钙化情况，但该检查应由接受过专业培训的人员进行。

测量阴茎的长度及详细记录斑块的位置和大小有助于制订治疗策略。在初次评估中，全面获取患者的性生活史同样关键。此外，必须评估是否存在 ED，因为 PD 通常与 ED 共存，且合并 ED 可能影响 PD 的治疗方案。值得注意的是，治疗 PD 引起的阴茎弯曲并不会改善阴茎的硬度。同样，详细了解阴茎弯曲的持续时间和稳定性，以及勃起和（或）性交时的疼痛情况，对于判断患者是否处于疾病活动期或稳定期非常重要。

治疗

活动期

PD 活动期是一个持续的生理过程，其间胶原蛋白的沉积不完全且易变。尽管曾多次尝试通过药物调节这一过程，但目前除了用于治疗与活动期疼痛相关的非甾体抗炎药（NSAID）外，尚无其他治疗被证明有效。在 PD 活动期，通常不推荐进行外科手术。虽然既往提出过多种可能预防或逆转阴茎弯曲的口服药物治疗方法，但目前这些治疗方案的证据仍不充分。最常用的口服药物（如维生素 E）已进行过多项观察性研究和随机对照试验，但均未能证明其在减少阴茎弯曲、疼痛或阻止病情进展方面的有效性。因此，活动期 PD 患者的主要治疗目标是使用 NSAID 来控制症状。

稳定期

对于处于 PD 稳定期的患者，如果阴茎弯曲度在至少 3 个月内保持稳定且在勃起时无明显疼痛，则治疗的目标是改善性功能和生活质量。在没有对患者造成困扰的情况下，没有立即干预 PD 的指征。治疗决策应

wishes and tailored according to degree of erectile function, tolerance of each intervention, and ability to undergo general anesthesia.

Intralesional injection therapy. There are currently two commonly used medications for PD that are directly injected into the fibrous plaque of patients and have been shown to be effective in improving curvature. Interferon-α was the first widely successful intralesional injection therapy used in PD patients. This medication functions by decreasing the rate of fibroblast proliferation within the tissues, thus decreasing the deposition of extracellular collagen. Interferon-α has been shown to have efficacy in improving both curvature and plaque size.

More recent, however, was the FDA approval of collagenase clostridium histolyticum (CCH) in 2013 for use in PD patients. This medication contains a collagenase enzyme that, when directly injected into Peyronie's lesions, enzymatically degrades interstitial collagen, improving curvature. The IMPRESS trial, which led to the FDA approval of CCH for PD patients, consisted of up to four 6-week cycles, with each cycle including two injections of CCH 24 to 72 hours apart. The treatment group, as compared to a saline control group, was found to fare significantly better, with a mean 34% improvement in curvature (17 degrees) in the treatment group as compared to 18% (9 degrees) in the control group. While this trial excluded individuals with curvatures of less than 30 degrees, as well as those with ventral curvatures and plaques, some providers have now extrapolated these data to treat individuals not initially eligible based on these inclusion criteria. Though no head-to-head trials have been conducted, CCH appears to be more effective at decreasing penile curvature than interferon-α.

While intralesional injection therapy is generally safe and minimally invasive, there are some associated risks. Patients who receive interferon-α are at significant risk of developing sinusitis, flulike symptoms, and penile swelling. CCH, on the other hand, has been associated with rare serious adverse events such as penile fracture, while the majority of patients developed mild adverse side effects such as pain, swelling, bruising, or painful erections. Lastly, patients may require up to 24 weeks of therapy to reach maximal improvement in curvature, which may dissuade some individuals.

Surgical therapy. The goal of surgical therapy for PD is to correct the penile deformity (curvature and/or hourglass) and allow the patient to return to satisfactory intercourse. For patients with PD who are either not interested in or not candidates for intralesional injection therapies there are three primary surgical options. The primary determinant of the surgical therapy offered is the degree of ED in the patient. Improvement of penile curvature in a patient who is otherwise unable to obtain a sufficient and satisfactory erection will improve that patient's quality of life. For patients with significant ED despite pharmacotherapy, placement of a penile prosthesis may be performed (as discussed previously), often with adjunct maneuvers discussed later to obtain straightening.

The most commonly performed procedure for men with PD is tunical plication. In this procedure, the convex side of the penis is shortened with placement of sutures directly in the tunica albuginea opposite the fibrous plaque on the contralateral side of the penis. This procedure may result in perceived penile shortening and is best reserved for men with sufficient preoperative stretched penile length, as well as for those with mild to moderate degrees of curvature. Plication techniques are unable to address hourglass or other indentation deformities but are unlikely to have any significant negative impact on erectile function.

An alternative approach, particularly for men with more significant curvatures or in those in whom a plication technique may have too significant of an impact on penile length, is plaque incision (or excision) and grafting. In this procedure, the PD plaque is identified and incised (or excised if extensively calcified). Incising the plaque relieves

TABLE 10.4   Symptoms of Lower Urinary Tract Syndrome

Overactive Bladder	Obstructive Voiding
Frequency	Hesitancy
Nocturia	Slow stream
Urgency	Stop-and-start voiding
Urge incontinence	Sensation of incomplete emptying

the tension that the fibrous plaque was applying to the penis causing it to curve, allowing it to return to its normal straight position without sacrificing length. The resultant defect in the tunica albuginea is then grafted using either autologous tissues (i.e., saphenous vein) or other graft materials (allograft, xenograft, or synthetic grafts have all been utilized). Importantly, this procedure can be used to correct hourglass and other indentation deformities that other techniques cannot. Although this procedure does maintain penile length, there are increased concerns related to postoperative ED, with up to 30% of men reporting new-onset or worsening ED after the procedure. However, overall, satisfaction and straightening rates are greater than 80% for both plication and grafting techniques.

BENIGN PROSTATIC HYPERPLASIA

Benign prostatic hyperplasia (BPH) is a nonmalignant enlargement of the prostate gland and is widely prevalent in the aging male patient. It is estimated that more than 90% of all men will develop histologic evidence of BPH during the course of their lifetime, with at least 50% of these men developing lower urinary tract symptoms (LUTS) that prompt them to seek medical care. Broadly speaking, LUTS can be divided into two groups: obstructive voiding symptoms and overactive bladder symptoms (Table 10.4).

Although most patients who seek medical care for BPH do so because of the associated LUTS, these same symptoms can also result from other illnesses such as diabetes mellitus, spine disease, Parkinson's disease, multiple sclerosis, and cerebrovascular disease (Fig. 10.3). It is important to evaluate all patients for these non–BPH-related conditions to ensure appropriate management is provided. It is also important to pay close attention to medication use, because a number of medications used in the elderly population can result in various urologic symptoms, including both obstructive and overactive bladder voiding symptoms. Lastly, BPH itself is a histologic diagnosis and does not in itself require intervention. Intervention is only indicated for individuals in which BPH is resulting in bothersome symptoms or complications related to impaired bladder emptying.

Pathophysiology

Prostate growth and the subsequent development of BPH occur under the influence of testosterone and the more metabolically active byproduct, dihydrotestosterone (DHT). Testosterone produced by the testes is converted to DHT by the action of the enzyme 5α-reductase within the prostate itself. DHT is the major intracellular androgen within the prostate and is believed to be responsible for the development and maintenance of the hyperplastic cell growth characteristics of BPH.

BPH develops predominantly in the periurethral prostatic tissue, referred to as the *transition zone* (Fig. 10.4). Tissue growth in this area leads to the phenomenon of bladder outlet obstruction (BOO), which causes LUTS. BOO occurs as a result of two mechanisms: first, mechanical obstruction from increased tissue volume in the periurethral zone of the prostate and, second, dynamic obstruction caused by decreased bladder neck relaxation during voiding and increased

基于患者的意愿，并根据患者的勃起功能、对各种治疗措施的耐受性及是否能进行全身麻醉来制订。

硬结内注射治疗　目前有两种治疗 PD 的主流药物，其可直接注射至纤维斑块中，并均已被证实能有效改善阴茎弯曲。干扰素 α 是首个在 PD 患者中成功广泛应用的硬结内注射药物，它可降低组织中成纤维细胞的增殖速度，减少细胞外胶原沉积，从而有效缩小斑块和改善阴茎弯曲程度。

2013 年 FDA 批准溶组织梭菌胶原酶（CCH）用于治疗 PD。该药物含有能够酶解间质胶原的胶原酶，直接注射到 PD 病变部位可改善阴茎弯曲。FDA 基于 IMPRESS 试验的结果批准了 CCH 用于治疗 PD，该试验包括 4 个周期的治疗，每个周期为 6 周，共注射 2 次 CCH，间隔 24～72 h。与生理盐水对照组相比，治疗组的平均阴茎弯曲改善率为 34%（17°），而对照组为 18%（9°）。尽管该试验排除了弯曲度＜30°及有腹侧弯曲和斑块的患者，但部分医生现在已将这些数据扩展至用于治疗最初不符合纳入标准的患者。虽然目前尚未进行 CCH 与干扰素 α 的直接对比试验，但初步数据显示，CCH 在减少阴茎弯曲度方面似乎更有效。

虽然硬结内注射治疗通常是安全且微创的，但也存在一定的风险。接受干扰素 α 治疗的患者发生鼻窦炎、流感样症状和阴茎肿胀的风险很大。此外，CCH 与罕见的严重不良事件（如阴茎折断）有关，但绝大多数患者仅出现轻微的不良反应，如疼痛、肿胀、瘀伤或痛性勃起。此外，患者可能需要长达 24 周的治疗才能实现阴茎弯曲度的最大改善，这可能会劝退一些患者。

外科治疗　PD 的外科治疗旨在纠正阴茎畸形［弯曲和（或）沙漏形］，使患者能够恢复满意的性生活。对于不愿意或不适合接受硬结内注射的患者，有 3 种主要的手术选择。选择的主要依据是患者的 ED 程度。对于勃起功能不佳的患者，矫正阴茎弯曲度能显著提高其生活质量。对于接受药物治疗后仍有显著 ED 的患者，可以考虑阴茎假体植入（见上文），通常会结合辅助操作（见下文）来实现矫直。

PD 患者最常进行的手术是白膜折叠术。该手术直接缝合阴茎纤维斑块对面的白膜，使阴茎的凸面缩短。这种手术可能导致阴茎缩短，因此最适合术前有足够阴茎拉伸长度和阴茎弯曲程度为轻中度的男性。这种技术无法解决沙漏形或其他凹陷畸形，但一般不会对勃起功能产生显著的负面影响。

另一种方法是斑块切开（或切除）和移植术，特别适用于弯曲程度较严重或白膜折叠术对阴茎长度影响较大的患者。该手术方法是定位并切开（大量钙化时切除）PD 斑块。切开斑块可缓解其对阴茎施加的张力，使阴茎恢复到正常的直立状态而不牺牲长度。然

表 10.4　下尿路综合征的症状

膀胱过度活动症状	梗阻性排尿症状
尿频	排尿踌躇
夜尿	尿流缓慢
尿急	尿流中断
急迫性尿失禁	尿不尽感

后，白膜的缺损部分通过自体组织（如隐静脉）或其他移植材料（同种异基因移植物、异种移植物或合成移植物均可用）进行移植修补。重要的是，这种方法可以纠正其他技术无法处理的沙漏形和其他凹陷畸形。虽然这种手术可以维持阴茎长度，但术后 ED 的风险增加，有高达 30% 的男性在手术后出现 ED 或 ED 加重。总体而言，白膜折叠术和移植术的满意度和矫直率均超过 80%。

良性前列腺增生

良性前列腺增生（BPH）是一种前列腺的非恶性增大，是老年男性的常见疾病。据估计，90% 以上的男性在其一生中会出现有组织学证据的 BPH，其中至少 50% 会出现下尿路症状（LUTS），并因此就医。广义上讲，LUTS 可分为两组症状群：梗阻性排尿症状和膀胱过度活动症状（表 10.4）。

尽管大多数 BPH 患者因 LUTS 就医，但其他疾病也可能出现 LUTS，如糖尿病、脊髓疾病、帕金森病、多发性硬化和脑血管疾病（图 10.3）。评估这些非 BPH 相关的疾病对制订合理的治疗方案至关重要。此外，还需要密切关注患者的用药史，因为老年人群使用的许多药物可能导致各种泌尿系统症状，包括梗阻性排尿症状和膀胱过度活动症状。BPH 是一种组织学诊断，其本身并不需要干预。只有在 BPH 导致降低患者生活质量的症状或与膀胱排空受损相关的并发症时才需要干预。

病理生理学

前列腺的生长和 BPH 的发生受睾酮及其活性更强的代谢产物双氢睾酮（DHT）的影响。由睾丸产生的睾酮在前列腺内通过 5α-还原酶的作用转化为 DHT。DHT 是前列腺的主要细胞内雄激素，被认为与 BPH 中细胞增生性生长特征的发展和维持有关。

BPH 主要发生在尿道周围的前列腺组织，即移行区（图 10.4）。该区域的组织增生会导致膀胱出口梗阻（BOO），从而引起 LUTS。BOO 的发生有两种机制：一种是由前列腺移行区组织体积增大而造成的机械性梗阻，另一种是由排尿时膀胱颈松弛减少及膀胱颈和前列腺平滑肌张力增加所引起的动态性梗阻。同样重

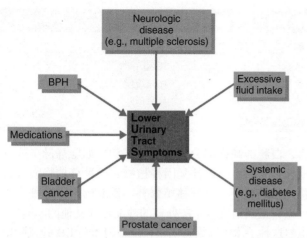

Fig. 10.3 Causes of lower urinary tract symptoms (LUTS). *BPH*, Benign prostatic hyperplasia.

smooth muscle tone in the bladder neck and prostate gland. Also important, but less well characterized, is the response of the detrusor muscle to the increase in outlet resistance provided by those two mechanisms. As bladder outlet resistance increases, the bladder responds by increasing the force of contraction. This added work results in physical and mechanical changes in bladder function over time and may contribute to the presence of overactive bladder symptomatology in patients with BOO.

Early in the course of BOO, the bladder is able to compensate to overcome the elevated outlet resistance; however, with persistent obstruction, the patient typically develops LUTS, particularly difficulty initiating the stream, weak stream, hesitancy, and intermittency. These symptoms frequently drive patients to seek medical care. Later during the course of the obstructive process, the bladder wall becomes thickened and loses compliance. The subsequent loss of compliance results in a decreased functional capacity of the bladder, which exacerbates the patient's overactive bladder symptoms such as urgency and frequency.

Diagnosis

The initial evaluation of a patient with LUTS suggestive of BPH should include a detailed medical history that focuses on the patient's urinary symptoms as well as the past medical history, including comorbid conditions and any previous surgical procedures, general health conditions, and history of alcohol and tobacco use. The assessment of symptoms can be facilitated with the use of the AUA Symptom Index (also known as the *International Prostate Symptom Score*, or IPSS). This is a self-administered, validated questionnaire consisting of seven questions related to the symptoms of BPH and BOO. The AUA Symptom Index classifies voiding symptoms as mild (0 to 7), moderate (8 to 19), or severe (20 to 35). Validated instruments such as the AUA Symptom Index are useful during the initial evaluation as an overall assessment of symptom severity and during follow-up visits to assess the effectiveness of any medical or surgical interventions.

A general physical examination should be performed that includes a DRE and a focused neurologic examination. Urinalysis, either by dipstick or by microscopic examination of urine sediment, is also mandatory to rule out hematuria and evidence of urinary tract infection. Glucosuria can be a significant finding, particularly if not previously identified, as this may indicate the presence of polyuria contributing to the patient's LUTS. The initial clinical practice guidelines for the diagnosis of BPH recommended a serum creatinine measurement to assess renal function in all patients with signs or symptoms suggestive

of BPH. However, this recommendation came under scrutiny because of its low yield for the detection of renal insufficiency secondary to obstructive uropathy. As such, serum creatinine measurement is no longer a routine part of the BPH work-up. According to the same clinical practice guidelines, PSA measurement is optional during the initial evaluation. PSA can function as a surrogate for prostate volume measurement in addition to being a screening test for prostate cancer. The Medical Therapy of Prostatic Symptoms (MTOPS) study, sponsored by the National Institutes of Health, demonstrated that PSA increases linearly with prostate volume and that a PSA level greater than 4 ng/mL conveys a 9% risk of requiring surgical therapy for benign disease over a 4.5-year period.

The following additional diagnostic tests should be considered when evaluating patients with BPH, specifically those in whom surgical therapy is being considered. Uroflowmetry is a noninvasive method of measuring urinary flow rate. The maximal urinary flow rate, Q_{max}, is considered the most useful measurement for identifying patients with BOO. However, a diminished Q_{max} alone is not diagnostic of BOO because patients with diminished flow rates may have such due to impaired bladder contraction rather than physical obstruction. Typical values range from 25 mL/second in a young man without BOO to 10 mL/second or slower in a man with significant BOO. Measurement of postvoid residual (PVR) urine may be accomplished by urethral catheterization or, preferably, by ultrasonography. Elevated PVR volumes indicate an increased risk for acute urinary retention and eventual need for surgical intervention. Elevated residuals, furthermore, put patients at risk for the formation of bladder stones, urinary tract infections, or renal deterioration with long-term retention. The MTOPS study demonstrated that 7% of men with PVR greater than 39 mL required surgical intervention over a 4.5-year period. Elevation of PVR to greater than 200 mL raises the question of functional impairment of the bladder and warrants further evaluation with urodynamic testing.

Routine evaluation of the upper urinary tracts (kidneys and ureters) with excretory urography or ultrasonography is not recommended for the average BPH patient unless there is concomitant urinary pathology (i.e., hematuria, urinary tract infection, renal insufficiency, a history of prior urologic surgery, or a history of nephrolithiasis). Likewise, transrectal ultrasonography (TRUS), CT or MRI imaging are not routinely recommended for medical therapy but should be considered in the preoperative assessment of prostate gland size prior to surgical intervention, as this may influence selection of technique.

Differential Diagnosis

A number of conditions can cause LUTS in the aging male. A DRE and PSA testing are helpful in distinguishing between BPH and prostate cancer, but neither is diagnostic. Early-stage prostate cancer is typically asymptomatic and patients can have both conditions concurrently. Although PSA testing is not sufficiently sensitive or specific to reliably differentiate BPH from prostate cancer, it is a useful tool to stratify a patient's risk for the presence of prostate cancer and assess the need for further prostate cancer evaluation. While controversy surrounding the use of PSA for prostate cancer screening persists, in general, patients between the ages of 40 and 55 at a higher risk for prostate cancer (i.e., African American men and/or those with a family history) and all men ages 55 to 69 should engage in shared decision making with their primary care providers to discuss the risks and benefits of prostate cancer screening and make an individualized decision on screening. Men with elevated PSAs or concerning DRE should be referred to a urologist for further evaluation and management.

Prostatitis is another condition that can cause LUTS. It may result from bacterial infection or from a nonbacterial inflammatory process, and the symptoms may substantially overlap those of BPH,

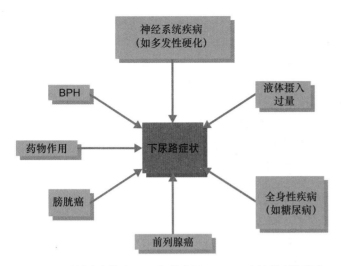

图 10.3 下尿路症状（LUTS）的病因。BPH，良性前列腺增生

要但尚未被充分阐述的机制是膀胱逼尿肌对以上两种机制所致膀胱出口阻力增加的反应。随着膀胱出口阻力的增加，膀胱会通过增加收缩力来做出反应。随着时间的推移，这种额外做功会导致膀胱功能发生物理和机械变化，并可能导致 BOO 患者出现膀胱过度活跃症状。

在 BOO 早期，膀胱尚能通过代偿机制克服出口阻力的增加；然而，随着梗阻的持续，患者通常会出现 LUTS，特别是排尿困难、尿无力、尿踌躇和尿流中断。这些症状常驱使患者就医。在 BOO 后期，膀胱壁增厚并失去顺应性。顺应性丧失导致膀胱的功能容量减少，从而加重患者的膀胱过度活动症状，如尿急和尿频。

诊断

对于提示 BPH 的 LUTS 患者，初步评估应包括详细的病史采集，重点关注患者的尿路症状及既往病史，包括共病情况、既往手术史、一般健康状况，以及吸烟和饮酒史。可以使用 AUA 症状指数［又称国际前列腺症状评分（IPSS）］进行 BPH 症状评估，该指数是经过验证的自评问卷，包括 7 个与 BPH 和 BOO 症状相关的问题。AUA 症状指数将排尿症状分为轻度（0～7 分）、中度（8～19 分）和重度（20～35 分）。在初次评估中，AUA 症状指数等经验证的工具可用于全面评估症状严重程度，并在随访中评估药物或手术治疗的效果。

一般体格检查应包括 DRE 和重点的神经系统检查。此外，还必须进行尿液分析（尿液检测试纸或尿沉渣镜检），以排除血尿和尿路感染。尿糖阳性是一个重要发现，尤其是在既往未发现的情况下，因为这可能提示患者的 LUTS 由多尿导致。早期临床指南推荐所有存在 BPH 症状或体征的患者均应检测血肌酐，以评估肾功能。然而，由于尿路梗阻引起肾功能不全的

比例较低，该建议受到质疑。因此，血肌酐不再作为 BPH 检查的常规项目。根据同一指南的建议，初次评估时可选择进行 PSA 检测。PSA 不仅可以作为前列腺体积测量的替代指标，也是前列腺癌的筛查项目。由美国国立卫生研究院资助的 MTOPS（Medical Therapy of Prostatic Symptoms）研究表明，PSA 水平与前列腺体积呈线性相关，且 PSA > 4 ng/ml 时，4.5 年内良性疾病需要手术治疗的风险为 9%。

在评估 BPH 患者，尤其是考虑手术治疗的患者时，应考虑进行以下额外的诊断性检查。尿流率测定是一种检测尿流速率的无创性检查。最大尿流率（Q_{max}）被认为是识别 BOO 最有用的参数。然而，单纯 Q_{max} 下降不能诊断 BOO，因为尿流率下降也可能由膀胱收缩功能受损而非物理性梗阻所致。在没有 BOO 的年轻男性中，Q_{max} 通常可达 25 ml/s，而在患有严重 BOO 的男性中，$Q_{max} \leq 10$ ml/s。可以通过导尿术或超声检查（首选）检测残余尿量（PVR）。PVR 增大提示急性尿潴留和最终需要手术治疗的风险增加。此外，PVR 增大会使患者面临膀胱结石、尿路感染或长时间尿潴留导致肾功能恶化的风险。MTOPS 研究表明，PVR > 39 ml 的男性中有 7% 在 4.5 年内需要手术治疗。PVR > 200 ml 时，需要进一步通过尿流动力学检查评估膀胱功能受损的可能性。

除非合并泌尿系统疾病（如血尿、尿路感染、肾功能不全、既往泌尿外科手术史或肾结石病史），否则不建议对一般 BPH 患者进行上尿路（肾和输尿管）的常规检查（如排泄性尿路造影或超声检查）。同样，在药物治疗时也不推荐常规进行经直肠超声检查（TRUS）、CT 或 MRI 检查，但在术前评估前列腺体积时应予以考虑，因为这可能会影响手术方案的选择。

鉴别诊断

许多疾病会导致老年男性出现 LUTS。DRE 和 PSA 检测有助于鉴别 BPH 和前列腺癌，但两者都不能作为确诊依据。早期前列腺癌通常无症状，且两种疾病可并存。虽然 PSA 在鉴别 BPH 和前列腺癌方面的敏感性和特异性均较低，但可用于前列腺癌的风险分层，并判断是否需要进一步进行前列腺癌的相关评估。虽然关于 PSA 用于前列腺癌筛查的争议仍然存在，但总体而言，前列腺癌风险较高［即非裔美国男性和（或）有家族史者］的 40～55 岁患者和所有 55～69 岁男性应与医生共同决策，讨论前列腺癌筛查的风险和获益，并做出个体化的筛查决策。PSA 水平升高或 DRE 异常的男性应转诊至泌尿外科进行进一步诊治。

前列腺炎也可引起 LUTS。它可能由细菌感染或非细菌性炎症引起，其症状可能与 BPH 基本重叠，尤其是在老年男性中。糖尿病、神经系统疾病（如帕金森

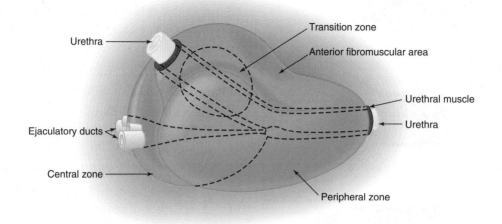

Fig. 10.4 Zonal anatomy of the prostate gland.

particularly in older men. Diabetes mellitus, neurologic diseases such as Parkinson's disease or cerebrovascular disease, and other conditions of the urinary tract, such as urethral strictures, may result in LUTS in patients with BPH. Finally, many medications, particularly those with significant anticholinergic side effects, can cause symptoms mimicking those associated with BPH.

Medical Management

Medical management is the preferred first-line treatment option for patients diagnosed with LUTS due to BPH, and most patients can be effectively managed with a minimum of side effects on medication alone. In general, medical management is initiated for patients with moderate to severe AUA symptom scores. However, in the absence of indications for surgery (refractory urinary retention, hydronephrosis with or without renal impairment, recurrent urinary tract infections, recurrent gross hematuria, or bladder calculi), the decision to embark on any course of therapy, medical or otherwise, is principally driven by the patient. Every patient has a different perception of his symptoms: nocturia twice nightly may be a minor nuisance for some but may represent a significant problem for others. There is no absolute AUA symptom score or other objective measure that dictates the need for initiation of therapy for symptomatic BPH. Each patient must be evaluated individually, and the treatment course must be tailored to the patient's individual situation.

α-Adrenergic Antagonists

α-Blockers are the most commonly prescribed medications for the treatment of LUTS associated with BPH. The bladder neck and prostate are richly innervated with α-adrenergic receptors, specifically α_{1a}-receptors, which constitute about 70% to 80% of the total number of α-receptors in these areas. α_{1b}-Receptors modulate vascular smooth muscle contraction and are located in the bladder neck and prostate to a lesser degree.

Doxazosin, terazosin, tamsulosin, and extended-release alfuzosin are long-acting α-receptor antagonists. These medications are typically administered once daily, usually at bedtime to minimize the potential side effect of orthostatic hypotension. They act through α_1-receptors and can cause vasodilation resulting in transient hypotension and lightheadedness. Blood pressure reduction is greater in patients with a history of hypertension (average reduction, 10 to 15 mm Hg)

relative to normotensive patients (average reduction, 1 to 4 mm Hg). Overall, 10% to 20% of patients experience some (often transient) side effects from these medications, including dizziness, asthenia, headaches, peripheral edema, and nasal congestion. Dose titration is recommended for doxazosin and terazosin to minimize occurrence of adverse effects and optimize the therapeutic response. Maximal response is usually seen within 1 to 2 weeks with doxazosin and within 3 to 6 weeks with terazosin. Overall, these drugs reduce symptom scores by 40% to 50% and improve urinary flow rates by 40% to 50% in about 60% to 65% of patients treated.

Tamsulosin is a selective α_{1a}-receptor antagonist with a long half-life. It has a significantly lower degree of nonspecific α-receptor binding compared with other α-receptor antagonists. Therefore, side effects such as postural hypotension and dizziness are less commonly seen. This drug does not appreciably affect blood pressure in hypertensive or normotensive patients. Maximal response is usually seen within 1 to 2 weeks after the initiation of therapy.

One notable side effect of this class of medications reported in a significant proportion of individuals is retrograde ejaculation. In this condition, the ejaculate is propelled across the bladder neck into the bladder, rather than out the urethra, as a result of the increased relaxation of the prostate and bladder neck tissues. While not medically dangerous, this can be disconcerting to many men who are unaware of this potential side effect. Tamsulosin and silodosin have been shown to have the highest rates of retrograde ejaculation of the regularly prescribed α-blockers.

5α-Reductase Inhibitors (Finasteride and Dutasteride)

Finasteride and dutasteride block the intracellular conversion of testosterone to DHT by inhibiting the action of the enzyme 5α-reductase. This results in an approximate 18% to 25% reduction in prostate gland size over 6 to 12 months. It is most effective in reducing symptoms and preventing disease progression in patients with large prostate glands (>40 g), although recent evidence suggests that symptomatic improvement and stabilization of disease progression may occur in treated men with prostates as small as 30 g. 5α-Reductase inhibition has also been shown to decrease the risk for urinary retention and subsequent surgical intervention, again predominantly in those patients with larger glands. Initial response is seen within 6 months, and maximal effect occurs 12 to 18 months after the initiation of therapy. Data from the MTOPS study demonstrated that combination therapy with

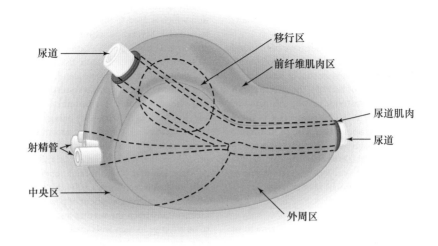

图 10.4 前列腺局部解剖学

病或脑血管病）和其他尿路疾病（如尿道狭窄）均可导致 BPH 患者出现 LUTS。许多药物，特别是具有明显抗胆碱能副作用的药物，也会引起类似 BPH 的症状。

药物治疗

药物治疗是确诊由 BPH 引起的 LUTS 患者首选的一线治疗方案，大多数患者仅通过药物治疗即可有效控制症状且副作用很少。通常情况下，AUA 症状评分为中重度的患者应进行药物治疗。然而，在没有手术指征（顽固性尿潴留、伴或不伴肾功能损害的肾积水、反复尿路感染、反复肉眼血尿或膀胱结石）的情况下，是否采取任何治疗措施（无论是药物治疗还是其他治疗）主要取决于患者的意愿。每位患者对其症状的感知不同：每晚两次夜尿对有些患者来说可能是轻微的困扰，但对其他患者来说可能是一个严重的问题。没有绝对的 AUA 症状评分或其他客观指标能决定是否需要对有症状的 BPH 进行治疗。必须单独评估每位患者，治疗方案必须根据患者的具体情况制订。

α 受体阻滞剂

α 受体阻滞剂是治疗 BPH 相关 LUTS 最常用的药物。膀胱颈和前列腺富含 α 受体，尤其是 α_{1a} 受体（占该区域 α 受体总数的 70% ~ 80%）。α_{1b} 受体调节血管平滑肌收缩，在膀胱颈和前列腺中的分布较少。

多沙唑嗪、特拉唑嗪、坦索罗辛和缓释阿夫唑嗪是长效 α 受体阻滞剂。这些药物通常每日睡前服用 1 次，以最大限度地减少体位性低血压的潜在副作用。它们通过 α_1 受体发挥作用，可能引起血管扩张，导致短暂的低血压和头晕。对于有高血压病史的患者，血压降幅较大（平均下降 10 ~ 15 mmHg），而对于血压正常的患者，血压降幅较小（平均下降 1 ~ 4 mmHg）。总体而言，10% ~ 20% 的患者会经历（通常是短暂的）副作用，包括头晕、乏力、头痛、外周水肿和鼻塞。为了减少不良反应的发生并优化治疗效果，建议对多沙唑嗪和特拉唑嗪进行剂量滴定。多沙唑嗪的最佳效果通常在 1 ~ 2 周出现，而特拉唑嗪则在 3 ~ 6 周出现。总体上，这些药物可以使 AUA 症状评分降低 40% ~ 50%，并使 60% ~ 65% 患者的尿流率提升 40% ~ 50%。

坦索罗辛是一种选择性 α_{1a} 受体阻滞剂，具有较长的半衰期。其与非特异性 α 受体结合的程度显著低于其他 α 受体阻滞剂，因此体位性低血压和头晕等副作用较少见。该药对高血压或血压正常患者的血压几乎没有影响。最佳效果通常在治疗开始后 1 ~ 2 周出现。

据报道，这类药物在相当一部分患者中的一个显著副作用是逆行射精。在这种情况下，由于前列腺和膀胱颈组织松弛程度增加，精液会被排入膀胱，而不是经尿道排出。虽然这种情况在医学上并不危险，但可能使许多不知道这种潜在副作用的男性感到不安。研究表明，在常用的 α 受体阻滞剂中，坦索罗辛和西洛多辛引起逆行射精的概率最高。

5α - 还原酶抑制剂（非那雄胺和度他雄胺）

非那雄胺和度他雄胺可通过抑制 5α - 还原酶的作用来阻断细胞内睾酮向 DHT 的转化。这类药物可在 6 ~ 12 个月使前列腺体积减小 18% ~ 25%。对于前列腺较大的患者（> 40 g），该类药物在缓解症状和预防疾病进展方面最为有效，虽然近期证据表明，对于前列腺仅为 30 g 的患者，治疗后也可改善症状和控制疾病进展。5α - 还原酶抑制剂还被证明可以降低尿潴留和后续手术干预的风险，尤其是在前列腺较大的患者中。治疗开始后，通常在 6 个月内可以观察到初步效果，最佳效果在 12 ~ 18 个月出现。MTOPS 研究数据显示，与单药治疗相比，α 受体阻滞剂联用 5α - 还

an α-blocker and a 5α-reductase inhibitor was more effective than single-agent therapy alone in men with large prostates. As such, many men are placed on concomitant therapy.

It should be noted that finasteride and dutasteride have been found to reduce serum PSA by about 50%. This must be taken into consideration when interpreting PSA values for prostate cancer screening in men taking these agents. After 6 months of therapy, the effective PSA level in a patient taking finasteride or dutasteride may be calculated by doubling the measured PSA value. Free PSA (the percentage of non–protein-bound PSA) is also reduced by about 50%. Use of finasteride or dutasteride may result in sexual dysfunction, including decreased erectile rigidity, decreased libido, and decreased ejaculate volume. ED caused by 5α-reductase inhibitor therapy is reversible and returns to baseline within 2 to 6 months after discontinuation of therapy.

Phosphodiesterase Type 5 Inhibitors

Although more often thought of as medications for the treatment of ED, sildenafil, vardenafil, and tadalafil have been shown to be efficacious in the treatment of urinary symptoms related to BPH. As previously discussed, these medications work by preventing the degradation of cGMP by PDE5. This results in lower intracellular calcium levels and, consequently, smooth muscle relaxation. This process works in the vasculature of the penis as well as the smooth muscle cells of the prostate, urethra, and bladder neck. A number of randomized, double-blind, placebo-controlled trials have shown significant improvements in LUTS in men treated with a once-daily regimen of one of these medications. Although it has not been conclusively shown that PDE5 inhibitors are more efficacious than α-blockers, it does appear that the combination of the two medications works better than either one of them alone. The common side effects of these medications are headache, nasal stuffiness, and facial flushing.

Anticholinergic Medications

For most men, symptoms of overactive bladder make up a large component of LUTS associated with BPH. As previously discussed, many men with long-standing BOO have symptoms of urgency, frequency, and nocturia. One of the best ways to treat these symptoms of overactive bladder is with the daily use of anticholinergic medications such as oxybutynin, tolterodine, or solifenacin. The use of anticholinergic medications in combination with α blockers has been shown to result in greater improvement in LUTS, quality of life, and AUA symptom scores in men with symptoms of overactive bladder due to BPH than use of either agent in monotherapy. The typical side effects of this class of medications include dry mouth, constipation, nausea, and impaired cognition. The risk of urinary retention related to the use of these medications in men appears to be minimal.

Surgical Management
Minimally Invasive Therapy

Although transurethral resection of the prostate (TURP) remains the standard for surgical treatment of BPH, substantial effort has been devoted to the development of less invasive and less morbid methods of treating patients with symptomatic BPH. This has led to a number of minimally invasive therapies, primarily using various energy platforms to cause tissue destruction within the prostate. These office-based techniques are best reserved for patients with smaller prostates and may transiently increase bladder outlet obstruction for 1 to 2 weeks due to postprocedure swelling. Maximal tissue reduction and treatment effect generally occur within 12 weeks.

Water vapor thermal therapy and transurethral microwave thermotherapy (TUMT) are the most widely used minimally invasive methods of treating symptomatic BPH. With water vapor therapy a hollow needle is placed in prostatic tissue under cystoscopic visualization which is used to inject steam. Surrounding tissue is immediately coagulated. Several puncture sites are chosen based on the prostatic anatomy. During TUMT, catheter-mounted transducers use microwave energy to heat prostatic tissue, resulting in coagulative necrosis and shrinkage of the prostate gland. The subsequent reduction in prostate transition zone volume results in an improvement in flow rates and symptom scores. Transurethral needle ablation (TUNA), which uses low-level radio frequency energy to effect similar changes within the prostate gland, is no longer recommended by the AUA guidelines. Water vapor thermal therapy and aquablation are both office-based procedures that have shown efficacy similar to TUMT in patients with prostates less than 80 g, although retreatment rates may be higher than with other interventions. Lastly, the prostatic urethral lift procedure, which involves the placement of permanent transprostatic implants to mechanically open the urethra and improve voiding, has been shown to be effective in men with small prostates and no appreciable median lobe.

The most common side effects of these treatments are temporary increases in overactive bladder symptoms, transient urinary retention, hematuria, and ejaculatory dysfunction. However, antegrade ejaculation is generally preserved in men undergoing both water vapor thermal therapy and the prostatic urethral lift procedures, so patients should be appropriately counseled. Late complications such as urethral strictures and ED have been reported but are significantly less common than with traditional surgical approaches. The major benefits of these less invasive therapies are the reduction in traditional surgical morbidities (e.g., bleeding) and risks associated with general or spinal anesthesia and decreased rates of long-term complications such as incontinence, ED, bladder neck contractures, and urethral strictures. Additionally, most of these procedures can be accomplished safely on an outpatient basis, either in the office or in an ambulatory surgical setting.

Success rates for minimally invasive therapies are intermediate between those achieved with medical management and those of traditional surgical therapy, with 65% to 75% of patients experiencing symptomatic improvement and improved flow rates. The long-term durability of these therapies appears to be good but is presently being evaluated.

Surgical Management

TURP remains the "gold standard" for the surgical management of symptomatic BPH. A TURP procedure involves removal of the transition zone of the prostate through the use of a scope passed through the urethra using a cutting electrocautery loop. The goals of the surgery are to reduce the transition zone prostate tissue to the level of the prostatic capsule and to create a smooth, open appearance of the prostatic urethra and bladder neck. Improvements in the conventional technique have included bipolar electrosurgical cutting, which allows the use of normal saline irrigation and eliminates the risks associated with the potential systemic absorption of hypotonic irrigation solutions.

Newer operating room–based therapies have evolved that produce end results similar to or better than those of TURP. Holmium laser enucleation (HoLEP) is a surgical technique performed by specially trained urologists, generally indicated for large size prostates (>80 g). In this procedure, the entirety of the prostatic adenoma is "enucleated" from the capsule of the prostate and then removed through the urethra after morcellation. Other procedures include various forms of vaporization of the transition zone tissue of the prostate. In contrast to the TURP and HoLEP, no pieces of prostate are removed with these procedures as the tissue is vaporized. The various vaporization procedures include potassium titanyl phosphate (KTP or GreenLight)

原酶抑制剂对于前列腺体积较大的患者更有效。因此，许多患者同时使用这两种药物治疗。

需要注意的是，非那雄胺和度他雄胺可使血清 PSA 水平降低约 50%。在对使用这些药物的患者进行前列腺癌筛查时，解读 PSA 值时必须考虑到这一点。治疗 6 个月后，服用非那雄胺或度他雄胺患者的有效 PSA 水平可通过将 PSA 测量值加倍来计算。游离 PSA（非蛋白结合 PSA 的百分比）也会减少约 50%。非那雄胺或度他雄胺可能导致性功能障碍，包括勃起硬度下降、性欲减退和射精量减少。由 5α - 还原酶抑制剂治疗引起的 ED 是可逆的，在停药后 2 ～ 6 个月可恢复到基线水平。

PDE5 抑制剂

尽管西地那非、伐地那非和他达拉非通常被认为是治疗 ED 的药物，但它们已被证明可有效治疗与 BPH 相关的尿路症状。如前所述，这些药物通过阻止 PDE5 降解 cGMP 来发挥作用，从而降低细胞内 Ca^{2+} 水平，引起平滑肌松弛。这一机制不仅在阴茎的血管中发挥作用，也在前列腺、尿道和膀胱颈的平滑肌细胞中起作用。多项随机、双盲、安慰剂对照试验表明，每日服用 1 次其中一种药物能显著改善男性的 LUTS。虽然尚未证明 PDE5 抑制剂比 α 受体阻滞剂更有效，但两者联合使用的效果似乎优于单药治疗。这些药物的常见副作用包括头痛、鼻塞和面部潮红。

抗胆碱能药

对于大多数 BPH 患者，LUTS 主要是膀胱过度活动症状。如前所述，许多长期存在 BOO 的男性会出现尿急、尿频和夜尿症状。治疗这些膀胱过度活动症状的最佳方式之一是每天使用抗胆碱能药，如奥昔布宁、托特罗定或索利那新。研究表明，相比于单药治疗，抗胆碱能药与 α 受体阻滞剂联合使用能显著改善由 BPH 引起的膀胱过度活动症状、生活质量和 AUA 症状评分。这类药物的典型副作用包括口干、便秘、恶心和认知功能损害。男性使用这类药物后出现尿潴留的风险很低。

外科治疗

微创治疗

尽管经尿道前列腺切除术（TURP）仍为 BPH 外科治疗的标准方法，但人们一直在努力开发创伤更小、病痛更少的方法来治疗症状性 BPH。由此产生了很多微创治疗，这些方法主要使用各种能量平台破坏前列腺组织。这些门诊技术最适用于前列腺较小的患者，由于术后组织水肿，可能会在术后 1 ～ 2 周短暂加重膀胱出口梗阻。最大的组织减少和治疗效果通常在 12 周内出现。

水蒸气热疗和经尿道微波热疗（TUMT）是治疗症状性 BPH 最常用的微创方法。水蒸气热疗是在膀胱镜引导下通过置入前列腺组织的空心针注入蒸汽，使周围组织立即凝固。可根据前列腺解剖学结构选择多个穿刺点。在 TUMT 过程中，导管上的换能器使用微波能量加热前列腺组织，导致凝固性坏死和前列腺缩小。前列腺移行区体积随之减小，从而使尿流率和症状评分得到改善。经尿道针刺消融术（TUNA）使用低频射频能量在前列腺腺体内产生类似的作用，但已不再被 AUA 指南推荐。水蒸气热疗和水消融均可在门诊实施，在前列腺＜ 80 g 的患者中显示出与 TUMT 相似的疗效，但再治疗率可能高于其他干预措施。此外，前列腺部尿道悬吊术是通过放置永久性经前列腺植入物来机械性打开尿道并改善排尿功能，已被证明对前列腺小且中叶不明显的男性有效。

这些治疗最常见的副作用是膀胱过度活动症状短暂加重、短暂性尿潴留、血尿和射精功能障碍。但是，接受水蒸气热疗和前列腺部尿道悬吊术的患者通常会保留顺行射精功能，因此应提前告知患者。虽然有晚期并发症（如尿道狭窄和 ED）的报道，但其发生率显著低于传统手术方法。这些微创治疗的主要优点是减小了传统手术并发症（如出血）和全身或脊髓麻醉相关的风险，并降低长期并发症（如尿失禁、ED、膀胱颈挛缩和尿道狭窄）的发生率。此外，大多数手术都可以在门诊或日间手术中心安全完成。

微创治疗的成功率介于药物治疗和传统手术治疗之间，65% ～ 75% 患者的症状和尿流率可得到改善。这些治疗的长期效果尚可，但仍在评估中。

手术治疗

TURP 仍然是手术治疗症状性 BPH 的"金标准"。TURP 通过经尿道插入的内窥镜，使用电灼切割环切除前列腺移行区组织。手术的目的是将前列腺移行区组织减少至前列腺包膜水平，从而创造光滑、开放的尿道前列腺部和膀胱颈部。传统技术的改进包括双极电外科切割，它允许使用生理盐水冲洗，消除了低渗冲洗溶液可能导致的全身性吸收风险。

目前已开发出基于手术室的新治疗方法，其效果与 TURP 相似甚至更好。钬激光前列腺剜除术（HoLEP）是一种由受过专业训练的泌尿科医生实施的手术，通常适用于前列腺较大的患者（＞ 80 g）。该手术是将整个前列腺从前列腺包膜中剜除，然后在粉碎后通过尿道取出。其他手术包括各种形式的前列腺移行区组织汽化。与 TURP 和 HoLEP 不同，这些手术不会切除任何前列腺组织，因为组织直接被汽化了。这些汽化手术包括磷酸钛氧钾（KTP 或绿色激光）激光治疗（又

TABLE 10.5	Success in Medical Versus Surgical Management of Benign Prostatic Hyperplasia				
Degree of Improvement	α_1-Blockers	Finasteride	TURP	TUIP	Open Surgery
Symptoms (%)	48	31	82	73	79
Flow rate (%)	40-50	17	120	100	185
Mean probability (%) of achieving the stated improvements	74	67	88	80	98

TUIP, Transurethral incision of the prostate; *TURP,* transurethral resection of the prostate.

laser therapy, also called photovaporization of the prostate, and bipolar plasma vaporization of the prostate (button TURP). Rates of urinary incontinence, retrograde ejaculation, and urethral stricture are all higher after operating room procedures than after office-based therapies. Perioperative morbidity, including the need for blood transfusion, although substantially decreased by technical improvements, is likewise higher after TURP and similar procedures. However, standard electrosurgical resection of the prostate (TURP) is the most effective surgical treatment for symptomatic BPH short of enucleation. Success rates, as measured by improved symptom scores and increased urinary flow rates, are 80% to 90% after TURP.

Transurethral incision of the prostate (TUIP) is a more limited surgical procedure, although still performed under anesthesia in the operating room, that consists of incising the bladder neck and proximal prostatic urethra. This procedure is generally reserved for men with smaller prostates (<30 g) who have significant LUTS. Although it is more invasive than the heat-based therapies, success rates approach those of TURP in properly selected patients. Morbidity after TUIP is significantly less than after TURP, but long-term durability of symptom relief is less than that seen with TURP.

Surgical enucleation (simple prostatectomy) is reserved for patients with very large glands. Traditionally performed via an open lower abdominal incision, this procedure involves incision into the bladder neck or the capsule of the prostate and then removal of the prostatic adenoma from within the prostatic capsule. While success rates are high, the rate of complications such as bleeding and incontinence is higher than with any of the other traditional surgical approaches (Table 10.5). With advancements in robotic technology, this surgery is now being performed with a robot-assisted laparoscopic approach that has significantly reduced the associated morbidity. For many centers, robot-assisted simple prostatectomy or HoLEP remain the mainstay for management of very large symptomatic prostates.

Conclusion

The management of LUTS resulting from BPH has undergone a dramatic shift from principally a surgical approach to more of a medical one. This evolution of care, coupled with the aging of the U.S. population, has resulted in a shift of care for these patients from the urologist to the primary care physician. In the absence of severe LUTS or indications for early surgical intervention, the primary care physician can now successfully manage most cases of mild to moderate BPH. If there is no or minimal response to therapy, a variety of minimally invasive and surgical options are now available that are all highly successful.

BENIGN SCROTAL DISEASES

Benign masses of the scrotum are some of the most common complaints of men presenting to their primary care providers. While serious concerns such as testicular cancer or an incarcerated inguinal hernia must always be considered, the majority of these masses

are benign. A thorough clinical history and physical exam alone will likely lead one to the correct diagnosis; scrotal ultrasound can be used to confirm a diagnosis or aid in finding the diagnosis for those with equivocal exam findings.

Varicocele

A scrotal varicocele is an abnormal dilation of the veins of the pampiniform plexus that run along the spermatic cord and can be palpated as a "bag of worms" with or without having the patient performing the Valsalva maneuver while standing. When examining a patient for any scrotal pathology, it is important to have the patient stand. A clinical varicocele is one that can be palpated on physical examination. Because the occurrence of varicoceles increases with age, the prevalence in the literature is highly variable. The prevalence of a unilateral palpable left-sided varicocele is between 6.5% and 22%, and that of bilateral palpable varicoceles ranges from 10% to 20%. The prevalence of an isolated right-sided palpable varicocele is less than 1%. However, because of a very rare association of isolated right-sided varicocele with retroperitoneal malignancy, many clinicians perform axial imaging on patients with a unilateral right-sided varicocele. In general, a left-sided varicocele does not have clinical significance unless it can be palpated on physical examination. A varicocele that is incidentally found during ultrasonography of the scrotum and is not palpable on examination is considered a subclinical varicocele and typically does not warrant intervention.

Palpable and nonpalpable varicoceles are most commonly found incidentally and, in most cases, have no clinical significance. However, palpable varicoceles can cause ipsilateral testicular atrophy, discomfort, and/or affect semen parameters. Therefore, it is important for the clinician to compare the size of the testicles in patients who desire future fertility. If the physical examination is unclear, scrotal ultrasonography can be used to accurately measure the size of both testicles. Any patient who desires future children and has a size discrepancy greater than 20% should be monitored closely and possibly referred to a urologist. Although varicoceles are most commonly found incidentally, they may also be found during a work-up for male factor infertility, scrotal pain, or asymptomatic testicular atrophy.

The pathophysiology of varicoceles is poorly understood but involves dilation of the internal spermatic vein and transmission of increased hydrostatic pressure across dysfunctional venous valves. Stasis of blood in the venous system disturbs the countercurrent heat exchange that is responsible for maintaining testicular temperature and may result in testicular parenchymal damage and impaired spermatogenesis.

Varicoceles are the most common cause of both primary male infertility (patient has fathered no children) and secondary male infertility (patient has fathered at least one child), accounting for 33% of cases. However, most men with palpable varicoceles are able to father children without difficulty. In a man with infertility and a palpable varicocele, semen analysis commonly reveals a low sperm count and

表 10.5　BPH 药物治疗与外科治疗的成功率

改善程度	α_1 受体阻滞剂	非那雄胺	TURP	TUIP	开放手术
症状（%）	48	31	82	73	79
尿流率（%）	40～50	17	120	100	185
达到预期改善程度的平均概率（%）	74	67	88	80	98

TUIP，经尿道前列腺切开术；TURP，经尿道前列腺切除术。

称前列腺光汽化术）和前列腺双极等离子汽化（button TURP）。这些手术的术后尿失禁、逆行射精和尿道狭窄的发生率均高于门诊手术。尽管技术改进已大大降低了围术期并发症（包括输血）的发生率，但 TURP 及类似手术后并发症的发生率仍然较高。然而，标准 TURP 是除前列腺摘除术外治疗症状性 BPH 最有效的手术。根据症状评分和尿流率的改善来衡量，TURP 的治疗成功率可达到 80%～90%。

经尿道前列腺切开术（TUIP）是一种更加微创的手术，虽然仍需在手术室麻醉下进行，手术过程包括切开膀胱颈和尿道前列腺部的近端。该手术通常适用于前列腺较小（< 30 g）且存在明显 LUTS 的男性。虽然其侵入性比热疗更大，但在经过适当选择的患者中，成功率接近 TURP。TUIP 后并发症的发生率显著低于 TURP，但症状缓解的长期持久性不及 TURP。

手术剜除（单纯前列腺切除术）适用于前列腺非常大的患者。此手术传统上通过开放性下腹部切口进行，包括切开膀胱颈或前列腺包膜，然后从前列腺包膜内部切除前列腺。虽然成功率较高，但并发症（如出血和尿失禁）的发生率高于其他传统手术方法（表 10.5）。随着机器人技术的进步，此类手术现在可通过机器人辅助腹腔镜方法进行，这大大降低了相关并发症的发生率。对于许多医疗中心而言，机器人辅助单纯前列腺切除术或 HoLEP 仍是处理前列腺体积非常大的症状性 BPH 患者的主要方法。

总结

针对 BPH 引起的 LUTS 的治疗已经发生了巨大的变化，从主要依赖手术治疗转变为更多采用药物治疗。这种治疗方式的演变，加之人口老龄化，导致对这些患者的治疗从泌尿科医生转向初级保健医生。在没有严重 LUTS 或不需要早期手术干预的情况下，初级保健医生可以成功治疗大多数轻中度 BPH 患者。如果治疗无效或效果不佳，目前有多种微创方法和手术方式可供选择，这些方法的成功率都很高。

良性阴囊疾病

阴囊良性肿块是男性向初级保健医生求诊时最常见的主诉之一。虽然必须考虑睾丸癌或嵌顿性腹股沟疝等严重情况，但绝大多数肿块是良性的。详尽的病史和体格检查通常能做出正确的诊断；阴囊超声可用于确诊或辅助诊断检查结果不明确的患者。

精索静脉曲张

精索静脉曲张是指沿精索走行的精索蔓状静脉丛的异常扩张，可在患者站立时（进行或不进行 Valsalva 动作）触及蚯蚓状团块。进行阴囊病变检查时，患者应保持站立位，这点很重要。具有临床意义的精索静脉曲张是指在体格检查时可触及的静脉曲张。由于静脉曲张的发生率随年龄升高，文献中其患病率差异很大。左侧单侧触及精索静脉曲张的患病率为 6.5%～22%，双侧触及精索静脉曲张的患病率为 10%～20%，右侧单侧触及精索静脉曲张的患病率低于 1%。然而，由于右侧单侧精索静脉曲张在极少数情况下与腹膜后恶性肿瘤有关，许多临床医生会对有右侧单侧精索静脉曲张的患者进行轴向影像学检查。通常情况下，体格检查时可触及的左侧精索静脉曲张才具有临床意义。通过阴囊超声偶然发现但在体格检查中无法触及的精索静脉曲张被认为是亚临床精索静脉曲张，通常无须干预。

精索静脉曲张（无论可否触及）通常是被偶然发现的，大多数情况没有临床意义。然而，可触及的精索静脉曲张可能导致同侧睾丸萎缩、不适和（或）影响精液质量。因此，对于未来有生育需求的患者，比较两侧睾丸的大小非常重要。如果体格检查结果不明确，可以使用阴囊超声准确测量两侧睾丸的大小。对于尚有生育需求且两侧睾丸大小差异超过 20% 的患者，应密切随访，并可转诊至泌尿科。尽管精索静脉曲张通常是被偶然发现的，但也可能在不育症、阴囊疼痛或无症状睾丸萎缩的检查过程中被发现。

精索静脉曲张的病理生理学机制尚不明确，但其涉及精索内静脉扩张和经过功能障碍的静脉瓣的静脉血压力增高。静脉系统中的血液淤滞会干扰维持睾丸温度的逆流热交换，可能导致睾丸实质损伤和影响精子发生。

精索静脉曲张是导致原发性男性不育症（即患者未曾生育子女）和继发性男性不育症（即患者至少有 1 名子女）最常见的原因，占所有病例的 33%。然而，大多数有可触及的精索静脉曲张的男性通常无生育困难。在不育症男性中，若发现可触及的精索静脉曲张，精液分

abnormal sperm morphology and motility. After surgical correction of a varicocele in a patient with infertility, semen parameters improve in 60% to 80% and subsequent pregnancy rates range from 20% to 60%.

Providers often perform scrotal ultrasonography on any patient with chronic testicular pain to determine the source. Varicoceles are commonly found during this evaluation, but usually only palpable (clinical) varicoceles are considered as a source of pain. If a nonpalpable varicocele is found on an ultrasound examination, the patient should not be told that it is the cause of his pain. However, patients with palpable varicoceles and chronic testicular pain should be referred for treatment, as more than 80% of these men will have improvement in their pain after surgical correction.

Common operative techniques for treatment of a varicocele include high retroperitoneal ligation of the internal spermatic vein, microsurgical inguinal and subinguinal varicocelectomy, laparoscopic varicocelectomy, and gonadal vein embolization. The inguinal approach using microscopic magnification has the highest success and lowest complication and recurrence rates. The most common complication is hydrocele formation, whereas a rare complication is inadvertent ligation of the testicular artery resulting in testicular atrophy and loss. Surgical intervention for subclinical (nonpalpable) varicoceles is not indicated.

Spermatocele (Epididymal Cyst)

Spermatoceles and epididymal cysts are dilations of the tubes that connect the testicle to the epididymis (ductuli efferentes). Although they are technically synonymous, many clinicians refer to small lesions as epididymal cysts and larger ones as spermatoceles. These cystic lesions are very common and are found in 29% of asymptomatic men on ultrasonography. After a vasectomy, 35% of men develop a new small spermatocele, suggesting that distal obstruction of the vasa likely contributes to their development.

On physical examination, spermatoceles are somewhat mobile, firm masses that are separate and distinguishable from the smooth border of the testicle. It may be possible to transilluminate larger lesions, but this is rarely performed in practice. Spermatoceles are filled with a clear fluid that usually contains abundant amounts of sperm. If the lesion cannot be transilluminated, it is advisable to perform an ultrasound study of the scrotum to distinguish a spermatocele from a solid mass or from other testicular lesions. Of note, should a solid mass be identified on the epididymis on imaging, the vast majority of solid masses of the epididymis are benign. However, referral to a urologist for risk evaluation is prudent. Small spermatoceles and epididymal cysts normally have no clinical significance and are typically not the source of a patient's chronic testicular pain. They can be surgically removed if they are large or are causing discomfort for the patient.

Acute Epididymitis

Acute epididymitis is a clinical syndrome that may manifest with fever, acute scrotal pain, and impressive swelling and induration of the epididymis. Epididymitis is most often caused by retrograde bacterial spread from the bladder or urethra into the vasa and then into the epididymides. In men younger than 35 years of age, the most common causative agents are those organisms associated with sexually transmitted infections—namely, *Neisseria gonococcus* and *Chlamydia trachomatis*. In older men, acute epididymitis is usually caused by a coliform bacteria such as *Escherichia coli* and often occurs in association other lower urinary tract infections or bladder outlet obstruction.

The most important consideration in diagnosing acute epididymitis is differentiating this disease from acute testicular torsion. Physical examination can be nonspecific, although focal epididymal swelling and tenderness are suggestive, and the presence of white cells and bacteria in the urine is indicative of an infectious etiology. Scrotal

ultrasonography with Doppler flow can be extremely helpful in differentiating acute epididymitis from torsion in difficult cases, as the epididymis will present with increased vascular flow (hyperemia) while torsion will show no or diminished flow within the testicle.

Patients with acute epididymitis have significant inflammation that can also involve the testicle (epididymo-orchitis). Patients with severe epididymitis involving the testicle are often systemically ill. In most instances, initial treatment should consist of antibiotics, nonsteroidal anti-inflammatory medications, and possibly oral narcotics. In some cases, broad-spectrum antibiotics or even hospital admission may be necessary. In general, patients younger than 35 years of age should be treated with ceftriaxone and doxycycline. Older patients are usually empirically treated with a fluoroquinolone for 2 to 4 weeks. Complications associated with acute epididymitis include abscess formation, reactive hydrocele formation, testicular infarction, infertility, and chronic epididymitis or orchalgia.

Hydrocele

A hydrocele is a sterile fluid collection located between the parietal and visceral layers of the tunica vaginalis of the scrotum. Noncommunicating hydroceles are commonly seen in adults and usually surround the testicle and spermatic cord. Communicating hydroceles are more common in children and actually represent indirect inguinal hernias. These communicating hydroceles contain only fluid and not bowel or fat because the opening into the peritoneal cavity is small. Communicating hydroceles can be distinguished from noncommunicating hydroceles on physical examination by gently pushing the fluid out of the scrotum and into the peritoneum, or by a history of fluctuation in size of the fluid collection throughout the day or with standing and lying down.

Patients with a noncommunicating hydrocele usually have complaints of heaviness in the scrotum, scrotal pain, or an enlarging scrotal mass. Usually the diagnosis is easily made based on the physical examination and transillumination of the scrotum. If the testis is not palpable, an ultrasound study may be performed to rule out a testicular tumor associated with a secondary or reactive hydrocele. Noncommunicating hydroceles are caused by increased secretion or decreased reabsorption of serous fluid by the tunica vaginalis. Infection, trauma, surgery, neoplastic disease, and lymphatic disease are causative in many adults, whereas the remainder of cases are idiopathic.

Asymptomatic hydroceles are benign and do not require treatment unless desired by the patient. Definitive treatment of symptomatic hydroceles requires surgical intervention. Although the recurrence rate is significantly higher with aspiration and sclerotherapy, this approach can be a good option in patients who are considered poor surgical candidates. Hydrocelectomy procedures involve drainage of the serous fluid with either excision of the redundant tunica vaginalis or plication of the sac without excision. After surgery, the rates of hydrocele recurrence and chronic pain are 9% and 1%, respectively.

Testicular Torsion

Testicular torsion is considered a true urologic emergency. The testicle receives its blood supply from the testicular artery (a branch of the aorta), the vasal artery (a branch of the inferior vesicle artery), and the cremasteric artery (a branch of the inferior epigastric artery). All three vessels are transmitted to the testicle through the spermatic cord. Torsion of the spermatic cord impairs arterial inflow as well as venous outflow. If detorsion is not performed within 6 to 8 hours, testicular infarction and hemorrhagic necrosis are likely to occur. Typically, patients are younger than 21 years of age, although testicular torsion can occur later in life. Delays in presentation and diagnosis are more

析常显示精子计数低、形态和活动力异常。对不育症患者进行精索静脉曲张手术治疗后，60%～80% 患者的精液质量会有所改善，后续的妊娠率为 20%～60%。

医生通常会对有慢性睾丸疼痛的患者进行阴囊超声检查以确定病因。超声检查中常发现精索静脉曲张，但通常只有可触及的精索静脉曲张被认为是疼痛的病因。如果在超声检查中发现无法触及的精索静脉曲张，不应告知患者这是导致其疼痛的原因。然而，对于有可触及的精索静脉曲张的慢性睾丸疼痛患者，应转诊治疗，因为超过 80% 的患者在手术治疗后疼痛会有所改善。

治疗精索静脉曲张的常见手术技术包括精索内静脉腹膜后高位结扎、经腹股沟和腹股沟下显微镜下精索静脉结扎术、腹腔镜精索静脉结扎术和经性腺静脉栓塞术。经腹股沟显微外科精索静脉结扎术的成功率最高，且并发症发生率和复发率最低。最常见的并发症是鞘膜积液，虽然意外结扎睾丸动脉极少见，但其可导致睾丸萎缩甚至坏死。亚临床精索静脉曲张不建议进行手术干预。

精液囊肿（附睾囊肿）

精液囊肿和附睾囊肿是指连接睾丸和附睾的管道（输精管）扩张。尽管两者之间并无差异，但许多临床医生将较小的囊肿称为附睾囊肿，较大的称为精液囊肿。这些囊肿很常见，在超声检查中，29% 的无症状男性存在这种病变。在进行输精管结扎术后，35% 的男性会出现小的新发精液囊肿，这表明输精管远端梗阻可能是这些囊肿发生的原因。

在体格检查中，精液囊肿通常为活动且质硬的包块，与睾丸的光滑边界有明显的分隔。较大的病变可能会透光，但在实际操作中很少进行透光试验。精液囊肿内充满清亮的液体，通常含有大量精子。如果病变不透光，建议进行睾丸超声检查，以鉴别精液囊肿与实质性肿块或其他睾丸病变。需要注意的是，影像学检查中发现的附睾实质性肿块绝大多数是良性的。然而，转诊至泌尿外科医生进行风险评估是谨慎的做法。通常情况下，小的精液囊肿没有临床意义，一般不是患者慢性睾丸疼痛的原因。如果囊肿较大或引起患者不适，可以考虑进行手术切除。

急性附睾炎

急性附睾炎是一种临床综合征，可表现为发热、急性阴囊疼痛，以及附睾明显肿胀和硬化。附睾炎最常见的病因是细菌从膀胱或尿道逆行传播到输精管，然后进入附睾。在 35 岁以下的男性中，最常见的致病菌是性传播感染相关病原体，即淋病奈瑟球菌和沙眼衣原体。在中老年男性中，急性附睾炎通常由大肠菌群细菌（如大肠埃希菌）引起，且常与其他下尿路感染或膀胱出口梗阻相关。

在诊断急性附睾炎时，最重要的是将其与急性睾丸扭转区分开来。虽然体格检查的特异性较低，但局部附睾肿胀和压痛具有提示作用，而尿液中有白细胞和细菌则提示感染性病因。在疑难病例中，阴囊超声检查配合多普勒血流检查非常有助于鉴别急性附睾炎和睾丸扭转，因为附睾炎表现为血流增加（充血），而睾丸扭转则表现为睾丸内无血流或血流减少。

急性附睾炎患者会出现明显的炎症，也可累及睾丸（附睾-睾丸炎）。累及睾丸的重度附睾炎患者常表现为全身不适。大多数情况下，初始治疗应包括抗生素、NSAID 和口服镇痛药。部分患者可能需要使用广谱抗生素甚至住院治疗。一般来说，35 岁以下患者应使用头孢曲松和多西环素进行治疗。中老年患者通常经验性使用氟喹诺酮治疗 2～4 周。急性附睾炎的并发症包括脓肿形成、反应性鞘膜积液形成、睾丸梗死、不育症、慢性附睾炎或睾丸疼痛。

鞘膜积液

鞘膜积液由阴囊鞘膜壁层和脏层之间的无菌性液体蓄积所致。非交通性鞘膜积液在成人中较为常见，通常包绕睾丸和精索。交通性鞘膜积液实则为腹股沟斜疝，在儿童中更为常见。由于通向腹膜腔的开口很小，交通性鞘膜积液只含有液体，而不包含肠道或脂肪。在体格检查时，可以通过轻压将积液从阴囊推向腹膜腔，或根据积液量在立位和卧位或一天中的变化来鉴别交通性和非交通性鞘膜积液。

非交通性鞘膜积液患者通常会感到阴囊沉重、阴囊疼痛或阴囊肿块增大等不适。通常根据体格检查和阴囊透光试验很容易确诊。若未能触及睾丸，可进行超声检查以排除睾丸肿瘤引起的继发性或反应性鞘膜积液。非交通性鞘膜积液由阴囊鞘膜分泌增加或吸收减少所致。感染、外伤、手术、肿瘤性疾病和淋巴系统疾病是许多成人鞘膜积液患者的病因，其他患者多由特发性病因导致。

无症状性鞘膜积液是良性的，除非患者有需求，否则无须治疗。症状性鞘膜积液需要手术治疗。虽然抽吸和硬化治疗的复发率较高，但对于不适合手术的患者来说，这可能是不错的选择。睾丸鞘膜积液切除术包括排出积液并切除多余的鞘膜或在不切除的情况下对鞘膜进行折叠。手术后，鞘膜积液的复发率和慢性疼痛的发生率分别为 9% 和 1%。

睾丸扭转

睾丸扭转为泌尿外科急症。睾丸的血液供应来自睾丸动脉（主动脉的分支）、输精管动脉（膀胱下动脉的分支）和提睾肌动脉（腹壁下动脉的分支），这三支血管通过精索进入睾丸。精索扭转会阻碍动脉血液流入和静脉血液回流。如果 6～8 h 不能解除扭转，睾丸可能发生梗死和出血性坏死。睾丸扭转的发病年龄通常在 21 岁以下，但也可能在其后发生。就诊延迟和诊断延迟常见于成人患者，通常与患者和医生因素均有关。急性睾丸扭转的典型体征和症状包括突发阴囊疼

common in the adult patient population and are often related to patient and physician factors.

The characteristic signs and symptoms of acute testicular torsion are the acute onset of scrotal pain, swelling, nausea, vomiting, loss of normal rugae of the scrotal skin, absent cremasteric reflex, and a high-riding, rotated, tender testicle. The diagnosis of testicular torsion remains a clinical one; however, in equivocal cases, if ultrasound equipment is readily available and obtaining an ultrasound does not negatively affect the patient promptly proceeding to the operating room, scrotal ultrasonography may be performed prior to surgery. In many cases, surgical exploration is undertaken when the index of suspicion is high but imaging is not available. Doppler ultrasonography is extremely useful in differentiating testicular torsion from other causes of acute scrotum, such as acute epididymitis, torsion of the appendix testis, and trauma, as previously discussed.

It is possible to untwist testicular torsion by manual manipulation of the testicle through the scrotum in the emergency room or in a physician's office. After giving the patient parenteral narcotics, the testicle can be untwisted by gently pulling down on it and, usually, rotating it laterally (like opening a book). If this is successful, the testicle will uncoil like a spring and fall into its normal position, with immediate relief of the patient's pain. Even if the procedure is successful, patients should still be taken to the operating room for bilateral orchiopexy to prevent future occurrences.

Important surgical principles include surgical detorsion and assessment of testicular viability in the operating room. If the testis is determined to be viable, bilateral orchiopexy is performed using the technique of three-point fixation (sutures placed medially, laterally, and inferiorly). In the presence of infarction, orchiectomy is recommended. Orchiopexy of the contralateral testicle is always performed simultaneously. When diagnosis and surgery occur in a timely fashion, testicular salvage rates approach 70%. Delayed surgical therapy significantly decreases the salvage rate to approximately 40%.

SUGGESTED READINGS

Alleman WG, Gorman B, King BF, et al: Benign and malignant epididymal masses evaluated with scrotal sonography: clinical and pathologic review of 85 patients, J Ultrasound Med 27:1195–1202, 2008.

Baillargeon J, Urban RJ, Ottenbacher KJ, et al: Trends in androgen prescribing in the United States, 2001 to 2011, JAMA Intern Med 173:1465–1466, 2013.

Bhasin S, Cunningham GR, Hayes FJ, et al: Testosterone therapy in men with androgen deficiency syndromes: an endocrine society clinical practice guideline, J Clin Endocrinol Metab 95:2536–2559, 2010.

Burnett AL, Nehra A, Breau RH, et al: Erectile dysfunction: AUA guideline, J Urol 200:633, 2018.

Capoccia E, Levine LA: Contemporary review of Peyronie's disease treatment, Curr Urol Rep 19:51, 2018.

Cappelleri JC, Rosen RC: The Sexual Health Inventory for Men (SHIM): a 5-year review of research and clinical experience, Int J Impotence Res 17:307–319, 2005.

Carson CC, Lue TF: Phosphodiesterase type 5 inhibitors for erectile dysfunction, Br J Urol Int 96:257–280, 2005.

Costa P, Potempa A-J: Intraurethral alprostadil for erectile dysfunction: a review of the literature, Drugs 72:2243–2254, 2012.

D'Amico AV, Chen MH, Roehl KA, et al: Preoperative PSA velocity and the risk of death from prostate cancer after radical prostatectomy, N Engl J Med 351:125–135, 2004.

Eggener SE, Roehl KA, Catalona WJ: Predictors of subsequent prostate cancer in men with a prostate specific antigen of 2.6 to 4.0 ng/ml and an initially negative biopsy, J Urol 174:500–504, 2005.

Feldman HA, Goldstein I, Hatzichristou DG, et al: Impotence and its medical and psychosocial correlates: results of the massachusetts male aging study, J Urol 151:54–61, 1994.

Ficarra V, Crestani A, Novara G, et al: Varicocele repair for infertility: what is the evidence? Curr Opin Urol 22:489–494, 2012.

Foster HE, Dahm P, Kohler TS, et al: Surgical management of lower urinary tract symptoms attributed to benign prostatic hyperplasia: AUA guideline amendment 2019, J Urol 202:592, 2019.

Gelbard M, Goldstein I, Hellstrom WJG, et al: Clinical efficacy, safety and tolerability of collagenase clostridium histolyticum for the treatment of Peyronie disease in 2 large double-blind, randomized, placebo controlled phase 3 studies, J Urol 190:199–207, 2013.

Kaplan SA, Roehrborn CG, Rovner ES, et al: Tolterodine and tamsulosin for treatment of men with lower urinary tract symptoms and overactive bladder: a randomized controlled trial, J Am Med Assoc 296:2319–2328, 2006.

Karmazyn B, Steinberg R, Kurareid L, et al: Clinical and radiographic criteria of the acute scrotum in children: a retrospective study in 172 boys, Pediatr Radiol 35:302–310, 2005.

Kostis JB, Jackson G, Rosen R, et al: Sexual dysfunction and cardiac risk (the second Princeton Consensus Conference), Am J Cardiol 96: 313–321, 2005.

Lowe FC, McConnell JD, Hudson PB, et al: for the Finasteride Study Group, Long-term 6-year experience with finasteride in patients with benign prostatic hyperplasia, Urology 61:791-796, 2003.

Lue TF: Erectile dysfunction, N Engl J Med 342:1802, 2000.

McConnell JD, Roehrborn CG, Bautista OM, et al, for the Medical Therapy of Prostatic Symptoms (MTOPS) Research Group: The long-term effect of doxazosin, finasteride, and combination therapy on the clinical progression of benign prostatic hyperplasia, N Engl J Med 349:2387-2398, 2003.

Meriggiola MC, Bremner WJ, Costantino A, et al: Low dose of cyproterone acetate and testosterone enanthate for contraception in men, Hum Reprod 13:1225–1229, 1998.

Morgentaler A, Caliber M: Safety of testosterone therapy in men with prostate cancer, Expert Opin Drug Saf 1, 2019.

Morgentaler A, Traish A, Hackett G, et al: Diagnosis and treatment of testosterone deficiency: updated recommendations from the lisbon 2018 international consultation for sexual medicine, Sex Med Rev, 2019.

Mulhall JP, Trost LW, Brannigan RE, et al: Evaluation and management of testosterone deficiency: AUA guideline, J Urol 200:423, 2018.

Nehra A, Alterowitz R, Culkin DJ, et al: Peyronie's disease: AUA guideline, J Urol 194:745, 2015.

Neiderberger C: Microsurgical treatment of persistent or recurrent varicocele, J Urol 173:2079–2080, 2005.

Nieschlag E, Swerdloff R, Behre HM, et al: Investigation, treatment, and monitoring of late-onset hypogonadism in males: ISA, ISSAM, and EAU recommendations, J Androl 27:135–137, 2006.

Rhoden EL, Morgentaler A: Risks of testosterone-replacement therapy and recommendations for monitoring, N Engl J Med 350:482–492, 2004.

Roehrborn CG, Kaplan SA, Jones JS, et al: Tolterodine extended release with or without tamsulosin in men with lower urinary tract symptoms including overactive bladder symptoms: effects of prostate size, Eur Urol 55:472–479, 2009.

Sessions AE, Rabinowitz R, Hulbert WC, et al: Testicular torsion: direction, degree, duration and disinformation, J Urol 169:663–665, 2003.

Shridharani A, Lockwood G, Sandlow J: Varicocelectomy in the treatment of testicular pain: a review, Curr Opin Urol 22:499–506, 2012.

Stewart CA, Yafi FA, Knoedler M, et al: Intralesional injection of interferon-α2b improves penile curvature in men with Peyronie's disease independent of plaque location, J Urol 194:1704–1707, 2015.

Svartberg J, Midtby M, Bønaa KH, et al: The associations of age, lifestyle factors and chronic disease with testosterone in men: the Tromsø Study, Eur J Endocrinol 149:145–152, 2003.

Wang C: Phosphodiesterase-5 inhibitors and benign prostatic hyperplasia, Curr Opin Urol 20:49–54, 2010.

Wu FCW, Tajar A, Beynon JM, et al: Identification of late-onset hypogonadism in middle-aged and elderly men, N Engl J Med 363:123–135, 2010.

Yafi FA, Pinsky MR, Sangkum P, et al: Therapeutic advances in the treatment of Peyronie's disease, Andrology 3:650, 2015.

痛、肿胀、恶心、呕吐、阴囊皮肤皱褶消失、提睾反射消失，以及睾丸呈高位扭转状态伴有触痛。睾丸扭转的诊断主要依靠临床表现，然而，在症状不明显的情况下，如果有超声设备，且超声检查不会延误患者迅速进行手术，可以在手术前进行阴囊超声检查。在许多情况下，当高度怀疑睾丸扭转但无法进行影像学检查时，应进行手术探查。如前所述，多普勒超声检查在鉴别睾丸扭转与其他急性阴囊疾病（如急性附睾炎、睾丸附件扭转和外伤）方面非常有用。

可在急诊室或门诊经阴囊对睾丸进行手法复位解除扭转。注射麻醉剂后，轻轻向下拉扯睾丸，并通常向侧面旋转（类似翻开一本书），以解除扭转。如果手法复位成功，睾丸会像弹簧一样解开，恢复到正常位置，患者的疼痛会立即缓解。即使手法复位成功，患者仍应立即送往手术室进行双侧睾丸固定术，以预防复发。

重要的手术原则包括手术解除扭转和手术室评估睾丸血运及活力。如果确定睾丸可存活，则进行双侧睾丸固定术，使用三点固定技术（内侧、外侧和下方缝合）。若发生睾丸梗死，建议行睾丸切除术。通常同时进行对侧睾丸固定术。若诊断和手术及时，睾丸挽救率可达到 70%。手术治疗延迟会显著降低挽救率（约 40%）。

推荐阅读

Alleman WG, Gorman B, King BF, et al: Benign and malignant epididymal masses evaluated with scrotal sonography: clinical and pathologic review of 85 patients, J Ultrasound Med 27:1195–1202, 2008.

Baillargeon J, Urban RJ, Ottenbacher KJ, et al: Trends in androgen prescribing in the United States, 2001 to 2011, JAMA Intern Med 173:1465–1466, 2013.

Bhasin S, Cunningham GR, Hayes FJ, et al: Testosterone therapy in men with androgen deficiency syndromes: an endocrine society clinical practice guideline, J Clin Endocrinol Metab 95:2536–2559, 2010.

Burnett AL, Nehra A, Breau RH, et al: Erectile dysfunction: AUA guideline, J Urol 200:633, 2018.

Capoccia E, Levine LA: Contemporary review of Peyronie's disease treatment, Curr Urol Rep 19:51, 2018.

Cappelleri JC, Rosen RC: The Sexual Health Inventory for Men (SHIM): a 5-year review of research and clinical experience, Int J Impotence Res 17:307–319, 2005.

Carson CC, Lue TF: Phosphodiesterase type 5 inhibitors for erectile dysfunction, Br J Urol Int 96:257–280, 2005.

Costa P, Potempa A-J: Intraurethral alprostadil for erectile dysfunction: a review of the literature, Drugs 72:2243–2254, 2012.

D'Amico AV, Chen MH, Roehl KA, et al: Preoperative PSA velocity and the risk of death from prostate cancer after radical prostatectomy, N Engl J Med 351:125–135, 2004.

Eggener SE, Roehl KA, Catalona WJ: Predictors of subsequent prostate cancer in men with a prostate specific antigen of 2.6 to 4.0 ng/ml and an initially negative biopsy, J Urol 174:500–504, 2005.

Feldman HA, Goldstein I, Hatzichristou DG, et al: Impotence and its medical and psychosocial correlates: results of the massachusetts male aging study, J Urol 151:54–61, 1994.

Ficarra V, Crestani A, Novara G, et al: Varicocele repair for infertility: what is the evidence? Curr Opin Urol 22:489–494, 2012.

Foster HE, Dahm P, Kohler TS, et al: Surgical management of lower urinary tract symptoms attributed to benign prostatic hyperplasia: AUA guideline amendment 2019, J Urol 202:592, 2019.

Gelbard M, Goldstein I, Hellstrom WJG, et al: Clinical efficacy, safety and tolerability of collagenase clostridium histolyticum for the treatment of Peyronie disease in 2 large double-blind, randomized, placebo controlled phase 3 studies, J Urol 190:199–207, 2013.

Kaplan SA, Roehrborn CG, Rovner ES, et al: Tolterodine and tamsulosin for treatment of men with lower urinary tract symptoms and overactive bladder: a randomized controlled trial, J Am Med Assoc 296:2319–2328, 2006.

Karmazyn B, Steinberg R, Kurareid L, et al: Clinical and radiographic criteria of the acute scrotum in children: a retrospective study in 172 boys, Pediatr Radiol 35:302–310, 2005.

Kostis JB, Jackson G, Rosen R, et al: Sexual dysfunction and cardiac risk (the second Princeton Consensus Conference), Am J Cardiol 96: 313–321, 2005.

Lowe FC, McConnell JD, Hudson PB, et al: for the Finasteride Study Group, Long-term 6-year experience with finasteride in patients with benign prostatic hyperplasia, Urology 61:791-796, 2003.

Lue TF: Erectile dysfunction, N Engl J Med 342:1802, 2000.

McConnell JD, Roehrborn CG, Bautista OM, et al, for the Medical Therapy of Prostatic Symptoms (MTOPS) Research Group: The long-term effect of doxazosin, finasteride, and combination therapy on the clinical progression of benign prostatic hyperplasia, N Engl J Med 349:2387-2398, 2003.

Meriggiola MC, Bremner WJ, Costantino A, et al: Low dose of cyproterone acetate and testosterone enanthate for contraception in men, Hum Reprod 13:1225–1229, 1998.

Morgentaler A, Caliber M: Safety of testosterone therapy in men with prostate cancer, Expert Opin Drug Saf 1, 2019.

Morgentaler A, Traish A, Hackett G, et al: Diagnosis and treatment of testosterone deficiency: updated recommendations from the lisbon 2018 international consultation for sexual medicine, Sex Med Rev, 2019.

Mulhall JP, Trost LW, Brannigan RE, et al: Evaluation and management of testosterone deficiency: AUA guideline, J Urol 200:423, 2018.

Nehra A, Alterowitz R, Culkin DJ, et al: Peyronie's disease: AUA guideline, J Urol 194:745, 2015.

Neiderberger C: Microsurgical treatment of persistent or recurrent varicocele, J Urol 173:2079–2080, 2005.

Nieschlag E, Swerdloff R, Behre HM, et al: Investigation, treatment, and monitoring of late-onset hypogonadism in males: ISA, ISSAM, and EAU recommendations, J Androl 27:135–137, 2006.

Rhoden EL, Morgentaler A: Risks of testosterone-replacement therapy and recommendations for monitoring, N Engl J Med 350:482–492, 2004.

Roehrborn CG, Kaplan SA, Jones JS, et al: Tolterodine extended release with or without tamsulosin in men with lower urinary tract symptoms including overactive bladder symptoms: effects of prostate size, Eur Urol 55:472–479, 2009.

Sessions AE, Rabinowitz R, Hulbert WC, et al: Testicular torsion: direction, degree, duration and disinformation, J Urol 169:663–665, 2003.

Shridharani A, Lockwood G, Sandlow J: Varicocelectomy in the treatment of testicular pain: a review, Curr Opin Urol 22:499–506, 2012.

Stewart CA, Yafi FA, Knoedler M, et al: Intralesional injection of interferon-α2b improves penile curvature in men with Peyronie's disease independent of plaque location, J Urol 194:1704–1707, 2015.

Svartberg J, Midtby M, Bønaa KH, et al: The associations of age, lifestyle factors and chronic disease with testosterone in men: the Tromsø Study, Eur J Endocrinol 149:145–152, 2003.

Wang C: Phosphodiesterase-5 inhibitors and benign prostatic hyperplasia, Curr Urol Rep 20:49–54, 2010.

Wu FCW, Tajar A, Beynon JM, et al: Identification of late-onset hypogonadism in middle-aged and elderly men, N Engl J Med 363:123–135, 2010.

Yafi FA, Pinsky MR, Sangkum P, et al: Therapeutic advances in the treatment of Peyronie's disease, Andrology 3:650, 2015.

SECTION IV

Diseases of Bone and Bone Mineral Metabolism

骨与骨矿物质代谢疾病

Normal Physiology of Bone and Mineral Homeostasis

Clemens Bergwitz, John J. Wysolmerski

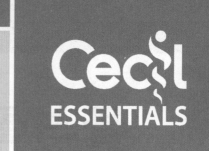

CALCIUM HOMEOSTASIS

Circulating free (or ionized) calcium concentrations are maintained within a narrow normal range by an intricate series of homeostatic mechanisms. Maintaining stable calcium levels is important for at least three reasons. First, calcium along with phosphorus forms *hydroxyapatite*, the major mineral contained within the skeleton. Hydroxyapatite provides structural integrity to bones and also provides a metabolic store of calcium to maintain circulating levels if calcium is not readily available from the environment. Reductions in the mineral content of the skeleton can impair its biomechanical integrity and result in fractures. Second, the circulating ionized calcium concentration influences membrane excitability in muscle and nervous tissue. An increase in serum calcium levels produces refractoriness to the stimulation of neurons and muscle cells, which could lead to muscular weakness and even coma. Conversely, a reduction in ionized calcium levels increases neuromuscular excitability, which can translate clinically into seizures or spontaneous muscle cramps and contractions referred to as *carpopedal spasm* or *tetany*. Finally, intracellular calcium contributes to a host of cellular functions, including enzymatic reactions, intracellular signaling, vesicular trafficking, and cytoskeletal organization to name a few. Therefore, all cells require a stable source of calcium in extracellular fluid for proper function. Physicians routinely use a variety of drugs that regulate channels and intracellular calcium concentrations to manipulate cellular function for the treatment of a wide variety of human diseases.

Total circulating calcium levels, which are customarily measured for diagnostic purposes, typically fall between 8.5 to 10.5 mg/dL (4 mg/dL = 1 mmol/L). Of this total value approximately 50% of calcium circulates as free or ionized calcium, 5% circulates as insoluble complexes such as calcium sulfate, phosphate, and citrate, and the remainder (45%) is bound to serum proteins, principally albumin. It is the free, ionized calcium that is important for physiologic processes or in pathophysiologic settings. While changes in the total calcium usually reflect changes in ionized calcium levels, in some instances, total serum calcium can change without a change in the ionized calcium level. For example, if the serum albumin level declines as a result of hepatic cirrhosis or the nephrotic syndrome, the total serum calcium also declines, but the ionized serum calcium concentration remains normal. Therefore, measuring the ionized serum calcium level directly or deriving it from formula 1 and 2 can be important clinically.

Formula 1 (Payne RB, Little AJ, Williams RB, Milner JR: Interpretation of serum calcium in patients with abnormal plasma proteins, Br Med J 4:643-646, 1973) is:

$$Ca_{Ad} \text{ (mmol/L)} = Ca_T \text{ (mmol/L)} + 0.025 \text{ (40-albumin, g/L)}$$

Formula 2 (Pfitzenmeyer P, Martin I, d'Athis P, et al: A new formula for correction of total calcium level into ionized serum calcium values in very elderly hospitalized patients, Arch Gerontol Geriatrics 45:151-157, 2007) is:

$$Ca^{2+} \text{ (mmol/L)} = 0.188 - 0.00469 \text{ protein (g/L)} \\ + 0.0110 \text{ albumin (g/L)} + 0.401 \, Ca_{Ad} \text{ (mmol/L)}.$$

An overview of calcium economy is represented in Fig. 11.1. As depicted, the circulating calcium level is influenced by a series of three major fluxes of calcium: (1) The net absorption of calcium from the diet in the gut, (2) the storage of calcium in and the liberation of calcium from the hydroxyapatite "warehouse" in the skeleton, and (3) the filtration and net excretion of calcium by the kidneys. Calcium homeostasis and disorders of calcium metabolism involve the hormonal regulation of fluxes between these three compartments.

Calcium Fluxes Into and Out of Extracellular Fluid
Intestinal Calcium Absorption

The average dietary calcium intake for an adult is approximately 1000 mg per day. About 300 mg of the total is absorbed (i.e., unidirectional absorption is about 30%), principally within the duodenum and proximal jejunum. However, about 150 mg of calcium per day is secreted by the liver (in bile), the pancreas (in pancreatic secretions), and the intestinal glands into the gut lumen. Thus, net absorption (called *fractional absorption*) of calcium is approximately 15% of intake and about 85% of calcium entering the gut lumen will be excreted in the feces each day.

The efficiency of calcium absorption is regulated at the level of the small intestinal epithelial cell, the enterocyte, by the active form of vitamin D, 1,25-dihydroxyvitamin D (1,25[OH]$_2$D), also called *calcitriol*. Increases in 1,25(OH)$_2$D enhance calcium absorption, and decreases in 1,25(OH)$_2$D reduce absorption of dietary calcium. Dietary calcium absorption can be increased over the short term by increasing calcium intake or by increasing plasma 1,25(OH)$_2$D concentrations, or both. Pathologic increases in serum calcium (i.e., hypercalcemia) can be caused by increases in circulating 1,25(OH)$_2$D (e.g., in sarcoidosis) or by excessive calcium intake (i.e., milk-alkali syndrome). Conversely, hypocalcemia can result from a decline in 1,25(OH)$_2$D (e.g., chronic renal failure, hypoparathyroidism, vitamin D deficiency).

骨和矿物质的生理稳态

夏维波 译 李梅 王鸥 审校 夏维波 通审

钙稳态

人体经过一系列复杂的体内平衡机制，将循环中游离钙（即离子钙）浓度维持在一个狭窄的正常范围内。保持稳定的钙浓度至少与3种重要生理学功能有关：第一，钙磷构成羟基磷灰石（骨骼中主要的矿物质成分）。羟基磷灰石不仅可维持骨结构的完整性，也是体内钙不足时维持循环钙浓度的代谢储存库。骨矿物质含量不足会损伤骨骼生物力学性能，并导致骨折。第二，循环离子钙浓度影响肌肉和神经组织的膜兴奋性。血清钙浓度升高会使神经元和肌肉细胞对刺激不敏感，导致肌无力，甚至昏迷。相反，离子钙浓度降低会增加神经肌肉兴奋性，在临床上表现为癫痫发作或自发性肌肉痉挛和收缩，即腕足痉挛或手足搐搦。第三，细胞内的钙参与许多细胞功能，包括酶促反应、细胞内信号转导、囊泡运输和细胞骨架组装等。因此，细胞的正常活动需要细胞外液中的钙保持稳定。临床上常用调节钙通道和细胞内钙浓度的药物来调控细胞功能，从而治疗疾病。

总血钙浓度的正常值范围为 8.5~10.5 mg/dl（4 mg/dl = 1 mmol/L）。其中，约50%以离子钙的形式存在，5%的钙以不溶性复合物的形式（如硫酸钙、磷酸钙和柠檬酸钙）循环，剩余的钙（45%）与血清蛋白质（以白蛋白为主）结合。离子钙参与重要的生理学和病理生理学过程。虽然总血钙浓度通常能反映离子钙浓度的变化，但在某些情况下，总血清钙浓度变化，但离子钙浓度不变。例如，肝硬化或肾病综合征可导致血清白蛋白下降，总血清钙浓度也下降，但离子钙浓度保持正常。因此，直接检测或通过公式1和公式2推导血清离子钙浓度具有重要的临床意义。

公式1（Payne RB，Little AJ，Williams RB，Milner JR：Interpretation of serum calcium in patients with abnormal plasma proteins，Br Med J 4：643-646，1973）：

校正血钙浓度（mmol/L）=测得的血钙（mmol/L）+ 0.025×［40－白蛋白（g/L）］

公式2（Pfitzenmeyer P，Martin I，d'Athis P，et al：A new formula for correction of total calcium level into ionized serum calcium values in very elderly hospitalized patients，Arch Gerontol Geriatrics 45：151-157，2007）：

血清离子钙［Ca^{2+}；（mmol/L）］= 0.188－0.00469×血清蛋白（g/L）＋0.0110×白蛋白（g/L）＋0.401×校正血钙浓度（mmol/L）

钙稳态调控如图 11.1 所示。循环钙浓度主要受3种钙流通的影响：①肠道对膳食钙的净吸收；②骨骼羟基磷灰石"仓库"中钙的储存和释放；③肾脏对钙的滤过和净排泄。这三部分钙流通间的激素调控决定了钙稳态或钙代谢紊乱。

钙吸收及排泄

肠钙吸收

成人每天平均膳食钙摄入量约为 1000 mg。其中约 300 mg 主要在十二指肠和近端空肠被吸收（即单向吸收约 30%）。然而，每天约有 150 mg 的钙由肝脏（经胆汁）、胰腺（经胰腺分泌物）和肠道腺体分泌至肠腔中。因此，钙的净吸收（即吸收率）约为摄入量的 15%，进入肠腔的剩余 85% 的钙随粪便排出体外。

活性维生素 D——1,25-二羟维生素 D［1,25（OH）$_2$D，即骨化三醇］，调节小肠上皮细胞的钙吸收率。提高 1,25（OH）$_2$D 水平可使膳食钙吸收增多，降低 1,25（OH）$_2$D 水平则使膳食钙吸收减少。通过增加钙摄入量和（或）提高血 1,25（OH）$_2$D 水平，可短期增加膳食钙吸收。血液中 1,25（OH）$_2$D 水平升高（如结节病）或钙摄入过多（如乳碱综合征）可导致高钙血症，相反，血液中 1,25（OH）$_2$D 水平降低（如慢性肾衰竭和甲状腺旁腺功能减退症）会导致低钙血症［译者注：原文中的维生素 D 缺乏症建议删除，因为缺乏维生素 D 时，血 1,25（OH）$_2$D 水平通常并不低］。

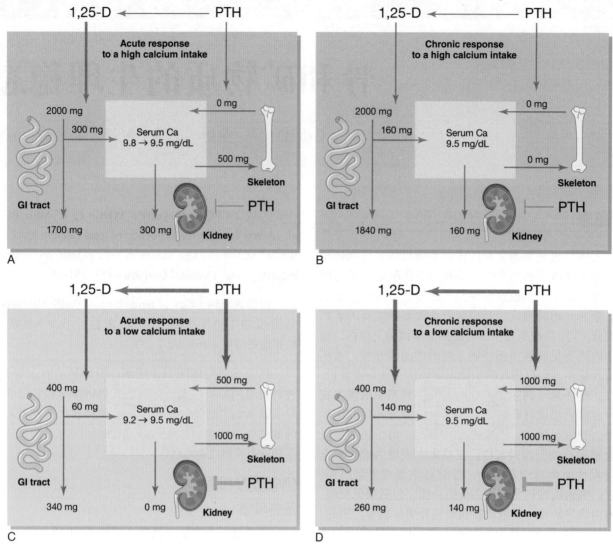

Fig. 11.1 Calcium homeostasis. (A) The acute response and (B) the chronic response to increases in calcium intake. (C) The acute response and (D) the chronic response to decreases in calcium intake. Details are provided in the text. *GI,* Gastrointestinal; *PTH,* parathyroid hormone; *1,25(OH)₂D,* 1,25-dihydroxycholecalciferol (calcitriol). SI conversion: 1 mg calcium = 0.4 mmol calcium.

Renal Calcium Handling

The filtered load of calcium by the kidneys is about 10,000 mg per day assuming a glomerular filtration rate (GFR) of 100 mL/min and serum calcium of 10 mg/dL, making the kidney the most important moment-to-moment regulator of the serum calcium concentration and, as a result, disordered renal calcium handling (e.g., thiazide diuretic use, hypoparathyroidism) can produce significant abnormalities in serum calcium homeostasis.

Of the 10,000 mg of calcium filtered at the glomerulus each day, about 9000 mg (90%) is reabsorbed *proximally* by the proximal convoluted tubule, the pars recta, and the thick ascending limb of Henle loop. This 90% is absorbed in conjunction/competition with sodium and chloride reabsorption and is not subject to regulation by parathyroid hormone (PTH). The remaining 10% (1000 mg) that arrives at the distal tubule is subject to regulation by PTH, which stimulates renal calcium reabsorption. The anticalciuric effect of PTH can be extremely efficient, and elevated PTH concentrations can essentially eliminate calcium

excretion into the urine. This action is a potent mechanism for retaining calcium under conditions of calcium deprivation (e.g., a low-calcium diet, vitamin D deficiency, intestinal malabsorption) and can contribute to hypercalcemia under pathologic conditions, as in primary hyperparathyroidism. The absence of PTH action, in turn, produces hypercalciuria and nephrolithiasis in hypoparathyroidism. Because of preserved PTH action at the distal tubules in pseudohypoparathyroidism, hypocalciuria characterizes this rare genetic condition, which is caused by end-organ resistance to PTH at the proximal tubules, leading to hypovitaminosis D and hypocalcemia despite often elevated PTH levels.

About 150 mg of calcium is excreted by the kidney in the final urine on a daily basis in a healthy individual. If the kidney filters 10,000 mg of calcium each day, and if 150 mg is excreted in the final urine, 9850 mg (98.5%) is reabsorbed at proximal and distal sites. Therefore, a healthy person is in zero calcium balance with respect to the outside world: intake (1000 mg/day) − output [(850 mg/day in feces) + (150 mg/day in urine)] = 0.

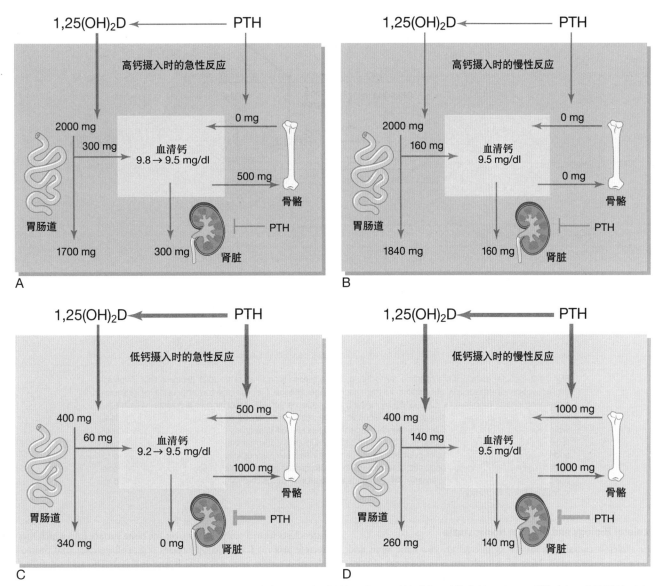

图 11.1　钙稳态。**A**. 高钙摄入时的急性反应。**B**. 高钙摄入时的慢性反应。**C**. 低钙摄入时的急性反应。**D**. 低钙摄入时的慢性反应。详见正文。PTH，甲状旁腺激素；1,25（OH）$_2$D，1,25- 二羟维生素 D（骨化三醇）。SI 换算：1 mg 钙 = 0.4 mmol 钙

肾脏的钙调节

若肾小球滤过率（GFR）为 100 ml/min，血清钙浓度为 10 mg/dl，则肾脏每天滤过的钙负荷约为 10 000 mg，故肾脏是随时调节血清钙浓度最重要的脏器。因此，肾脏的钙调节异常（如使用噻嗪类利尿剂、甲状旁腺功能减退症）可引起血钙稳态的严重失衡。

在肾小球每天滤过的 10 000 mg 钙中，约 9000 mg（90%）被近曲小管、近直小管、髓袢升支粗段重吸收。这 90% 钙的重吸收与钠和氯的重吸收相关，且不受甲状旁腺激素（PTH）的调节。到达远端小管的剩余 10%（1000 mg）的钙受 PTH 的调节，PTH 可刺激肾脏重吸收钙。PTH 水平升高可强效减少尿钙排泄。这是钙缺乏时（如低钙饮食、维生素 D 缺乏症、肠道吸收不良等）维持血钙浓度的有效机制，这一机制在病理情况下会导致高钙血症（如原发性甲状旁腺功能亢进症等）。PTH 作用缺失（如甲状旁腺功能减退症等）会导致高钙尿症和肾结石。在假性甲状旁腺功能减退症这一罕见遗传病中，由于 PTH 对远端小管的作用保留，故其特征为低钙尿症，但由于近端小管对 PTH 抵抗，尽管患者的 PTH 水平升高，仍会出现 1,25（OH）$_2$D 水平降低和低钙血症。

生理状态下，健康个体每天约有 150 mg 钙通过肾脏在终尿中排出。如果肾脏每天滤过 10 000 mg 钙，且 150 mg 在终尿中排出，则 9850 mg 钙（98.5%）在近端小管和远端小管被重吸收。因此，健康个体与外界处于零钙平衡：钙摄入（1000 mg/d）－钙排出［（粪便中 850 mg/d）＋（尿液中 150 mg/d）］＝ 0。

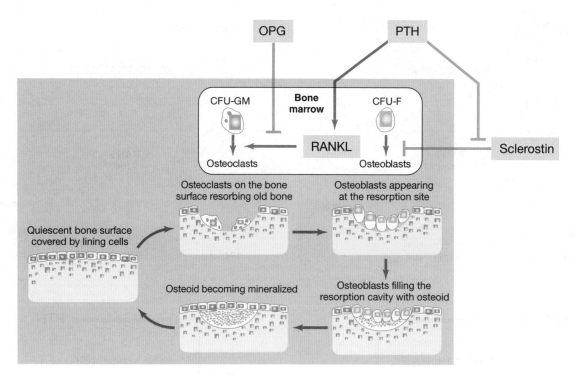

Fig. 11.2 Cellular components of bone remodeling. Bone remodeling is a continuous process that involves the activation of osteoclast precursors in the macrophage lineage (i.e., colony-forming units of granulocyte-macrophage progenitors [CFU-GM]) by RANKL that become actively resorbing osteoclasts, which tunnel into the bone surface to dig resorption lacunae. Bone resorption can be inhibited by bisphosphonates, which are toxic to osteoclasts, or by antibody drugs that inhibit RANKL, such as the decoy receptor osteoprotegerin (OPG). Osteoblast precursors in the fibroblast–bone marrow stromal cell lineage (CFU-F) then appear and become active at the sites of prior resorption, and they secrete new osteoid, which later mineralizes to fill the lacunae created by osteoclastic bone resorption. Both processes are stimulated by PTH, which inhibits the bone formation inhibitor sclerostin. PTH analogs and antibody drugs that inhibit sclerostin can be used to stimulate bone formation.

Skeletal Biology and Calcium Homeostasis

The skeleton contains about 1.2 kg of calcium in a male adult and 1.0 kg in a female adult. Most of this calcium is in the form of crystal hydroxyapatite, a calcium phosphate salt. Calcium contributes in an important way to the structural integrity of the skeleton and, in turn, the skeleton serves as a quantitatively large reservoir (i.e., a sink) for adding and removing calcium to and from the extracellular fluid (ECF) compartment at appropriate times.

The adult skeleton is composed of two types of bone: cortical (or lamellar) bone and trabecular (or cancellous) bone. Cortical bone predominates in the skull and the shafts of long bones, and trabecular bone predominates at other sites, such as the distal radius, the vertebral bodies, and the trochanters of the hip.

Bone is not an inert tissue; rather, it is continually turning over. The adult skeleton is completely remodeled every 3 to 10 years. Remodeling is perhaps best appreciated by recalling that orthopedic surgeons routinely and intentionally set fractures imperfectly, knowing that the normal processes of bone remodeling will restore the bone's original shape with the passage of time.

The cells that regulate bone turnover can be divided into those that remove old bone, those that provide new bone (Fig. 11.2) (see Chapter 13), and those that regulate these two processes. Cells that remove, or resorb, old bone are osteoclasts. These cells are large, metabolically active, multinucleated cells derived from the fusion of circulating macrophages. Following attachment to the surface of bone, osteoclasts form a sealing zone over the bone surface into which they secrete protons (i.e., acid), proteases (e.g., collagenase), and proteoglycan-digesting enzymes (e.g., hyaluronidase). The acid solubilizes hydroxyapatite crystals, releasing calcium, and the enzymes digest bone proteins and proteoglycans (e.g., collagen, osteocalcin, osteopontin), which constitute the nonmineral, or osteoid, component of bone. Osteoclasts move along the surface of trabecular bone plates and drill tunnels in cortical bone, periodically releasing the digested contents within their sealed zones into the bone marrow space and thereby creating resorption pits, called Howship's lacunae, on the trabecular bone surface. The released calcium contributes to the ECF calcium pool, and the released proteolytic products, such as deoxypyridinoline cross-links (i.e., collagen fragments and hydroxyproline), can be used clinically as indices of bone resorption.

New bone formation is accomplished by osteoblasts, which are derived from marrow stromal cells or bone surface lining cells. Osteoblasts synthesize and secrete the components of the nonmineral phase of bone, called osteoid. The components are mostly proteins and include collagen, osteopontin, osteonectin, osteocalcin, proteoglycans, and a plethora of growth factors, including transforming growth factor-β and insulin-like growth factor-I. Osteoblasts also produce alkaline phosphatase, which inactivates the mineralization inhibitor pyrophosphate, and type 1 collagen, which forms cable-like structures in bone matrix, and they also facilitate the deposition of hydroxyapatite between these proteinaceous cables. Both the bone-specific

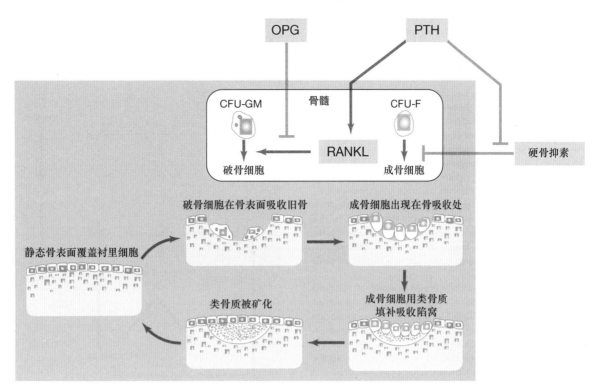

图 11.2　骨重建的细胞模式图。骨重建是一个持续的过程，涉及巨噬细胞谱系中破骨细胞前体细胞［即粒细胞-巨噬细胞祖细胞集落形成单位（CFU-GM）］被 RANKL 激活，成为活跃的、有吸收能力的破骨细胞，进入骨表面形成吸收陷窝。骨吸收可被双膦酸盐（破骨细胞抑制剂）或 RANKL 抗体［如诱饵受体（骨保护素）］抑制。随后，成纤维细胞集落形成单位（CFU-F）中的成骨细胞前体细胞出现在既往的吸收部位并活化，分泌新的类骨质，这些类骨质随后被矿化，填补破骨细胞骨吸收形成的腔隙。PTH 可刺激这两个过程，抑制硬骨抑素（骨形成抑制剂）的作用。PTH 类似物和抑制硬骨抑素的抗体可用于刺激骨骼形成

骨骼生物学和钙稳态

成年男性骨骼中的钙含量约为 1.2 kg，女性约为 1.0 kg。这些钙大部分以羟基磷灰石晶体（一种磷酸钙盐）的形式存在。钙对骨骼的结构完整性发挥重要作用，而骨骼也是一个容量可观的钙库（即钙池），可以适时向细胞外液释放或移除钙。

成人骨骼由两种类型的骨组成：皮质骨（或板层骨）和小梁骨（或松质骨）。皮质骨主要见于颅骨和长骨骨干，而小梁骨主要见于其他部位，如桡骨远端、椎体和股骨粗隆。

骨不是一种惰性组织，骨转换是持续进行的。成人骨骼每 3～10 年会完全重建 1 次。得益于骨重建，骨科医生无须完美固定骨折处，因为随着时间的推移，骨重建过程会使骨骼恢复至最初的形状。

调节骨转换的细胞可分为移除旧骨的细胞和产生新骨的细胞（图 11.2）（见第 13 章），以及调控这两个过程的细胞。清除或吸收旧骨的细胞是破骨细胞。这些细胞是由循环中巨噬细胞融合而成的大的、代谢活跃的多核细胞。破骨细胞附着在骨表面后，在骨表面

形成一个封闭区，并向封闭区内分泌质子（即酸）、蛋白酶（如胶原酶）和蛋白聚糖消化酶（如透明质酸酶）。酸能溶解羟基磷灰石晶体，释放钙；酶能消化骨蛋白和蛋白聚糖（如胶原蛋白、骨钙蛋白、骨桥蛋白），这些是骨的非矿物质或类骨质成分。破骨细胞沿着骨小梁板层表面移动，在皮质骨上钻出隧道，周期性地将封闭区内消化的内容物释放到骨髓中，在骨小梁表面形成吸收小坑（即吸收陷窝）。其释放的钙进入细胞外液钙池，释放的蛋白质水解产物［如脱氧吡啶啉交联物（如胶原蛋白碎片、羟脯氨酸）］在临床上可作为反映骨吸收的指标。

新骨的形成由成骨细胞完成，其来源于骨髓基质细胞或骨表面衬里细胞。成骨细胞合成并分泌骨的非矿物质成分，即类骨质。这些成分主要为蛋白质（包括胶原蛋白、骨桥蛋白、骨粘连蛋白、骨钙蛋白、蛋白聚糖）和大量生长因子（包括转化生长因子 -β 和胰岛素样生长因子 -Ⅰ）。成骨细胞还可产生碱性磷酸酶（使骨矿化抑制剂焦磷酸盐失活）和 Ⅰ 型胶原蛋白（形成骨基质中的条索状结构），从而促进羟基磷灰石在这

isoform of alkaline phosphatase and procollagen can be used clinically as indices of bone formation. Maintaining the correct balance between protein and mineral in bone provides the combination of compliance and toughness needed to withstand the biomechanical forces encountered by the skeleton.

In the past decade, attention has focused on a third, previously underappreciated bone cell type, the osteocyte. These cells are descendants of osteoblasts and are embedded into the mineralized phase of bone. Osteocytes physically connect with one another and to cells at the mineral surface through long dendritic processes. The dendritic processes extensively permeate the mineralized phase of bone through an elaborate canalicular network. Osteocytes serve a critical role in sensing biomechanical strain within bone, and through their cellular extensions to the bone surface, they communicate signals that attract, activate, or repress osteoclasts and osteoblasts. In this way, they determine which areas of the skeleton require new bone formation and which need to be targets of osteoclastic bone resorption, a critical function for proper structural remodeling of bone tissue.

Bone remodeling involves the coordinated removal of old bone through osteoclastic bone resorption stimulated by receptor activator of nuclear factor κB ligand (RANKL) followed by the formation of new bone via osteoblastic bone formation. This process occurs in discrete locations called bone remodeling units, the locations of which, as described previously, are likely dictated by osteocytes. In adults, skeletal homeostasis requires the careful balancing of osteoclast and osteoblast activities so that the same amount of bone that is removed by osteoclasts is replaced by osteoblasts. This is accomplished by a complex, and only partly understood, three-way series of communications between osteoclasts, osteoblasts, and osteocytes, that are modulated by systemic hormones. Altering the relative activities of these cells can result in the net movement of calcium out of or into the skeleton on a physiologic basis but a prolonged imbalance of osteoclastic and osteoblastic activities can result in disease. For example, excessive bone remodeling leads to osteoporosis, while absent bone remodeling leads to adynamic bone disease, both conditions that can predispose to fractures. Bone remodeling is also exploited therapeutically. Anabolic agents for osteoporosis, such as sclerostin inhibitors or parathyroid hormone and parathyroid hormone-related protein analogues stimulate the activity of osteoblasts to produce new bone. In contrast, antiresorptive agents, such as estrogens, estrogen-like drugs, bisphosphonates, and RANKL inhibitors, reduce bone resorption to improve bone mass and bone mechanical properties.

Bone remodeling is important for systemic calcium homeostasis. Osteoclasts are mobilized to release calcium from the skeleton in times of need in order to maintain a normal serum calcium concentration and prevent hypocalcemia. Conversely, unmineralized osteoid produced by osteoblasts serves to deposit excess calcium to prevent hypercalcemia. Under normal circumstances, osteoclasts result in the release of about 500 mg of calcium per day from the skeleton to the ECF compartment. At the same time, osteoblasts produce osteoid that mineralizes at a rate such that about 500 mg of ECF calcium is deposited in the skeleton at new sites. From the perspective of the normal homeostatic fluxes shown in Fig. 11.1, the skeleton is in zero calcium balance with the ECF, and the whole organism is in zero calcium balance with the external environment.

Considering the complexity of this calcium homeostatic system and the importance of maintaining tight control of serum calcium levels, an obvious need exists for systemic regulation and integration of the calcium fluxes across the GI, skeletal, and renal compartments. The two key metabolic regulatory hormones that coordinate these activities are PTH and the active form of vitamin D, 1,25(OH)$_2$D.

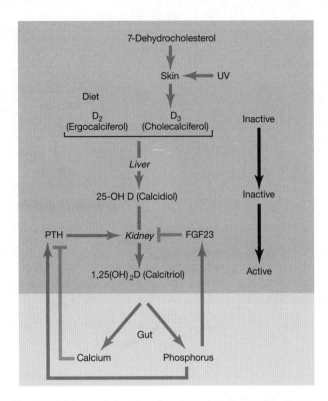

Fig. 11.3 Calcium and phosphate homeostasis are co-regulated by parathyroid hormone (PTH). PTH is secreted as an 84-amino-acid protein, which is cleaved in the liver to derivative amino-terminal and carboxyl-terminal (C-term) forms. Actions of the amino-terminally intact forms of PTH are listed in Table 11.1. It stimulates synthesis of the active form of 1,25(OH)$_2$D, 1,25-dihydroxycholecalciferol, from its biologically inactive precursors, vitamin D$_2$ and D$_3$, which are either produced in the skin or absorbed from the diet in the gastrointestinal (GI) tract, and 25-hydroxylated in the liver and kidney. 1,25(OH)$_2$D stimulates absorption of calcium and phosphate from the diet in the GI tract. Different from PTH, fibroblast growth factor 23 (FGF23) stimulates renal phosphate excretion and inhibits the last step (1α hydroxylation) of vitamin D activation. Although both PTH and FGF23 lower phosphate levels, PTH primarily responds to changes in circulating calcium levels, while FGF23 responds to alterations in phosphate levels. Their different actions on vitamin D synthesis reflect their different primary functions since PTH increases 1,25 vitamin D levels to help restore low calcium levels towards normal and FGF23 suppresses 1,25 vitamin D levels to help restore elevated phosphate levels towards normal.

Regulatory Hormones
Parathyroid Hormone

PTH is a peptide hormone produced by the four parathyroid glands (Fig. 11.3 and Table 11.1). These glands are located behind the normal thyroid lobes, with two on the right and two on the left. Through the calcium sensor—a G protein–coupled receptor for calcium that is located on the surface of the parathyroid cell—the serum ionized calcium concentration is continuously monitored. In this exquisitely sensitive system, minor (e.g., 0.1 mg/dL) reductions in serum ionized calcium lead to PTH secretion, and minor increments in serum calcium lead to suppression of PTH secretion.

PTH is secreted as an 84-amino-acid peptide hormone that is rapidly (half-life of about 3 to 5 minutes) cleaved by the Kupffer cells in the liver into an active amino-terminal form and an inactive carboxyl-terminal fragment. Continuous monitoring of the serum calcium concentration by the parathyroid glands, the immediate secretion of PTH in response

些蛋白条索间沉积。骨特异性碱性磷酸酶和前胶原蛋白均可作为临床上反映骨形成的指标。保持骨骼中蛋白质和矿物质间的正常平衡，可提供骨承受生物机械力时所需的弹性和韧性。

在过去的 10 年里，研究焦点集中在既往未被重视的第 3 种细胞类型：骨细胞。这类细胞由成骨细胞生成，被包埋在矿化骨内。骨细胞通过长的树突相互连接，并与矿化表面的细胞连接。这些树突通过精细的管状网络在骨骼矿化期提供广泛的通透性。骨细胞在感知骨内生物力学应力中发挥关键作用，它们通过向骨表面细胞扩散信息来传递信号，从而吸引、激活或抑制破骨细胞和成骨细胞。通过这种方式，骨细胞能确定需要新骨形成和破骨细胞骨吸收的区域，这是骨组织正常重建的关键功能。

骨重建包括通过核因子 κB 受体激活蛋白配体（RANKL）刺激破骨细胞吸收旧骨，以及通过成骨细胞形成新骨。该过程发生在骨重建单位，其位置可能由骨细胞决定。成人骨稳态需要破骨细胞和成骨细胞活性的精细平衡，从而使破骨细胞移除的旧骨被相同数量成骨细胞形成的新骨所取代。该过程由破骨细胞、成骨细胞和骨细胞的细胞间信息传递来完成，其受全身激素的调控，目前仅部分调控机制被阐明。改变这些细胞的相对活性可在生理学基础上导致钙向骨骼内或骨骼外的净转移，但长期破骨细胞和成骨细胞活性不平衡可导致疾病。例如，过度的骨重建会导致骨质疏松症，而缺乏骨重建会导致无动力性骨病，两种情况均可能导致骨折。骨重建的机制可用于治疗。促骨形成药物（如硬骨抑素抑制剂或甲状旁腺激素和甲状旁腺激素相关蛋白类似物）可刺激成骨细胞活性而产生新骨。相反，抗骨吸收药物（如雌激素、雌激素样药物、双膦酸盐和 RANKL 抑制剂）可减少骨吸收，改善骨量和骨的力学性能。

骨重建对维持全身钙稳态至关重要。破骨细胞会在需要时被动员，从而及时从骨骼中释放钙，以维持正常血钙浓度，防止低钙血症。相反，由成骨细胞产生的未矿化类骨质则能沉积多余的钙，防止高钙血症。在生理学条件下，破骨细胞每天将约 500 mg 的钙从骨骼释放到细胞外液。同时，成骨细胞产生类骨质的矿化过程可使约 500 mg 的钙从细胞外液沉积至新骨上。从正常稳态钙流通的角度看（图 11.1），骨骼与细胞外液之间，以及整个机体与外部环境之间均处于零钙平衡状态。

考虑到钙稳态系统的复杂性和严格控制血清钙浓度的重要性，需要系统调节和整合胃肠道、骨骼和肾脏间的钙流通。其中两个关键的代谢调控激素是甲状旁腺激素和活性维生素 D［即 1,25（OH）$_2$D］。

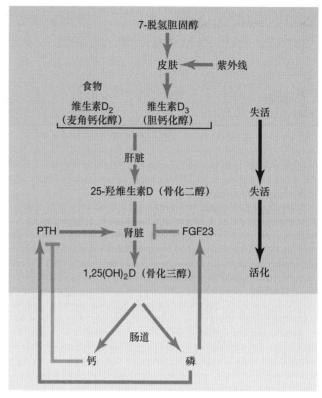

图 11.3　体内钙稳态和磷稳态受甲状旁腺激素（PTH）的共同调节。PTH 是一种由 84 个氨基酸组成的蛋白质，在肝脏中分解，衍生为 N- 末端片段和 C- 末端片段两种形式。PTH 的 N- 末端的功能见表 11.1，它促进活性维生素 D［1,25（OH）$_2$D］的生成。1,25（OH）$_2$D 的前体是肠道从饮食中吸收的维生素 D$_2$、皮肤生成的维生素 D$_3$、肝脏和肾脏中的 25- 羟维生素 D。1,25（OH）$_2$D 可促进胃肠道从食物中吸收钙和磷。与 PTH 不同，成纤维细胞生长因子 23（FGF23）可促进肾磷排泄，抑制维生素 D 活化的最后一步（1α 羟基化）。虽然 PTH 和 FGF23 都能降低血磷浓度，但 PTH 主要对血钙浓度变化做出反应，FGF23 则主要对血磷浓度的变化做出反应。低钙血症时，PTH 通过增加 1,25（OH）$_2$D 的合成来保持血钙浓度，而高磷血症时，FGF23 通过抑制 1,25（OH）$_2$D 使血磷浓度恢复正常

调节激素

甲状旁腺激素

PTH 是由 4 个甲状旁腺产生的肽类激素（图 11.3 和表 11.1）。甲状旁腺位于正常甲状腺叶的后面，左右各有两个。通过位于甲状旁腺细胞表面的钙感受器（钙的 G 蛋白偶联受体）来持续监测血清离子钙浓度。在这个非常敏感的系统中，血清离子钙浓度的轻微降低（如 0.1 mg/dl）即可刺激 PTH 分泌，而轻微升高可抑制 PTH 分泌。

PTH 是一种由 84 个氨基酸组成的肽类激素，可迅速（半衰期为 3～5 min）被肝脏 Kupffer 细胞分解为活性氨基末端和非活性羧基末端片段。甲状旁腺对血钙浓度进行持续监测，在低钙血症时迅速分泌 PTH，

TABLE 11.1	Hormone Actions							
Hormone	S-CA	U-CA	P-Pi	U-Pi	S-1,25(OH)$_2$-D	S-Mg	U-Mg	Other
PTH	↑	↓	↓	↑	↑	=	=	Stimulates bone remodeling, induces hypotension
FGF23	=/↓	=/↓	↓	↑	↓	=	=	Inhibits growth plates resulting in short stature, causes left ventricular hypertrophy
1,25(OH)$_2$D	↑	↑	↑	↑	↓	=	=	Inhibits PTH secretion and stimulates FGF23 synthesis
EGF1	=/↓	=/↑	=	=	=/↓	↑	↓	

EGF1, Epidermal growth factor 1; *FGF23*, fibroblast growth factor 23; *PTH*, parathyroid hormone; *1,25(OH)$_2$D*, 1,25-dihydroxy vitamin D.

to hypocalcemia, and the rapid clearance of PTH after secretion enable the parathyroid gland and PTH to regulate serum calcium rapidly and with remarkable precision.

PTH targets three organs, two directly and one indirectly. In the kidney, PTH stimulates calcium reabsorption in the distal tubule inhibiting urinary calcium excretion. PTH also inhibits phosphate and bicarbonate reabsorption by the proximal tubules, which induces phosphaturia and hypophosphatemia and proximal renal tubular acidosis, respectively. PTH also stimulates the production of the active form of vitamin D, 1,25(OH)$_2$D by the renal tubules. These actions of PTH on the kidney are rapid and direct.

The second PTH target is the skeleton. PTH can mobilize calcium immediately from the skeleton through the activity of osteoclasts and osteocytes, without activating bone formation, which is important for the rapid delivery of calcium to the ECF. If PTH is elevated over days to weeks, it also stimulates the activity of osteoblasts directly and through inhibition of sclerostin release by osteocytes to produce new bone. This type of prolonged elevation in PTH stimulates bone resorption in excess of bone formation to maintain a net release of skeletal calcium to the ECF, enabling the skeleton to help prevent hypocalcemia in states of nutritional calcium deficiency, malabsorption or vitamin D deficiency.

The third target organ is the intestine, which PTH affects indirectly. By increasing renal synthesis of 1,25(OH)$_2$D, PTH can lead to increased intestinal calcium absorption to supply more calcium to the ECF from the diet, a response that is not immediate but occurs over several days of PTH stimulation. Seen in concert, PTH is secreted in response to hypocalcemia, and the actions of PTH combine to restore a low serum calcium concentration to normal by preventing renal calcium losses, by releasing calcium from the skeleton, and by indirectly stimulating (through 1,25[OH]$_2$D) increases in intestinal calcium absorption.

Vitamin D

Vitamin D occurs in two forms: ergocalciferol (vitamin D$_2$) and cholecalciferol (vitamin D$_3$) (Fig. 11.3 and Table 11.2). Both substances are inactive precursors. One (D$_3$) is derived principally from skin exposed to sunlight and the other (D$_2$) is derived from plant sterols in the diet. Either D$_2$, D$_3$ or both can be found in multivitamins and commercial dietary supplements.

Both precursors are constitutively converted to their respective 25-hydroxyvitamin D (25[OH]D) derivatives in the liver through the actions of the enzyme vitamin D 25-hydroxylase (CYP2R1). 25(OH)D is also called calcidiol and has 1000-fold lower affinity to the vitamin D receptor (VDR) when compared to 1,25(OH)$_2$D, but it is a helpful clinical laboratory measure of the vitamin D status (i.e., repletion or deficiency) of patients with hypocalcemia, osteomalacia or rickets, osteoporosis, intestinal malabsorption, and other similar conditions. Furthermore, severe liver disease such as cirrhosis prevents this 25-hydroxylation and leads to a vitamin D–deficiency syndrome called hepatic osteodystrophy.

25(OH)D is converted, or activated, in the renal proximal tubule by the enzyme 25-hydroxyvitamin D$_3$ 1α-hydroxylase (CYP27B1) to the active form of the vitamin, 1,25(OH)$_2$D, which is also called calcitriol.

PTH increases 1,25(OH)$_2$D levels by stimulating its formation through the activity of CYP27B1 while also inhibiting its degradation through the activity of another enzyme, CYP24A1 (24-hydroxylase), which converts 1,25(OH)$_2$D to its inactive metabolite, 24,25(OH)$_2$D. The primary action of 1,25(OH)$_2$D is to regulate intestinal calcium absorption. PTH, through 1,25(OH)$_2$D, indirectly regulates calcium absorption from the diet by the intestine. The hypocalcemia of hypoparathyroidism is a result, in part, of inadequate intestinal calcium absorption. Conversely, hyperparathyroidism is associated with hypercalciuria and nephrolithiasis, both of which directly result from increases in circulating 1,25(OH)$_2$D levels. Therefore, measurement of 1,25(OH)$_2$D can be used as an index of parathyroid function and intestinal calcium absorption.

Because of some affinity to the vitamin D receptor, high doses of calcidiol can be used to treat hypoparathyroidism. However, 1α-hydroxylated versions (i.e., hectoral), which can be 25-hydroxylated by CYP2R1 in the liver or calcitriol, have become standard of care for these disorders (see Table 11.2).

Calcitonin

Calcitonin is produced by the parafollicular or C cells of the thyroid gland in response to hypercalcemia. It was once viewed as an essential calcium-regulating hormone. Pharmacologic doses of calcitonin reduce serum calcium levels by inhibiting osteoclastic bone resorption, which is used in the emergency setting along with hydration to rapidly treat life-threatening hypercalcemia, but this effect wears off quickly due to tachyphylaxis (i.e., desensitization of osteoclasts). Little evidence exists that calcitonin has homeostatic relevance in humans, although it appears to contribute to the regulation of calcium and skeletal homeostasis during reproductive cycles in female rodents.

Integration of Calcium Homeostasis

Ingestion of a greater than normal dietary calcium load (see Fig. 11.1A) leads to a mild rise in the serum calcium level. The rise in calcium is sensed by the parathyroid glands that suppress PTH secretion causing a rapid and marked increase in renal calcium excretion by the distal tubule. It also immediately decreases osteoclastic activity, which slows continued bone resorption but allows continued calcium entry from the ECF into unmineralized osteoid. These two effects produce a rapid, short-term reduction in serum calcium to normal levels. However, if the high-calcium diet is maintained over the long term, these adaptations are insufficient. Continued renal calcium wasting leads to hypercalciuria (with nephrolithiasis and nephrocalcinosis), and unopposed osteoblastic bone formation leads to excessive skeletal mineralization (i.e., osteopetrosis).

Two additional responses (see Fig. 11.1B) are required to prevent the long-term adverse effects of a high-calcium diet. First, subacute or chronic suppression of PTH reduces circulating 1,25(OH)$_2$D. This reduces the efficiency of calcium absorption from the intestine, calcium entry into the ECF, and urinary calcium excretion. Second, a chronic decrement in PTH leads to a chronic decline in osteoblastic activity. No osteoid is formed, and the ability to deposit calcium into the skeleton is decreased.

表 11.1　激素的主要作用

激素	S-CA	U-CA	P-Pi	U-Pi	S-1,25(OH)$_2$D	S-Mg	U-Mg	其他
PTH	↑	↓	↓	↑	↑	=	=	刺激骨重建，诱发低血压
FGF23	= / ↓	= / ↓	↓	↑	↓	=	=	抑制生长板导致身材矮小，导致心左心室肥大
1,25(OH)$_2$D	↑	↑	↑	↑		=	=	抑制 PTH 分泌，刺激 FGF23 合成
EGF1	= / ↑	= / ↑	=	=	= / ↓	=	↓	

CA，钙；EGF1，表皮生长因子 1；FGF23，成纤维细胞生长因子 23；Pi，磷；PTH，甲状旁腺激素；S，血清；U，尿；1,25(OH)$_2$D，1,25-二羟维生素 D。

并在分泌后快速清除 PTH，从而保证了甲状旁腺和 PTH 对血钙的快速、精准调节。

PTH 有 3 个靶器官，其中 2 个是直接作用，1 个是间接作用。在肾脏中，PTH 可刺激远端小管重吸收钙，并抑制尿钙排泄。PTH 还能抑制近端肾小管对磷酸盐和碳酸氢盐的重吸收，分别引起磷酸盐尿、低磷血症和近端肾小管性酸中毒。PTH 还可刺激肾小管产生 1,25(OH)$_2$D。PTH 对肾脏的这些作用迅速且直接。

PTH 的第 2 个靶器官是骨骼。PTH 可通过破骨细胞和骨细胞的活性从骨骼中快速动员钙，而不激活骨形成，这对于钙快速输送到细胞外液中很重要。如果 PTH 水平升高维持数天至数周，可直接刺激成骨细胞的活性，并通过抑制骨细胞释放硬骨抑素来促进新骨形成。这种 PTH 水平持续升高会刺激骨吸收大于骨形成，可维持骨骼钙释放到细胞外液，从而防止膳食钙缺乏、吸收不良或维生素 D 缺乏症所致的低钙血症。

PTH 的第 3 个靶器官是肠道，其作用是间接的。通过增加肾脏合成 1,25(OH)$_2$D，PTH 可使肠道的钙吸收增加，从膳食中为细胞外液提供更多的钙。这一反应不是即刻发生，而是在 PTH 水平升高数天后发生。同时，低钙血症时 PTH 分泌，PTH 可通过减少肾钙流失、从骨骼中释放钙、间接增加肠道钙吸收 [通过 1,25(OH)$_2$D] 等方式将血钙浓度恢复至正常水平。

维生素 D

维生素 D 以两种形式存在：麦角钙化醇（维生素 D$_2$）和胆钙化醇（维生素 D$_3$）（图 11.3 和表 11.2）。这两种物质均为无活性的前体。维生素 D$_3$ 主要源自暴露于阳光照射的皮肤，维生素 D$_2$ 来源于饮食中的植物固醇。复合维生素和市售的膳食补剂常含有维生素 D$_2$ 或维生素 D$_3$。

两种前体在肝脏经维生素 D 25- 羟化酶（CYP2R1）不断转化为相应的 25- 羟维生素 D [25(OH)D] 衍生物。25(OH)D 又称骨化二醇，其对维生素 D 受体（VDR）的亲和力是 1,25(OH)$_2$D 的 1/1000，但有助于实验室检测低钙血症、骨软化症、佝偻病、骨质疏松症、肠道吸收不良等患者的维生素 D 营养状况（如正常或缺乏）。此外，肝硬化等严重的肝脏疾病会阻止 25- 羟基化过程，导致维生素 D 缺乏，即肝性骨营养不良。

25(OH)D 在肾近端小管中被 1α- 羟化酶（CYP27B1）转化或活化为 1,25(OH)$_2$D，即骨化三醇。PTH 通过刺激 CYP27B1 促进 1,25(OH)$_2$D 形成，提高血 1,25(OH)$_2$D

水平，同时通过抑制 CYP24A1（24- 羟化酶）来抑制其降解，该酶可将 25(OH)D [译者注：原文的 1,25(OH)$_2$D 有误] 转化为无活性的代谢产物 24,25(OH)$_2$D。1,25(OH)$_2$D 的主要作用是调节肠道钙吸收。PTH 通过 1,25(OH)$_2$D 间接调节肠道对膳食钙的吸收。甲状旁腺功能减退症的低钙血症是由肠道钙吸收不足所致。相反，甲状旁腺功能亢进症出现的高钙尿症和肾结石是由循环 1,25(OH)$_2$D 水平升高直接引起。因此，1,25(OH)$_2$D 可作为甲状旁腺功能和肠道钙吸收的指标。

由于对 VDR 具有一定亲和力，高剂量的 25(OH)D 可用于治疗甲状旁腺功能减退症。然而，1α- 羟维生素 D 类似物（如 Hectoral）可通过肝脏中的 CYP2R1 进行 25- 羟化或直接使用 1,25(OH)$_2$D，这是该病目前的标准治疗（表 11.2）。

降钙素

降钙素由甲状腺的滤泡旁细胞或 C 细胞产生，以应对高钙血症。它曾被认为是一种重要的钙调节激素。药理剂量的降钙素可通过抑制破骨细胞骨吸收来降低血钙浓度，紧急情况下可联用水化，从而迅速治疗危及生命的高钙血症，但这种效应会由于快速耐受而很快消失（破骨细胞脱敏）。尽管降钙素似乎有助于调节雌性大鼠生殖周期中的钙稳态和骨骼稳态，但很少有证据表明降钙素与人体稳态有关。

钙稳态整合

摄入量超过正常膳食钙负荷（图 11.1A）会导致血清钙浓度轻度升高。甲状旁腺感应到钙浓度升高，抑制 PTH 的分泌，进而导致远端小管肾钙排泄迅速而显著增加。高血钙还能立即降低破骨细胞活性，从而减缓骨吸收，但钙仍能从细胞外液持续进入未矿化的类骨质。这两种作用可使血清钙在短期内迅速降至正常水平。然而，如果长期维持高钙饮食，则这些适应作用不足以代偿。持续肾钙排泄增多可导致高钙尿症（伴有肾结石和肾钙盐沉着症），缺乏对抗的成骨细胞性骨形成会导致过度的骨骼矿化（即骨硬化症）。

两个额外的反应可用于防止高钙饮食的长期副作用（图 11.1B）。首先，亚急性或慢性抑制 PTH 可减少循环 1,25(OH)$_2$D，降低了肠道吸收钙、钙进入细胞外液和尿钙排泄的效率。其次，PTH 水平慢性降低可导致成骨细胞活性缓慢下降。没有类骨质形成，钙质沉积到骨骼的能力也会下降。

TABLE 11.2	Phosphate and Vitamin D Metabolite Preparations		
Phosphate Preparations	**Phosphorus Content**	**Potassium (K) Content**	**Sodium (Na) Content**
Neutra-Phos powder (for mixing with liquid)	250 mg/packet	270 mg	164 mg
Neutra-Phos-K powder (for mixing with liquid)	250 mg/packet	556 mg	0 mg
K-Phos Original tablet (to mix in liquid, acidifying)	114 mg/tablet	144 mg	0 mg
K-Phos MF tablet (mixing not required, acidifying)	126 mg	45 mg	67 mg
K-Phos #2 (double strength of K-Phos MF)	250 mg	90 mg	133 mg
K-Phos Neutral tablet (nonacidifying, mixing not required)	250 mg	45 mg	298 mg
Phospho-Soda solution (small doses may be given undiluted)	127 mg/mL	0 mg/mL	152 mg/mL
Joule's solution (prepared by compounding pharmacies)	30 mg/mL	0 mg/mL	17.5–20 mg/mL

Vitamin D and Related Agents	Available Preparations
Vitamin D	
Calciferol (Drisdol)	Solution: 8000 IU/mL
	Tablets: 25,000 and 50,000 IU
Dihydrotachysterol	
DHT (Hytakerol)	Solution: 0.2 mg/mL
	Tablets: 0.125, 0.2, and 0.4 mg
1,25 Dihydroxyvitamin D	
Calcitriol (Rocaltrol)	0.25 and 0.5 μg capsules and 1 μg/mL solution
Calcijex	Ampules for IV use containing 1 or 2 μg of drug per mL
1α-Hydroxyvitamin D	
Alfacalcidol	0.25, 0.5, and 1 μg capsules
	Oral solution (drops): 2 μg/mL
	Solution for IV use: 2 μg/mL
Vitamin D Analogues	
Paricalcitol (Zemplar)	1 and 2 mcg capsules
	2 and 5 mcg/mL injectable solution
Doxercalciferol (Hectoral)	0.5, 1, and 2.5 μg capsules
	2 mcg/mL injectable solution

SI conversion: 1 mg phosphorus = 0.32 mmol phosphorus, 1 μg vitamin D = 40 IU vitamin D.
From Carpenter TO, Imel EA, Holm IA, Jan de Beur SM, Insogna KL. A clinician's guide to X-linked hypophosphatemia. J Bone Miner Res. 2011 Jul;26(7):1381-8. https://doi.org/10.1002/jbmr.340. Epub 2011 May 2.

Conversely, during brief periods of dietary calcium deficiency (see Fig. 11.1C), as occurs between meals, the serum calcium level declines almost imperceptibly and PTH levels rise, which immediately reduces renal calcium excretion. At the same time, an acute activation of osteoclasts and osteocytes delivers skeletal calcium into the ECF. The combination of reduced urinary calcium loss and increased skeletal calcium efflux rapidly returns blood calcium to normal.

Over the longer term, the initial response is inadequate and leads to skeletal demineralization. A longer-term solution is required, and the adaptation is 2-fold (see Fig. 11.1D). First, a chronic low calcium intake, as may occur in a person with lactose intolerance, leads to a chronic elevation in PTH, and over a matter of days to weeks, this leads to an increase in the 1,25(OH)$_2$D level, which increases the efficiency of calcium absorption from the intestine (i.e., increase in the fractional absorption of calcium) to compensate for the reduction in dietary intake. Second, chronically elevated PTH leads to an increase in osteoblast activity to match the increased osteoclastic activity. In this steady-state adaptation to a low-calcium diet, PTH levels are elevated, and coupled increases in osteoclastic and osteoblastic activities take place (i.e., increased bone turnover), but net skeletal calcium losses are negligible or normal. These physiologic adaptations hold for mild reductions in dietary calcium but in cases of severe calcium restriction or malabsorption, chronic and more significant elevations in PTH can lead to an imbalance of greater bone resorption than bone formation and chronic bone loss.

From an evolutionary standpoint, as life moved from a calcium-rich marine environment to a terrestrial setting in which calcium availability was unpredictable, a complex, elegant regulatory mechanism evolved that permitted survival without requiring intentional behavioral adaptations to the vagaries of calcium supply. As discussed in Chapter 12, disorders that cause hypercalcemia or hypocalcemia are always caused by abnormalities at the interfaces of the ECF with the intestine, kidney, and skeleton. The physician needs only to recall these homeostatic premises to dissect the pathophysiologic process with precision, enabling her or him to treat the underlying disorder effectively.

PHOSPHATE HOMEOSTASIS

Phosphorus is an inorganic element, abbreviated as P in physical chemistry literature. The biologically relevant molecule is the negatively charged, divalent phosphate ion (HPO_4^{2-}), also referred to as inorganic phosphate (Pi). Phosphate is an important physiologic buffer, and at neutral pH in blood, it is apportioned between HPO_4^{2-} (divalent) and $H_2PO_4^-$ (monovalent) species. Clinical laboratories use differing methods to measure either phosphate (colorimetric assays) or phosphorus (flame photometry), but phosphate measurements are converted to phosphorus (1 mg/

表 11.2　磷酸盐和维生素 D 制剂

磷酸盐制剂	磷含量	钾含量	钠含量
中性磷酸盐粉末（与液体混合）	每包 250 mg	每包 270 mg	每包 164 mg
中性磷酸盐钾粉末（与液体混合）	每包 250 mg	每包 556 mg	每包 0 mg
磷酸-钾片剂（与液体混合，需酸化）	每片 114 mg	每片 144 mg	每片 0 mg
磷酸-钾 MF 片剂（不需与液体混合，需酸化）	126 mg	45 mg	67 mg
磷酸-钾 #2（是磷酸-钾 MF 片剂药效的 2 倍）	250 mg	90 mg	133 mg
中性磷酸-钾片剂（无须与液体混合，无须酸化）	250 mg	45 mg	298 mg
碳酸氢钠-磷酸盐溶液（小剂量无须稀释）	127 mg/ml	0 mg/ml	152 mg/ml
Joule 溶液（由药店配置）	30 mg/ml	0 mg/ml	17.5 ～ 20 mg/ml

维生素 D 及其类似物制剂	可选剂型
维生素 D	
维生素 D_2（Drisdol）	溶液：8000 IU/ml 片剂：25 000 IU、50 000 IU
双氢速固醇	
DHT（Hytakero）	溶液：0.2 mg/ml 片剂：0.125 mg、0.2 mg、0.4 mg
1,25- 二羟基维生素 D	
骨化三醇（Rocaltrol）	胶囊：0.25 μg、0.5 μg；溶液：1 μg/ml
骨化三醇注射液	静脉注射用安瓿，每毫升含药物 1 ～ 2 μg
1α- 羟维生素 D	
阿法骨化醇	胶囊：0.25 μg、0.5 μg、1 μg 口服溶液（滴）：2 μg/ml 注射液：2 μg/ml
维生素 D 类似物	
帕立骨化醇（Zemplar）	胶囊：1 μg、2 μg 注射液：2 μg/ml、5 μg/ml
度骨化醇（Hectoral）	胶囊：0.5 μg、1 μg、2.5 μg 注射液：2 μg/ml

SI 换算：1 mg 磷 = 0.32 mmol 磷，1 μg 维生素 D = 40 IU 维生素 D。
引自 Carpenter TO，Imel EA，Holm IA，Jan de Beur SM，Insogna KL. A clinician's guide to X-linked hypophosphatemia. J Bone Miner Res. 2011 Jul；26（7）：1381-8. https://doi.org/10.1002/jbmr.340. Epub 2011 May 2.

相反，短时间内（如两餐间）膳食钙缺乏（图 11.1C）时，血清钙浓度的下降难以察觉，PTH 水平上升，肾钙排泄立即减少。同时，破骨细胞和骨细胞的快速激活可将骨钙输送到细胞外液。减少尿钙流失和增加骨骼钙外排可使血清钙浓度迅速恢复正常。

长期缺钙时，上述初始急性反应并不足以应对，可导致骨骼去矿化。这需要一个长期的适应方案，其适应性包括两个方面（图 11.1D）。首先，慢性低钙摄入（如乳糖不耐受患者）可导致 PTH 水平慢性升高。在数天至数周导致 1,25（OH）$_2$D 水平升高，增加肠道钙吸收的效率（即提高钙的吸收率），以代偿膳食摄入量的减少。其次，PTH 水平慢性升高导致成骨细胞活性增加，与破骨细胞活性增加相匹配。在这种对低钙饮食的稳态适应中，PTH 水平升高，破骨细胞和成骨细胞活性同时增加（即骨转换率增加），但净骨骼钙损失可以忽略不计。这些生理性适应仅出现在膳食钙摄入轻度减少的情况下，但在严重钙限制或吸收不良的情况下，PTH 水平长期显著升高，可导致骨吸收大于

骨形成，引发慢性骨丢失。

从进化的角度看，当生命从钙质丰富的海洋环境转移到钙质供应不可预测的陆地环境时，进化出能根据钙供应的变化而进行复杂且精细的调节机制，即可使机体得以生存。正如第 12 章所讨论的，引起高钙血症或低钙血症的疾病通常是由细胞外液与肠、肾和骨骼之间的相互作用异常所引起。医生只需要记住这些稳态调控，就能精确剖析病理生理学过程，从而有效地治疗潜在疾病。

磷稳态

磷是一种无机元素（在物理和化学文献中简写为 P）。与生物学相关的分子是带负电荷的二价磷酸离子（HPO_4^{2-}），又称无机磷酸盐（Pi）。磷酸盐是一种重要的生理缓冲剂，在血液的中性 pH 值下，它有 HPO_4^{2-}（二价）和 $H_2PO_4^-$（一价）两种存在形式。临床上可使用不同的方法来检测磷酸盐（比色法）或磷（火焰光度法），但磷酸盐检测值可转换为磷（1 mg/dl 磷酸盐含

dL phosphate contains 0.32 mmol/L phosphate, which is equal to 0.32 mmol/L phosphorus). Physicians need to be aware that phosphorus preparations often list the mass of the phosphate salt, which includes oxygen, sodium, and potassium (see Table 11.2). Phosphorus content varies for the specific preparation being prescribed, which should be considered in consultation with the pharmacist and hospital formulary.

Pi participates in the regulation of an enormous number of biologic processes fundamental to life. They include being an integral component of the DNA double helix, shuttling oxygen from hemoglobin to cells and vice versa using 2,3-diphosphoglycerate (2,3-DPG), intracellular signaling through kinases that attach phosphate groups to other molecules, facilitating critical intracellular messenger systems such as cyclic monophosphate (cAMP) and inositol phosphates, maintaining basic intracellular redox status through the nicotinamide adenine dinucleotide phosphate (NADP-NADPH) system, and serving as the gateway to the glucose metabolic pathway through glucose 6-phosphate.

Most phosphorus is intracellular as Pi or organophosphate. In addition to its critical intracellular roles, Pi has a key extracellular role. The anion pairs with calcium in the hydroxyapatite crystal lattice that provides structural integrity to the skeleton (discussed earlier). As with calcium, phosphate is critical to skeletal strength, and disorders of phosphorus homeostasis, such as hypophosphatemic rickets, lead to pathologic skeletal fractures. The skeleton also serves as a major storage site for phosphate that is accessed in times of severe phosphate deficiency.

The broad intracellular roles for Pi have two corollaries. First, clinically significant intracellular Pi deficiency may exist without marked hypophosphatemia. Second, life-threatening Pi deficiency is often unrecognized because its manifestations (i.e., reduced levels of consciousness, hypotension, respirator dependence, and muscular weakness) are nonspecific but common in intensive care unit settings. Astute clinicians learn to recognize general debility as a potential sign of Pi deficiency. Pi repletion in this setting may produce dramatic results.

In contrast to regulation of the serum calcium concentration, which is very tight, the regulation of the serum phosphate concentration is relatively lax. Serum phosphate levels are maintained in a range between 2.5 and 4.5 mg/dL, which is broader than the range of normal calcium concentrations. Furthermore, the normal range of infants is higher, between 3.5 and 5.5 mg/dL, and decreases to the adult range in the first few years of life. Even so, the regulation of the extracellular Pi concentrations is no less important, because hypophosphatemia and hyperphosphatemia can both cause disease. Pi is abundant in most diets, and only 33% of intestinal Pi absorption is regulated, principally by 1,25(OH)$_2$D, while 67% occurs in an unregulated fashion. Conversely, its excretion is tightly regulated in the renal proximal tubules by PTH and fibroblast growth factor 23 (FGF23).

Fig. 11.4 outlines the main fluxes of phosphate that define the circulating level as well as overall phosphate economy. The box represents the ECF, and as with calcium, it has interfaces with the GI tract, kidney, and skeleton. Because most phosphate is contained within cells, the phosphate black box has a quantitatively significant interface with the intracellular compartment.

Intestinal Phosphate Absorption

A normal diet contains about 1200 to 1600 mg of phosphorus, and about two thirds of this amount, or 800 to 1200 mg, is absorbed each day. This fixed fractional absorption of about 67% occurs in the duodenum and jejunum. In the normal world of phosphate abundance, this intake is more than ample. Under conditions of dietary phosphorus deficiency, as occurs in chronic alcoholism, intensive care units, intestinal malabsorption, or phosphate-binding antacid use, failure of adequate phosphorus absorption presents a physiologic challenge for which no physiologic remedy exists.

Skeletal Phosphate Fluxes

As with calcium, osteoclastic bone resorption and osteoblastic new bone formation (see Fig. 11.2) lead to skeletal phosphate exit or entry, respectively. Under pathophysiologic conditions, skeletal phosphate fluxes may become important. For example, skeletal destruction in multiple myeloma or severe immobilization syndromes leads to hypercalcemia and hyperphosphatemia, which can cause nephrocalcinosis and renal failure. Conversely, osteoblastic metastases in prostate and breast cancers as well as the hungry bone syndrome after parathyroidectomy can cause clinically significant hypophosphatemia. Although phosphorus has been viewed as a passive passenger with calcium in the calcium regulatory process, recent insights suggest that FGF23, whose levels are determined by phosphate concentrations, stimulates bone matrix mineralization independently of calcium by suppressing osteopontin and by stimulating alkaline phosphatase activity.

Intracellular-Extracellular Phosphate Fluxes

Phosphate shuttles from extracellular to intracellular compartments. This issue becomes important in certain clinical situations. For example, in the setting of metabolic acidosis, phosphate leaves the intracellular compartment and may lead to hyperphosphatemia, whereas under conditions of alkalosis, serum phosphate concentrations decline, and hypophosphatemia develops as phosphate enters the intracellular compartment.

The intracellular phosphate level has important clinical implications, in part, in the settings of crush injury (i.e., rhabdomyolysis) and tumor lysis syndrome. In both conditions, large intracellular loads of phosphate are delivered into the ECF and result in hypocalcemia, seizures, nephrocalcinosis, and renal failure. Conversely, glucose shifts phosphate into cells as glucose 6-phosphate, and overzealous intravenous or oral caloric restitution in the undernourished patient can result in severe hypophosphatemia and sudden death.

Renal Phosphate Handling

The most important mechanism for maintaining a normal serum phosphorus concentration is the regulation of renal phosphorus excretion. As with calcium, phosphate is filtered by the glomerulus, and 90% is reabsorbed (i.e., tubular reabsorption of filtered phosphate [TRP]). The remaining 10% is excreted (i.e., fractional excretion of phosphorus [FE$_{Pi}$]). The FE$_{Pi}$ can be calculated in a spot urine sample using formula 3:

$$FE_{Pi} = (urine\ Pi\ [mg/dL]\ /\ urine\ creatinine\ [mg/dL])$$
$$(serum\ creatinine\ [mg/dL]\ /\ serum\ phosphorus\ [mg/dL])$$

The TRP is simple to calculate using formula 4:

$$TRP = 1 - FE_{Pi}\ (expressed\ in\ \%,\ when\ multiplied\ by\ 100)$$

The renal handling of phosphorus is best considered as a tubular maximum (Tm)–regulated process. The TmP/GFR is normally identical to a normal serum phosphorus concentration in blood, 2.5 to 4.5 mg/dL. If the serum phosphate concentration rises above this level, phosphaturia occurs, and as a result the serum phosphorus returns to the normal range. If the serum phosphate concentration declines below this level, filtered phosphate is entirely reabsorbed as TRP approaches 100%. Thus, the TmP/GFR can be considered as a dam in the phosphate reservoir, over which excess phosphate spills and whose level controls the concentration of serum phosphorus. The TmP/GFR is not fixed but can be moved upward or downward, depending on metabolic needs and prevailing metabolic conditions (described later).

有 0.32 mmol/L 磷酸盐，等于 0.32 mmol/L 磷）。医生需要意识到，磷酸盐制剂通常会列出磷酸盐的量，这包括氧气、钠和钾（表 11.2）。磷酸盐含量因具体制剂而异，应结合药剂师建议和医院配方使用。

磷参与调节大量对生命至关重要的生物学过程。磷是 DNA 双螺旋结构的组成部分；形成 2,3- 二磷酸甘油酸（2,3-DPG），与血红蛋白结合调节组织供氧；通过激酶将磷酸基团与其他分子连接，进行细胞内信号传导；形成胞内关键信使系统，如环磷酸腺苷（cAMP）和磷酸肌醇；通过氧化型-还原型辅酶 II 系统（NADP-NADPH）维持细胞内基本的氧化还原状态；通过葡萄糖 6- 磷酸作为葡萄糖代谢途径的开关。

大多数磷以无机磷酸盐或有机磷酸盐的形式存在于细胞内。除了关键的细胞内作用外，无机磷酸盐还具有重要的细胞外作用。磷酸盐与钙结合形成的羟基磷灰石晶体保障了骨骼的结构完整性（如前所述）。与钙相同，磷酸盐对骨骼强度至关重要，磷稳态失衡会导致病理性骨折（如低血磷性佝偻病）。骨骼也是磷酸盐的重要储存库，在严重磷酸盐缺乏时发挥作用。

磷在细胞内的广泛作用有两个必然结果。首先，有临床意义的细胞内磷缺乏可能不伴有明显的低磷血症。其次，危及生命的磷缺乏症常被忽视，因其症状（如意识水平降低、低血压、呼吸机依赖和肌无力）无特异性，但在重症监护病房中很常见。敏锐的医生会将虚弱视为磷缺乏的征兆。在这种情况下，补磷可能会产生显著疗效。

与对血钙浓度的严格调控不同，机体对血磷浓度的调控相对宽松。正常血清磷浓度为 2.5 ～ 4.5 mg/dl，这比血钙浓度的正常范围更宽。此外，婴儿的血磷正常值较高（3.5 ～ 5.5 mg/dl），并在出生后最初数年逐渐降至成人范围。即便如此，细胞外磷浓度的调节也同样重要，因为低磷血症和高磷血症都可能导致疾病。大多数饮食中都富含磷，肠道吸收的磷中只有 33% 受到调节［主要由 1,25（OH）₂D 调节］，而 67% 的磷不受调节。相反，磷在肾近端小管的排泄受 PTH 和 FGF23 的严格调节。

图 11.4 列出了决定循环磷浓度和内环境总体磷浓度的主要磷流通。方框代表细胞外液，与钙相同，磷与胃肠道、肾脏和骨骼交互作用。由于大多数磷酸盐在细胞内，因此机体含磷量与细胞内液密切相关。

肠道磷吸收

正常饮食中含有 1200 ～ 1600 mg 磷，每天约 2/3（即 800 ～ 1200 mg）被吸收。其中，约 67% 的固定吸收发生在十二指肠和空肠。在磷酸盐丰富的生理情况下，该摄入量是绰绰有余的。在膳食磷缺乏的情况下（如长期酗酒、危重症、肠道吸收不良或使用结合磷酸盐的抗酸剂），由于没有生理补救机制，磷吸收不足会影响躯体健康。

骨骼磷流通

与钙相同，破骨细胞骨吸收和成骨细胞新骨形成（图 11.2）分别会导致骨骼磷酸盐的外流和内流。在病理生理情况下，骨骼磷酸盐流通极为重要。例如，多发性骨髓瘤的骨骼破坏或严重的制动综合征可导致高钙血症和高磷血症，从而导致肾钙盐沉着症和肾衰竭。相反，前列腺癌和乳腺癌的骨转移及甲状旁腺切除术后的骨饥饿综合征可引起临床显著的低磷血症。尽管磷在钙调节过程中被视为被动变化指标，但近期研究表明，FGF23（其水平由磷酸盐浓度决定）可通过抑制骨桥蛋白、刺激碱性磷酸酶活性来促进骨基质矿化，而不依赖于钙。

细胞内外磷流通

磷酸盐可在细胞外和细胞内流动。这一点在某些临床情况中很重要。例如，在代谢性酸中毒的情况下，磷酸盐离开细胞内液可能导致高磷血症，而在碱中毒的情况下，随着磷酸盐进入细胞内液，血清磷浓度下降，从而发生低磷血症。

细胞内磷酸盐水平具有重要的临床意义，尤其在挤压损伤（如横纹肌溶解）和肿瘤溶解综合征时。在这两种情况下，大量的细胞内磷酸盐负荷被输送到细胞外液，导致低钙血症、癫痫发作、肾钙盐沉着症和肾衰竭。相反，葡萄糖可将磷酸盐带入细胞转化为葡萄糖 6- 磷酸，营养不良患者过度静脉或口服营养补充可导致严重的低磷血症和猝死。

肾磷调节

保持血磷浓度最重要的机制是调节肾磷排泄。与钙相同，磷酸盐被肾小球滤过，90% 被重吸收［即肾小管重吸收滤过的磷酸盐（TRP）］。剩余 10% 被排出体外［即磷排泄分数（FE_pi）］。单次尿标本的 FE_pi 可用公式 3 计算：

$$FE_{pi} = [（尿磷酸盐（mg/dl）/ 尿肌酐（mg/dl）） × [血清肌酐（mg/dl）/ 血清磷酸盐（mg/dl）]$$

标本的 TRP 可用公式 4 计算：

$$TRP（肾小管重吸收磷） = 1 - FE_{pi}（乘以 100 以 \% 表示）$$

肾磷调节被认为是与肾小管最大转运率（Tm）相关的可调节过程。TmP/GFR（肾磷阈）通常与正常血磷浓度相同，为 2.5 ～ 4.5 mg/dl。如果血清磷浓度超过该范围，则可出现磷酸盐尿，使血清磷恢复至正常范围。如果血清磷酸盐水平低于该范围，则滤过的磷酸盐几乎完全被重吸收（TRP 接近 100%）。因此，TmP/GFR 可被视为磷储备库的闸门，超过 TmP/GFR 时磷酸盐溢出，其水平控制着血清磷浓度。TmP/GFR 不是固定的，可以上调或下调，这取决于代谢需要和代谢情况（见下文）。

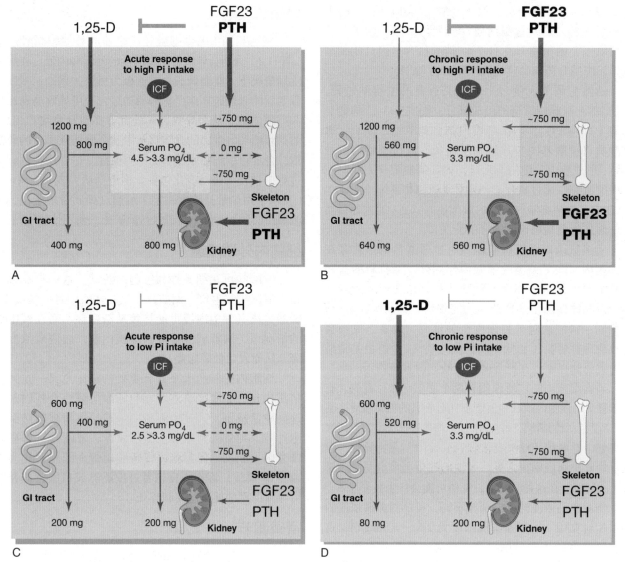

Fig. 11.4 Phosphate homeostasis. (A) The acute response and (B) the chronic response to increases in phosphate intake. (C) The acute response and (D) the chronic response to decreases in phosphate intake. Details are provided in the text. *FGF23,* Fibroblast growth factor 23; *GI,* gastrointestinal; *ICF,* intracellular fluid; *PTH,* parathyroid hormone; *1,25(OH)₂D,* 1,25-dihydroxycholecalciferol (calcitriol). SI conversion: 1 mg phosphorus = 0.32 mmol phosphorus.

The TRP can be used to derive TmP/GFR from the nomogram of Bijvoet, which is shown in Fig. 11.5. Determining renal handling of Pi by calculation of TRP and deriving TmP/GFR proves enormously useful in clinical practice because it is the central starting point for determining whether hypophosphatemia is principally renal or nonrenal in origin.

Regulatory Hormones
Fibroblast Growth Factor

In addition to PTH, which has long been appreciated to be phosphaturic, experimental dietary phosphorus deprivation in laboratory animals and humans leads to a PTH-independent increase in the TmP/GFR, and high-phosphate feeding results in a PTH-independent decline in the TmP/GFR. Over the past two decades, the principal phosphaturic hormone or phosphatonin responsible for regulating renal phosphate handling was identified as fibroblast growth factor 23 (FGF23). FGF23 also affects calcium regulatory hormones; however, the principle regulator of FGF23 is phosphate, while the principle

regulator of PTH is calcium. FGF23 together with FGF19 and FG21 define a family of evolutionarily conserved endocrine fibroblast growth factors. FGF23 elicits its phosphaturic actions in the renal proximal and distal tubules by activation of a co-receptor complex composed of FGFR1c and alpha klotho (aKL). It also acts in an aKL-independent fashion to suppress CYP27B1 and stimulate CYP24A1, leading to inactivation of 1,25(OH)₂D. This requires two different receptors, FGFR3 and FGFR4. The net effect of these actions is a decrease of serum phosphorus. FGF23 also suppresses PTH, stimulates bone mineralization, and inhibits erythropoietin-mediated synthesis of red blood cells, which are less well-understood actions.

FGF23 is produced by osteoblasts and osteocytes. Its gene expression is stimulated by a number of factors including 1,25(OH)₂D and bone matrix factors, for example phosphate-regulating neutral endopeptidase, X-linked (PHEX), the gene mutated in X-linked hypophosphatemia (XLH). Phosphate stimulates FGF23 secretion on the posttranslational level, presumably by increasing activity of the o-glycosylase, GALNT3, which prevents FGF23 inactivation. Mutations

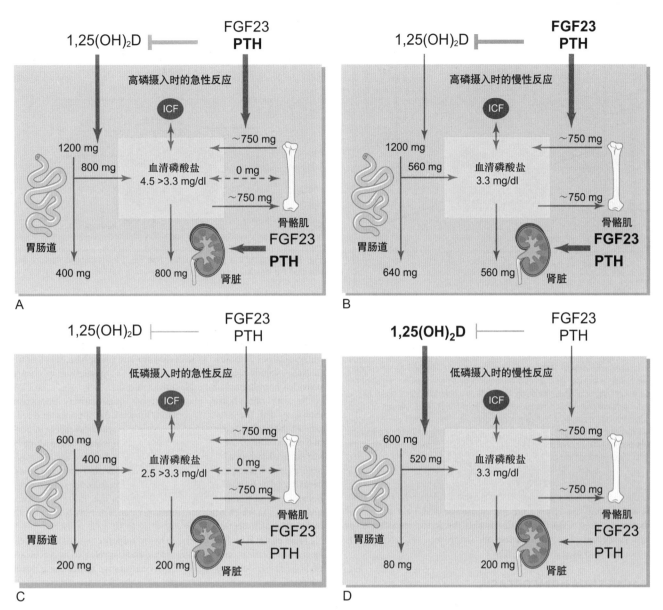

图 11.4 磷稳态。**A**. 高磷摄入时的急性反应。**B**. 高磷摄入时的慢性反应。**C**. 低磷摄入时的急性反应。**D**. 低磷摄入时的慢性反应。详见正文。FGF23，成纤维细胞生长因子 23；ICF，细胞内液；PTH，甲状旁腺激素；1,25（OH）$_2$D，骨化三醇。SI 转换：1 mg 磷 = 0.32 mmol 磷

可利用 TRP 在 Bijvoet 列线图中得到 TmP/GFR（图 11.5）。通过计算 TRP 和 TmP/GFR 来确定肾磷阈值在临床实践中非常有用，因为它可用于判断低磷血症主要是肾源性还是非肾源性。

调节激素
成纤维细胞生长因子

除了 PTH 具有促尿磷排泄作用外，在实验动物和人类中进行的实验性饮食磷剥夺也会导致 PTH 非依赖性 TmP/GFR 升高，而高磷酸盐喂养会导致 PTH 非依赖性 TmP/GFR 下降。在过去的 20 年中，研究发现的主要促尿磷排泄激素或调磷因子是 FGF23。FGF23 也可影响钙调节激素，但 FGF23 主要调节磷酸盐，而 PTH 主要调节钙。FGF23 与 FGF19、FGF21 共同组成

进化保守的分泌性成纤维细胞生长因子家族。FGF23 通过激活由 FGFR1c 和 α-klotho 组成的共受体复合物，在肾近端小管和远端小管中发挥促尿磷排泄作用。FGF23 也可通过不依赖于 α-klotho 的方式与 FGFR3、FGFR4 结合，抑制 CYP27B1 活性、增加 CYP24A1 活性，使 1,25（OH）$_2$D 失活，最终导致低磷血症。FGF23 还能抑制 PTH，刺激骨矿化和抑制促红细胞生成素介导的红细胞生成。

FGF23 由成骨细胞和骨细胞生成。FGF23 的基因表达受多种因子的刺激，包括 1,25（OH）$_2$D 和骨基质因子 [如 X 染色体连锁的磷酸盐调节内肽酶（PHEX），PHEX 基因突变会导致 X 连锁低血磷性佝偻病（XLH）]。磷酸盐在翻译后水平促进 FGF23 的分泌，可能是通过增加 O- 糖基化酶（GALNT3）的活性，从而阻止 FGF23 失

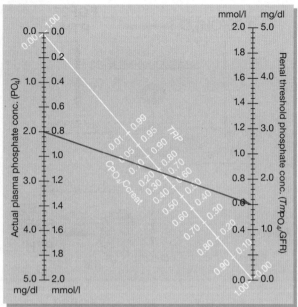

Fig. 11.5 Nomogram shows the tubular maximum for the phosphorus glomerular filtration rate (TmP-GFR). It allows conversion of the fractional excretion of phosphorus (or its inverse, the tubular reabsorption of filtered phosphate [TRP]) into the TmP-GFR. The TRP is calculated, and a line is drawn (*red arrow*) extending from the serum phosphorus level (*left vertical line*), through the TRP (*middle diagonal line*), to the *right vertical line*, which represents the TmP/GFR. TmP values are provided in millimolar and milligram per deciliter units. TmP values below 1.0 mmol or 2.5 mg/dL are abnormal in the setting of hypophosphatemia and indicate renal phosphate wasting. C_{creat}, Creatinine concentration; C_{PO4}, phosphate concentration.

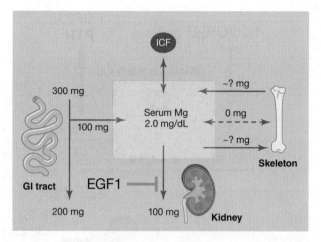

Fig. 11.6 Magnesium homeostasis. See Fig. 11.1 for nomenclature and the text for details.

in the o-glycosylation site of FGF23 stabilize and thereby increase its bioactivity and are responsible for autosomal dominant hypophosphatemic rickets (ADHR). FGF23 is also the factor responsible for most paraneoplastic hypophosphatemic syndromes, also referred to as tumor-induced osteomalacia (TIO).

MAGNESIUM HOMEOSTASIS

Magnesium is a divalent cation and its homeostasis parallels phosphorus homeostasis. Like Pi, magnesium is principally intracellular, with concentrations inside the cell that far exceed those outside the cell. Both substances govern key intracellular regulatory processes. In the case of magnesium, these processes include fundamental events such as DNA replication and transcription, translation of RNA, the use of adenosine triphosphate as an energy source, and regulated peptide hormone secretion.

Both substances are abundant inside all kinds of cells. Because they are well supplied in vegetarian and carnivorous diets, little evolutionary pressure exists to develop a complex regulatory network and, as with phosphate, serum magnesium concentrations are not tightly regulated. Because magnesium is principally intracellular, measurement of serum levels may provide false estimates of actual total body and intracellular magnesium status. Because magnesium is essential for fundamental processes such as gene transcription and cellular energy use, life-threatening magnesium deficiency is often unrecognized because its symptoms are nonspecific: weakness, respirator dependence, diffuse neurologic syndromes (including seizures), and cardiovascular collapse.

Magnesium has a molecular weight of 24 (1 mole = 24 g), and because it is divalent, one equivalent is 12 g. Blood magnesium

measurements are often provided in milligrams per deciliter (mg/dL) or milliequivalents per liter (mEq/L); oral magnesium supplements are expressed in milligrams per tablet or milliequivalents per vial; and urinary magnesium excretion values are given in milliequivalents or milligrams per 24 hours. As with calcium and phosphate, it is helpful to examine daily magnesium fluxes. In Fig. 11.6, magnesium values are provided in milligram and milliequivalent units.

As with phosphorus, magnesium has quantitatively important interfaces with the intestine, skeleton, intracellular supplies, and kidney. At the level of the intestine, magnesium is widely available in normal diets and about one third of what is ingested is absorbed in a largely unregulated fashion. In normal circumstances, because dietary magnesium is abundant, magnesium deficiency does not occur. However, deficiency due to insufficient dietary absorption may occur with alcoholism, proton pump inhibitor or cyclosporin use, in intensive care unit settings in which adequate nutrition often is not provided, or with intestinal malabsorption.

Magnesium is incorporated into hydroxyapatite crystals in the skeleton as mineralization of osteoid occurs, and it is released by osteoclastic bone resorption (see Fig. 11.3). In quantitative terms, these fluxes are small.

Many instances of magnesium deficiency are caused by excessive renal losses. Functional examples include the magnesuria that accompanies saline infusions, aminoglycoside, diuretic, or alcohol use, and secondary hyperaldosteronism states such as cirrhosis and ascites. Genetic magnesium deficiency occurs as a result of mutations in claudin 16 and 19 (*CLCN16* and *CLCN19*), both of which encode for paracellular calcium and magnesium channels in the thick ascending limb, and transient receptor potential melastatin 6 (TRPM6) in the distal renal tubules. Gitelman-like hypomagnesemia occurs with several of the Bartter syndromes.

As with calcium and phosphorus, the fractional excretion of magnesium (FE_{Mg}) can be calculated, and it should be used as an index of whether the kidney is appropriately conserving magnesium in states of hypomagnesemia or whether renal magnesium wasting is the cause of the hypomagnesemia. The normal FE_{Mg} is 2% to 4%. Hypomagnesemic individuals have FE_{Mg} values below 1% to 2%.

Like phosphate, magnesium homeostasis can best be viewed as a renal Tm-regulated process (see "Renal Phosphate Handling"), with the renal Tm for magnesium set at a fixed level of about 2.2 mg/dL. In this scenario, abundant dietary magnesium exists, and excessive magnesium intake is managed by spillage of excess magnesium into urine when the Tm of 2.2 mg/dL is exceeded. Conversely, in settings

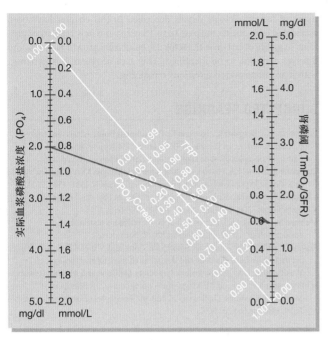

图 11.5　肾磷阈（TmP/GFR）列线图。利用肾磷排泄率和肾小管重吸收滤过的磷酸盐（TRP）可换算 TmP/GFR。计算所得 TRP，并绘制一条从实际血浆磷酸盐浓度（左竖线），通过 TRP（中间对角线），向右延伸的线（红线），表示 TmP/GFR。TmP 值以 mmol/L 和 mg/dl 为单位，TmP < 1.0 mmol（2.5 mg/dl）为异常情况（低血症），表明肾磷消耗。C_{creat}，肌酐清除率（原文有误）；C_{PO4}，磷酸盐清除率（原文有误）

活。FGF23 的 O-糖基化位点突变可使其生物活性增加，导致常染色体显性遗传性低血磷性佝偻病（ADHR）。FGF23 也是多数低血磷性副肿瘤综合征（即肿瘤性骨软化症）的致病因素。

镁稳态

镁是一种二价阳离子，镁稳态与磷平行。与磷相同，镁主要存在于细胞内，细胞内镁浓度远远超过细胞外浓度。这两种物质都在细胞内调节过程中发挥重要作用。镁调控基本细胞生命活动，如 DNA 复制和转录、RNA 翻译、利用腺苷三磷酸（ATP）作为能量来源，以及调节肽类激素分泌。

镁和磷在各种细胞中都很丰富。它们在素食和肉类食物中供应充足，几乎没有建立复杂调节网络的进化压力。此外，与磷酸盐相同，血清镁浓度不受严格调控。由于镁主要存在于细胞内，测定血清浓度可能会对实际的全身和细胞内镁浓度产生错误评估。镁对基因转录和细胞能量代谢等基本过程至关重要，但危及生命的镁缺乏常被忽视，因为它的症状无特异性，包括虚弱、呼吸机依赖、弥漫性神经系统综合征（包括癫痫发作）和心血管系统衰竭。

镁的分子量是 24（1 mol = 24 g），由于镁离子为二

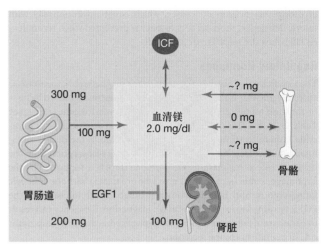

图 11.6　镁稳态。术语见图 11.1 及正文

价，故 1 个当量为 12 g。血镁浓度检测值通常以 mg/dl 或 mmol/L 表示；口服镁补充剂以毫克/片或毫当量/瓶表示；尿镁排泄值以毫当量或 mg/24 h 表示。与钙和磷酸盐相同，检测每日镁流通很有帮助。在图 11.6 中，血镁浓度检测值的单位为毫克和毫当量。

与磷相同，镁的含量与肠道、骨骼、细胞内供应和肾脏关系密切。在肠道吸收方面，镁在日常饮食中广泛存在，约 1/3 的镁以基本不受调控的方式被吸收。在正常情况下，由于膳食镁含量丰富，因此不会发生镁缺乏。然而，在酗酒、使用质子泵抑制剂或环孢素、重症监护病房治疗期间没有提供足够营养或肠道吸收不良等情况下，由于膳食镁补充不足，可导致镁缺乏。

当类骨质矿化时，镁被包入骨骼的羟基磷灰石晶体中，并通过破骨细胞的骨吸收释放出来（图 11.3）。从数量上讲，这些流通很小。

许多酶缺乏是由肾丢失过多引起的。例如，伴随生理盐水输注、氨基糖苷、利尿剂或饮酒所致的尿镁排泄过多，以及继发性醛固酮增多症（如肝硬化和腹腔积液）。遗传性镁缺乏是 CLCN16 和 CLCN19 基因突变的结果，这两种基因编码髓袢升支粗段的细胞旁钙镁通道及远曲小管的细胞顶端 M 型瞬时受体电位通道 6（TRPM6）。Gitelman 样低镁血症可见于多种巴特综合征（Bartter 综合征）。

与钙和磷相同，镁排泄分数（FE_{Mg}）可经计算得出，并作为低镁血症状态下肾重吸收镁是否适量、肾镁排泄与低镁血症的关系的判定指标。FE_{Mg} 的正常值为 2% ~ 4%。低镁患者的 FE_{Mg} 可低于 1% ~ 2%。

与磷酸盐相同，镁稳态也是与肾阈值相关的调控过程（见上文"肾磷调节"），肾脏中镁的阈值约为 2.2 mg/dl 的固定水平。因此，当膳食镁含量丰富或镁摄入过量而超过这一阈值时，过量的镁会溢入尿液中。

of dietary magnesium deficiency, which equate evolutionarily with caloric deficiency, short-term deficiency is prevented when serum levels fall below the renal Tm of 2.0 mg/dL.

Regulatory Hormones

The significance of hormonal regulators for magnesium homeostasis is currently unclear. Isolated recessive hypomagnesemia is caused by loss-of-function mutations in the epidermal growth factor gene (*EGF1*; see Table 11.1). EGF1 is magnesiotropic as it acts in an autocrine or paracrine fashion to stimulate expression of TRPM6 in the distal convoluted tubules of the kidneys, which increases Mg reabsorption from the urine. Its role as magnesiotropic hormone is further supported by the hypomagnesemia in cancer patients who are treated with the chimeric human/mouse anti-EGF antibody cetuximab or with inhibitors of the EGFR tyrosine kinase (i.e., erlotinib). Magnesium deficiency can result in parathyroid failure and therefore hypocalcemia due to its important role in peptide hormone secretion.

PROSPECTUS FOR THE FUTURE

Although it may seem that calcium, PTH, vitamin D, magnesium, and phosphorus homeostasis and skeletal biology are well understood, many of the physiologic details described in this chapter have been elucidated only during the past 10 to 15 years, and new regulatory proteins (e.g., fibroblast growth factor 23, epidermal growth factor 1) and diseases continue to be identified. This area of research is dynamic, with many unanswered questions remaining.

SUGGESTED READINGS

Carpenter TO, Bergwitz C, Insogna K: Phosphorus homeostasis and related clinical disorders. In Bilezikian JP, Martin TJ, Clemens TL, Rosen CJ, editors: Principles of bone biology, ed 4, 2019, Elsevier Inc., p. 469.

Carpenter TO, Imel EA, Holm IA, Jan de Beur SM, Insogna KL: A clinician's guide to X-linked hypophosphatemia, J Bone Miner Res 26(7):1381–1388, 2011.

Chande S, Bergwitz C: Role of phosphate sensing in bone and mineral metabolism, Nat Rev Endocrinol 14(11):637–655, 2018.

Melmed S, Polonsky KS, Larsen PR, et al: In Williams textbook of endocrinology, ed 12, Philadelphia, 2012, Saunders.

Rosen CJ, editor: The American Society for Bone and Mineral Research primer on metabolic bone diseases and disorders of mineral metabolism, ed 8, Washington, D.C., 2013, American Society for Bone and Mineral Research.

Schlingmann KP, Konrad M: Magnesium homeostasis. In Bilezikian JP, Martin TJ, Clemens TL, Rosen CJ, editors: Principles of bone biology, ed 4, 2019, Elsevier Inc., p. 509.

相反，与热量摄入不足相同，膳食中镁缺乏时血清镁浓度会降至 2.0 mg/dl 以下，来预防短期的缺镁。

调节激素

　　激素调节对于镁稳态的意义目前尚不清楚。表皮生长因子基因（*EGF1*；表 11.1）的功能缺失突变可引起常染色体隐性遗传性低镁血症。EGFl 以自分泌或旁分泌的方式促进肾远端小管中 TRPM6 的表达，从而增加尿液中镁的重吸收。接受嵌合人 / 小鼠抗 EGF 抗体西妥昔单抗或 EGFR 酪氨酸激酶抑制剂（如厄洛替尼）治疗的肿瘤患者会出现低镁血症，这进一步支持了 EGFl 的调镁激素作用。由于镁在肽类激素分泌中的重要作用，其缺乏可导致甲状旁腺功能衰竭，从而导致低钙血症。

未来展望

　　虽然钙、PTH、维生素 D、镁和磷的稳态与骨骼生物学似乎已被很好地阐释，但本章中提及的许多生理学细节仅在过去 10 ～ 15 年才被研究清楚，新的调控蛋白（如 FGF23、EGF1）及疾病不断被发现。该领域的研究持续进展，但仍有许多问题悬而未决。

推荐阅读

Carpenter TO, Bergwitz C, Insogna K: Phosphorus homeostasis and related clinical disorders. In Bilezikian JP, Martin TJ, Clemens TL, Rosen CJ, editors: Principles of bone biology, ed 4, 2019, Elsevier Inc., p. 469.

Carpenter TO, Imel EA, Holm IA, Jan de Beur SM, Insogna KL: A clinician's guide to X-linked hypophosphatemia, J Bone Miner Res 26(7):1381–1388, 2011.

Chande S, Bergwitz C: Role of phosphate sensing in bone and mineral metabolism, Nat Rev Endocrinol 14(11):637–655, 2018.

Melmed S, Polonsky KS, Larsen PR, et al: In Williams textbook of endocrinology, ed 12, Philadelphia, 2012, Saunders.

Rosen CJ, editor: The American Society for Bone and Mineral Research primer on metabolic bone diseases and disorders of mineral metabolism, ed 8, Washington, D.C., 2013, American Society for Bone and Mineral Research.

Schlingmann KP, Konrad M: Magnesium homeostasis. In Bilezikian JP, Martin TJ, Clemens TL, Rosen CJ, editors: Principles of bone biology, ed 4, 2019, Elsevier Inc., p. 509.

Disorders of Serum Minerals

Emily M. Stein, Yi Liu, Elizabeth Shane

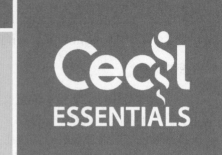

INTRODUCTION

This chapter will provide an overview of the metabolic disorders that can impact serum calcium, phosphorus, and magnesium. We will review those disorders that manifest in both excess and deficiency. Please refer to Chapter 11 for descriptions of normal calcium, phosphorus, and magnesium metabolism. We will briefly review the pathophysiology of these disorders, the signs and symptoms, and strategies for treatment. When evaluating a patient, it is critical to consider the broad differential diagnosis for each metabolic abnormality. For all of the metabolic disturbances, the severity of presentation can vary dramatically depending not only on the magnitude of the abnormal value but also on the acuity with which it develops. Patients with chronic abnormalities may have very few symptoms, whereas those with more acute changes are more likely to be symptomatic. Even among patients who have multiple conditions that may result in metabolic disturbances, the most common diagnoses are still most likely. For example, a patient with a history of malignancy who develops hypercalcemia may have humoral hypercalcemia of malignancy, but primary hyperparathyroidism (HPT) should also be considered.

DISORDERS OF CALCIUM METABOLISM

Hypercalcemia

Pathophysiology

Serum calcium is tightly regulated by the movement of ionized calcium between the skeleton, intestines, kidney, and serum binding proteins. Hypercalcemia develops when there are abnormalities in the movement of calcium between the extracellular fluid (ECF) and one of these compartments or when there is abnormal binding of calcium to serum proteins. Hypercalcemia causes hyperpolarization of neuromuscular cell membranes, which become refractory to stimulation and can result in several symptoms, including neuropsychiatric disturbances, gastrointestinal abnormalities, renal dysfunction, musculoskeletal symptoms, and cardiovascular disease.

The physiologic black box described in Chapter 11 should be considered when diagnosing or treating patients with hypercalcemia. Causes of hypercalcemia can be grouped into factitious disorders (e.g., abnormalities in serum proteins), parathyroid mediated, non-parathyroid mediated, medication related, and miscellaneous disorders. The differential diagnosis for hypercalcemia is outlined in Table 12.1.

Symptoms and Signs

Calcium is included in the standard basic metabolic panel, and as a result asymptomatic hypercalcemia is often discovered by routine laboratory testing. Whether a patient develops symptoms depends on several factors, including the degree of hypercalcemia and the rapidity with which it develops. Typically, when absolute serum calcium is above 13 mg/dL patients are symptomatic. A gradual increase in serum calcium, even into the severe range above 15 mg/dL, may cause fewer symptoms then a rapid rise to 13 mg/dL. The overall health status and age of the person with hypercalcemia influence the severity of symptoms. Symptoms can be most severe in elderly patients.

Hypercalcemia can cause smooth muscle hypoactivity, resulting in constipation and ileus. Pancreatitis and peptic ulcer, although less commonly seen, can occur in patients with severe hypercalcemia. Hypercalcemia is also associated with neurologic dysfunction, which can range in severity from mild confusion to coma. Renal impairment can result from hypercalcemia through several mechanisms. Hypercalcemia causes afferent arteriolar vasoconstriction and activation of the calcium receptor in the distal nephron, which reduces the glomerular filtration rate (GFR). It can also cause a form of nephrogenic diabetes insipidus with associated polydipsia and polyuria. As a result, the ECF volume is reduced and the GFR further lowered. Hypercalcemia can directly cause kidney damage through deposition of calcium phosphate crystals into the renal interstitium (i.e., nephrocalcinosis or interstitial nephritis) as well as into the urine leading to nephrolithiasis and obstructive uropathy. Hypercalcemia can have severe adverse effects on the heart, including arrhythmias. Abnormalities on electrocardiogram include shortening of the QTc interval, prolonged PR interval, widened QRS complex and bradycardia. ST elevations mimicking myocardial infarctions have also been reported. Muscular weakness is also frequently seen among hypercalcemia patients.

Differential Diagnosis

Hyperproteinemia. Approximately 50% of circulating calcium is bound to serum albumin and other proteins. Increases in serum proteins lead to an artifactual increase in total, but not ionized, serum calcium concentrations. This increase is commonly observed in settings of volume depletion and dehydration. Patients with hypercalcemia as a result of hyperproteinemia do not display signs or symptoms. Treatment should be avoided in this setting as it might actually result in hypocalcemia.

Parathyroid hormone–related hypercalcemia

Hyperparathyroidism. Both primary and tertiary hyperparathyroidism are characterized by hypercalcemia. Patients who have secondary hyperparathyroidism (SHPT) in response to other abnormalities, such as vitamin D deficiency, calcium deficiency, or chronic kidney disease, will have serum calcium values that are frankly low or in the low-normal range. However, it is important to note that these disorders can coexist. Full consideration of a patient's comorbidities and laboratory test results may be necessary for making the proper diagnosis or combination of diagnoses.

Primary hyperparathyroidism. Primary hyperparathyroidism (PHPT), due to overproduction of parathyroid hormone (PTH) from

血清矿物质疾病

姜艳 译 李梅 审校 夏维波 通审

引言

本章将概述影响血清钙、磷和镁的代谢性疾病。请参考第 11 章中关于正常钙、磷和镁代谢的内容，本章将介绍表现为这些矿物质过多和过少的疾病，并简要回顾这些疾病的病理生理学、体征和症状及治疗策略。在评估患者时，对每种代谢异常疾病进行全面的鉴别诊断十分重要。对于所有代谢异常疾病，临床表现的严重程度不仅取决于血清矿物质水平的异常程度，还取决于变化的速度。慢性代谢异常的患者症状可能很少，而变化越迅速的患者症状可能越多。虽然多种因素可造成患者代谢紊乱，但常根据可能性最大的病因做出诊断。例如，有恶性肿瘤病史的患者出现高钙血症时，可能是恶性肿瘤的体液性高钙血症，但也需考虑原发性甲状旁腺功能亢进症（PHPT）的可能性。

钙代谢疾病

高钙血症

病理生理学

血清钙浓度受到在骨骼、肠道、肾脏和血清结合蛋白之间移动的离子钙的严格调控。当钙在细胞外液（ECF）及上述组分之间发生移动异常或钙与血清蛋白结合异常时，将发生高钙血症。高钙血症可导致神经肌肉细胞膜超极化，从而对刺激的反应减弱，并引起多种症状，包括神经精神紊乱、胃肠道异常、肾功能不全、肌肉骨骼症状和心血管疾病。

在诊断或治疗高钙血症患者时，应考虑第 11 章所述的生理性情况。高钙血症的病因可分为人为性疾病（如血清蛋白异常）、甲状旁腺介导的疾病、非甲状旁腺介导的疾病、药物相关疾病和其他疾病。表 12.1 列出了高钙血症的鉴别诊断。

症状和体征

常规代谢检查包含血钙检测，因此常规实验室检查通常能发现无症状的高钙血症。患者是否出现症状取决于多个因素，其中包括高钙血症的严重程度和进展速度。一般来说，当血清钙浓度绝对值 > 13 mg/dl 时，患者会出现症状。若患者的血清钙浓度缓慢升高，则血清钙浓度 > 15 mg/dl 时出现的症状也可能少于快速上升至 13 mg/d。高钙血症患者的全身健康状况和年龄会影响症状的严重程度。老年患者的症状可能最严重。

高钙血症可造成平滑肌运动减少，导致便秘和肠梗阻。胰腺炎和消化性溃疡较少见，可见于严重高钙血症患者。高钙血症还与神经系统功能障碍有关，严重程度可从轻度意识模糊到昏迷。高钙血症可通过多种机制导致肾损害。高钙血症引起入球小动脉收缩并激活远端肾单位的钙受体，从而降低肾小球滤过率（GFR）。高钙血症还可引起肾性尿崩症，伴有多饮和多尿，从而使 ECF 容量减少，GFR 进一步降低。高钙血症可造成磷酸钙结晶沉积到肾间质（即肾钙盐沉着症或间质性肾炎）和尿液中，引起肾结石和尿路梗阻，直接导致肾损害。高钙血症可对心脏产生多种严重不良影响，包括心律失常。心电图异常包括 QTc 间期缩短、PR 间期延长、QRS 波增宽及心动过缓。也有报道出现疑似心肌梗死的 ST 段抬高。高钙血症患者还常表现为肌无力。

鉴别诊断

高蛋白血症 血液循环中约 50% 的钙与血清白蛋白和其他蛋白质相结合。血清蛋白质增加可使血清总钙浓度增加，而血清离子钙浓度并不增加。在容量减少和脱水的情况下通常可观察到血清钙浓度升高。高蛋白血症导致的高钙血症患者没有任何体征和症状，此种情况无须治疗，以免造成低钙血症。

甲状旁腺激素相关的高钙血症

甲状旁腺功能亢进症（HPT） 原发性和三发性甲状旁腺功能亢进症均表现为特征性的高钙血症。其他疾病（如维生素 D 缺乏症、钙缺乏或慢性肾脏病）导致的继发性甲状旁腺功能亢进症（SHPT）患者的血清钙浓度明显低于正常值或为正常值下限。然而，值得注意的是，这些病因可同时存在。充分考虑患者的共病情况和实验室检查结果是做出正确诊断或综合诊断的必要条件。

原发性甲状旁腺功能亢进症（PHPT） PHPT 是由异常的甲状旁腺产生过多甲状旁腺激素（PTH）所致，

TABLE 12.1   Disorders Associated With Hypercalcemia

PTH-Related Hypercalcemia	Non-PTH Mediated Hypercalcemia
Primary hyperparathyroidism	Malignancy-associated hypercalcemia
Tertiary hyperparathyroidism	Humoral hypercalcemia of malignancy
Familial hypocalciuric hypercalcemia or familial benign hypercalcemia	Hypercalcemia caused by 1,25-dihydroxyvitamin D_3 (1,25[OH]$_2$D$_3$)–secreting lymphomas
	Hypercalcemia caused by direct skeletal invasion
	Granulomatous disorders
	Sarcoid
	Berylliosis
	Foreign body
	Tuberculosis
	Coccidioidomycosis
	Blastomycosis
	Histoplasmosis
	Granulomatous leprosy
	Eosinophilic granuloma
	Histiocytosis
	Inflammatory bowel disease
	Endocrine disorders other than hyperparathyroidism
	Hyperthyroidism
	Pheochromocytoma
	Addisonian crisis
	Vasoactive intestinal peptide–producing tumor (VIPoma); watery diarrhea, hypokalemia, and achlorhydria (WDHA) syndrome
	Milk-alkali syndrome
	Total parenteral nutrition (TPN)
	Calcium-containing TPN in patients with decreased glomerular filtration rate
	Chronic TPN in patients with short-bowel syndrome
	Immobilization plus high bone turnover (risk is particularly high in individuals with the following)
	Juvenile skeleton
	Paget's disease
	Myeloma and breast cancer with bone metastases
	Mild primary hyperparathyroidism
	Secondary hyperparathyroidism (e.g., from continuous ambulatory peritoneal dialysis)
	Medications
	Thiazides
	Aminophylline
	Lithium
	Estrogen/antiestrogen in breast cancer with bone metastases (estrogen flare)
	Vitamin D and derivatives (calcitriol, dihydrotachysterol)
	Vitamin A (including retinoic acid derivatives)
	Foscarnet
	Anabolic agents (teriparatide, abaloparatide)

abnormal parathyroid glands, is by far the most common cause of hypercalcemia among otherwise healthy outpatients. In approximately 85% of patients with HPT, a single parathyroid adenoma is responsible for excess PTH secretion, while in about 15% there is hyperplasia of multiple glands. Rarely, HPT may result from parathyroid carcinoma. The diagnosis of HPT is relatively straightforward in patients who have hypercalcemia in the setting of a frankly elevated serum PTH. It is important to note, however, that in a patient with normal parathyroid gland function, PTH synthesis and secretion should be suppressed by hypercalcemia. Therefore, a PTH level within the normal range should be considered inappropriately high in the setting of hypercalcemia and may indicate underlying hyperparathyroidism. Concurrent vitamin D deficiency, which predisposes to hypocalcemia, can mask elevated calcium levels in patients with HPT; in such cases, hypercalcemia may become apparent only after vitamin D is repleted. Other typical biochemical features of HPT include hypophosphatemia, increased 1,25(OH)$_2$D and chloride levels, and a reduction in serum bicarbonate.

Many patients diagnosed with PHPT are asymptomatic and have serum calcium in the mildly elevated range. Because serum calcium is typically included in chemistry panels, this diagnosis is frequently made when hypercalcemia is found during routine laboratory testing. Less frequently, patients may present with symptoms including osteoporosis, bone pain, and nephrolithiasis. Kidney stones are most often comprised of calcium oxalate and, less commonly, calcium phosphate. Osteoporosis is common among patients with HPT. In the classic densitometric pattern of HPT, bone mineral density (BMD) is relatively preserved at the spine, lower at the hip, and particularly low at the ⅓ radius. This is because the ⅓ radius is a predominantly cortical site, which is susceptible to the effects of excess PTH. Though rarely seen today, severe HPT can cause the classic skeletal manifestations known as *osteitis fibrosa cystica* in which there are bone cysts and "brown tumors," which are collections of osteoclasts intermixed with fibrous tissue and poorly mineralized woven bone (see Chapter 13). Some patients with HPT may develop renal disease as a result of the mechanisms described earlier.

Rarely, HPT can occur as part of one of the multiple endocrine neoplasia (MEN) syndromes. It is associated with pituitary and pancreatic neuroendocrine tumors (MEN 1) and with pheochromocytomas and medullary carcinoma of the thyroid (MEN 2).

Tertiary hyperparathyroidism. Tertiary HPT refers to HPT-associated hypercalcemia that occurs in the setting of prolonged stimulation of the parathyroid glands. Chronic hypocalcemic stimulation of the parathyroids eventually leads to hyperplasia. The abnormal glands stop responding appropriately to elevations in serum calcium, ultimately resulting in hypercalcemia. This is typically seen in patients with chronic renal failure and can be seen after renal transplantation.

Familial hypocalciuric hypercalcemia. Familial hypocalciuric hypercalcemia (FHH), or *familial benign hypercalcemia*, is an autosomal dominant genetic disorder caused by heterozygous inactivating mutations of the calcium sensing receptor. As a result of the defect, the parathyroid glands interpret normal serum calcium levels as low, increase PTH in response, and serum calcium rises. PTH in this disorder is in the high-normal to slightly high range. Hypercalcemia is typically mild, in the range of 11 to 12 mg/dL. Abnormal calcium receptors are also expressed in the kidney, leading to inappropriate renal conservation of calcium and hypocalciuria, further exacerbating hypercalcemia. With the exception of the hypocalciuria, patients with FHH have biochemical profiles similar to those with PHPT. However, affected individuals are asymptomatic and do not develop adverse sequelae from FHH. It is critical to distinguish the two disorders, particularly in patients being considered for parathyroidectomy, because patients with FHH do not require any intervention. In contrast to the mild presentation of heterozygous individuals, homozygous patients usually develop severe hypercalcemia in infancy, requiring urgent total parathyroidectomy.

表 12.1　高钙血症的相关疾病

PTH 相关的高钙血症	非 PTH 介导的高钙血症
原发性甲状旁腺功能亢进症	恶性肿瘤相关高钙血症
三发性甲状旁腺功能亢进症	恶性肿瘤体液性高钙血症
家族性低尿钙高血钙症或家族性良性高钙血症	分泌 1,25(OH)₂D₃ 的淋巴瘤引起的高钙血症
	直接骨骼侵犯引起的高钙血症
	肉芽肿性疾病
	结节病
	铍中毒
	异物
	结核
	球孢子菌病
	芽生菌病
	组织胞浆菌病
	肉芽肿性麻风
	嗜酸细胞肉芽肿
	组织细胞增多症
	炎症性肠病
	甲状旁腺功能亢进症以外的内分泌疾病
	甲状腺功能亢进症
	嗜铬细胞瘤
	Addison 病危象
	产生血管活性肠肽的肿瘤（VIP 瘤）；水样腹泻、低钾血症和胃酸缺乏（WDHA）综合征
	乳碱综合征
	全肠外营养（TPN）
	肾小球滤过率降低的患者使用含钙 TPN
	短肠综合征患者长期使用 TPN
	制动且高骨转换（以下情况的风险尤其高）
	青少年
	骨佩吉特病（Paget 骨病）
	骨髓瘤和乳腺癌骨转移
	轻度原发性甲状旁腺功能亢进症
	继发性甲状旁腺功能亢进症（如持续非卧床腹膜透析）
	药物
	噻嗪类药物
	氨茶碱
	锂剂
	乳腺癌骨转移患者使用雌激素/抗雌激素药物（雌激素剧变）
	维生素 D 及其衍生物（骨化三醇、二氢速固醇）
	维生素 A（包括维甲酸衍生物）
	膦甲酸
	促骨形成药物（特立帕肽、阿巴洛肽）

这是其他方面健康状况良好的门诊患者发生高钙血症的最常见病因。约 85% 的 HPT 患者由单个甲状旁腺腺瘤分泌过多 PTH 所致，约 15% 的患者由多个甲状旁腺增生所致，甲状旁腺癌是罕见的 HPT 病因。当患者出现高钙血症且血清 PTH 水平显著升高时，HPT 的诊断相对简单。然而，需要注意的是，对于甲状旁腺功能

正常的患者，PTH 的合成和分泌应能被高钙血症所抑制。因此，在高钙血症的情况下，PTH 水平正常应被认为是不适当的高水平，并提示可能存在 HPT。患者合并维生素 D 缺乏症时易导致低钙血症，这可能掩盖 HPT 引发的血钙浓度升高。在这种情况下，只有在补充维生素 D 之后，高钙血症才会显现。HPT 的其他典型生化特征包括低磷血症、血 1,25(OH)₂D 及血氯浓度升高、血清碳酸氢盐浓度降低。

许多被诊断为 PHPT 的患者并无症状，且血钙浓度仅轻度升高。由于常规的生化检查项目中包含血清钙，因此是在常规实验室检查发现高钙血症时才做出诊断。少数情况下，患者可表现为骨质疏松症、骨痛和肾结石等。肾结石的成分通常是草酸钙，少数是磷酸钙。HPT 患者常出现骨质疏松症。典型的 HPT 骨密度（BMD）变化模式是椎体的 BMD 相对正常，髋部的 BMD 较低，桡骨下 1/3 处的 BMD 更低。这是因为桡骨下 1/3 处主要是皮质骨，容易受到过多 PTH 的影响。虽然目前已非常少见，但严重 HPT 可导致典型的骨骼表现，即囊性纤维性骨炎（包含骨囊肿和"棕色瘤"），这是由破骨细胞混合纤维组织和矿化不良的编织骨组成（见第 13 章）。一些 HPT 患者可能因上述机制而出现肾病。

罕见情况下，HPT 可作为多发性内分泌腺瘤病（MEN）综合征的一部分，可伴有垂体和胰腺神经内分泌肿瘤（MEN 1）及嗜铬细胞瘤和甲状腺髓样癌（MEN 2）。

三发性甲状旁腺功能亢进症　三发性 HPT 是指在甲状旁腺长期刺激的情况下发生的 HPT 相关性高钙血症。长期低血钙对甲状旁腺的刺激最终会导致甲状旁腺增生。异常的腺体对血清钙浓度升高缺乏正常的适当反应，最终导致高钙血症。这通常见于慢性肾衰竭患者，也可见于肾移植后。

家族性低尿钙高血钙症　家族性低尿钙高血钙症（FHH）或家族性良性高钙血症是一种常染色体显性遗传病，由钙敏感受体的杂合失活突变引起。由于这种缺陷，甲状旁腺将正常血清钙浓度感知为低血钙浓度，并相应增加 PTH 分泌，使血清钙浓度升高。该病患者的 PTH 水平处于正常值上限或轻度升高。高钙血症通常为轻度（11～12 mg/dl）。异常的钙受体也在肾脏中表达，导致肾脏对钙的不适当保留和尿钙减少，进一步加剧高钙血症。除尿钙减少外，FHH 患者的生化检查与 PHPT 患者相似。然而，FHH 患者无症状，且不会出现不良后果。由于 FHH 患者不需要任何干预措施，因此区分这两种疾病至关重要，特别是在考虑患者是否需要进行甲状旁腺切除术时。与杂合子 FHH 患者（症状表现轻微）不同，纯合子患者通常在婴儿期即发生严重高钙血症，需要紧急进行甲状旁腺全切除术。

Nonparathyroid hormone–mediated hypercalcemia

Malignancy-associated hypercalcemia. The most common cause of hypercalcemia among hospitalized patients is malignancy. Cancer may lead to hypercalcemia through several mechanisms, the majority of which are PTH independent. Hypercalcemia typically occurs in patients with end-stage malignancies and progresses rapidly. Approximately 50% of patients die within 30 days of developing malignancy-associated hypercalcemia (MAHC). Hypercalcemia usually occurs in patients with large tumor burdens but can also be seen in patients who have small neuroendocrine tumors, such as islet cell tumors and bronchial carcinoids. Tumors that commonly cause hypercalcemia include breast, renal, squamous cell, ovarian carcinomas, multiple myeloma, and lymphoma.

Humoral hypercalcemia of malignancy (HHM) results from excessive secretion of parathyroid hormone–related protein (PTHrP) by tumor cells. This is the most common cause of MAHC, accounting for approximately 80% of cases. PTHrP acts on the same receptor as PTH and can induce similar systemic effects. PTHrP mimics the actions of PTH on the kidney to promote calcium retention and on the skeleton to activate osteoclasts and induce bone resorption. PTHrP is typically produced at low levels in healthy individuals; however, excess levels can cause significant hypercalcemia. Patients with HHM have elevations in PTHrP and reductions in the levels of PTH, 1,25-dihydroxyvitamin D_3 (1,25[OH]$_2$D), and serum phosphorus (see Chapter 11). Tumors classically associated with HHM include squamous cell carcinomas (i.e., larynx, lung, cervix, and esophagus), renal, ovarian, and breast carcinomas. In HHM, hypercalcemia typically occurs in the absence of skeletal metastases. If tumor resection or ablation is possible, hypercalcemia will reverse.

Another etiology of MAHC is local tumor invasion of the skeleton, a process called *local osteolytic hypercalcemia* (LOH). LOH accounts for approximately 20% of patients with MAHC. In contrast to HHM, these patients often have extensive skeletal metastases. The primary tumor is most commonly breast cancer or a hematologic neoplasm such as multiple myeloma, leukemia, or lymphoma. Local factors secreted by tumors in the bone marrow induce osteoclastic bone resorption. These include PTHrP, macrophage inflammatory protein 1α (MIP-1α), receptor-activating nuclear factor-κB ligand (RANKL), interleukin-6, and interleukin-1. Typically, patients with LOH have both hypercalcemia and hyperphosphatemia as a result of excess bone resorption. PTH, PTHrP and 1,25(OH)$_2$D levels are reduced, reflecting appropriate suppressive responses to hypercalcemia

A third, rare, form of MAHC is secretion of 1,25(OH)$_2$D by lymphomas and dysgerminomas. The increased 1,25(OH)$_2$D leads to intestinal calcium hyperabsorption as well as bone resorption. This condition is mechanistically similar to the hypercalcemia that occurs in granulomatous disease (see below).

Granulomatous diseases. Another type of PTH-independent hypercalcemia occurs in patients with granulomatous disease including sarcoidosis, tuberculosis, and fungal infections (see Table 12.1). The granulomas in these conditions contain the 1α-hydroxylase enzyme and therefore have the ability to convert inactive 25-hydroxyvitamin D to its active metabolite, 1,25(OH)$_2$D. Hypercalcemia results from intestinal calcium hyperabsorption and to a lesser extent, 1,25(OH)$_2$D-induced bone resorption. As a result of increased 1α-hydroxylase activity, patients with these disorders are susceptible to developing hypercalcemia when exposed to sunlight, ultraviolet radiation, or relatively trivial quantities of dietary vitamin D. The excess 1,25(OH)$_2$D results in an elevated serum phosphorus and suppression of endogenous PTH. The combined hypercalcemia and hyperphosphatemia can result in nephrocalcinosis and renal failure.

Other endocrine disorders. Although HPT is most common, other endocrine disorders can cause hypercalcemia as well. Hyperthyroidism can cause mild hypercalcemia through an increase in bone resorption driven by elevated thyroid hormone. This can occur in up to half of patients with this disorder. Serum calcium in these patients is usually below 11 mg/dL.

Hypercalcemia can also be seen in patients with pheochromocytoma. In patients with pheochromocytoma as part of MEN 2, hypercalcemia can result directly from PHPT, which is also part of this syndrome. In other patients, hypercalcemia is due to PTHrP secretion by the pheochromocytoma. Hypercalcemia has also been reported in patients with hypoadrenalism and those with VIPomas, a type of islet cell tumor.

Milk-Alkali syndrome. As reviewed in Chapter 11, absorption of calcium from the diet is usually well regulated. However, ingestion of very large quantities of calcium, particularly from supplements, can exceed the regulatory ability of this system and result in hypercalcemia. This can occur in patients ingesting large quantities of calcium carbonate or other calcium-containing antacids for peptic ulcer disease. This condition, known as milk-alkali syndrome, consists of the triad of hypercalcemia, metabolic alkalosis, and acute kidney injury. Severe hypercalcemia is common and may lead to renal failure. Calcium intake in patients with milk-alkali syndrome typically exceeds 4 g/day and can be in the 10- to 20-g/day range.

Parenteral nutrition. Patients receiving both enteric and parenteral nutrition can develop hypercalcemia. Hypercaloric enteric feeding regimens may contain large quantities of calcium, which can lead to a form of milk-alkali syndrome. Patients with renal impairment are at particular risk for developing hypercalcemia in this setting. Hypercalcemia has also been described in patients treated with total parenteral nutrition (TPN). In some cases, hypercalcemia results from large amounts of calcium, vitamin D, or aluminum in the TPN solution. Often patients who develop hypercalcemia have short-bowel syndrome and are on long-term TPN.

Immobilization. Hypercalcemia can occur in the setting of immobilization. Immobilization activates osteoclast mediated bone resorption and inhibits osteoblast activity, uncoupling bone turnover. As a result, there is substantial, rapid movement of calcium from the skeleton into the ECF. This condition is associated with hypercalciuria and calcium nephrolithiasis. It can result in severe skeletal demineralization if untreated. Typically, for immobilization-related hypercalcemia to occur, patients must be completely immobilized for weeks and have a concurrent underlying predisposition to hypercalcemia because of high bone turnover. This condition is most commonly seen in young adults or children, patients with HPT, Paget's disease, skeletal metastases or multiple myeloma. The most effective treatment for immobilization-related hypercalcemia is resumption of active weight bearing. Hydration and antiresorptive medications, if hypercalcemia is severe, can be used to lower serum calcium as well.

Medications. Drugs that may cause hypercalcemia include thiazide diuretics, lithium, aminophylline, theophylline, vitamins D and A, foscarnet, and osteoanabolic agents like teriparatide and abaloparatide.

Treatment of Hypercalcemia

Patients with mild, asymptomatic hypercalcemia may not require immediate treatment. For severe (Ca >14 mg/dL) or symptomatic hypercalcemia, the initial treatment includes intravenous hydration, calcitonin, and antiresorptive agents like bisphosphonates or denosumab. Volume expansion with isotonic saline is usually initiated first. Loop diuretics should be avoided unless patients have volume overload or heart failure. Subcutaneous calcitonin, which has a rapid onset of action, is usually administered in addition to fluids for the first

非甲状旁腺激素介导的高钙血症

恶性肿瘤相关高钙血症（MAHC）　住院患者发生高钙血症最常见的病因是恶性肿瘤。癌症可通过多种机制导致高钙血症，其中绝大多数不依赖 PTH。高钙血症通常发生于恶性肿瘤终末期患者，且进展迅速。约 50% 的患者会在发生 MAHC 后 30 天内死亡。高钙血症常见于肿瘤负荷大的患者，但也可见于小的神经内分泌肿瘤患者，如胰岛细胞肿瘤和支气管类癌。可引起高钙血症的常见肿瘤包括乳腺癌、肾癌、鳞状细胞癌、卵巢癌、多发性骨髓瘤和淋巴瘤。

恶性肿瘤体液性高钙血症（HHM）由肿瘤细胞过度分泌 PTH 相关蛋白（PTHrP）引起。这是 MAHC 最常见的病因，约占 80%。PTHrP 与 PTH 作用于同一受体，并可产生类似的全身效应。PTHrP 可模拟 PTH 对肾脏的作用，促进钙的重吸收，在骨骼中可激活破骨细胞并促进骨吸收。健康个体 PTHrP 的生成水平通常很低，生成过量会导致显著的高钙血症。HHM 患者的 PTHrP 水平升高，PTH、1,25（OH)$_2$D 和血清磷浓度降低（见第 11 章）。通常与 HHM 相关的肿瘤包括鳞状细胞癌（如喉癌、肺癌、宫颈癌和食管癌），肾癌、卵巢癌和乳腺癌。HHM 患者的高钙血症通常发生在肿瘤尚未发生骨转移时，如果肿瘤被切除或消除，高钙血症能够被逆转。

MAHC 的另一个病因是局部肿瘤侵犯骨骼，这一过程被称为局部溶骨性高钙血症（LOH）。LOH 约占 MAHC 患者的 20%。与 HHM 不同，这些患者通常有广泛的肿瘤骨转移。最常见的原发肿瘤是乳腺癌或血液系统肿瘤，如多发性骨髓瘤、白血病和淋巴瘤。骨髓内的肿瘤分泌局部因子诱导破骨细胞骨吸收。这些因子包括 PTHrP、巨噬细胞炎症蛋白 1α（MIP-1α）、核因子 κB 受体激活蛋白配体（RANKL）、IL-6 和 IL-1。由于过度的骨吸收，LOH 患者常表现为高钙血症和高磷血症。患者的 PTH、PTHrP 和 1,25（OH)$_2$D 水平因高钙血症的抑制而降低。

第 3 个罕见的 MAHC 病因是由淋巴瘤和无性细胞瘤分泌 1,25（OH)$_2$D。1,25（OH)$_2$D 增多可导致肠道钙吸收过多和骨吸收增加。这种情况与肉芽肿性疾病引起高钙血症的机制类似（见下文）。

肉芽肿性疾病　肉芽肿性疾病导致的高钙血症是另一种非 PTH 介导的高钙血症，可见于结节病、结核和真菌感染等肉芽肿性疾病患者（表 12.1）。肉芽肿含有 1α-羟化酶，可将无活性的 25-羟维生素 D 转化为有活性的 1,25（OH)$_2$D。1,25（OH)$_2$D 使肠道过度吸收钙，并在一定程度上增加骨吸收，导致高钙血症。由于 1α-羟化酶的活性增加，肉芽肿性疾病患者在日光暴露、紫外线辐射或给予相对少量的膳食维生素 D 时，容易出现高钙血症。过量的 1,25（OH)$_2$D 可导致血清磷浓度升高和内源性 PTH 受抑制。高钙血症合并高磷血症可导致肾钙盐沉着症和肾衰竭。

其他内分泌疾病　虽然 HPT 最常见，但其他内分泌疾病也可引起高钙血症。甲状腺功能亢进症可通过甲状腺激素水平升高引起骨吸收增加，进而引起轻度高钙血症。多达 1/2 的甲状腺功能亢进症患者会出现这种情况。这些患者通常血清钙浓度 < 11 mg/dl。

嗜铬细胞瘤患者也可出现高钙血症。当患者的嗜铬细胞瘤是 MEN 2 的一部分时，高钙血症可直接由 PHPT 引起，这也是该综合征的一部分。在其他患者中，高钙血症也可由嗜铬细胞瘤分泌 PTHrP 所致。肾上腺皮质功能减退症和 VIP 瘤（一种胰岛细胞肿瘤）患者也可发生高钙血症。

乳碱综合征　如第 11 章所述，膳食钙的吸收通常受到严格调控。然而，摄入非常大量的钙（特别是补充剂中的钙）可能会超过系统的调控能力，并导致高钙血症。这可能见于摄入大量碳酸钙或其他用于治疗消化性溃疡的含钙抗酸剂的患者。这种情况被称为乳碱综合征，由高钙血症、代谢性碱中毒和急性肾损伤三联征组成。严重高钙血症常见并可能导致肾衰竭。乳碱综合征患者的钙摄入量通常超过 4 g/d，范围可在 10 ～ 20 g/d。

肠外营养　接受肠内和肠外营养的患者均可出现高钙血症。高能量的肠内营养方案可能含有大量的钙，这可导致乳碱综合征。在这种情况下，肾功能损害患者尤其易出现高钙血症。接受全肠外营养（TPN）治疗的患者也有出现高钙血症的报道。在一些情况下，高钙血症由 TPN 溶液中大量的钙、维生素 D 或铝引起。出现高钙血症的患者通常伴有短肠综合征，并长期接受 TPN。

制动　制动情况下可发生高钙血症。制动会激活破骨细胞介导的骨吸收，同时抑制成骨细胞活性，使骨转换失偶联。因此，大量的钙从骨骼快速进入 ECF。这种情况与高钙尿症和钙质肾结石有关。如果不及时治疗，会引起严重的骨骼去矿化。通常情况下，发生制动相关的高钙血症需要患者经历数周的完全制动，且由于骨转换率高而有高钙血症的潜在易感性。这种情况最常见于年轻成人或儿童，以及 HPT、Paget 骨病、肿瘤骨转移或多发性骨髓瘤患者。对于制动相关的高钙血症，最有效的治疗方法是恢复主动负重。如果高钙血症很严重，可同时给予水化和抗骨吸收药物来降低血清钙浓度。

药物　可能导致高钙血症的药物包括噻嗪类利尿剂、锂剂、氨茶碱、茶碱、维生素 D 和维生素 A、膦甲酸和促骨形成药物（如特立帕肽和阿巴洛肽）。

高钙血症的治疗

轻度、无症状性高钙血症不需要立即治疗。对于严重（血钙 > 14 mg/dl）或症状性高钙血症，初始治疗方案包括静脉水化、降钙素和抗骨吸收药物（如双膦酸盐或地舒单抗）。通常先使用等张生理盐水进行扩容。除非患者出现容量超负荷或心力衰竭，应避免使用袢利尿剂。皮下注射降钙素起效迅速，通常作为第 1 个 48 h 中除补液外的治疗措施。但是，由于降钙素治

48 hours. However, because tachyphylaxis develops rapidly to calcitonin therapy, it should be discontinued after 24 to 48 hours. Concurrent use of intravenous bisphosphonates, preferably zoledronic acid, is often needed, particularly in patients with hypercalcemia of malignancy. Denosumab is an alternative option for patients who are refractory to bisphosphonates or have renal dysfunction that precludes bisphosphonate use. These medications have a slower onset of action, so it is important to treat concurrently with fluids and calcitonin when rapid correction of the calcium is required. Cinacalcet, a calcimimetic agent typically used in patients with secondary HPT from chronic kidney disease (CKD), can also be used to treat severe hypercalcemia from tertiary HPT or due to parathyroid carcinoma. Glucocorticoids are the preferred treatment for hypercalcemia due to overproduction of 1,25-vitamin D related to granulomatous disease or lymphomas. In cases of severe hypercalcemia that are refractory to medical treatment, or in patients with advanced CKD, dialysis against a low or zero calcium bath can be performed.

Therapy for hypercalcemia should ultimately be directed at reversing the underlying pathophysiologic abnormality. Patients with symptomatic primary HPT should undergo parathyroidectomy. For asymptomatic patients with PHPT, indications for surgery include osteoporosis, kidney stones, reduced renal function, and a serum calcium concentration greater than 1 mg/dL above normal. Other patients may be monitored conservatively. In patients who are unwilling or unable to undergo surgery, medical management of hypercalcemia may be attempted using bisphosphonates. As above, familial hypocalciuric hypercalcemia does not require treatment.

Treatment of hypercalcemia related to granulomatous diseases focuses on correcting the underlying disorder. Measures include a low dietary calcium intake, low vitamin D intake, limiting sun exposure, and hydration. If hypercalcemia is severe, glucocorticoids can be used. Disorders associated with increased intestinal calcium absorption (e.g., sarcoid, milk-alkali syndrome, 1,25[OH]$_2$D$_3$-secreting lymphomas) should be treated by having patients limit intake of both calcium and vitamin D. Medications that induce hypercalcemia should be discontinued.

Hypocalcemia
Pathophysiology

Hypocalcemia can be caused by several mechanisms. Apparent hypocalcemia can result from a reduction in serum proteins that bind calcium, typically albumin. In these patients, ionized calcium and calcium corrected for albumin will be normal. Increased serum phosphate can cause hypocalcemia via an increase in the calcium-phosphate solubility product. Increased renal calcium excretion or a reduction in intestinal calcium absorption can cause hypocalcemia. Hypocalcemia can also result from loss of calcium from the ECF into the skeleton, which can occur in the setting of some malignancies, after parathyroidectomy (hungry bone syndrome), or with certain medications, including bisphosphonates, denosumab, chelating agents, and foscarnet. Many disorders that cause severe hypocalcemia do so by impacting several of these processes simultaneously. In order to provide effective treatment, all of the mechanisms through which a disorder is causing hypocalcemia should be considered and addressed. Hypocalcemia leads to a reduction in the potential difference across cell membranes, producing hyperexcitability in neuromuscular cells which can spontaneously fire (see Chapter 11).

Symptoms and Signs

The seminal signs of hypocalcemia on physical exam relate to neuromuscular hyperexcitability. Hypocalcemia can cause paresthesias, seizures, and skeletal muscle contractions (i.e., carpal spasm, pedal spasm, or tetany). The *Trousseau sign* describes spontaneous contraction of the forearm muscles in response to inflation of a blood pressure cuff around the upper arm to above systolic pressure. The *Chvostek sign* describes twitching of the facial muscles that is elicited by gentle tapping of the facial nerve as it exits the parotid gland. On an electrocardiogram, hypocalcemia can manifest as a prolonged QTc interval. Patients with hypocalcemia may also have more general symptoms such as fatigue, weakness, and abdominal pain. As with hypercalcemia, the severity of symptoms will relate to both the severity and chronicity of hypocalcemia.

Differential Diagnosis

Disorders that may lead to hypocalcemia are summarized in the following sections and Table 12.2.

Hypoalbuminemia. The majority of serum calcium is bound to albumin. Low serum albumin will lead to a low measured total calcium although ionized values will be normal. This is commonly seen in patients with cirrhosis, nephrotic syndrome, malnutrition, and severe burns. The formula commonly used to correct serum calcium for low serum albumin levels is: corrected calcium = measured total calcium + (0.8 × [4.0 − measured albumin]). This formula should be used to confirm the presence of hypocalcemia.

Hypoparathyroidism. In hypoparathyroidism, low levels of parathyroid hormone result in hypocalcemia through decreased intestinal calcium absorption and reduced calcium reabsorption in the distal renal tubule. Hypoparathyroidism most commonly occurs as a complication of neck surgery or as a consequence of autoimmune disease. Postoperative hypoparathyroidism typically occurs after thyroid, parathyroid, or laryngeal surgery. Autoimmune hypoparathyroidism can occur as a single entity or as part of autoimmune polyglandular syndrome, where it can be associated with primary adrenal insufficiency (Addison's disease), type 1 diabetes, autoimmune thyroid disease, vitiligo, and mucocutaneous candidiasis. Other less common causes of hypoparathyroidism include congenital hypoparathyroidism as part of DiGeorge syndrome, isolated parathyroid failure, or genetic mutations. Rarely, infiltrative conditions including sarcoidosis, hemochromatosis, HIV, and malignancy (i.e., breast cancer) can cause hypoparathyroidism.

The diagnosis of hypoparathyroidism is made by finding an inappropriately low serum PTH in a patient with hypocalcemia. The phosphorus concentration is usually high normal or frankly elevated, and plasma 1,25(OH)$_2$D concentrations are reduced. Prolonged hypoparathyroidism may be associated with asymptomatic basal ganglia calcification on computed tomography scans and plain radiographs of the skull.

Treatment for hypoparathyroidism has historically been directed at increasing intestinal calcium absorption through the use of large doses of calcium (up to 6 to 8 g of elemental calcium per day) along with active vitamin D (1,25[OH]$_2$D) in doses of 0.25 to 1.0 μg/day. With this regimen it is possible to induce sufficient intestinal calcium hyperabsorption to overwhelm the ability of the kidney to excrete it. However, this treatment can exacerbate hypercalciuria leading to nephrocalcinosis and nephrolithiasis, making it critical to monitor 24-hour urinary calcium. Thiazide diuretics can be used as adjunctive treatment to stimulate renal calcium reabsorption, reduce hypercalciuria, and raise serum calcium. Treatment should be aimed at maintaining serum calcium concentration in the low-normal range.

The approval of recombinant PTH 1-84 by the FDA for chronic hypoparathyroidism has provided an important option for treatment that lowers the risk of some of the adverse effects of high dose calcium and calcitriol.

Pseudohypoparathyroidism. In the group of disorders known as pseudohypoparathyroidism, patients are resistant to the actions of PTH. In these disorders, resistance may result from several different inactivating mutations in the signal-transducing protein G$_{s\alpha}$. The most

疗可产生快速耐药反应，因此应在 24 ～ 48 h 后停用。患者（特别是 MAHC 患者）通常需要同时静脉使用双膦酸盐，首选唑来膦酸。地舒单抗是双膦酸盐效果不佳或因肾功能不全而无法使用双膦酸盐患者的替代选择。这些药物起效较慢，因此当需要快速纠正血钙时，与补液和降钙素同时使用十分重要。西那卡塞是一种拟钙剂，通常用于慢性肾脏病（CKD）继发性 HPT 的患者，也可用于治疗三发性 HPT 或甲状旁腺癌引起的严重高钙血症。对于因肉芽肿性疾病或淋巴瘤引起1,25（OH）$_2$D 过量生成导致的高钙血症患者，首选糖皮质激素治疗。对于药物治疗无效的严重高钙血症或晚期 CKD 患者，可采用低钙或零钙透析液进行透析。

高钙血症的治疗最终应能够逆转潜在的病理生理学异常。有症状的 PHPT 患者应进行甲状旁腺切除术。对于无症状的 PHPT 患者，手术指征包括骨质疏松症、肾结石、肾功能下降和血清钙浓度高于正常水平 1 mg/dl 以上。其他患者也可进行保守性观察。对于不愿或不能接受手术的患者，可尝试使用双膦酸盐进行药物治疗。如上所述，家族性低尿钙高血钙症患者不需要进行治疗。

肉芽肿性疾病相关高钙血症的治疗应注重纠正潜在疾病。治疗措施包括低膳食钙摄入、低维生素 D 摄入、限制阳光暴露和注意水化。如果高钙血症很严重，可使用糖皮质激素。

对于与肠道钙吸收增加相关的疾病［如结节病、乳碱综合征、分泌 1,25（OH）$_2$D 的淋巴瘤］，治疗措施为限制钙和维生素 D 的摄入。应停用引起高钙血症的药物。

低钙血症

病理生理学

多种机制可引发低钙血症。结合钙的血清蛋白质（通常是白蛋白）减少可导致明显的低钙血症。患者的离子钙和白蛋白校正钙浓度正常。血磷浓度升高可通过增加钙-磷可溶性产物而导致低钙血症。肾钙排泄增加或肠道钙吸收减少均可导致低钙血症。低钙血症也可能是由于 ECF 中的钙进入骨骼，这可能见于部分恶性肿瘤、甲状旁腺切除术后（骨饥饿综合征）或使用某些药物（包括双膦酸盐、地舒单抗、螯合剂和膦甲酸）。许多导致严重低钙血症的疾病可同时影响上述多种机制。为了提供有效的治疗，应考虑和处理疾病引起低钙血症的所有机制。低钙血症可导致细胞膜间的电位差减小，使神经肌肉细胞的兴奋性增高，出现自发放电表现（见第 11 章）。

症状和体征

在体格检查中，低钙血症的重要体征与神经肌肉过度兴奋有关。低钙血症可引起感觉异常、癫痫发作和骨骼肌收缩（即腕关节痉挛、足部痉挛或手足搐搦）。束臂征（Trousseau 征）可见上臂受血压袖带束缚至收缩压以上时前臂肌肉出现自发的收缩反应。面神经叩击征（Chvostek 征）可见轻轻叩击耳前（即面神经腮腺部位）引起面部肌肉的抽搐反应。在心电图上，低钙血症可表现为 QTc 间期延长。低钙血症患者也可出现全身症状，如疲劳、乏力和腹痛。与高钙血症相同，症状的严重程度与低钙血症的严重程度和进展速度有关。

鉴别诊断

可能导致低钙血症的疾病见下文和表 12.2。

低白蛋白血症　绝大多数的血清钙与白蛋白结合。血清白蛋白降低会引起总血清钙浓度降低，而离子钙浓度正常。这常见于肝硬化、肾病综合征、营养不良和严重烧伤的患者。血清白蛋白水平低时，计算校正血清钙的常用公式是：校正血清钙＝测定的总血清钙＋［0.8×（4.0－测定的白蛋白）］。该公式可用于确认是否存在低钙血症。

甲状旁腺功能减退症　甲状旁腺功能减退症时，低水平的 PTH 可通过降低肠道钙吸收和减少远端肾小管的钙重吸收而引起低钙血症。甲状旁腺功能减退症最常见的病因是颈部手术或自身免疫病。术后甲状旁腺功能减退症通常发生在甲状腺、甲状旁腺或喉部手术后。自身免疫性甲状旁腺功能减退症可以是独立疾病或作为自身免疫性多内分泌腺综合征的一部分，可伴有原发性肾上腺皮质功能不全（Addison 病）、1 型糖尿病、自身免疫性甲状腺疾病、白癜风和黏膜皮肤念珠菌病。其他导致甲状旁腺功能减退症的少见病因包括作为 DiGeorge 综合征一部分的先天性甲状旁腺功能减退症、孤立性甲状旁腺功能衰竭或基因突变。罕见病因包括浸润性疾病［包括结节病、血色病、HIV 感染和恶性肿瘤（如乳腺癌）］。

当低钙血症患者伴有不适当的血清 PTH 水平降低时，可诊断甲状旁腺功能减退症。血磷水平通常处于正常值上限或超过正常范围，血浆 1,25（OH）$_2$D 水平降低。长期甲状旁腺功能减退症可能伴有 CT 和头颅 X 线平片显示的无症状基底节钙化。

甲状旁腺功能减退症的治疗是通过使用大剂量钙（元素钙剂量上限为 6 ～ 8 g/d）和活性维生素 D［1,25（OH）$_2$D；0.25 ～ 1.0 μg/d］来增加肠道钙吸收。该方案可能使肠道钙吸收显著增加并超过肾钙排泄能力。然而，这种治疗可加重高钙尿症，导致肾钙盐沉着症和肾结石，因此监测 24 h 尿钙水平至关重要。噻嗪类利尿剂可作为辅助治疗，促进肾钙重吸收、减少高钙尿症，并提高血清钙浓度。治疗目标应将血清钙浓度维持在正常值下限。

FDA 已批准重组 PTH 1-84 用于治疗慢性甲状旁腺功能减退症，其为减少大剂量钙和骨化三醇引起的不良反应提供了重要的治疗选择。

假性甲状旁腺功能减退症　假性甲状旁腺功能减退症是一组疾病，患者对 PTH 的作用不敏感。这种激素不敏感可能由信号传导蛋白 G$_{s\alpha}$ 的多种失活突变引

TABLE 12.2 Differential Diagnosis of Hypocalcemia

Hypoparathyroidism
  Surgical
  Idiopathic and autoimmune
  Infiltrative diseases
  Wilson's disease (copper)
  Hemochromatosis
  Sarcoidosis
  Metastatic (breast) cancer
  Congenital
  Isolated, sporadic
  DiGeorge syndrome
  Infant of mother with hyperparathyroidism
Hereditary
  X-linked
  Parathyroid gland calcium receptor (Gα11 subunit)–activating mutations
  Parathyroid hormone (PTH) signal peptide mutation
  GCM2 (formerly *GCMB*) mutation
Pseudohypoparathyroidism
  Type Ia: multiple hormone resistance, Albright hereditary osteodystrophy
  Type Ib: PTH resistance without other abnormalities
  Type Ic: specific PTH resistance, resulting from defect in catalytic subunit of PTH-receptor complex
  Type II: specific PTH resistance, postreceptor defect of adenylyl cyclase, undefined
Vitamin D disorders
  Absent ultraviolet exposure
  Vitamin D deficiency
  Fat malabsorption
  Vitamin D–dependent rickets, renal 1α-hydroxylase deficiency, 1,25-dihydroxyvitamin D–receptor defects
  Chronic renal failure
  Hepatic failure

Hypoalbuminemia
Sepsis
Hypermagnesemia and hypomagnesemia
Rapid bone formation
  Hungry bone syndrome after parathyroidectomy or thyroidectomy
  Osteoblastic metastases
  Vitamin D therapy of osteomalacia, rickets
Hyperphosphatemia
  Crush injury, rhabdomyolysis
  Renal failure
  Tumor lysis
  Excessive phosphate (PO_4) administration (PO, IV, PR)
Medications
  Mithramycin, plicamycin
  Bisphosphonates
  Denosumab
  Calcitonin
  Fluoride
  Ethylenediaminetetraacetic acid (EDTA)
  Citrate
  Intravenous contrast
  Foscarnet
  Cisplatin
Pancreatitis
  Hypoalbuminemia
  Hypomagnesemia
  Calcium soap formation

---

common form of pseudohypoparathyroidism, Type Ia, also known as *Albright hereditary osteodystrophy,* is associated with resistance to multiple hormones and has a classic phenotype: short stature, shortened fourth and fifth metacarpals and metatarsals, obesity, mental retardation, subcutaneous calcifications, and café au lait spots. Laboratory studies in these patients demonstrate hypocalcemia and hyperphosphatemia similar to hypoparathyroidism. However, PTH levels are paradoxically elevated. Treatment involves supplementation with calcium and active vitamin D analogs.

Vitamin D deficiency. Sufficient vitamin D is necessary for maintenance of serum calcium. Active vitamin D, 1,25(OH)$_2$D, is required for intestinal calcium absorption. In order to maintain sufficient vitamin D levels, individuals must have adequate intake of vitamin D from diet and supplements or sufficient sunlight exposure for cutaneous manufacture of vitamin D. As calcium and vitamin D are absorbed from the small intestine, patients with inflammatory gastrointestinal disease, including celiac disease or short-bowel syndrome, or prior upper intestinal surgery are at risk for vitamin D deficiency and hypocalcemia. Patients with hepatic disease commonly have vitamin D deficiency, due in part to impaired 25-hydroxylation. Because the majority of conversion of 25-hydroxyvitamin D to 1,25(OH)$_2$D occurs in the kidney (see Chapter 11), patients with reduced kidney function often have low 1,25(OH)$_2$D, which can cause reduced intestinal absorption of vitamin D and hypocalcemia. Severe vitamin D deficiency can result in osteomalacia or rickets (see Chapter 13). Certain genetic syndromes affecting vitamin D conversion or causing vitamin D resistance can result in severe hypocalcemia.

Long-term, high-dose treatment with older antiseizure medications such as phenytoin or phenobarbital or their derivatives may lead to hypocalcemia and osteomalacia.

Sepsis. Sepsis from both gram-positive and gram-negative organisms has been associated with hypocalcemia. The mechanisms for this are poorly understood. Although hypocalcemia occurring in the setting of sepsis is typically mild, its presence is associated with a poor prognosis.

Magnesium disorders. Hypocalcemia can result from low magnesium levels. This occurs most commonly in patients with alcoholism, malnutrition, intestinal malabsorption, and cisplatin-based chemotherapy. Magnesium deficiency causes a form of functional hypoparathyroidism that is due to decreased PTH secretion and resistance to PTH at the kidney and skeleton. These abnormalities can be quickly reversed with magnesium replacement. Paradoxically, in rare instances, hypermagnesemia can cause hypocalcemia. Magnesium, like calcium, is a divalent cation. In very high concentrations, it can mimic the actions of calcium and suppress PTH, causing hypoparathyroidism and hypocalcemia.

Hyperphosphatemia. Phosphate binds calcium avidly and therefore, excess can cause hypocalcemia. This can be seen in disorders that cause severe hyperphosphatemia including rhabdomyolysis (e.g., crush injuries), renal failure, and tumor lysis syndrome. Severe hyperphosphatemia can also be caused by ingestion of large amounts of phosphate-containing purgatives in preparation for colonoscopy, inadvertent perforation of the rectum during the administration of phosphate enemas, and administration of large doses of intravenous

表 12.2 低钙血症的鉴别诊断

甲状旁腺功能减退症	低白蛋白血症
手术后	感染中毒症
特发性和自身免疫性	高镁血症和低镁血症
浸润性疾病	快速骨形成
肝豆状核变性（Wilson 病）（铜）	甲状旁腺切除术或甲状腺切除术后骨饥饿综合征
血色病	成骨性骨转移
结节病	维生素 D 治疗骨软化症、佝偻病
转移癌（乳腺癌）	高磷血症
先天性	挤压伤、横纹肌溶解
孤立性、散发性	肾衰竭
DiGeorge 综合征	肿瘤溶解
母亲患有甲状旁腺功能亢进症的婴儿	过度补磷（磷酸盐）（口服、静脉输液、灌肠）
遗传性	药物
X 连锁遗传	普卡霉素
甲状旁腺钙受体（Gα11 亚基）激活性突变	双膦酸盐
甲状旁腺激素（PTH）信号肽突变	地舒单抗
GCM2（既往被称为 GCMB）突变	降钙素
假性甲状旁腺功能减退症	氟化物
Ⅰa 型：多激素抵抗、Albright 遗传性骨营养不良	乙二胺四乙酸（EDTA）
Ⅰb 型：PTH 抵抗而无其他异常	柠檬酸
Ⅰc 型：特异性 PTH 抵抗，由 PTH 受体复合物的催化亚基缺陷引起	静脉造影剂
Ⅱ型：特异性 PTH 抵抗，腺苷酸环化酶的受体后缺陷，未明确	膦甲酸
维生素 D 相关疾病	顺铂
无紫外线暴露	胰腺炎
维生素 D 缺乏症	低白蛋白血症
脂肪吸收不良	低镁血症
维生素 D 依赖性佝偻病、肾 1α- 羟化酶缺陷、1,25- 二羟维生素 D 受体缺陷	钙皂形成
慢性肾衰竭	
肝衰竭	

起。最常见的假性甲状旁腺功能减退症类型是 Ⅰa 型，又称 Albright 遗传性骨营养不良，与多种激素抵抗有关，患者具有典型的临床表型：身材矮小、第 4 和第 5 掌骨和跖骨缩短、肥胖症、智力低下、皮下钙化和咖啡斑。实验室检查可显示与甲状旁腺功能减退症类似的低钙血症和高磷血症，但患者的 PTH 水平反常性升高。治疗包括补充钙和活性维生素 D 类似物。

维生素 D 缺乏症 充足的维生素 D 是维持血清钙浓度所必需的。肠道钙吸收需要 $1,25(OH)_2D$ 的作用。为了保证充足的维生素 D，个体必须从饮食和补充剂中充分摄入足够的维生素 D，或皮肤接受充分的阳光照射以自身合成维生素 D。由于钙和维生素 D 在小肠被吸收，炎症性胃肠疾病（包括乳糜泻、短肠综合征）和上部小肠手术史的患者有发生维生素 D 缺乏症和低钙血症的风险。肝病患者通常合并维生素 D 缺乏症，部分原因是 25- 羟化作用受损。由于绝大部分 25- 羟维生素 D 在肾脏转化为 $1,25(OH)_2D$（见第 11 章），肾功能下降的患者通常 $1,25(OH)_2D$ 水平较低，进而导致肠道对维生素 D 的吸收减少和低钙血症。严重维生素 D 缺乏症可导致骨软化症或佝偻病（见第 13 章）。某些影响维生素 D 转化或引起维生素 D 抵抗的遗传综

合征可造成严重低钙血症。长期大剂量使用传统抗癫痫药（如苯妥英或苯巴比妥及其衍生物）可能导致低钙血症和骨软化症。

感染中毒症 由革兰氏阳性和革兰氏阴性菌引起的感染中毒症均可出现低钙血症。其发病机制尚不清楚。虽然感染中毒症引起的低钙血症通常较轻微，但与不良预后相关。

镁代谢疾病 低镁血症可导致低钙血症。常见于酒精中毒、营养不良、肠道吸收不良和接受以顺铂为基础的化疗的患者。镁缺乏会导致功能性甲状旁腺功能减退症，这是由 PTH 分泌减少及肾脏和骨骼对 PTH 抵抗所致。这些异常可通过镁替代治疗而迅速逆转。相反，在极少数情况下，高镁血症也会导致低钙血症。镁和钙均为二价阳离子，在非常高的浓度下，镁可以模拟钙的作用，抑制 PTH，导致甲状旁腺功能减退症和低钙血症。

高磷血症 磷酸盐与钙紧密结合，因此磷过量会导致低钙血症。导致严重高磷血症的疾病［包括横纹肌溶解（如挤压伤）、肾衰竭和肿瘤溶解综合征］均可引起低钙血症。严重高磷血症也可能是由于在准备结肠镜检查时摄入大量含磷酸盐的泻药、在使用磷酸盐灌肠的过程中意外发生直肠穿孔及静脉输注大量的磷。

phosphate. In these examples, the onset of hyperphosphatemia is acute, and hypocalcemia is immediate and severe. Seizures can occur as the earliest manifestation. Treatment involves reducing the serum phosphorus level. Intravenous calcium should not be given to hyperphosphatemic patients because calcium-phosphate salts can precipitate into soft tissues.

Recalcification and rapid bone formation. Increased rates of skeletal mineralization that exceed the rate of bone resorption lead to net calcium entry into the skeleton and can cause hypocalcemia. This classically occurs in patients with hyperparathyroidism following parathyroidectomy, a situation known as "hungry bone syndrome." In these patients, preoperative rates of bone turnover are very high but formation and resorption are coupled. Postoperatively, as PTH acutely drops, so do rates of osteoclastic bone resorption. However, an elevated rate of bone remineralization continues. As a result of this imbalance, there is a net influx of calcium and phosphorus into the skeleton. This disorder can persist for weeks after surgery and may require very high doses of calcium and vitamin D metabolites to treat. Hypocalcemia from rapid skeletal uptake can also occur in the setting of extensive osteoblastic bone metastases, most commonly observed in prostate or breast cancer.

Pancreatitis. In patients with pancreatitis, fatty acid soaps are formed by lipases released from the inflamed pancreas. The free lipases then autodigest omental and retroperitoneal fat into negatively charged ions that tightly bind calcium in the ECF, resulting in hypocalcemia. The hypocalcemia is reversible by calcium infusion and self-terminates when pancreatitis improves. The development of hypocalcemia in patients with pancreatitis is a poor prognostic sign.

Medications. Several medications can cause hypocalcemia, including those used to treat hypercalcemia and osteoporosis such as bisphosphonates, denosumab, and cinacalcet. Fluoride compounds (e.g., anesthetic gas), chelating agents such as ethylenediaminetetraacetic acid (EDTA) and citrate in stored blood products, radiographic intravenous contrast agents, the antiviral drug foscarnet, and chemotherapy including cisplatin, 5-fluorouracil, and leucovorin can all cause hypocalcemia. Patients with undiagnosed vitamin D deficiency may be particularly susceptible to developing hypocalcemia when they receive one of these medications.

DISORDERS OF PHOSPHATE METABOLISM

Hyperphosphatemia
Pathophysiology

Phosphate plays a key role in many ubiquitous cellular processes, including DNA synthesis and replication, energy generation and use, oxygen uptake and delivery by erythrocytes, and maintenance of the redox state (see Chapter 11). Hyperphosphatemia can develop due to one of three mechanisms: decreased renal excretion, increased phosphate load in the acute setting, and redistribution to the extracellular space. Chronic hyperphosphatemia can lead to soft tissue calcifications. Most diets naturally contain substantial quantities of phosphate, which is cleared by the kidney. However, as GFR declines below 20 to 30 mg/dL, the renal capacity to excrete phosphate diminishes. Patients with stage 4 and 5 CKD (GFR below 30 mL/min) often have some degree of hyperphosphatemia. As detailed above, excess phosphate will avidly bind calcium, and can cause hypocalcemia.

Symptoms and Signs

Hyperphosphatemia is usually identified incidentally on routine blood tests. There are no specific symptoms or signs.

Differential Diagnosis

The differential diagnosis of hyperphosphatemia is detailed in the following sections and in Table 12.3.

TABLE 12.3 Causes of Hyperphosphatemia
Artifactual
Hemolysis
Increased gastrointestinal intake
Rectal enemas
Oral Phospho-Soda purgatives
Gastrointestinal bleeding
Large phosphate loads
K-Phos
Blood transfusions
Redistribution to the extracellular space
Tumor lysis syndrome
Rhabdomyolysis (crush injury)
Hemolysis
Reduced renal clearance
Chronic or acute renal failure
Hypoparathyroidism
Acromegaly
Tumoral calcinosis

Pseudohyperphosphatemia. Hyperphosphatemia may occur artifactually as a result of hemolysis of red blood cells in blood collection tubes. This effect is also commonly seen with potassium, another ion with high intracellular concentrations. Hemolysis should be considered as a cause when unexplained hyperphosphatemia and hyperkalemia occur concurrently. In this circumstance, a new blood sample should be obtained and the levels repeated.

Reduced renal clearance. Renal clearance of phosphate is the main mechanism for maintaining phosphate homeostasis. Acute and chronic kidney disease can cause hyperphosphatemia. Parathyroid hormone promotes phosphate excretion in the proximal nephron. Therefore, patients who have hypoparathyroidism tend to have high-normal or frankly elevated serum phosphate values.

In *tumoral calcinosis*, the ability of the kidney to clear phosphate is defective, either because of genetic mutations in proteins involved in renal phosphate clearance or from advanced CKD. This reduced clearance leads to chronic hyperphosphatemia and the accumulation of calcium-phosphate salts around large joints of the appendicular skeleton. Children and adolescents have higher serum phosphate concentrations than adults and are more prone to this condition.

Increased gastrointestinal intake. Hyperphosphatemia can occur in the setting of excess oral phosphate loads. This most commonly occurs in patients using phosphate-containing purgatives as preparation for colonoscopy. Inadvertent perforation of the rectum during the administration of a Phospho-Soda enema, with delivery of large amounts of phosphate directly into the peritoneal cavity, can also cause hyperphosphatemia. Bleeding from the upper GI tract can also lead to delivery of a large GI phosphate load that is absorbed systemically, therefore leading to hyperphosphatemia.

Systemic phosphate loads. A large phosphate load delivered into the ECF through intravenous medications, or endogenous sources such as muscle or tumor necrosis, can result in hyperphosphatemia. Hyperphosphatemia is often seen in patients who receive large doses of potassium phosphate for hypokalemia (see Chapter 11).

Redistribution to the extracellular space. Hyperphosphatemia may result from the rapid destruction of large amounts of tissue. In tumor lysis syndrome, large tumors respond to chemotherapy with massive cell death and can release substantial amounts of phosphate. This is commonly seen with treatment of Burkitt lymphoma. In acute rhabdomyolysis, phosphate is released from damaged skeletal muscle.

在这些情况下，高磷血症呈急性发生，低钙血症可迅速发生且病情严重。癫痫发作可能是首发症状。治疗包括降低血清磷浓度。高磷血症患者不能采用静脉注射钙治疗，因为钙-磷酸盐可沉积到软组织中。

再矿化和快速骨形成　骨矿化的速率增加超过骨吸收的速率会使钙进入骨骼，并导致低钙血症。这通常发生在甲状旁腺功能亢进症患者行甲状旁腺切除术后，被称为"骨饥饿综合征"。这些患者术前的骨转换非常高，但骨形成和骨吸收是同步的。在术后，随着PTH水平急剧下降，破骨细胞的骨吸收率快速下降，而骨骼再矿化仍继续升高，钙和磷流入骨骼。这种状况可在术后持续数周，可能需要非常大剂量的钙和维生素 D 代谢产物来治疗。快速骨骼摄取引起的低钙血症也可发生在广泛成骨性骨转移中，最常见于前列腺癌或乳腺癌。

胰腺炎　胰腺炎症可释放脂肪酶形成脂肪酸皂。游离脂肪酶随后将大网膜和腹膜后的脂肪自体消化为带有负电荷的离子，并与 ECF 中的钙紧密结合，导致低钙血症。低钙血症可通过输注钙而获得逆转，并在胰腺炎改善时自行终止。胰腺炎患者发生低钙血症提示预后不良。

药物　多种药物可导致低钙血症，包括用于治疗高钙血症和骨质疏松症的药物，如双膦酸盐、地舒单抗和西那卡塞。氟化物化合物（如麻醉气体）、螯合剂［如储存血液制品的乙二胺四乙酸（EDTA）和柠檬酸］、静脉用影像学造影剂、抗病毒药物（膦甲酸）及化疗药物（如顺铂、5-氟尿嘧啶和亚叶酸）均可引起低钙血症。未诊断的维生素 D 缺乏症患者在接受这些药物治疗时更易出现低钙血症。

磷代谢紊乱

高磷血症

病理生理学

磷在许多细胞过程中发挥关键作用，包括 DNA 合成和复制、能量产生和利用、红细胞的氧摄取和传递，以及维持氧化还原状态（见第 11 章）。高磷血症的发生有以下 3 种机制：肾脏排泄减少、急性状况下磷酸盐负荷增加和细胞外部位再分布。慢性高磷血症可导致软组织钙化。绝大多数饮食中含有足量的磷，其进入体内后可被肾脏排出。然而，当 GFR 降至 20 ～ 30 mg/dl 以下时，肾脏排泄磷的能力减弱。4 期和 5 期慢性肾脏病（CKD）（GFR < 30 ml/min）的患者常有一定程度的高磷血症。如上所述，过量的磷酸盐可过多地结合钙，并引起低钙血症。

症状和体征

高磷血症通常是在常规血液化验中被偶然发现的。患者没有特殊的症状或体征。

表 12.3　高磷血症的病因
人为因素
溶血
胃肠道摄入增加
直肠灌肠剂
口服含磷酸盐的泻药
消化道出血
磷酸盐负荷增加
磷酸钾
输血
细胞外部位再分布
肿瘤溶解综合征
横纹肌溶解（挤压伤）
溶血
肾排泄减少
慢性或急性肾衰竭
甲状旁腺功能减退症
肢端肥大症
肿瘤性钙质沉着

鉴别诊断

高磷血症的鉴别诊断见下文和表 12.3。

假性高磷血症　高磷血症可由人为因素造成采血管中的血细胞发生溶血所致。这种现象也常见于另一种细胞内浓度较高的离子——钾。当高磷血症和高钾血症同时出现且无法解释时，溶血是需要考虑的一个原因。在这种情况下，需要重新获得新的血液样本并重复化验。

肾脏排泄减少　肾脏排泄磷是维持磷稳态的主要机制。急性和慢性肾脏病可引起高磷血症。PTH 能够促进近端肾单位对磷的排出，因此，甲状旁腺功能减退症患者的血清磷浓度通常为正常值上限或超过正常范围。

当出现肿瘤性钙质沉着时，肾脏排泄磷的能力受损，原因包括参与肾脏磷排泄的蛋白质发生基因突变和晚期 CKD。这种排泄减少可导致慢性高磷血症，并造成钙-磷酸盐在四肢骨的大关节周围沉积。儿童和青少年的血清磷浓度高于成人，故更易出现这种情况。

胃肠道摄入增加　口服过量磷酸盐可导致高磷血症。最常发生于因准备结肠镜检查而使用含磷酸盐的泻药的患者。在使用磷酸钠灌肠剂时发生直肠意外穿孔可使大量磷酸盐直接进入腹膜腔，导致高磷血症。上消化道出血也可导致胃肠道大量磷负荷并被机体吸收，从而造成高磷血症。

全身磷酸盐负荷　静脉使用药物或内源性因素（肌肉或肿瘤坏死等）可使大量磷酸盐进入 ECF，导致高磷血症。高磷血症常见于因治疗低钾血症而使用大剂量磷酸钾的患者（见第 11 章）。

细胞外部位再分布　高磷血症可能由大量组织的快速破坏所致。肿瘤溶解综合征时，大体积的肿瘤对化疗有反应，产生大量细胞死亡并释放大量的磷，常见于伯基特淋巴瘤的治疗。在急性横纹肌溶解中，磷可从受损的骨骼肌中释放出来。严重溶血时，储存在

In severe hemolysis, phosphate stored in red blood cells is released and moves to the extracellular space. In each of these conditions, renal impairment is also common and the excess phosphate combined with worsening renal dysfunction can result in progressive renal failure, severe hypocalcemia, seizures, and even death.

Hypophosphatemia
Symptoms and Signs

Because phosphate plays such a ubiquitous and critical role in cellular processes, low phosphate levels can be life threatening. Hypophosphatemia can result in generalized, nonspecific symptoms and signs ranging from generalized weakness and malaise, to hypotension, respiratory failure, congestive heart failure, and coma. Hypophosphatemia often occurs in critically ill patients. These patients are at high risk because of limited oral nutrition, as well as exposure to intravenous diuretics and saline infusions that accelerate renal phosphate losses. With correction of serum phosphate, patients can have complete recovery of mental status and respiratory capacity.

Chronic hypophosphatemia leads to defects in skeletal mineralization, a phenomenon called *rickets* in children or *osteomalacia* in adults. These syndromes produce weakness, bone pain, bowing of the long bones, and fractures or pseudofractures (see Chapter 13). Hypophosphatemia can go unnoticed if phosphate is not routinely checked because symptoms are nonspecific. Under-mineralization can cause low bone mineral density and patients with osteomalacia may be mistaken for having osteoporosis if not properly identified. This is a critical distinction because osteoporosis treatment can actually exacerbate the underlying mineralization disorder. As with acute hypophosphatemia in critically ill patients, patients with chronic hypophosphatemia will dramatically improve with correction of phosphate. Bone pain resolves and wheelchair-bound patients can regain full ambulatory ability.

Differential Diagnosis

Hypophosphatemia can result from excessive renal phosphate loss, decreased intestinal absorption, or intracellular shifts of phosphate from the ECF (Table 12.4). Once a low serum phosphate has been found, urine collection for measurement of the maximum tubular reabsorption of phosphate (TmP) can help to identify the cause (see Chapter 11). In the setting of a low serum phosphate, renal reabsorption should be high as a compensatory response. A low TmP in a patient with hypophosphatemia is therefore indicative of a renal deficit.

Excessive renal phosphate losses. Patients with hypophosphatemia resulting from renal losses will have a low TmP. Inappropriately increased renal phosphate excretion may be due to the presence of a circulating factor versus an intrinsic defect in renal phosphate reabsorption. PTH is phosphaturic, and HPT can cause hypophosphatemia in patients with normal renal function. Hypophosphatemia can be seen in patients with PHPT and in SHPT due to vitamin D deficiency and calcium malabsorption. Vitamin D deficiency can lead to decreased gastrointestinal calcium absorption and secondary HPT, resulting in increased urinary phosphate excretion. A low serum phosphate level may be the first clue to severe vitamin D deficiency. PTHrP is also phosphaturic, and as a result, patients with humoral hypercalcemia of malignancy are commonly hypophosphatemic.

Certain genetic disorders may lead to severe renal phosphate wasting (see Chapter 13). Most of these genetic disorders result in elevated levels of fibroblast growth factor 23 (FGF23), a circulating protein that both inhibits intestinal phosphate absorption and decreases renal phosphate reabsorption, resulting in hypophosphatemia. These disorders include X-linked hypophosphatemia (XLH), also called *vitamin*

TABLE 12.4 **Causes of Hypophosphatemia**
Inadequate phosphate (PO_4) intake
Starvation
Malabsorption
PO_4-binding antacid use
Alcoholism
Renal PO_4 losses
Primary, secondary, or tertiary hyperparathyroidism
Humoral hypercalcemia of malignancy (parathyroid hormone–related protein)
Diuretics, calcitonin
X-linked hypophosphatemic rickets
Autosomal dominant hypophosphatemic rickets
Oncogenic osteomalacia
Fanconi syndrome
Alcoholism
Excessive skeletal mineralization
Hungry bone syndrome after parathyroidectomy
Osteoblastic metastases
Healing osteomalacia, rickets
PO_4 shift into extracellular fluid
Recovery from metabolic acidosis
Respiratory alkalosis
Starvation refeeding, intravenous glucose

D–resistant rickets, in which there is an inactivating mutation in the enzyme PHEX that regulates FGF23. In autosomal dominant hypophosphatemic rickets (ADHR), there are mutations in FGF23 that disrupt its breakdown. Oncogenic osteomalacia or *tumor-induced osteomalacia* is an acquired renal phosphate-wasting syndrome. In this disorder, mesenchymal tumors secrete excess amounts of FGF23. Acquired or inherited diffuse proximal renal tubular disorders, such as Fanconi syndrome, may lead to hypophosphatemia as a result of renal phosphate wasting.

Thiazide and loop diuretics are potent phosphaturic agents, and their use without phosphate replacement therapy can lead to hypophosphatemia. Excessive ethanol can also have this effect. Tenofovir, an antiretroviral medication that is increasingly used for the treatment and prevention of HIV infection, can also induce renal phosphate wasting. In some cases, tenofovir can cause Fanconi syndrome, with renal loss of glucose, uric acid, amino acids, and bicarbonate in addition to phosphate. As a result of significant phosphate loss, these patients can present with bone pain, weakness, and fractures because of skeletal demineralization and osteomalacia.

Decreased intestinal absorption. Hypophosphatemia that results from inadequate phosphate intake will be associated with a high TmP. Because most foods are rich in phosphate, it is rare for an individual with a normal diet to develop phosphate deficiency. However, deficiency can occur in settings of severe caloric deprivation, such as anorexia nervosa, prisoner-of-war camps, prolonged critical illness, malabsorption syndromes, and chronic alcoholism. In the first three disorders, caloric intake is low and little phosphate is consumed. Conversely, in alcoholism, overall caloric intake may be high but is primarily derived from alcohol, which does not contain phosphate. The use of phosphate-binding antacids such as aluminum hydroxide gels may lead to severe phosphate deficiency, hypophosphatemia, and osteomalacia.

Intracellular phosphate shift. Phosphate can be shifted from serum into the intracellular compartment as a result of increased formation of phosphorylated carbohydrate compounds. Insulin increases the rate of glucose uptake into cells and its subsequent phosphorylation to

红细胞中的磷酸盐被释放出来并转移到细胞外部位。在这些情况下，肾损害也很常见，磷过多合并肾功能不全恶化可导致进行性肾衰竭、严重低钙血症、癫痫发作，甚至死亡。

低磷血症

症状和体征

由于磷在细胞中发挥非常广泛和重要的作用，低磷血症可能危及生命。低磷血症可导致非特异性的全身症状和体征，从全身乏力和不适到低血压、呼吸衰竭、充血性心力衰竭和昏迷。危重症患者常发生低磷血症。这些高危患者由于摄入营养有限、静脉应用利尿剂和生理盐水，导致肾脏磷酸盐丢失加速。通过纠正血清磷浓度，患者的精神状态和呼吸功能可完全恢复。

慢性低磷血症会导致骨矿化障碍，这种现象在儿童期被称为佝偻病，在成人期被称为骨软化症。这些疾病表现为乏力、骨痛、长骨弯曲变形、骨折或假骨折（见第 13 章）。由于症状缺乏特异性，如果不常规检查血磷浓度，低磷血症可能会被忽视。骨骼矿化不足可造成骨密度降低，若未正确识别，骨软化症可能被误诊为骨质疏松症。鉴别诊断很重要，因为骨质疏松症的治疗实际上会加剧潜在的矿化障碍。与危重症患者的急性低磷血症相同，慢性低磷血症患者在血磷浓度被纠正后，病情可明显改善。骨痛逐渐缓解，需要使用轮椅的患者可完全恢复行动能力。

鉴别诊断

低磷血症可由肾脏磷排泄增加、肠道吸收减少或磷从 ECF 转移至细胞内引起（表 12.4）。一旦发现低磷血症，收集尿液测定肾小管最大磷重吸收（TmP）有助于明确病因（见第 11 章）。在低磷血症时，肾脏的磷重吸收应增加，这是一种代偿性反应。因此，当低磷血症伴随 TmP 降低时，提示患者存在肾功能不全。

肾脏排泄增加　因肾脏排泄增加导致低磷血症的患者的 TmP 降低。不适当的肾脏排泄增加可能是由于存在循环因子，而不是由肾脏磷酸盐重吸收的内在缺陷所致。PTH 可促进尿磷酸盐排出，因此 HPT 可导致肾功能正常的患者出现低磷血症。PHPT 或由维生素 D 缺乏症和钙吸收不良造成 SHPT 的患者均可出现低磷血症。维生素 D 缺乏症可导致胃肠道钙吸收减少和 SHPT，使尿磷酸盐排泄增加。低磷血症可能是严重维生素 D 缺乏症的第一个线索。PTHrP 也能促进尿磷酸盐排泄，因此，恶性肿瘤体液性高钙血症的患者通常出现低磷血症。

某些遗传病可造成严重肾脏磷酸盐丢失（见第 13 章）。其中许多疾病可引起成纤维细胞生长因子 23（FGF23）水平升高，FGF23 是一种循环蛋白，可抑制肠道磷酸盐吸收并降低肾脏磷酸盐的重吸收，从而导致低磷血症。这些遗传病包括 X 连锁低血磷性佝偻病

表 12.4　低磷血症的病因

磷酸盐（PO₄）不适当摄入
　饥饿
　吸收不良
　应用可结合 PO₄ 的抗酸剂
　酒精中毒
肾脏磷酸盐丢失
　原发性、继发性或三发性甲状旁腺功能亢进症
　恶性肿瘤体液性高钙血症（甲状旁腺激素相关蛋白）
　利尿剂、降钙素
　X 连锁低血磷性佝偻病
　常染色体显性遗传性低血磷性佝偻病
　肿瘤性骨软化症
　范科尼综合征
　酗酒
骨矿化过度
　甲状旁腺切除术后的骨饥饿综合征
　成骨性骨转移
　骨软化症、佝偻病恢复过程中
PO₄ 转移至细胞外液
　代谢性酸中毒恢复
　呼吸性碱中毒
　饥饿再喂养、静脉应用葡萄糖

（XLH），又称为维生素 D 抵抗性佝偻病，由 FGF23 的调节酶 PHEX 发生失活突变所致。在常染色体显性遗传性低血磷性佝偻病（ADHR）中，FGF23 发生突变，使其降解受到破坏。肿瘤性骨软化症是一种获得性肾脏磷酸盐丢失综合征，由间叶性肿瘤分泌过量的 FGF23 所致。获得性或遗传性弥漫性近端肾小管疾病（如范科尼综合征）可导致肾脏磷酸盐丢失，引发低磷血症。

噻嗪类和袢利尿剂是强效的促尿磷酸盐排泄的药物，若使用药物后未进行磷酸盐补充，可引起低磷血症。过量的乙醇也可产生相同效果。替诺福韦是一种抗逆转录病毒药物，越来越多地被用于预防和治疗 HIV 感染，它也可引起肾脏磷酸盐丢失。在一些病例中，替诺福韦可引发范科尼综合征，导致肾脏除排泄磷酸盐外，还会排泄葡萄糖、尿酸、氨基酸和碳酸氢盐。由于显著的磷酸盐丢失，这些患者可因骨矿化不良和骨软化症而出现骨痛、乏力和骨折。

肠道吸收减少　因磷酸盐摄入不足导致低磷血症的患者的 TmP 升高。因为大多数食物富含磷酸盐，故饮食正常的个体很少发生磷缺乏。然而，磷缺乏可见于严重能量剥夺的情况，如神经性厌食、战俘营、长期危重疾病、吸收不良综合征和长期酗酒。在前 3 种情况中，患者能量摄入很低，磷酸盐摄入极少。相反，酗酒患者的总能量摄入可能很高，但主要来自于酒精，其中不含磷酸盐。使用与磷酸盐相结合的抗酸剂（如氢氧化铝凝胶）可能导致严重的磷缺乏、低磷血症和骨软化症。

细胞内磷酸盐转移　磷酸化碳水化合物形成增加时，磷酸盐可从血清转移到细胞内。胰岛素可促进细胞摄取葡萄糖，葡萄糖随后被磷酸化，形成 6-磷酸葡

glucose-6-phosphate. Patients with diabetic ketoacidosis require phosphate repletion to avoid hypophosphatemia. In the setting of significantly depleted phosphate reserves, rapid consumption of oral carbohydrates or parenteral glucose can precipitate profound hypophosphatemia and sudden death due to respiratory or circulatory failure.

Increased bone mineralization rates may result in large amounts of phosphate entering the skeleton and hypophosphatemia. One example is the hungry bone syndrome that occurs after parathyroidectomy when there is an acute drop in PTH and in bone resorption (see section on hypocalcemia). Hypophosphatemia as a result of increased skeletal uptake can also be seen in patients with osteoblastic metastases and after treatment of vitamin D–deficient rickets or osteomalacia from vitamin D deficiency.

Treatment

Oral phosphate replacement is the optimal method for correction of hypophosphatemia. Phosphate is usually provided in two to four divided doses of 2000 to 4000 mg/day. Doses greater than 1000 to 2000 mg/day can cause diarrhea and other gastrointestinal side effects, particularly at initiation. Gradual increases in doses may be helpful for minimizing GI effects. Intravenous phosphate should be given only to patients for whom oral administration is not an option. Intravenous dosages up to 500 to 800 mg/day may be required. Frequent monitoring of serum phosphate, calcium, and creatinine levels is necessary. Burosumab, a monoclonal antibody to FGF23, was recently approved by the FDA to treat XLH.

DISORDERS OF MAGNESIUM METABOLISM

Hypermagnesemia
Symptoms and Signs

Clinically significant hypermagnesemia is uncommon. The most common symptom is drowsiness. On exam, patients have hyporeflexia and if untreated, eventual neuromuscular, respiratory, and cardiovascular collapse. Hypermagnesemia can also lead to hypocalcemia through effects on PTH (see "Hypocalcemia" section).

Differential Diagnosis

Hypermagnesemia is typically encountered in two settings: patients with severe renal failure who receive magnesium-containing antacids and in women who receive large doses of intravenous magnesium sulfate for eclampsia or preeclampsia (Table 12.5). Mild hypermagnesemia is common in patients on dialysis, but severe hypermagnesemia occurs only in the settings of renal failure accompanied by parenteral or oral magnesium salt administration, such as the use of magnesium-containing antacids or phosphate binders. In women being treated for eclampsia, hypermagnesemia occurs but is rarely severe, as patients are typically closely monitored by labs and physical exam.

Hypomagnesemia
Symptoms and Signs

Hypomagnesemia is common, particularly among critically ill patients in the ICU setting. As with hypophosphatemia, it is not always detected. Magnesium is key to many biologic processes, and hypomagnesemia may cause hypocalcemia, seizures, and paresthesias as well as many neuromuscular, cardiovascular, and respiratory symptoms.

Differential Diagnosis

The differential diagnosis of hypomagnesemia is reviewed in the following sections and in Table 12.5.

Inadequate intake. Inadequate intake of magnesium is common among alcoholics and other malnourished individuals. It may occur as

---

TABLE 12.5 Causes of Hypermagnesemia and Hypomagnesemia

Hypermagnesemia
  Renal failure accompanied by magnesium antacid use
  Parenteral magnesium sulfate administration for eclampsia
Hypomagnesemia
  Inadequate intake
  Starvation
  Malabsorption
  Alcoholism
  Vomiting, nasogastric suction
  Excessive renal losses
  Diuretics
  Saline infusion
  Secondary aldosteronism
  Cirrhosis
  Congestive heart failure
  Osmotic diuresis, hyperglycemia
  Cisplatin, aminoglycoside antibiotics, amphotericin
  Hypokalemia
  Hypercalcemia, hypercalciuria
  Proximal tubular diseases
  Genetic defects

---

part of an intestinal malabsorption syndrome and in association with continuous vomiting or nasogastric suctioning.

Excessive renal losses. Excessive renal losses of magnesium are common in clinical practice. Thiazide and loop diuretics cause renal magnesium losses, and saline infusions can have a similar effect. Aldosterone can induce renal magnesium loss. This can be seen in patients with primary hyperaldosteronism and more commonly in the secondary hyperaldosteronism from cirrhosis, volume depletion, and congestive heart failure. Osmotic diuresis can cause renal magnesium loss as well, which is commonly seen in patients with poorly controlled diabetes mellitus. Certain nephrotoxic drugs such as cisplatin, aminoglycoside antibiotics, and amphotericin induce proximal renal tubular injury and severe renal magnesium wasting. Hypokalemia, hypercalcemia, and hypercalciuria can also lead to increased renal magnesium excretion. In diseases that lead to proximal tubular injury, such as Fanconi syndrome and interstitial nephritis, magnesium wasting can occur.

Treatment

Magnesium can be replaced intramuscularly or intravenously. A typical treatment regimen is 24 to 48 mEq (3 to 6 g) of magnesium sulfate given over 24 hours. Oral magnesium salts such as magnesium oxide are also available; however, oral dosing is limited to mild cases requiring low doses because of the cathartic effects of high doses of oral magnesium.

SUGGESTED READINGS

Bilezikian JP, Bandeira L, Khan A, et al: Hyperparathyroidism, Lancet 391(10116):168–178, 2018.

Bilezikian JP, editor: The American Society for Bone and Mineral Research primer on metabolic bone diseases and disorders of mineral metabolism. Regulation of calcium homeostasis, ed 9, Orlando, FL, 2019, American Society for Bone and Mineral Research, pp 165–172.

Bilezikian JP, editor: The American Society for Bone and Mineral Research primer on metabolic bone diseases and disorders of mineral metabolism.

萄糖。糖尿病酮症酸中毒患者需要补充磷酸盐，以避免发生低磷血症。在磷酸盐储备明显耗竭时，快速口服碳水化合物或肠外应用葡萄糖可导致严重低磷血症，从而造成患者呼吸或循环衰竭，引发猝死。

骨矿化加快可导致大量的磷酸盐进入骨骼而引发低磷血症。一个例证是甲状旁腺切除术后 PTH 水平和骨吸收快速下降，发生骨饥饿综合征（见上文"低钙血症"）。肿瘤发生成骨性骨转移的患者及维生素 D 缺乏症导致的佝偻病和骨软化症患者，在使用维生素 D 治疗后可出现骨骼摄取磷增加导致的低磷血症。

治疗

口服补充磷酸盐治疗是纠正低磷血症的最佳方法。磷酸盐的补充剂量为 2000 ～ 4000 mg/d，分 2 ～ 4 次口服。剂量超过 1000 ～ 2000 mg/d 时，可出现腹泻和其他胃肠道不良反应，尤其在起始服药时。逐渐增加剂量可减少药物对胃肠道的影响。不能口服的患者可选择静脉应用磷酸盐。静脉应用的最高剂量为 500 ～ 800 mg/d。必须监测血清磷酸盐、血清钙和血清肌酐水平。布罗索尤单抗（FGF23 的单克隆抗体）近期被 FDA 批准用于治疗 XLH。

镁代谢疾病

高镁血症

症状和体征

临床上显著的高镁血症并不常见。最常见的症状是嗜睡。患者在体格检查时可出现反射减退。如果不治疗，最终会出现神经肌肉功能障碍、呼吸衰竭和心血管衰竭。高镁血症也可通过影响 PTH 而导致低钙血症（见上文"低钙血症"）。

鉴别诊断

高镁血症通常见于两种情况：严重肾衰竭患者使用含镁抗酸剂，子痫或先兆子痫女性患者静脉使用大剂量硫酸镁（表 12.5）。透析患者常出现轻度高镁血症，但严重的高镁血症仅发生在肾衰竭患者口服或肠外使用镁盐（如使用含镁抗酸剂或磷结合剂）的情况下。接受治疗的子痫患者可发生高镁血症，但严重者极少，因为患者通常正在接受体格检查和实验室检查的密切监测。

低镁血症

症状和体征

低镁血症很常见，特别是在 ICU 的危重患者中。与低磷血症相同，低镁血症不易被发现。镁对于许多生物学过程非常重要，低镁血症可导致低钙血症、癫痫发作和感觉异常，以及许多神经肌肉、心血管和呼吸系统症状。

鉴别诊断

低镁血症的鉴别诊断见下文表 12.5。

表 12.5　高镁血症和低镁血症的病因
高镁血症
肾衰竭患者使用含镁抗酸剂
子痫患者使用肠外硫酸镁治疗
低镁血症
摄入不足
饥饿
吸收不良
酒精中毒
呕吐、鼻胃管引流
肾丢失增多
利尿剂
生理盐水输注
继发性醛固酮增多症
肝硬化
充血性心力衰竭
渗透性利尿、高血糖
顺铂、氨基糖苷类抗生素、两性霉素
低钾血症
高钙血症、高钙尿症
近端小管疾病
遗传缺陷

摄入不足　酗酒和营养不良的个体常存在镁摄入不足。低镁血症可作为肠吸收不良综合征的一部分，也可见于持续性呕吐或鼻胃管引流的患者。

肾脏排泄增多　在临床实践中，肾脏镁丢失增加较常见。噻嗪类利尿剂和袢利尿剂会导致肾脏镁丢失，生理盐水也有类似的效果。醛固酮可引起肾脏镁丢失，可见于原发性醛固酮增多症，更常见于肝硬化、容量不足和充血性心力衰竭引起的继发性醛固酮增多症。渗透性利尿也可导致肾脏镁丢失，常见于血糖控制不佳的糖尿病患者。一些肾毒性药物（如顺铂、氨基糖苷类抗生素和两性霉素）可导致近端肾小管损伤和严重的肾脏镁丢失。低钾血症、高钙血症和高尿钙症也可导致肾脏镁排泄增加。引起近端肾小管损伤的疾病（如范科尼综合征和间质性肾炎）可引起肾脏镁丢失。

治疗

可通过肌内注射或静脉注射来补充镁。经典的治疗方案是在 24 h 内给予 12 ～ 24 mmol（3 ～ 6 g）硫酸镁。还可选择口服镁制剂（如氧化镁），但由于口服大剂量镁剂可引起腹泻，口服制剂仅用于需要小剂量补充的轻度低镁血症患者。

推荐阅读

Bilezikian JP, Bandeira L, Khan A, et al: Hyperparathyroidism, Lancet 391(10116):168–178, 2018.

Bilezikian JP, editor: The American Society for Bone and Mineral Research primer on metabolic bone diseases and disorders of mineral metabolism. Regulation of calcium homeostasis, ed 9, Orlando, FL, 2019, American Society for Bone and Mineral Research, pp 165–172.

Bilezikian JP, editor: The American Society for Bone and Mineral Research primer on metabolic bone diseases and disorders of mineral metabolism.

Magnesium homeostasis, ed 9, Orlando, FL, 2019, American Society for Bone and Mineral Research, pp 173–179.

Bilezikian JP, editor: The American Society for Bone and Mineral Research primer on metabolic bone diseases and disorders of mineral metabolism. Primary Hyperparathyroidism, ed 9, Orlando, FL, 2019, American Society for Bone and Mineral Research, pp 619–628.

Bilezikian JP, editor: The American Society for Bone and Mineral Research primer on metabolic bone diseases and disorders of mineral metabolism. Non-Parathyroid hypercalcemia, ed 9, Orlando, FL, 2019, American Society for Bone and Mineral Research, pp 639–645.

Bilezikian JP, editor: The American Society for Bone and Mineral Research primer on metabolic bone diseases and disorders of mineral metabolism. Disorders of Phosphate Homeostasis, ed 9, Orlando, FL, 2019, American Society for Bone and Mineral Research, pp 674–683.

Bilezikian JP, editor: The American Society for Bone and Mineral Research primer on metabolic bone diseases and disorders of mineral metabolism.

Disorders of mineral metabolism in childhood, ed 9, Orlando, FL, 2019, American Society for Bone and Mineral Research, pp 705–712.

Christov M, Juppner H: Insights from genetic disorders of phosphate homeostasis, Semin Nephrol 33:143–157, 2013.

Kinoshita Y, Fukumoto S: X-Linked hypophosphatemia and FGF23-related hypophosphatemic diseases: prospect for new treatment, Endocr Rev 39(3):274–291, 2018.

Nazeri AS, Reilly Jr RF: Hereditary etiologies of hypomagnesemia, Nat Clin Pract Nephrol 4:80–89, 2008.

Nesbitt MA, Hanan FM, Howles SA, et al: Mutations affecting G-protein subunit alpha-11 in hypercalcemia and hypocalcemia, N Engl J Med 368:2476–2486, 2013.

Stewart AF: Translational implications of the parathyroid calcium receptor, N Engl J Med 351:324–326, 2004.

Zagzag J, Hu MI, Fisher SB, et al: Hypercalcemia and cancer: differential diagnosis and treatment, CA Cancer J Clin 68(5):377–386, 2018.

Magnesium homeostasis, ed 9, Orlando, FL, 2019, American Society for Bone and Mineral Research, pp 173–179.

Bilezikian JP, editor: The American Society for Bone and Mineral Research primer on metabolic bone diseases and disorders of mineral metabolism. Primary Hyperparathyroidism, ed 9, Orlando, FL, 2019, American Society for Bone and Mineral Research, pp 619–628.

Bilezikian JP, editor: The American Society for Bone and Mineral Research primer on metabolic bone diseases and disorders of mineral metabolism. Non-Parathyroid hypercalcemia, ed 9, Orlando, FL, 2019, American Society for Bone and Mineral Research, pp 639–645.

Bilezikian JP, editor: The American Society for Bone and Mineral Research primer on metabolic bone diseases and disorders of mineral metabolism. Disorders of Phosphate Homeostasis, ed 9, Orlando, FL, 2019, American Society for Bone and Mineral Research, pp 674–683.

Bilezikian JP, editor: The American Society for Bone and Mineral Research primer on metabolic bone diseases and disorders of mineral metabolism.

Disorders of mineral metabolism in childhood, ed 9, Orlando, FL, 2019, American Society for Bone and Mineral Research, pp 705–712.

Christov M, Juppner H: Insights from genetic disorders of phosphate homeostasis, Semin Nephrol 33:143–157, 2013.

Kinoshita Y, Fukumoto S: X-Linked hypophosphatemia and FGF23-related hypophosphatemic diseases: prospect for new treatment, Endocr Rev 39(3):274–291, 2018.

Nazeri AS, Reilly Jr RF: Hereditary etiologies of hypomagnesemia, Nat Clin Pract Nephrol 4:80–89, 2008.

Nesbitt MA, Hanan FM, Howles SA, et al: Mutations affecting G-protein subunit alpha-11 in hypercalcemia and hypocalcemia, N Engl J Med 368:2476–2486, 2013.

Stewart AF: Translational implications of the parathyroid calcium receptor, N Engl J Med 351:324–326, 2004.

Zagzag J, Hu MI, Fisher SB, et al: Hypercalcemia and cancer: differential diagnosis and treatment, CA Cancer J Clin 68(5):377–386, 2018.

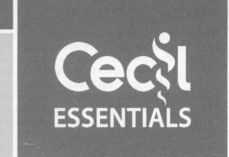

Metabolic Bone Diseases

Marcella D. Walker, Thomas J. Weber

INTRODUCTION

Metabolic bone disease (MBD) is an umbrella term that describes a heterogeneous group of skeletal disorders due to focal or diffuse alterations in bone remodeling and/or mineralization, often with associated abnormalities in mineral metabolism. Bone mineral density (BMD) is usually affected, although in some cases is normal. Etiology varies by disorder but includes metabolic, pathophysiologic, nutritional, genetic, toxic, infectious, and other causes. This family of disorders encompasses common conditions such as osteoporosis (see Chapter 14), less common conditions such as osteomalacia, as well as rare disorders including osteopetrosis. This chapter provides an overview with a focus on the more common diseases (Table 13.1). Normal skeletal homeostasis and histopathology are reviewed in Chapter 11 and Fig. 13.1A.

The clinical presentation of MBD is variable, ranging from asymptomatic incidental findings on laboratory tests, or radiographs, to disabling bone pain, muscle weakness, skeletal deformity, and fractures. Common laboratory and radiologic tests are useful in the evaluation of MBD and can often be diagnostic (Table 13.2 and 13.3). The "gold standard" for assessing both static and dynamic bone metabolism, although rarely required based on clinical history, remains tetracycline-labeled undecalcified bone biopsy of the anterior iliac crest. Bone biopsy allows assessment of osteoclast and osteoblast activity as well as osteoid mineralization. Undecalcified sections (see Fig. 13.1A to F) are necessary because the acid-mediated decalcification performed during routine pathology removes calcium and cannot distinguish between mineralized mature bone and unmineralized osteoid that may be normal or pathologic. Because tetracycline is incorporated into hydroxyapatite crystals as osteoid mineralizes and fluoresces under fluorescence microscopy, administration to patients before biopsy allows evaluation of the rates and effectiveness of bone formation and mineralization (see Fig. 13.1B and F).

PAGET'S DISEASE OF BONE

Paget's disease, or *osteitis deformans*, is the second most common MBD after osteoporosis, affecting 2% to 3% of adults over age 55 years in the United States. Incidence varies geographically and by race/ethnicity (most frequent in those of European descent) and may be declining. Paget's disease is usually a focal disorder of bone remodeling, in contrast to many others, such as osteoporosis, that affect the entire skeleton. Paget's disease may be *monostotic* or *polyostotic* (affecting one vs. multiple bones). Original lesions may expand, but new lesions rarely develop. It may involve any skeletal site, but the pelvis, vertebrae, skull, femur, and tibia are most commonly affected.

Paget's disease is characterized by an increase in bone resorption by abnormal osteoclasts, followed by rapid formation of poorly organized,

structurally weak "woven" bone (see Fig. 13.1C). The markedly increased osteoblast activity accounts for the typical sclerotic lesions observed on plain radiographs (Fig. 13.2A to C), the increased uptake of radionuclide on bone scan (see Fig. 13.2D), and the concomitant increase in serum levels of alkaline phosphatase, the latter of which is a protein byproduct of bone formation and the biochemical hallmark of Paget's disease. The pathogenesis of Paget's disease is unknown, but both genetic variants and viruses may contribute. Up to 30% with Paget's have a familial history and several genes have been implicated, including *SQSTM1*, *ZNF687*, *CSF-1*, *RANK*, and *PML* among others. Evidence suggests Paget's disease may result from chronic paramyxovirus infection with measles, respiratory syncytial virus or canine distemper virus.

Most patients are asymptomatic and diagnosed incidentally, either by increased serum alkaline phosphatase level on routine testing or on radiographs obtained for other reasons. Depending on the location and extent of lesions, however, patients may have bone pain, skeletal deformities including long bone bowing, fractures, osteoarthritis, and signs of nerve compression (e.g., deafness, spinal stenosis). Rare sequelae include hypercalcemia (in immobilized patients) and high-output cardiac failure. Because pagetic lesions are highly vascular, the skin over affected bones may be warm. The most feared (rare) complication is development of osteosarcoma in a pagetic lesion (<1%).

Paget's disease is typically diagnosed using biochemical markers of bone turnover and radiologic studies. In most patients, elevated total serum alkaline phosphatase is an adequate and sensitive indicator of disease activity. However, the serum level of bone-specific alkaline phosphatase may be a more sensitive indicator in those with low disease activity or if hepatic-derived alkaline phosphatase levels are low. A bone scan at diagnosis defines the location and extent of pagetic lesions (see Fig. 13.2D). Radiographs of the affected areas can confirm Paget's disease and are useful for evaluating complications and local disease progression (see Fig. 13.2A to C).

Therapeutic goals include relief of symptoms and prevention of complications. Indications for treatment include alleviating symptoms (e.g., bone pain, headache, neurologic complications), decreasing blood flow preoperatively to minimize bleeding during elective surgery involving a pagetic site, managing hypercalcemia, and preventing future complications of progressive local disease (bowing of the long bones, hearing loss due to temporal bone involvement, and neurologic complications from foramen magnum or vertebral involvement). Moderate quality evidence exists only for pain reduction with bisphosphonate therapy.

Treatment of Paget's disease involves a combination of nonpharmacologic (i.e., physical therapy) and pharmacologic therapy, including antiresorptive agents and analgesics. Bisphosphonates, the mainstay of treatment, decrease bone resorption at pagetic sites by

代谢性骨病

王鸥 译 姜艳 审校 夏维波 通审

引言

代谢性骨病（MBD）是一个总称，描述了局部或弥漫性骨重建和（或）矿化改变导致的一组异质性骨骼疾病，通常伴有矿物质代谢异常。患者的骨密度（BMD）通常受损，但在某些情况下是正常的。MBD的病因各异，包括代谢性、病理生理性、营养性、遗传性、中毒性、感染性及其他原因。这组疾病包括常见的疾病（如骨质疏松症）（见第 14 章）、较少见的疾病（如骨软化症）及罕见疾病（如骨硬化症）。本章主要介绍较常见的疾病（表 13.1）。正常骨稳态和组织病理学见第 11 章和图 13.1A。

MBD 的临床表现多变，范围可从无症状而在实验室检查或影像学检查中偶然被发现，到导致活动受限的骨痛、肌无力、骨畸形及骨折。常见的实验室和影像学检查可用于评估 MBD，且常具有诊断价值（表 13.2 和表 13.3）。用于评估静态和动态骨代谢的"金标准"仍然是四环素标记的非脱钙髂前上棘骨活检，尽管基于临床病史极少需要这种检查。骨活检可用于评估破骨细胞和成骨细胞活性及类骨质矿化。由于在常规病理学检查中酸介导的脱钙会去除钙质，因而不能区分矿化的成熟骨和正常或病理性的未矿化类骨质，必须采用非脱钙切片来评估（图 13.1A ~ F）。由于四环素在类骨质矿化过程中会被整合入焦磷酸盐结晶并在荧光显微镜下发出荧光，在患者进行骨活检之前使用四环素可用于评估骨形成和矿化的速率和有效性（图 13.1B 和 F）。

骨佩吉特病

骨佩吉特病（Paget 骨病）或畸形性骨炎是 MBD 的第二大病因，仅次于骨质疏松症，美国 55 岁以上成人的患病率为 2% ~ 3%。骨佩吉特病的发病率因地域和种族而异（欧洲裔最为常见），且可能呈下降趋势。与其他累及整体骨骼的疾病（如骨质疏松症）不同，骨佩吉特病通常表现为局灶性骨重建异常。骨佩吉特病可分为单骨型或多骨型（影响单块骨 vs. 多块骨）。原有病灶可以扩大，但极少出现新的病灶。骨佩吉特病可累及任何部位的骨骼，但骨盆、椎体、颅骨、股骨和胫骨最常受累。

骨佩吉特病的特征是破骨细胞异常导致的骨吸收增加，继之以组织紊乱、结构脆弱的"编织"骨的快速形成（图 13.1C）。成骨细胞活性显著增加可在 X 线平片上表现为典型的硬化性改变（图 13.2A ~ C），在骨显像中表现为放射性摄取增高（图 13.2D），且血清碱性磷酸酶水平同步升高，后者为骨形成中的蛋白中间产物及骨佩吉特病的生化特征。骨佩吉特病的发病机制未明，但遗传变异及病毒可能均有参与。高达 30% 的患者有家族史，目前已发现多种相关基因，包括 SQSTM1、ZNF687、CSF-1、RANK 和 PML 等。有证据显示，慢性副黏病毒（如麻疹病毒、呼吸道合胞病毒或犬瘟热病毒）感染可导致骨佩吉特病。

大多数骨佩吉特病患者无症状，是因常规化验发现血清碱性磷酸酶水平升高或其他原因行影像学检查而意外确诊。然而，根据病变部位及范围，患者也可出现骨痛，骨畸形（如长骨弯曲），骨折，骨关节炎及神经受压症状（如耳聋、椎管狭窄）。罕见并发症包括高钙血症（见于制动患者）和高排出量心力衰竭。由于病变部位血供丰富，受累骨骼表面皮温升高。最严重的罕见并发症是在病变骨骼部位发生骨肉瘤（＜ 1%）。

骨佩吉特病通常通过骨转换生化标志物及影像学检查做出诊断。在大多数患者中，血清总碱性磷酸酶水平升高是反映疾病活动度的充分且敏感的标志物。但是，骨特异性血清碱性磷酸酶可能在疾病活动度低或肝源性碱性磷酸酶水平低的患者中更为敏感。诊断时的骨显像可显示病变部位及范围（图 13.2D）。受累区域的 X 线检查可确诊骨佩吉特病，并可用于评估并发症及局部病变进展（图 13.2A ~ C）。

治疗目标包括缓解症状和预防并发症。治疗适应证包括缓解症状（如骨痛、头痛、神经系统并发症），减少术前血流以减少择期手术（包括病变部位）中的出血，治疗高钙血症，以及预防进展性局灶病变的远期并发症（长骨弯曲、颞骨受累导致的听力丧失、枕骨大孔或椎体受累导致的神经系统并发症）。目前仅有支持使用双膦酸盐减轻疼痛的中等质量证据。

骨佩吉特病的治疗包括非药物治疗（如物理治疗）和药物治疗（包括骨吸收抑制剂和镇痛药）的联合治疗。双膦酸盐是治疗的基石，可通过抑制破骨细胞而

TABLE 13.1   Conditions, Diseases, and Medications That Cause or Contribute to Metabolic Bone Disease

Osteoporosis (see also Chapter 14)
Paget's disease of the bone
Osteomalacia and rickets
   Vitamin D syndromes
   Hypophosphatemic syndromes
   Hypophosphatasia
   Medications (anticonvulsants, aluminum)
   Metabolic acidosis
Hyperparathyroid bone disease
Renal osteodystrophy/transplantation osteoporosis
Genetic diseases
   Low bone mass phenotypes
     • Osteogenesis imperfecta
     • Osteoporosis-pseudoglioma syndrome
     • X-linked osteoporosis
   High bone mass phenotypes
     • Osteopetrosis
     • Autosomal dominant (LRP-5)
     • Van Buchem disease and sclerosteosis
   Disorganized skeletal development
     • Fibrous dysplasia
Infiltrative diseases
   Multiple myeloma
   Mastocytosis
   Lymphoma, leukemia
   Sarcoid
   Malignant histiocytosis
   Gaucher's disease
   Hemolytic diseases (e.g., thalassemia, sickle cell anemia)

inhibiting osteoclasts. Intravenous zoledronic acid is the first-line treatment and leads to more rapid and sustained normalization of alkaline phosphatase than oral bisphosphonates. Surgery may be needed for an impending or complete fracture through pagetic bone, realignment of arthritic joints, and total joint arthroplasty in affected hips or knees.

OSTEOMALACIA AND RICKETS

Although common in the United States and throughout the world, osteomalacia and rickets are often underappreciated and overlooked. Osteomalacia and rickets are essentially the same disorders, but by definition, rickets occurs in children with open growth plates (i.e., epiphyses), and osteomalacia occurs in adults who are skeletally mature. The fundamental abnormality in these disorders is an inability to mineralize (i.e., form hydroxyapatite crystals) osteoid, the precursor to mineralized bone. Although osteoid is produced, there is a defect in the mineralization process. This results in the accumulation of characteristic thick osteoid seams on bone biopsy (see Fig. 13.1E and F) and a reduction in the bone mineral content that renders it mechanically inferior, leading to stress or pseudofractures, frank fractures, bowing of the long bones, and other skeletal deformities (Fig. 13.3A to C).

Mineralization disorders are due to disturbances in vitamin D, calcium, phosphorus or inhibitors of mineralization/matrix development. Vitamin D deficiency (low 25-hydroxyvitamin D level) is the most common cause of rickets and osteomalacia and is usually due to poor intake or malabsorption, but impaired hepatic production, excessive renal loss, and accelerated catabolism of vitamin D can occur in advanced liver disease, nephrotic syndrome, and with anticonvulsant use, respectively. Mutations in P450 enzymes regulating vitamin D metabolism (1α-hydroxylase and 25-hydroxylase) and the vitamin D receptor (VDR) are much rarer causes of rickets and osteomalacia.

Hypophosphatemic disorders are less frequent causes of osteomalacia, but often present with more severe symptoms. These conditions include inherited or acquired disorders, like X-linked hypophosphatemic rickets (XLH) and tumor-induced osteomalacia, respectively, due to altered metabolism or over-production of a "phosphatonin" protein, fibroblast growth factor 23 (FGF23), as well as other renal phosphate-wasting conditions such as Fanconi syndrome.

Toxins interfering with mineralization, including aluminum, fluoride, and heavy metals (e.g., cadmium), can also cause osteomalacia. In addition, because calcium salts are acid soluble, chronic metabolic acidoses can result in osteomalacia or rickets. Mutations in tissue nonspecific alkaline phosphatase (TNSALP) result in skeletal over-accumulation of the naturally occurring mineralization inhibitor, pyrophosphate, causing hypophosphatasia (HPP). HPP, which is life-threatening in neonates due to respiratory failure from lack of rib mineralization, presents less severely in adults with bone pain, lower extremity stress fractures, and dental disease/tooth loss, though it can be a source of significant morbidity. Finally, osteomalacia is rarely due to inherent defects in bone matrix, such as in type VI *osteogenesis imperfecta (OI)*.

In children, rickets presents with decreased longitudinal growth, widening of the long bone metaphyses (wrists, tibias), and bowing but may also include dental and other skeletal sequelae (i.e., rachitic rosary from enlargement of the costochondral junctions). In adults, osteomalacia presents with bone pain, proximal muscle weakness, fractures, and difficulty walking. The diagnosis of osteomalacia is suggested by the above symptoms and signs. Biochemistries, particularly serum phosphorus, vitamin D (25-hydroxyvitamin D_3 and $1,25[OH]_2D_3$), parathyroid hormone (PTH), and alkaline phosphatase reflect the underlying pathobiology. Inappropriate phosphaturia with a low tubular maximum for phosphorus or glomerular filtration rate, measured with a fasting 2-hour urine phosphorus and creatinine (see Chapter 12), typifies renal phosphate-wasting disorders.

The characteristic radiologic signs of osteomalacia are stress fractures, also known as Looser's zones or Milkman's pseudofractures, primarily in weight-bearing bones. They can be identified by plain radiographs, but computed tomography (CT), MR or whole body bone scintigraphy may be required (Fig. 13.3C).

BMD, measured by dual-energy x-ray absorptiometry or DXA, is usually low, although often is erroneously assumed to be due to osteoporosis. Given this, and that some osteoporosis treatments (i.e., bisphosphonates) can worsen osteomalacia, the physician should review the list in Table 13.1 and exclude alternative mineralization disorders prior to recommending conventional osteoporosis treatments. Finally, although the diagnosis of osteomalacia can often be made clinically, definitive diagnosis in uncertain cases relies on tetracycline-labeled undecalcified bone biopsy, which quantitates the degree of mineralization defect (see Fig. 13.1E and F).

Treatment of rickets or osteomalacia is dependent on underlying etiology. Ergocalciferol or cholecalciferol with supplemental calcium leads to fracture healing and reduced pain in severe vitamin D deficiency. Oral phosphorous salts and activated vitamin D

表 13.1　导致或参与发生代谢性骨病的情况、疾病及药物

骨质疏松症（见第 14 章）

骨佩吉特病

骨软化症和佝偻病
　　维生素 D 相关综合征
　　低磷血症相关综合征
　　低磷酸酯酶症
　　药物（抗惊厥药、铝剂）
　　代谢性酸中毒

甲状旁腺功能亢进性骨病

肾性骨营养不良 / 移植相关骨质疏松症

遗传病
　　低骨量表型
　　● 成骨不全
　　● 骨质疏松症-假神经胶质瘤综合征
　　● X 连锁骨质疏松症
　　高骨量表型
　　● 骨硬化症
　　● 常染色体显性遗传（LRP-5）
　　● Van Buchem 病及硬化性骨病
　　骨骼发育紊乱
　　● 纤维性结构不良

浸润性疾病
　　多发性骨髓瘤
　　肥大细胞增多症
　　淋巴瘤、白血病
　　结节病
　　恶性组织细胞增生症
　　戈谢病（Gaucher 病）
　　溶血性疾病（如地中海贫血、镰状细胞贫血）

降低病变部位的骨吸收。静脉使用唑来膦酸为一线治疗，与口服双膦酸盐相比，其能更迅速、更持久地使碱性磷酸酶水平恢复正常。对于即将发生或已经发生骨折的病变骨、关节炎（修复术）及受累髋关节或膝关节（全关节置换术），可能需要手术治疗。

骨软化症和佝偻病

虽然骨软化症和佝偻病在美国和全球均很常见，但其经常被低估和忽视。骨软化症和佝偻病本质上是一种疾病，从定义上，佝偻病发生于生长板（即骨骺）开放的儿童，骨软化症见于骨骼成熟的成人。这些疾病的基础改变是类骨质（矿化骨质的前体）的矿化（即形成焦磷酸盐结晶）障碍。尽管产生了类骨质，但患者的矿化过程存在缺陷。这会导致骨活检可见特征性的厚的类骨质堆积（图 13.1E ～ F）和骨矿物质含量减少，使其机械性能较差，导致应力性骨折或假骨折、真性骨折、长骨弯曲和其他骨骼畸形（图 13.3A ～ C）。

矿化异常性疾病的病因包括维生素 D 缺乏症、钙磷代谢紊乱或矿化 / 基质生成抑制物。维生素 D 缺乏症（25- 羟维生素 D 水平低）是佝偻病和骨软化症最常见的病因，通常由摄入不足或吸收不良导致，但也可见于肝脏合成受损（见于进展期肝病）、肾脏丢失增多（见于肾病综合征）及维生素 D 分解代谢加速（应用抗癫痫药物）。调节维生素 D 代谢的 P450 酶（1α - 羟化酶和 25- 羟化酶）和维生素 D 受体（VDR）基因突变是佝偻病和骨软化症非常罕见的病因。

低血磷性疾病是较少见的骨软化症病因，但通常症状更严重。这组疾病包括遗传性疾病［如 X 连锁低血磷性佝偻病（XLH）］或获得性疾病（如肿瘤性骨软化症），由"调磷因子"FGF23 代谢异常或合成过多和其他失磷性肾病（如范科尼综合征）导致。

铝、氟、重金属（如镉）等毒素可干扰矿化，导致骨软化症。此外，由于钙盐可溶于酸，慢性代谢性酸中毒可导致骨软化症或佝偻病。组织非特异性碱性磷酸酶（TNSALP）突变会导致自然形成的矿化抑制物焦磷酸盐的蓄积，引起低磷酸酯酶症（HPP）。新生儿 HPP 可因肋骨不能矿化导致呼吸衰竭而危及生命，成人 HPP 患者的症状较轻，可表现为骨痛、下肢应力性骨折和牙齿疾病 / 牙齿脱落，但可显著增加并发症。骨软化症的罕见病因还包括骨基质遗传缺陷［如 Ⅵ 型成骨不全（OI）］。

在儿童中，佝偻病表现为影响纵向生长，长骨干骺端（腕骨、胫骨）增宽和弯曲，但也可导致牙齿和其他骨骼后遗症（即肋软骨连接处增大导致的串珠肋）。在成人中，骨软化症表现为骨痛、近端肌无力、骨折和行走困难。上述症状及体征可提示骨软化症的诊断。生化指标反映了潜在的病理生理学机制，尤其是血清磷、维生素 D［25- 羟维生素 D 和 1,25（OH)$_2$D$_3$］、PTH 和碱性磷酸酶。测定空腹 2 h 尿磷和肌酐（见第 12 章）时出现异常磷酸盐尿伴随肾小管最大磷重吸收降低或肾小球滤过率降低，是失磷性肾病的典型表现。

骨软化症的影像学特征性表现为应力性骨折，又称 Looser 区或 Milkman 假骨折，主要出现在负重骨。可通过 X 线平片识别，但有时也需要进行 CT、MRI 或全身骨显像（图 13.3C）。

应用双能 X 射线吸收法（DXA）测量的 BMD 通常较低，患者常被误诊为骨质疏松症。由于某些骨质疏松症的治疗（即双膦酸盐）可加重骨软化症，因此内科医生需要回顾表 13.1，在推荐传统骨质疏松症治疗前先排除其他矿化异常性疾病。虽然骨软化症的诊断常为临床诊断，但疑诊病例的确诊仍有赖于四环素标记的非脱钙骨活检，以定量分析矿化缺陷的程度（图 13.1E ～ F）。

佝偻病或骨软化症的治疗取决于潜在病因。严重维生素 D 缺乏症者使用维生素 D$_2$ 或维生素 D$_3$ 联合补充钙剂可促使骨折愈合，减轻骨痛。口服磷酸盐和活性维生素 D 类似物（如骨化三醇）可改善低血磷性佝

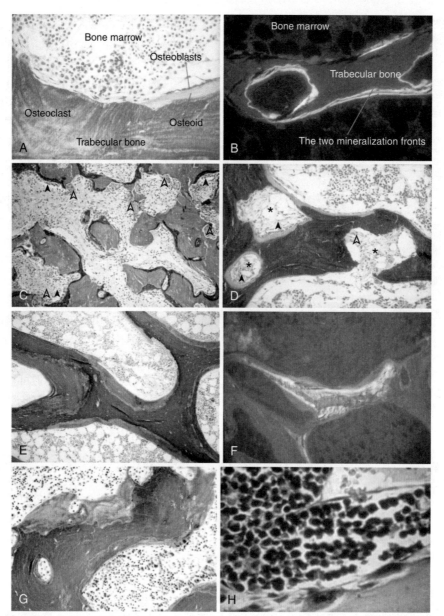

Fig. 13.1 (A) Normal bone histology, showing a normal bone-remodeling unit as seen in an undecalcified human anterior iliac crest biopsy. On the left, a multinucleated osteoclast has moved across the mineralized trabecular bone surface over the previous week or two, resorbing (removing) old bone. On the extreme right, the bone surface is covered by osteoid secreted by the overlying osteoblasts. In between the osteoclast- and osteoblast-covered surfaces of the trabecular bone are a large number of flat, fibroblastoid cells referred to as *lining cells*. No osteocytes are visible in this section. (B) Tetracycline labeling of a bone biopsy from a patient with hyperparathyroid bone disease. Notice the bright yellow parallel lines on the trabecular bone surface. These lines represent the two sets of tetracycline labeling, which occurred 14 days apart. From these sets, the mineralization rate can be described in micrometers (microns) per day, the so-called *mineral apposition rate*, and it is increased dramatically in this example, as is typical of hyperparathyroid bone disease. Contrast with example F, which has no tetracycline labeling. (C) Paget's disease. Enormous and abundant highly multinucleated osteoclasts *(open arrowheads)* are resorbing trabecular bone, and a comparably enormous number of osteoblasts *(closed arrowheads)* are making new but disorganized bone. The marrow space is replaced by fibrous cells. (D) Primary hyperparathyroidism has the classic features of osteitis fibrosa cystica. Far more osteoid and osteoblasts *(closed arrowheads)* and osteoclasts *(open arrowhead)* exist than in the normal example (A). Three large microcysts *(asterisks)* have been created by aggressive osteoclastic bone resorption. These microcysts account for the *cystica* component of osteitis fibrosa cystica. The marrow space, particularly within the microcysts, is filled with fibroblasts, which make up the *fibrosa* component of osteitis fibrosa cystica. (E) Osteomalacia or rickets. Notice the abundant quantities of partially and chaotically mineralized osteoid *(orange)*. These seams are the thick osteoid seams and represent osteoid that has been produced by osteoblasts but that cannot mineralize, which is the signature defect in osteomalacia and rickets. (F) Tetracycline labeling reveals a complete absence of mineralization, diagnostic of osteomalacia or rickets. Compare with example B. (G) Renal osteodystrophy. This photomicrograph of a biopsy from a patient on dialysis demonstrates many of the classic features of renal osteodystrophy, including evidence of aggressive osteoclastic bone resorption (i.e., numerous osteoclastic lacunae on the bone surface compared with the smooth surfaces in example A) and abundant, partially and chaotically mineralized areas of osteoid *(orange)*. (H) Infiltrative bone disease as exemplified by multiple myeloma. The bone marrow is replaced by plasma cells, and two large osteoclasts in lacunae are actively resorbing the trabecular bone surface.

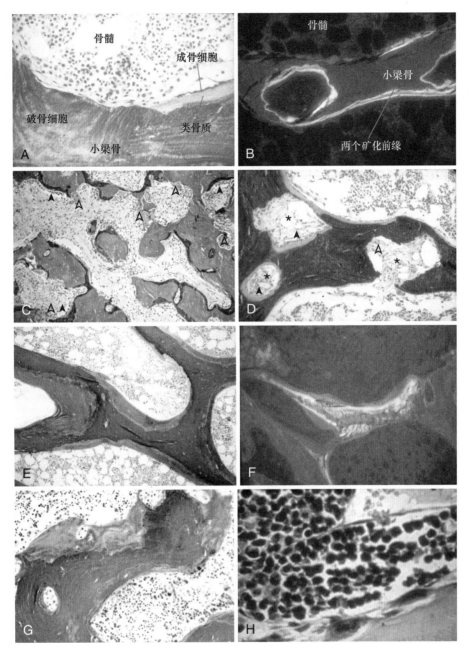

图 13.1 A. 正常骨活检，在人体髂前上棘活检非脱钙切片中可见正常的骨重建单位。图左侧可见 1 个多核破骨细胞已在 1～2 周前经过矿化的小梁骨表面，吸收（去除）旧骨。图最右侧可见骨表面覆有成骨细胞分泌的类骨质。在破骨细胞和成骨细胞覆盖的小梁骨表面，可见大量扁平的成纤维样细胞，即衬里细胞。该切片中未见骨细胞。B. 甲状旁腺功能亢进性骨病患者间隔 14 天进行四环素标记的骨活检。可见小梁骨表面有明亮的黄色平行线，代表间隔 14 天的两组四环素标记。根据这套切片，可用 μm/d 来描述矿化速率（即矿盐沉积速率），本例患者的矿化速率显著加快，这是甲状旁腺功能亢进性骨病的典型表现。本例与 F 图的病例不同，后者未观察到四环素标记。C. 骨佩吉特病。可见大量高度多核的破骨细胞（空心箭头）正在吸收小梁骨，相当数量的成骨细胞（实心箭头）正在形成新的结构紊乱的骨。骨髓腔被纤维细胞替代。D. 原发性甲状旁腺功能亢进症患者具有囊性纤维性骨炎的典型特征。相较于正常情况（图 A），本例有更多的类骨质、成骨细胞（实心箭头）和破骨细胞（空心箭头）。进行性破骨细胞骨吸收形成了 3 个大的微囊（*），即囊性纤维性骨炎中的囊性组分。骨髓腔（尤其是微囊内的骨髓腔）被成纤维细胞充填，构成了囊性纤维性骨炎的纤维组分。E. 骨软化症或佝偻病。可见大量不完全矿化或矿化紊乱的类骨质（橙色）。厚的类骨质层代表成骨细胞产生类骨质但未能矿化，这是骨软化症和佝偻病的特征性缺陷。F. 四环素标记显示完全未矿化（相较于图 B），这对骨软化症或佝偻病有诊断意义。G. 肾性骨营养不良。来自透析患者的活检光镜照片显示肾性骨营养不良的许多典型特征，包括进行性破骨细胞骨吸收（即骨表面大量破骨细胞陷窝，相较于图 A 中的光滑表面）和大量的部分矿化和矿化紊乱的类骨质区域（橙色）。H. 浸润性骨病，以多发性骨髓瘤为例。骨髓被浆细胞替代，陷窝中可见 2 个大的破骨细胞正在吸收小梁骨表面

analogues, such as calcitriol, improve osteomalacia in hypophos-phatemic rickets, although targeted reduction of FGF23 levels with a monoclonal antibody also improves bone pain and fracture healing in XLH. Treatment of children with HPP using recombinant TNSALP can be life-saving and markedly reduces pain and disability. Identification and withdrawal of drugs/toxins causing inhibition of mineralization generally improves osteomalacic symptoms. Treatment of these diseases is gratifying because the responses are often dramatic with restoration of normal function in patients who were severely disabled.

HYPERPARATHYROID BONE DISEASE

Hyperparathyroid bone disease can be a major cause of skeletal morbidity, though the clinical presentation varies widely, depending on the nature and severity of the underlying parathyroid disorder. Patients with primary hyperparathyroidism (PHPT), characterized by elevated serum calcium and PTH levels from a parathyroid adenoma or hyperplasia, typically have no symptoms related to accelerated bone remodeling from excess PTH. However, in many patients, osteopenia or osteoporosis can be detected by DXA, which often shows bone loss at the cortical-rich proximal one third radius and proximal femur and

sparing of the cancellous-rich lumbar spine. Fracture risk, particularly risk for vertebral fractures, is also increased in PHPT, but many vertebral fractures are clinically occult (i.e., only identified by spine imaging).

Secondary hyperparathyroidism (SHPT), which is a physiologic PTH elevation occurring in response to hypocalcemia and/or 25-hydroxyvitamin D_3 deficiency, is also associated with bone loss from cortical-rich sites. SHPT is almost always present in advanced chronic kidney disease (CKD) as a result of chronic hypocalcemia, hyperphosphatemia, and low calcitriol (1,25[OH]$_2$D$_3$) levels, as well as in malabsorptive states such as gastric bypass. Tertiary hyperparathyroidism is characterized by hypercalcemia and elevated PTH resulting from long-standing SHPT, usually from end-stage renal disease (ESRD). In tertiary hyperparathyroidism, chronic parathyroid stimulation results in hyperplasia or adenomas and autonomous gland function.

In patients with chronically, markedly elevated PTH levels, severe hyperparathyroid bone disease, known as *osteitis fibrosa cystica* (OFC), may develop. OFC was common among patients with PHPT in the United States before the onset of routine biochemical screening that began in the 1970s but occurs in fewer than 2% of patients today. OFC remains frequent in regions of the world where calcium is not routinely measured. Today, OFC is typically seen in the context of severe, prolonged, and uncontrolled secondary and tertiary hyperparathyroidism (from ESRD) and parathyroid carcinoma. OFC, a *high turnover* skeletal disease, is characterized by coupled increases in osteoclastic bone resorption and osteoblastic osteoid synthesis, accelerated rates of bone mineralization accompanied by microcysts in the cortex and trabeculae (the *cystica* of OFC), and increased numbers of fibroblasts and marrow stroma (the *fibrosa* of OFC) (see Fig. 13.1B and D). Levels of markers of bone formation (i.e., alkaline phosphatase and osteocalcin) and resorption (i.e., N-terminal and C-terminal telopeptides) are usually increased, reflecting the bone histology. The radiologic hallmarks of OFC are salt-and-pepper demineralization of the calvarium, resorption of the tufts of the terminal phalanges and distal clavicles, subperiosteal resorption of the radial aspect of the cortex of the second phalanges (Fig. 13.4), and Brown tumors (i.e., collections of osteoclasts that produce gross lytic lesions) of the pelvis and long bones. Patients with OFC may have bone pain or fractures.

The treatment involves normalizing or lowering elevated PTH concentrations. In patients with OFC, curative parathyroidectomy normalizes biochemistries and leads to resolution of the radiologic

---

TABLE 13.2 Diagnostic Studies in the Evaluation of Metabolic Bone Disease

Laboratory Evaluation
    Serum calcium, phosphate, magnesium
    Alkaline phosphatase (total and bone-specific)
    Vitamin D metabolites (25-hydroxyvitamin D and 1,25-dihydroxyvitamin D)
    Creatinine
    Parathyroid hormone
    24-hour urine calcium and creatinine
    Fasting 2-hour urine phosphorus and creatinine
    Markers of bone formation and resorption
Imaging
    Radiographs
    DXA
    Technetium-99 bone scan
Pathology
    Tetracycline-labeled bone biopsy

TABLE 13.3 Biochemical Hallmarks of Various Metabolic Bone Diseases

	Calcium	Phosphate	PTH	25-Hydroxy Vitamin D	1,25-Dihydroxyvitamin D	Alkaline Phosphatase
Vitamin D deficiency with osteomalacia	Low or low normal	Low or low normal	High	Low	High or high normal	High
Renal phosphate wasting with osteomalacia	Normal	Low	Normal or high	Normal	Low or low normal	High
Paget's disease	Normal	Normal	Normal or high	Dependent on intake; Often low	Normal	High
Primary/hyperparathyroidism	High	Low or low normal	High	Dependent on intake; Often low	High or high normal	High or high normal

偻病的骨软化，应用靶向降低 FGF23 水平的单克隆抗体也能改善 XLH 患者的骨痛和骨折愈合。使用重组 TNSALP 可挽救 HPP 儿童患者的生命，并显著改善疼痛和活动受限。识别和停用导致矿化抑制的药物 / 毒素通常可改善骨软化症状。这些疾病的治疗效果令人满意，因为患者的治疗反应通常非常明显，严重活动障碍的患者也能够恢复正常功能。

甲状旁腺功能亢进性骨病

甲状旁腺功能亢进性骨病是骨骼合并症的主要原因，但患者的临床表现差异很大，因其甲状旁腺疾病的特征和严重程度而异。原发性甲状旁腺功能亢进症（PHPT）患者以甲状旁腺腺瘤或增生导致的血清钙和 PTH 水平升高为特征，通常没有过量 PTH 导致骨重建加速的相关症状；然而，DXA 检查可发现许多患者存在骨量减少或骨质疏松症，常表现为在以皮质骨为主的桡骨近端 1/3 和近端股骨的骨丢失，而富含松质骨的腰椎骨量正常。PHPT 患者的骨折（尤其是椎体骨折）

表 13.2　评估代谢性骨病的诊断性检查
实验室评估
血清钙、磷酸盐、镁
碱性磷酸酶（总碱性磷酸酶和骨特异性碱性磷酸酶）
维生素 D 代谢产物［25- 羟维生素 D 和 1,25（OH）$_2$D］
肌酐
甲状旁腺激素
24 h 尿钙、肌酐
空腹 2 h 尿磷、肌酐
骨形成和骨吸收的标志物
影像学检查
X 线检查
DXA
锝 99- 骨扫描
病理学检查
四环素标记的骨活检

风险增加，但很多椎体骨折无临床症状（即仅在椎体影像学检查时发现）。

继发性甲状旁腺功能亢进症（SHPT）是由于低钙血症和（或）25- 羟维生素 D 缺乏引起的 PTH 生理性升高，也与富含皮质骨部位的骨丢失相关。SHPT 主要见于进展期慢性肾脏病（CKD），由慢性低钙血症、高磷血症及 1,25（OH）$_2$D 水平降低导致，也可见于吸收不良性疾病，如胃旁路手术。三发性甲状旁腺功能亢进症以高钙血症和 PTH 水平升高为特征，由长期 SHPT 导致，通常见于终末期肾病（ESRD）。在三发性甲状旁腺功能亢进症中，对甲状旁腺的慢性刺激会导致增生或腺瘤，并影响腺体的自主功能。

在长期 PTH 水平显著升高的患者中，可发生严重的甲状旁腺功能亢进性骨病，又称囊性纤维性骨炎（OFC）。美国在 20 世纪 70 年代开始常规生化筛查以前，OFC 在 PHPT 患者中很常见，但目前仅见于不足 2% 的患者。在一些未常规筛查血钙的国家中，OFC 仍然常见。目前，OFC 通常见于严重、长期且未控制的 SHPT 和三发性甲状旁腺功能亢进症（由 ESRD 所致）和甲状旁腺癌。OFC 是一种高骨转换性骨病，其特征是破骨细胞的骨吸收和成骨细胞的类骨质形成同步增加，骨矿化速率增加伴随皮质骨和小梁骨中的微囊（OFC 中的囊性组分），以及成纤维细胞数量增加和骨髓基质增加（OFC 中的纤维组分）（图 13.1B 和 D）。骨形成指标（即碱性磷酸酶和骨钙蛋白）和骨吸收指标（即 N- 末端和 C- 末端交联肽）的水平通常升高，反映了骨的组织学改变。OFC 的影像学特征包括颅骨椒盐征、远端指骨末端和锁骨远端的骨吸收、第 2 指骨桡侧皮质的骨膜下骨吸收（图 13.4），以及骨盆和长骨棕色瘤（即破骨细胞聚集产生大的溶骨性病变）。OFC 患者可出现骨痛或骨折。

治疗目标包括降低 PTH 水平或使其恢复正常。在 OFC 患者中，成功的甲状旁腺手术可使生化指标恢复正常，影像学改变减轻。在没有 OFC 但有骨量减少或

表 13.3　代谢性骨病的生化特征						
	钙	磷酸盐	PTH	25- 羟维生素 D	1,25（OH）$_2$D	碱性磷酸酶
维生素 D 缺乏症伴骨软化症	低或正常偏低	低或正常偏低	高	低	高或正常	高
肾性失磷伴骨软化症	正常	低	正常或高	正常	低或正常偏低	高
骨佩吉特病	正常	正常	正常或高	取决于摄入情况；通常低	正常	高
原发性甲状旁腺功能亢进症	高	低或正常偏低	高	取决于摄入情况；通常低	高或正常偏高	高或正常偏高

signs. In hyperparathyroid patients without OFC but with osteopenia or osteoporosis, BMD typically increases robustly after parathyroidectomy, particularly in the lumbar spine. If the hypercalcemia is mild and BMD is normal, no treatment may be required. Medical therapy with cinacalcet, a *calcimimetic* (mimics the action of calcium at the calcium-sensing receptor) can be used to lower PTH levels in those with parathyroid carcinoma who have failed surgical resection and patients with severe hypercalcemia due to primary or tertiary hyperparathyroidism who are not surgical candidates. Hypocalcemia may occasionally occur after parathyroidectomy in patients with more severe disease, a condition known as *hungry bone syndrome* (see Chapter 12).

SHPT due to vitamin D deficiency is treated with oral vitamin D_3 (cholecalciferol) or D_2 (ergocalciferol). SHPT from ESRD can be treated with a combination of the active form of vitamin D (1,25[OH]$_2$D$_3$ [calcitriol] or analogues), calcium supplementation, phosphate binders, and cinacalcet, depending on the clinical situation.

Infrequently, parathyroidectomy is needed for severe hyperparathyroid bone disease related to SHPT.

RENAL OSTEODYSTROPHY

Renal osteodystrophy (ROD) refers to changes in bone turnover, mineralization, and morphology that occur in CKD. ROD is typically associated with abnormalities in serum calcium, phosphate, PTH, FGF23 or vitamin D metabolism and also may be accompanied by vascular and soft tissue calcification. The term *chronic kidney disease–mineral and bone disorder (CKD-MBD)* describes the systemic disorder encompassing both the mineral and bone metabolism abnormalities in CKD.

ROD may occur as early as stage 2 CKD and is prevalent among those with stage 4 to 5 CKD. Furthermore, even mild and moderate CKD confers an increased risk of fracture. The pathophysiology of ROD is complex and related to alterations in both hormonal and

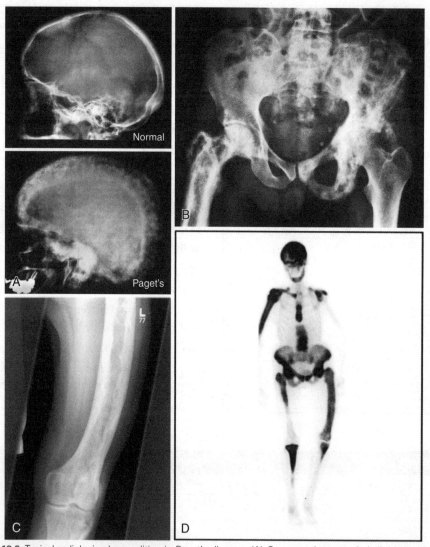

Fig. 13.2 Typical radiologic abnormalities in Paget's disease. (A) Compare the normal skull *(top)* with the skull *(bottom)* with the classic cotton-wool appearance, an expanded calvarium, and osteosclerosis of the petrous bones. (B) Classic asymmetrical involvement of the pelvis with a mixture of lytic and blastic lesions. (C) Bowing deformity of the femur with a markedly thickened cortex. (D) A whole-body radionuclide scan demonstrates polyostotic Paget's disease.

骨质疏松症的甲状旁腺功能亢进症患者中，甲状旁腺切除术后 BMD 通常显著升高，尤其是腰椎部位。轻度高钙血症且 BMD 正常时，不需要治疗。甲状旁腺癌手术失败、PHPT 或三发性甲状旁腺功能亢进症导致的重度高钙血症但不能手术者，可使用西那卡塞（一种拟钙剂，可模拟离子钙对钙敏感受体的作用）来降低 PTH 水平。病情较严重的患者在甲状旁腺切除术后偶可发生低钙血症，即骨饥饿综合征（见第 12 章）。

口服维生素 D₃（胆钙化醇）或维生素 D₂（麦角钙化醇）可治疗维生素 D 缺乏导致的 SHPT。ESRD 导致的 SHPT 可根据临床情况使用活性维生素 D［1，25（OH）₂D］、钙补充剂、磷结合剂和西那卡塞的联合治疗。少数情况下，需要采用甲状旁腺切除术治疗 SHPT

相关的重度甲状旁腺功能亢进性骨病。

肾性骨营养不良

肾性骨营养不良（ROD）是指 CKD 中发生的骨转换、矿化及形态学改变。ROD 通常与血清钙、磷酸盐、PTH、FGF23 或维生素 D 代谢产物水平异常相关，常伴有血管和软组织钙化。慢性肾脏病矿盐骨代谢紊乱（CKD-MBD）这一名词描述了 CKD 患者矿盐和骨代谢异常的系统性病变。

ROD 在 CKD 2 期即可出现，在 CKD 4 ～ 5 期常见。此外，即使是轻中度 CKD 也可导致骨折风险增加。ROD 的病理生理学机制复杂，与激素和矿盐代谢的改变

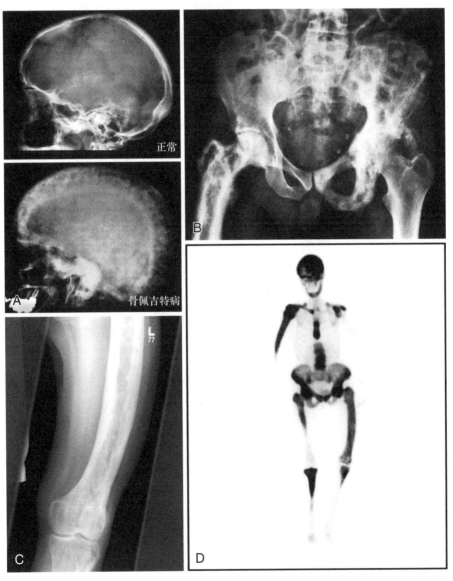

图 13.2　骨佩吉特病的典型影像学异常。**A**. 与正常颅骨（上）相比，病变颅骨（下）有典型的棉花团样表现，伴有颅骨膨胀和岩骨骨硬化。**B**. 骨盆典型的非对称性受累，溶骨性和成骨性病变混合存在。**C**. 股骨弯曲畸形，骨皮质显著增厚。**D**. 全身核素扫描显示多骨型骨佩吉特病

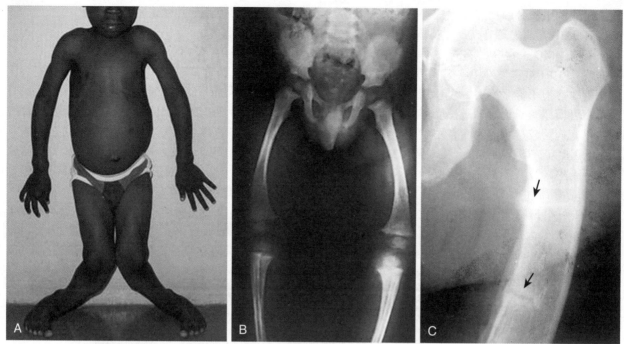

Fig. 13.3 (A) A typical example of rickets, with bowing of the femurs and tibias, wrist enlargement due to metaphyseal flaring and rachitic rosary, and enlargement of the costochondral junctions of the ribs. (From Thacher TD, Pludowski P, Shaw NJ, Mughal MZ, Munns CF, Högler W. Nutritional rickets in immigrant and refugee children. Public Health Rev. 2016 Jul 22;37:3. (B) A skeletal radiograph of a child with rickets. The weight-bearing bones of the lower extremities are bowed, and the epiphyses are open, mottled, and overgrown. (C) Looser's zones or pseudofractures *(arrows)* are characteristic of osteomalacia or rickets. The closed epiphyses indicate the patient is an adult. This radiograph is diagnostic of osteomalacia.)

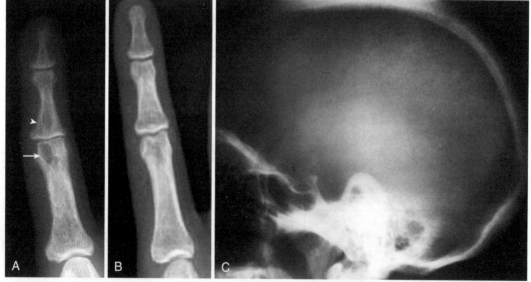

Fig. 13.4 Skeletal radiographic changes of hyperparathyroidism. (A) A hand film from a patient with primary hyperparathyroidism. The *arrow* indicates a typical giant cell tumor (brown tumor), which is a collection of osteoclasts that lead to macrocystic changes in bone. The *arrowhead* indicates the irregular radial surface of a phalanx resulting from subperiosteal bone resorption, which is typical of hyperparathyroidism. The brown tumor and the subperiosteal resorption refill and disappear when the offending parathyroid tumor or hyperplasia is resected. (B) Radiograph of a normal hand for comparison. No brown tumors are seen, and the phalangeal periosteal surfaces are smooth. (C) The classic salt-and-pepper appearance of the skull in hyperparathyroidism. The periosteal surfaces of the inner and outer cortices or tables of the calvarium are indistinct as a result of subperiosteal bone resorption. The lateral view of the calvarium is hazy and indistinct, showing micropunctations. (Courtesy J. Towers, MD, and D. Armfield, MD, University of Pittsburgh, Pittsburgh, Penn.)

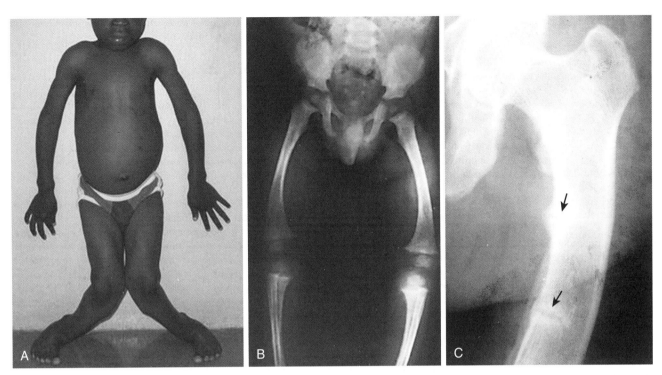

图 13.3 **A**. 典型的佝偻病，股骨和胫骨弯曲，干骺端膨大导致腕关节膨大，肋骨的骨软骨连接处膨大导致串珠肋（引自 Thacher TD，Pludowski P，Shaw NJ，Mughal MZ，Munns CF，Högler W. Nutritional rickets in immigrant and refugee children. Public Health Rev. 2016 Jul 22；37：3）。**B**. 佝偻病儿童患者的骨骼 X 线片。下肢负重骨弯曲，骨骺开放，呈斑驳样过度增生。**C**. Looser 区或假骨折（箭头）是骨软化症或佝偻病的特征。骨骺关闭提示为成年患者，故诊断为骨软化症

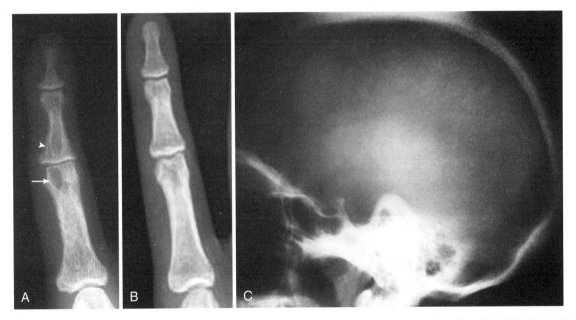

图 13.4 甲状旁腺功能亢进症的骨骼影像学改变。**A**. 原发性甲状旁腺功能亢进症患者的手部图像。箭头所指为典型的巨细胞瘤（棕色瘤），是由破骨细胞聚集导致的骨囊样改变。短箭头所指为骨膜下骨吸收导致的指骨桡侧不规则表面，是甲状旁腺功能亢进症的典型改变。切除甲状旁腺肿瘤或增生后，棕色瘤和骨膜下吸收可被再充填而消失。**B**. 用于对比的正常手部图像。无棕色瘤，指骨骨膜下表面平滑。**C**. 甲状旁腺功能亢进症典型的颅骨椒盐征。颅骨内外皮质或骨板的骨膜下表面由于骨膜下骨吸收而模糊不清。颅骨侧位相显示模糊不清，呈微粒样（引自 J. Towers，MD，and D. Armfield，MD，University of Pittsburgh，Pittsburgh，Penn.）

mineral metabolism. In early CKD, reduced phosphorous excretion leads to increased production and circulating levels of FGF23. SHPT results from hypocalcemia due to hyperphosphatemia and its precipitation with phosphate into soft tissues as well as defective renal $1,25[OH]_2D_3$ production (see Chapters 12).

Several types of ROD can occur and are classified as high-turnover (OFC), low-turnover (adynamic bone disease or ABD), osteomalacia, or mixed ROD. Tetracycline-labeled transiliac bone biopsy is the only way to reliably distinguish which type of ROD is present, though levels of PTH and alkaline phosphatase may provide noninvasive guidance (typically high in OFC). OFC and osteomalacia were common in the past, but their prevalence has declined while that of ABD has increased. The reasons for this, and the exact mechanisms leading to development of one type of ROD versus another, are not entirely clear, but may be related to degree of PTH elevation and other pathogenic factors.

As noted previously, OFC is due to excessive PTH secretion that causes marked increases in bone turnover, demineralization, and fracture. OFC may respond dramatically to $1,25(OH)_2D_3$, cinacalcet, or both. Intravenous etelcalcetide, a newer calcimimetic, may be more effective. In contrast, ABD is characterized by little or no osteoblastic or osteoclastic activity or osteoid on bone biopsy. The condition results from excessive treatment with $1,25[OH]_2D_3$ or calcium-phosphate binders that are believed to cause "over-suppression" of PTH, although other factors may contribute as well. Patients may have bone pain, fractures, hypercalcemia, and vascular calcification. Treatment centers on reducing the dose of active vitamin D analogs, cinacalcet or other measures. Though an intuitive choice of treatment, little data confirm that osteoanabolic agents, such as PTH analogues, are beneficial in the treatment of ABD.

Severe osteomalacia, now uncommon in CKD, is characterized by bone pain, low BMD, and thickened osteoid seams with a mineralization defect on bone biopsy (see Fig. 13.1E). A major contributor to osteomalacia in the past was aluminum bone deposition from now obsolete aluminum-containing phosphate binders. More subtle defects in mineralization can be seen, however, even in early CKD from increased phosphorous and FGF23. CKD-associated osteomalacia may respond to $1,25[OH]_2D_3$ replacement. Mixed ROD is much less common and can be characterized by either high- or low-turnover bone disease along with osteomalacia (see Fig. 13.1G).

TRANSPLANTATION OSTEOPOROSIS

Patients who have undergone organ transplantation often have osteoporosis and are at high risk for fracture. Post-transplant use of immunosuppressive drugs, particularly glucocorticoids, leads to rapid bone loss. Glucocorticoids increase bone resorption, reduce bone formation, decrease gastrointestinal calcium absorption, and increase renal calcium excretion, leading to marked bone loss, and often fracture, within 6 months of initiation. Tacrolimus and cyclosporine have also been associated with bone loss.

Decreased BMD may, however, be present before transplantation as a result of organ failure and its treatment, malnutrition or malabsorption, inactivity, or hypogonadism. For example, those with primary biliary cirrhosis have reduced osteoblast function and low-turnover osteoporosis due to cholestatic toxins. Patients with cystic fibrosis have calcium and vitamin D malabsorption, malnutrition, and low weight. In those with end-stage lung or cardiac disease, physical inactivity contributes. Patients with ESRD who undergo renal transplantation often have ROD. Screening of patients at risk for transplant osteoporosis is paramount. Pretransplant DXA, measurement of vitamin D, and spine imaging is recommended. Early intervention with osteoporosis

therapies in those at high risk for fracture or post-transplant bone loss may prevent post-transplant fractures.

GENETIC DISEASES

Monogenic disorders that lead to abnormal BMD (low or high) or focal skeletal disease are uncommon, but their discovery has advanced our understanding of basic skeletal biology and in turn led to the development of new therapeutic agents for osteoporosis.

The most common monogenic disorder causing low BMD is OI, the severity of which is dependent on the underlying gene involved. OI most often results from mutations in the genes for type I collagen, although defects in collagen processing and mineralization may also cause disease. Patients with OI generally have very low BMD with marked skeletal fragility and deformities but may also have involvement of collagen-containing tissues including the tendons, skin, eyes, and teeth (dentogenesis imperfecta). A much rarer but mechanistically important monogeneic form of low BMD is the osteoporosis-pseudoglioma syndrome, characterized by autosomal dominant, severe osteoporosis with blindness. This disease results from inactivating mutations in the low-density lipoprotein receptor–related protein 5 gene (LRP5), which acts in the osteoblast WNT-signaling pathway to increase bone formation. A missense mutation in WNT has also been described in a family with early-onset osteoporosis.

In contrast, activating mutations in LRP5 lead to an autosomal-dominant form of very high BMD. Mutations in the gene encoding an inhibitor of the WNT signaling pathway, sclerostin, also lead to increased bone formation and high bone mass phenotypes, such as Van Buchem disease and sclerosteosis. These latter discoveries have led to the development of a monoclonal antibody against sclerostin for the treatment of osteoporosis.

In contrast to the disorders that affect bone formation, osteopetrosis, or "marble bone disease," refers to a group of disorders resulting from mutations that impair osteoclastic bone resorption. Although osteopetrosis is associated with increased skeletal mass, fracture risk is increased, presumably due to a change in material properties or "brittleness" that results in reduced bone strength. The clinical presentation is variable depending on the underlying genetic etiology, but the features may include skeletal deformity/short stature, recurrent and poorly healing fractures, macrocephaly, dental abnormalities, overgrowth of neural foramina with nerve paralysis, and impaired hematopoiesis due to bone overgrowth crowding out the bone marrow space. Radiographic findings are diagnostic and indicate generalized sclerosis, a "bone in bone" appearance (from remaining primary spongiosa or calcified cartilage), rugger-jersey vertebrae, flaring of the long bone metaphyses (Erlenmeyer flask deformity) and calvarial and basilar thickening (Fig. 13.5A to C). There is no established treatment for osteopetrosis.

Genetic bone diseases can also present with focal skeletal lesions. Fibrous dysplasia (FD) is a rare condition characterized by fibro-osseous lesions within the skeleton and sometimes extra-skeletal manifestations. It is due to activating mutations in the GNAS gene, encoding the alpha subunit of the stimulatory G protein involved in cyclic adenosine monophosphate (cAMP) production and signaling that causes abnormal differentiation of osteoblasts and osteocytes. Mutations occur post-zygotically and are not inherited, resulting in a somatic mosaicism, with the extent of disease dependent on the timing of the mutation in development. Abnormal osteoblasts secrete a disorganized fibrotic bone matrix resulting in irregular trabeculae enmeshed within a fibrous stroma of spindle-shaped cells, as well as cytokines that result in bone resorption within lesions. Abnormal bone mineralization also

相关。在早期 CKD，磷排泄减少导致 FGF23 合成增加及循环水平升高。SHPT 是由于高磷血症导致低钙血症、钙与磷酸盐沉淀于软组织中及肾脏合成 $1,25(OH)_2D_3$ 减少（见第 12 章）。

ROD 可分为高转换型（OFC）、低转换型［无动力性骨病（ABD）］、骨软化型或混合型 ROD。四环素标记的髂前上棘骨活检是目前唯一能可靠鉴别 ROD 类型的方法，但 PTH 和碱性磷酸酶水平也具有提示作用（在 OFC 时通常升高）。OFC 和骨软化症在过去较常见，但其患病率逐渐下降，而 ABD 的患病率升高。这种改变的原因及特定类型 ROD 的确切机制尚不完全清楚，但可能与 PTH 水平升高的程度和其他致病因素相关。

如前所述，OFC 是由于过量的 PTH 分泌导致骨转换水平显著升高、脱矿及骨折。OFC 对 $1,25(OH)_2D_3$ 和（或）西那卡塞的治疗反应良好。静脉应用维拉卡肽（一种新的拟钙剂）可能更有效。相反，ABD 的特征是骨活检中很少或无成骨细胞或破骨细胞活性或类骨质，这是由于 $1,25(OH)_2D_3$ 和含钙的磷结合剂过量治疗导致对 PTH 的"过度抑制"，但也可能有其他因素参与。患者可能出现骨痛、骨折、高钙血症及血管钙化。治疗的关键在于减少活性维生素 D 类似物、西那卡塞或其他药物的剂量。虽然在直觉上是有效治疗选择，但几乎没有数据证实骨形成促进剂（如 PTH 类似物）可有效治疗 ABD。

严重骨软化症目前在 CKD 中已不常见，其特征是骨痛、低 BMD、骨活检中类骨质层增厚伴矿化缺陷（图 13.1E）。既往骨软化症的主要原因是使用含铝的磷结合剂（目前已不再应用）使铝沉积在骨中。但是，即使是在早期 CKD，也可出现血磷浓度和 FGF23 水平升高导致的轻微矿化缺陷。$1,25(OH)_2D_3$ 替代对于 CKD 相关的骨软化症有效。混合型 ROD 较少见，特征为高转换型或低转换型骨病伴骨软化（图 13.1G）。

移植性骨质疏松症

接受器官移植的患者常出现骨质疏松症，骨折风险增加。移植后使用免疫抑制药物（尤其是糖皮质激素）可导致快速骨丢失。糖皮质激素可增加骨吸收、减少骨形成、减少胃肠道钙吸收，并增加肾脏钙排泄，在起始用药 6 个月内导致显著的骨丢失，并常导致骨折。他克莫司和环孢素也与骨丢失相关。

但是，BMD 降低可能出现在移植之前，由器官功能衰竭及其治疗、营养不良或吸收不良、活动减少或性腺功能减退导致。例如，原发性胆汁性肝硬化患者由于存在胆汁淤积性毒素，可出现成骨细胞功能降低及低骨转换性骨质疏松。囊性纤维化患者存在钙磷吸收不良、营养不良及低体重。终末期心肺疾病患者体力活动减少。ESRD 进行肾移植者通常合并 ROD。筛查有移植性骨质疏松症风险的患者至关重要。推荐在移植前进行 DXA、维生素 D 测定及脊柱影像学检查。早期对骨折或移植后骨丢失风险高的患者进行抗骨质疏松症治疗可预防移植后骨折的发生。

遗传病

导致 BMD 异常（降低或升高）或局灶性骨骼疾病的单基因疾病并不常见，但其发现促进了人们对基础骨骼生物学的理解，进而研发新的骨质疏松症治疗药物。

最常见的导致低 BMD 的单基因疾病是成骨不全（OI），其严重程度取决于受累基因。OI 最常见于编码 I 型胶原蛋白的基因突变，但是胶原蛋白加工过程及矿化缺陷也可致病。OI 患者通常表现为 BMD 极低、骨脆性明显增加及骨畸形，也可累及含有胶原蛋白的组织［如肌腱、皮肤、眼和牙齿（牙本质发生不全）］。骨质疏松症-炎性假瘤综合征是一种非常罕见但在机制上很重要的低 BMD 的单基因疾病，其特征是呈常染色体显性遗传、严重骨质疏松症和失明。该病是由低密度脂蛋白受体相关蛋白 5 基因（LRP5）的失活性突变所致，LRP5 作用于成骨细胞 WNT 信号通路以增加骨形成。在一个早发性骨质疏松症家系中还发现了 WNT 的一种错义突变。

相反，LRP5 的激活性突变导致呈常染色体显性遗传的极高 BMD。编码 WNT 信号通路抑制因子硬骨抑素的基因突变也可导致骨形成增加和高骨量表型，如 Van Buchem 病和硬化性骨病。这一发现促进了硬骨抑素单克隆抗体的研发，其可用于治疗骨质疏松症。

与影响骨形成的疾病相反，骨硬化症（又称"大理石骨病"）是指由影响破骨细胞骨吸收的基因突变所致的一组疾病。尽管骨硬化症患者的骨量增加，但骨折风险增加，这可能是由于材料特性或骨脆性改变导致骨强度下降。骨硬化症的临床表现多样，其取决于致病基因，特征包括骨畸形 / 身材矮小、反复及不易愈合的骨折、大头畸形、牙齿异常、神经孔过度生长伴神经麻痹，以及造血功能受损（由于骨过度生长导致骨髓空间受压）。X 线检查具有诊断价值，表现为弥漫性骨硬化、"骨中骨"外观（来自残余的海绵状原始软骨或钙化软骨）、夹心椎、长骨干骺端增宽（锥形瓶畸形）、颅骨基底增厚（图 13.5A ～ C）。目前尚无针对骨硬化症的有效治疗。

遗传性骨病也可表现为局灶性骨骼病变。纤维性结构不良（FD）是一种罕见疾病，以骨组织内纤维骨性病变为特征，有时伴有骨外表现。FD 是由编码刺激性 G 蛋白 α 亚单位的 GNAS 基因激活性突变导致，该蛋白参与环磷酸腺苷（cAMP）合成及信号传导，GNAS 突变可导致成骨细胞和骨细胞的异常分化。突变发生在合子后阶段，不具有遗传性，形成体细胞嵌合体，病变范围取决于突变发生的时期。异常的成骨细胞可分泌结构紊乱的纤维性骨基质，形成嵌入梭形细胞纤维基质中的不规则的骨小梁，并可分泌细胞因子，

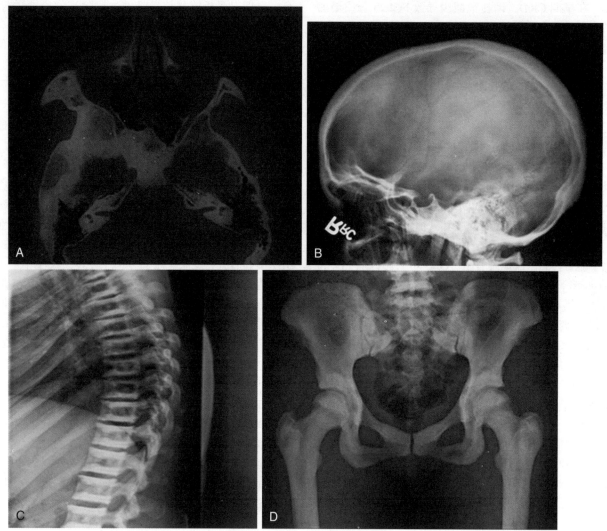

Fig. 13.5 (A) Head/face CT from a patient with fibrous dysplasia indicating expansion of the right maxilla; the cortex is intact but there are multiple lucent and sclerotic areas and some areas of ground-glass appearance; there is narrowing of the right maxillary sinus. (B–D) indicate diagnostic radiographic findings in a patient with "adult" osteopetrosis. There is generalized sclerosis. (B) The calvarium is thickened due to osteopetrosis. (C) The typical "Rugger-Jersey" spine due to bands of calcified primary spongiosa. (D) Endobones *(arrow)* or a "bone in bone" appearance can be seen in the pelvis due to calcified cartilage deposited during endochondral bone formation.

occurs locally and sometimes systemically, related to over-production of FGF23.

FD can involve one (monostotic) or multiple (polystotic) bones but can rarely affect the entire skeleton (pan ostotic). The presentation of FD varies from incidentally discovered asymptomatic radiographic findings to severe disability from fractures, pain, and skeletal deformity. FD most often affects the skull and femur, though the spine, ribs, and pelvis are commonly involved as well. Radiographically, FD lesions appear as expansile, deforming, medullary lesions with cortical thinning and overall "ground-glass" appearance (Fig. 13.5D) but can evolve over time and become sclerotic. Diagnosis is often made radiologically with plain films or CT. Bone biopsy is infrequently required. As in Paget's disease, extent of disease is best assessed with technetium-99 scan. FD also may be associated with extra-skeletal features including café au lait spots and/or hyperfunctioning endocrinopathies (McCune-Albright syndrome), resulting from mutant progeny cells within extraskeletal tissues. Skeletal malignancies are a

rare complication of FD. Depending on the extent of disease, management may include analgesia, physical therapy, orthopedic surgery for proximal femur or spine disease, monitoring for cranial nerve deficits, treatment of endocrinopathies and mineral disturbances, and bisphosphonates, though there are limited data regarding efficacy of the latter.

ISCHEMIC AND INFILTRATIVE DISEASES

Bone disease may also develop from ischemia or infiltration of the skeleton. Ischemic injury may develop due to drugs/toxins (excess glucocorticoids/alcohol), hemoglobinopathies, glycogen storage disorders (e.g. Gaucher's disease) and excess radiation, among other causes. Radiographs may show focal or diffuse changes in BMD, as well as bone collapse. In multiple myeloma, malignant infiltration of the bone marrow by plasma cells results in excessive osteoclast activation, severe osteoporosis, and commonly hypercalcemia (see Fig. 13.1H). Systemic mastocytosis, another lymphoproliferative disease that can

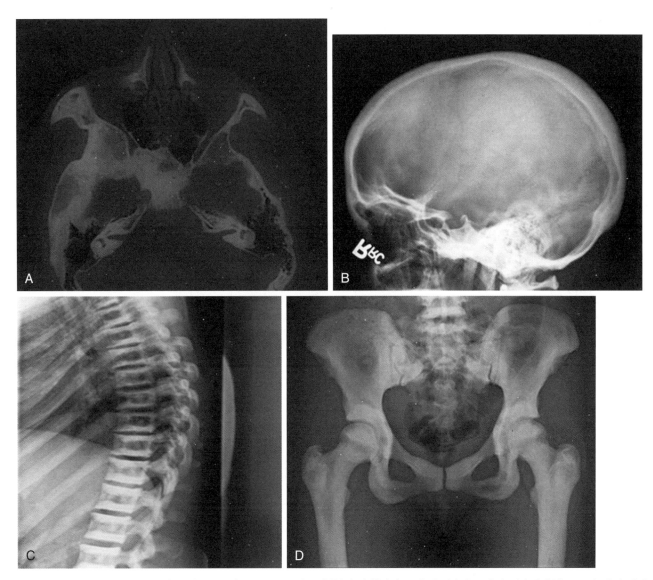

图 13.5　A. 纤维性结构不良患者的头颅 / 面部 CT，显示右上颌骨膨胀样改变，皮质不完整，多发透亮和硬化区，部分磨玻璃样区；右上颌窦变窄。B ~ D 显示一例"成人"骨硬化症患者具有诊断意义的影像学表现。可见弥漫性硬化。B. 骨硬化症导致的颅骨增厚。C. 原始海绵状软骨钙化带导致的典型夹心椎（"Rugger-Jersey"）改变。D. 骨盆的骨内骨或"骨中骨"改变，由软骨内骨形成时遗留的软骨钙化所致

导致病变部位的骨吸收。骨矿化异常可发生在局部，有时也可为全身性，与 FGF23 的过量生成相关。

　　FD 可累及单块（单骨型）或多块（多骨型）骨骼，极少数可累及所有骨骼（泛骨型）。FD 的症状范围可从偶然发现的无症状性影像学异常，到骨折、疼痛及骨畸形导致的严重活动受限。FD 最常累及颅骨和股骨，但脊椎、肋骨、骨盆也是常见的受累部位。在 X 线片上，FD 病变呈膨胀性、畸形的髓质病变，伴有皮质变薄和整体"磨玻璃"样外观（图 13.5D），但随时间延长也可演变为硬化性改变。诊断通常根据 X 线平片或 CT 的影像学表现。FD 很少需要骨活检。与骨佩吉特病类似，首选锝-99 扫描评估 FD 的病变范围。FD 的骨外表现包括牛奶咖啡斑和（或）内分泌腺体功能亢进（McCune-Albright 综合征），这是由骨外组织的突变后代细胞导致。骨骼恶性病变是 FD 的罕见并

发症。根据病变范围，治疗方法包括镇痛、物理治疗、近端股骨或椎体病变的骨科手术、监测颅神经功能受损、治疗内分泌疾病及矿盐紊乱、双膦酸盐，但后者的疗效数据很少。

缺血性疾病和浸润性疾病

　　骨病也可源于骨骼的缺血性或浸润性病变。药物 / 毒物（过量糖皮质激素 / 乙醇）、血色病、糖原贮积病（如戈谢病）及过量辐射等可导致缺血性损伤。X 线片可显示局灶性或弥漫性 BMD 改变和骨塌陷。在多发性骨髓瘤中，浆细胞对骨髓的恶性浸润导致过度的破骨细胞活化、重度骨质疏松症，常出现高钙血症（图13.1H）。系统性肥大细胞增多症（另一种淋巴增殖性疾病）可累及多个器官，包括皮肤（色素性荨麻疹）、

affect multiple organs including the skin (urticaria pigmentosa), liver, spleen, and lymph nodes, may cause focal osteolytic lesions as well as diffuse osteoporosis and fractures. These and other infiltrative disorders can lead to diffuse osteopenia, bone pain, and fractures, and should be considered in unexplained osteoporosis.

SUGGESTED READINGS

Bilezikian JP: Primer on the metabolic bone diseases and disorders of mineral metabolism, ed 9, Ames Iowa, 2018, J Wiley & Sons and American Society for Bone and Mineral Research.

Christov M, Pereira R, Wesselig-Perry K: Bone biopsy in renal osteodystrophy: continued insights into a complex disease, Curr Opin Nephrol Hypertens 22:210–215, 2013.

Corral-Gudino L, Tan AJ, Del Pino-Montes J, Ralston SH: Bisphosphonates for Paget's disease of bone in adults, Cochrane Database Syst Rev 12:CD004956, 2017.

Khosla S, Westendorf JJ, Oursler MJ: Building bone to reverse osteoporosis and repair fractures, J Clin Invest 118:421–428, 2008.

Lindsay R, Cosman F, Zhao H, et al: A novel tetracycline labeling strategy for longitudinal evaluation of the short term effects of anabolic therapy with a single iliac crest bone biopsy, J Bone Miner Res 21:366–373, 2006.

Moe S, Drueke T, Cunningham J, et al: Definition, evaluation and classification of renal osteodystrophy: a position statement from Kidney Disease: Improving Global Outcomes (KIDIGO), Kidney Int 69:1945–1953, 2006.

Ralston SH: Paget's disease of bone, N Engl J Med 368:644–650, 2013.

Stewart AF: Translational implications of the parathyroid calcium receptor, N Engl J Med 351:324–326, 2004.

肝脏、脾和淋巴结，可导致局部溶骨性病变、弥漫性骨质疏松症和骨折。上述疾病和其他浸润性疾病均可导致弥漫性骨量减少、骨痛和骨折，在原因未明的骨质疏松症中应予以考虑。

推荐阅读

Bilezikian JP: Primer on the metabolic bone diseases and disorders of mineral metabolism, ed 9, Ames Iowa, 2018, J Wiley & Sons and American Society for Bone and Mineral Research.

Christov M, Pereira R, Wesselig-Perry K: Bone biopsy in renal osteodystrophy: continued insights into a complex disease, Curr Opin Nephrol Hypertens 22:210–215, 2013.

Corral-Gudino L, Tan AJ, Del Pino-Montes J, Ralston SH: Bisphosphonates for Paget's disease of bone in adults, Cochrane Database Syst Rev 12:CD004956, 2017.

Khosla S, Westendorf JJ, Oursler MJ: Building bone to reverse osteoporosis and repair fractures, J Clin Invest 118:421–428, 2008.

Lindsay R, Cosman F, Zhao H, et al: A novel tetracycline labeling strategy for longitudinal evaluation of the short term effects of anabolic therapy with a single iliac crest bone biopsy, J Bone Miner Res 21:366–373, 2006.

Moe S, Drueke T, Cunningham J, et al: Definition, evaluation and classification of renal osteodystrophy: a position statement from Kidney Disease: Improving Global Outcomes (KIDIGO), Kidney Int 69:1945–1953, 2006.

Ralston SH: Paget's disease of bone, N Engl J Med 368:644–650, 2013.

Stewart AF: Translational implications of the parathyroid calcium receptor, N Engl J Med 351:324–326, 2004.

Osteoporosis

Susan L. Greenspan, Mary P. Kotlarczyk

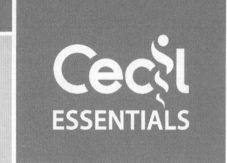

INTRODUCTION

Osteoporosis, the most common disorder of bone and mineral metabolism, affects about 50% of women and 20% of men older than 50 years. The National Institutes of Health Consensus Development Panel on Osteoporosis Prevention defines osteoporosis as a skeletal disorder characterized by compromised bone strength, predisposing a person to an increased risk of fracture. Bone strength has two major components: bone density and bone quality. Bone density reflects the peak adult bone mass and the amount of bone lost in adulthood. Bone quality is determined by bone architecture, bone geometry, bone turnover, mineralization, and damage accumulation (i.e., microfractures) (Fig. 14.1).

DEFINITION AND EPIDEMIOLOGY

In the United States, 2 million osteoporotic fractures occur each year. There are almost 300,000 hip fractures annually, which are associated with a mortality rate of more than 20% during the first year. The mortality rate is higher in men than in women. More than 40% of patients with hip fracture are unable to return to their previous ambulatory state, and about 20% of them are placed in long-term care facilities. When defined by bone mineral densitometry, 44 million Americans have low bone mass, and 10 million have osteoporosis. Although morbidity is less with vertebral fractures, the 5-year mortality rate is similar to that for hip fractures. Only one third of radiologically diagnosed vertebral fractures receive medical attention.

PATHOLOGY AND RISK FACTORS

Peak bone mass is determined primarily by genetic factors. Men have a higher bone mass than women, and African American and Hispanic individuals have a higher bone mass than white individuals. Other factors that contribute to the development of peak bone mass include nutrition and calcium intake, physical activity, timing of puberty, chronic illness, smoking, and use of medications that harm bone such as glucocorticoids.

The causes of bone loss in adults are multifactorial. The pattern of bone loss is different in women than in men, and bone loss is greater in sites rich in trabecular bone (e.g., spine) than cortical bone (e.g., femoral neck) (Fig. 14.2). Women lose significantly more trabecular bone than men. Estrogen deficiency during menopause contributes significantly to bone loss in women, and they may lose 1% to 5% of bone mass per year in the first few years after menopause. Women continue to lose bone mass throughout the remainder of their lives, with another acceleration of bone loss occurring after age 75 years. The mechanism of this accelerated loss in old age is not clear.

Multiple causes of secondary bone loss contribute to osteoporosis and fractures. Medications that commonly cause bone loss include glucocorticoids, antiseizure medications, excess thyroid hormone, heparin, androgen deprivation therapy, aromatase inhibitors, and depo-medroxyprogesterone. Endocrine diseases resulting in female or male hypogonadism also lead to bone loss. Hyperparathyroidism, hyperthyroidism, and hypercortisolism commonly cause bone loss, as can vitamin D deficiency. Gastrointestinal problems can contribute to decreased absorption of calcium and vitamin D (Table 14.1). Risk factors for falls (e.g., age, poor vision, previous falls, immobility, orthostatic hypotension, cognitive impairment, vitamin D insufficiency, poor balance, gait problems, weak muscles, sarcopenia) also contribute to fractures.

CLINICAL PRESENTATION

Unlike many other chronic diseases with multiple signs and symptoms, osteoporosis is considered a silent disease until fractures occur. Whereas 90% of hip fractures occur after a fall, two thirds of vertebral fractures are silent and occur with minimal stress, such as lifting, sneezing, and bending. An acute vertebral fracture may result in significant back pain that decreases gradually over several weeks with analgesics and physical therapy. Patients with significant vertebral osteoporosis may have height loss, kyphosis, and severe cervical lordosis, also known as a *dowager's hump*. Prolonged bisphosphonate use (>5 years) may result in an atypical femoral fracture, which may manifest as unilateral or bilateral thigh pain and result in a femoral shaft fracture with no or minimal trauma.

Bone Mineral Density and Other Bone Mass Assessments

In 1994, the World Health Organization (WHO) developed a classification system for osteoporosis and low bone mass based on data from white, postmenopausal women (Table 14.2). Osteoporosis is defined as a bone mineral density less than or equal to 2.5 standard deviations (SDs) below young adult peak bone mass (T-score ≤ −2.5 SD). Low bone mass (i.e., osteopenia) is defined as a bone mass measurement between 1.0 and 2.5 SDs below adult peak bone mass (T-score between −1.0 and −2.5 SD). Normal bone mineral density is defined as assessments at or above 1.0 SD below adult peak bone mass (T-score ≥ −1.0 SD).

The standard for assessing bone mineral density is dual-energy x-ray absorptiometry (DXA), which has excellent precision and accuracy. Measurements are made at the hip and spine, and in about 30% of cases, discordance is found between these measurements (Fig. 14.3). Classification should be made only if two or more vertebrae are available for analysis on spine images because of the high error rate when a single vertebra is assessed. Classification is based on the lowest value (i.e., total spine, total hip, or femoral neck).

In patients with hyperparathyroidism, in which cortical bone loss is often seen, forearm DXA using the one third distal radius site should

骨质疏松症

李梅 译 王鸥 姜艳 审校 夏维波 通审

引言

骨质疏松症是最常见的骨和矿盐代谢性疾病，累及约50%的50岁以上女性和20%的50岁以上男性。美国国立卫生研究院骨质疏松症预防共识委员会将骨质疏松症定义为以骨强度下降为特征，导致骨折风险增加的骨骼疾病。骨强度取决于两个重要部分：骨密度和骨质量。骨密度反映成年后的峰值骨量和成年期骨丢失量。骨质量取决于骨结构、骨几何形态、骨转换、矿化程度和损伤积累情况（即微小骨折）（图14.1）。

定义和流行病学

在美国，每年发生200万例骨质疏松症性骨折。每年约有30万例髋部骨折，髋部骨折后第1年的死亡率超过20%，男性死亡率高于女性。超过40%的髋部骨折患者无法恢复到以前的活动状态，约20%的患者需长期居住在护理机构中。根据骨密度测定结果，4400万美国人存在低骨量，其中1000万人罹患骨质疏松症。尽管椎体骨折的发生率低于髋部骨折，但其5年死亡率与髋部骨折相似。在影像学诊断的椎体骨折患者中，仅有1/3接受了药物治疗。

病理学和危险因素

峰值骨量主要由遗传因素决定。男性的骨量高于女性，非裔美国人和西班牙裔人群的骨量高于白人。其他影响峰值骨量的因素包括营养和钙的摄入、运动、青春期开始时间、慢性疾病、吸烟和使用损害骨骼的药物（如糖皮质激素）。

成人的骨量丢失由多因素导致。女性与男性的骨量丢失模式不同，富含松质骨部位（如脊柱）的骨量丢失较皮质骨（如股骨颈）更显著（图14.2）。女性松质骨的丢失较男性更显著。绝经期雌激素缺乏可导致女性骨量丢失加快，在绝经开始的前几年内，女性每年可丢失1%～5%的骨量；之后表现为持续性骨量丢失，且75岁以后骨量丢失再次加速，但老年期骨量丢失加速的机制尚不明确。

多种导致骨量丢失的继发性病因会导致骨质疏松症和骨折。常引起骨量丢失的药物包括糖皮质激素、抗癫痫药、过量的甲状腺激素、肝素、雄激素剥夺治疗、芳香化酶抑制剂和醋酸甲羟孕酮。可导致女性或男性性腺功能减退的内分泌疾病也会引起骨量丢失，如甲状旁腺功能亢进症、甲状腺功能亢进症、皮质醇增多症和维生素D缺乏症。胃肠道疾病可导致钙和维生素D吸收减少（表14.1）。跌倒相关危险因素也会增加骨折风险，如年龄、视力欠佳、既往跌倒史、行动不便、体位性低血压、认知障碍、维生素D不足、平衡能力欠佳、步态异常、肌无力、肌肉减少症等。

临床表现

与具有多种症状和体征的其他慢性疾病不同，骨质疏松症是一种隐匿性疾病，直至出现骨折才被发现。90%的髋部骨折出现在跌倒后，而2/3的椎体骨折是在轻微外力（如提重物、打喷嚏和弯腰时）下隐匿地发生。急性椎体骨折可引发明显的背部疼痛，通过数周的镇痛治疗和物理治疗可逐渐减轻。严重椎体骨质疏松症的患者可出现身高变矮、脊柱后凸和严重颈椎前凸，即"驼背"。长期双膦酸盐治疗（＞5年）可能导致非典型股骨骨折，表现为单侧或双侧大腿疼痛，在无外力或轻微创伤下引发股骨干骨折。

骨密度和其他骨量评估方法

1994年，世界卫生组织（WHO）基于白人绝经女性的数据，建立了骨质疏松症和低骨量的诊断标准（表14.2）。骨质疏松症的定义为骨密度低于正常年轻成人峰值骨量均值的2.5个标准差（SD）及以上（T值≤−2.5 SD）。低骨量（即骨量减少）的定义为骨密度测量值比正常年轻成人峰值骨量的均值低1.0～2.5个标准差（T值为−1.0 SD～−2.5 SD）。正常骨密度定义为骨密度测量值不低于正常年轻成人峰值骨量的1.0个标准差（T值≥−1.0 SD）。

骨密度评估的标准方法是双能X射线吸收法（DXA），该方法具有高精确性和高准确性。测量部位选择髋部和腰椎，约30%的病例存在测量部位结果不一致（图14.3）。由于评估单个椎体的误差率较高，脊柱图像中有多个椎体（≥2个）可供分析时才能进行诊断。骨质疏松症的诊断应依据全部椎体、全髋或股骨颈部位的最低骨密度值。

对于患有甲状旁腺功能亢进症的住院患者，还应评估皮质骨的丢失，应采用前臂DXA测量桡骨远端

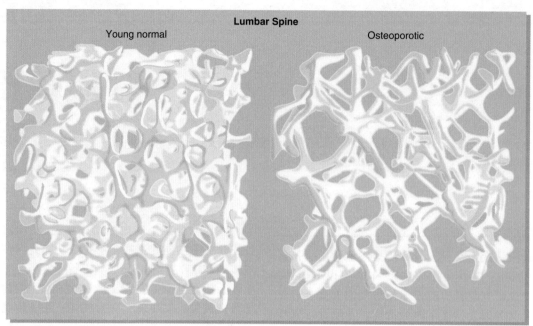

Fig. 14.1 Three-dimensional reconstruction by microcomputed tomography of a lumbar spine sample from a young adult normal woman and from a woman with postmenopausal osteoporosis. In the osteoporotic woman, bone mass is reduced and microarchitectural bone structure is deteriorated. Whereas the platelike structure in the normal case is very isotropic, the structure in the osteoporotic case shows preferential loss of horizontal struts; the plates have become rods that are thin and farther apart, and there is a concomitant loss of trabecular connectivity. These changes lead to a reduction in bone strength that is more than would be predicted by the decrease in bone mineral density. (From Riggs BL, Khosla S, Melton LJ 3rd: Sex steroids and the construction and conservation of the adult skeleton, Endocr Rev 23:279-302, 2002; Courtesy Ralph Mueller, PhD, Swiss Federal Institute of Technology [ETH] and University of Zurich, Switzerland.)

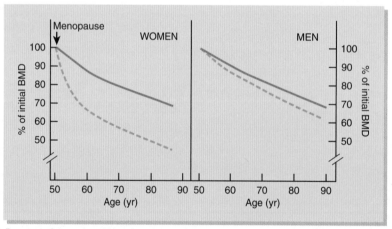

Fig. 14.2 Patterns of age-related bone loss in women and in men. *Dashed lines* represent trabecular bone, and *solid lines* represent cortical bone. The figure is based on multiple cross-sectional and longitudinal studies using dual-energy x-ray absorptiometry. *BMD,* Bone mineral density. (From Khosla S, Riggs BL: Pathophysiology of age-related bone loss and osteoporosis, Endocrinol Metab Clin North Am 34:1015-1030, 2005.)

also be assessed. Forearm assessments may be helpful in older patients who often have falsely elevated bone mineral density measurements at the spine as a result of atypical calcifications from degenerative joint disease, sclerosis, or aortic calcifications or in obese patients whose weight exceeds the table limit.

Bone mineral density can be measured by hip or spine quantitative computed tomography (QCT). However, less normative data are available for hip QCT, vertebral precision is inferior to that of DXA,

and radiation doses are significantly higher than those of DXA. Single-photon absorptiometry of the forearm and peripheral measures, such as heel ultrasound, have also been used to assess bone mass. However, the WHO classification should be used only with the central DXA measurements.

The National Osteoporosis Foundation (NOF) recommends obtaining a bone mineral density assessment in all women 65 years old or older, men aged 70 or older regardless of risk factors, and in adults

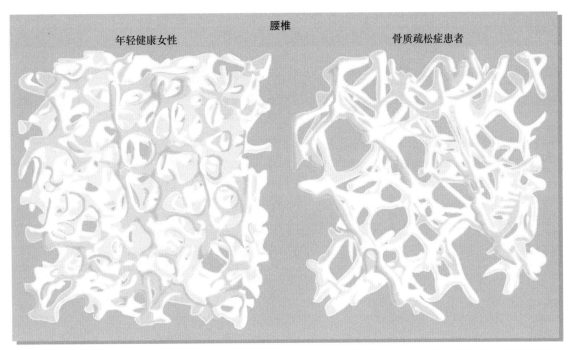

图 14.1 通过显微计算机断层成像（microcomputed tomography）对年轻健康女性和绝经后骨质疏松症女性的腰椎样本进行三维重建。在骨质疏松症女性中，可见椎体骨量减少，骨微结构受损。正常情况下的骨骼板状结构具有很强的各向同性，而在骨质疏松症的情况下，骨结构的水平支柱先消失；板状结构变为更薄、间距更大的杆状结构，同时骨小梁连接性下降。这些改变导致的骨强度下降程度超过了骨密度降低所预测的下降程度［引自 Riggs BL，Khosla S，Melton LJ 3rd：Sex steroids and the construction and conservation of the adult skeleton，Endocr Rev 23：279-302，2002；Courtesy Ralph Mueller，PhD，Swiss Federal Institute of Technology（ETH）and University of Zurich，Switzerland.］

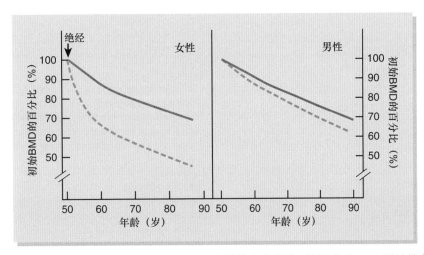

图 14.2 男女性的年龄相关骨量丢失模式。虚线代表小梁骨，实线代表皮质骨。该图基于 DXA 测量骨密度的多项横断面和纵向研究。BMD，骨密度（引自 Khosla S，Riggs BL：Patho-physiology of age-related bone loss and osteoporosis，Endocrinol Metab Clin NorthAm 34：1015-1030，2005.）

1/3 部位的骨密度。由于退行性关节病所致的非典型钙化、硬化症或主动脉钙化，老年患者的腰椎骨密度测量值可呈假性升高，前臂骨密度评估可能对这些患者和体重超过 DXA 仪器承重限制的肥胖症患者有帮助。

骨密度还可通过髋部或脊柱定量 CT（QCT）进行测量。然而，髋部 QCT 缺乏正常参考值，椎体测量精度低于 DXA，而辐射剂量显著高于 DXA。前臂单光子吸收法和外周测量法（如跟骨超声）也可测量骨量。然而，WHO 的诊断标准仅基于 DXA 测量的中轴骨骨密度。

美国国家骨质疏松基金会（NOF）建议，≥ 65 岁的女性、≥ 70 岁的男性及 ≥ 50 岁伴有骨折史的成人，无论是否存在危险因素，均应进行骨密度测量。此外，50 ～ 69 岁有骨折危险因素的绝经后女性和男性，以及

TABLE 14.1 Conditions, Diseases, and Medications That Cause or Contribute to Osteoporosis and Fractures

Lifestyle Factors
Alcohol abuse
Excessive thinness
Excess vitamin A
Falling
High salt intake
Immobilization
Inadequate physical activity
Low calcium intake
Smoking (active or passive)
Vitamin D insufficiency

Genetic Factors
Cystic fibrosis
Ehlers-Danlos syndrome
Gaucher's disease
Glycogen storage diseases
Hemochromatosis
Homocystinuria
Hypophosphatasia
Hypophosphatemia
Idiopathic hypercalciuria
Marfan syndrome
Osteogenesis imperfecta
Parental history of hip fracture or osteoporosis
Porphyria

Hypogonadal States
Anorexia nervosa and bulimia
Athletic amenorrhea
Hyperprolactinemia
Male hypogonadism
Panhypopituitarism
Premature and primary ovarian failure
Secondary gonadal failure
Turner's syndrome, Klinefelter syndrome

Endocrine Disorders
Cushing's syndrome
Diabetes mellitus (types 1 and 2)
Hyperparathyroidism
Thyrotoxicosis

Gastrointestinal Disorders
Celiac disease
Gastric bypass and bariatric surgery
Gastrointestinal surgery
Inflammatory bowel disease
Malabsorption
Pancreatic disease
Primary biliary cirrhosis

Hematologic Disorders
Hemophilia
Leukemia and lymphomas
Monoclonal gammopathies
Multiple myeloma
Sickle cell disease
Systemic mastocytosis
Thalassemia

Rheumatologic and Autoimmune Diseases
Ankylosing spondylitis
Lupus
Rheumatoid arthritis
Other rheumatic and autoimmune diseases

Neurologic Disorders
Epilepsy
Multiple sclerosis
Muscular dystrophy
Parkinson's disease
Spinal cord injury
Stroke

Miscellaneous Conditions and Diseases
Human immunodeficiency virus (HIV) infection/acquired immunodeficiency syndrome (AIDS)
Alcoholism
Amyloidosis
Chronic metabolic acidosis
Chronic obstructive lung disease
Congestive heart failure
Depression
End-stage renal disease
Hypercalciuria
Idiopathic scoliosis
Post-transplantation bone disease
Sarcoidosis
Weight loss

Medications
Aluminum (in antacids)
Anticoagulants (heparin)
Anticonvulsants
Aromatase inhibitors
Barbiturates
Cancer chemotherapeutic drugs
Cyclosporine and tacrolimus
Depo-medroxyprogesterone (premenopausal contraception)
Glucocorticoids ($\geq$5 mg/day of prednisone or equivalent for $\geq$3 mo)
Gonadotropin-releasing hormone (GnRH) antagonists and agonists
Lithium
Methotrexate
Parenteral nutrition
Proton pump inhibitors
Selective serotonin reuptake inhibitors
Tamoxifen (premenopausal use)
Thiazolidinediones (e.g., Actos, Avandia)
Thyroid hormones (in excess)

Modified from National Osteoporosis Foundation: Clinician's Guide to Prevention and Treatment of Osteoporosis; 2020 (in press). Available at https://cdn.nof.org/wp-content/uploads/2016/01/995.pdf.

表 14.1 导致骨质疏松症和骨折的情况、疾病和药物

生活方式因素
酒精滥用
过度消瘦
维生素 A 摄入过多
跌倒
盐摄入过多
制动
运动不足
低钙摄入
主动或被动吸烟
维生素 D 不足

遗传因素
囊性纤维化
Ehlers-Danlos 综合征
戈谢病
糖原贮积病
血色病
同型胱氨酸尿症
低磷酸酯酶症
低磷血症
特发性高钙尿症
马方综合征
成骨不全
父母有髋部骨折或骨质疏松症病史
卟啉病

性腺功能减退状态
神经性厌食和贪食
运动性闭经
高催乳素血症
男性性腺功能减退
全垂体功能减退
卵巢早衰和原发性卵巢功能衰竭
继发性性腺功能衰竭
Turner 综合征、Klinefelter 综合征

内分泌疾病
库欣综合征
糖尿病（1 型和 2 型）
甲状旁腺功能亢进症
甲状腺毒症

胃肠道疾病
乳糜泻
胃旁路手术和减重术
胃肠道手术
炎症性肠病
吸收不良
胰腺疾病
原发性胆汁性肝硬化

血液系统疾病
血友病
白血病和淋巴瘤
单克隆免疫球蛋白病
多发性骨髓瘤
镰状细胞病
系统性肥大细胞增多症
地中海贫血

风湿性疾病和自身免疫病
强直性脊柱炎
系统性红斑狼疮
类风湿关节炎
其他风湿性疾病和自身免疫病

神经系统疾病
癫痫
多发性硬化症
肌营养不良
帕金森病
脊髓损伤
卒中

其他疾病和情况
人类免疫缺陷病毒（HIV）感染 / 艾滋病（AIDS）
酒精中毒
淀粉样变性
慢性代谢性酸中毒
慢性阻塞性肺疾病
充血性心力衰竭
抑郁症
终末期肾病
高钙尿症
特发性脊柱侧凸
器官移植后骨病
结节病
体重减轻

药物
铝（抑酸剂中）
抗凝剂（肝素）
抗惊厥药
芳香化酶抑制剂
巴比妥类药物
恶性肿瘤化疗药物
环孢素和他克莫司
醋酸甲羟孕酮（用于绝经前避孕）
糖皮质激素（相当于泼尼松 ≥ 5 mg/d，持续 ≥ 3 个月）
促性腺激素释放激素（GnRH）拮抗剂和激动剂
锂剂
甲氨蝶呤
肠外营养
质子泵抑制剂
选择性 5- 羟色胺再摄取抑制剂
他莫昔芬（用于绝经前）
噻唑烷二酮类（如盐酸吡格列酮、马来酸罗格列酮）
甲状腺激素（过量）

改编自 National Osteoporosis Foundation：Clinician's Guide to Prevention and Treatment of Osteoporosis；2020（in press）. Available at https:// cdn.nof.org/wp-content/uploads/2016/01/995.pdf.

TABLE 14.2   World Health Organization Classification for Osteoporosis

Classification	Criteria for Bone Mineral Density
Normal	At or above −1.0 SD of young adult peak mean value
Low bone mass (osteopenia)	Between −1.0 and −2.5 SD of young adult peak mean value
Osteoporosis	At or below −2.5 SD of young adult peak mean value

SD, Standard deviation.

age 50 and older who have a fracture. They also suggest screening younger postmenopausal women and men age 50 to 69 with clinical risk factors for a fracture and adults with a condition or on a medication associated with low bone mass or bone loss (Table 14.3). This recommendation differs from 2018 US Preventive Services Task Force (USPSTF) guidelines that recommend screening women age 65 and older and younger women at risk (using screening tools) but did not endorse screening for men. The guidelines of the NOF concur with the Endocrine Society and International Society for Clinical Densitometry. Reference databases are available for white, African American, Asian and Hispanic men and women.

FRAX, a fracture risk assessment tool, predicts the 10-year risk for hip or any major osteoporotic fracture for women and men between 40 and 90 years of age. The FRAX for the individual patient incorporates femoral neck T-score, age, gender, height, weight, and specific risk factors, including history of adult fracture, parental hip fracture, current smoking, glucocorticoid use, rheumatoid arthritis, alcohol (three drinks or more per day), and secondary osteoporosis. The fracture risk prediction is specific for race and country and should be used for patients *not* on therapy.

Bone mineral density determined by DXA usually can be monitored after 2 years of therapy, depending on the site to be assessed and the type of therapy prescribed. For example, trabecular bone, which has greater surface area and is more metabolically active than cortical bone, is more likely to show improvements with stronger-acting antiresorptive agents. Changes in bone mass with potent antiresorptive therapy are more prominent in the spine compared with other areas. Seeing no changes in forearm bone mineral density over time is common despite good precision. Although the heel has a high percentage of trabecular bone, precision is poor, and monitoring should not be done at this site.

All patients with osteoporosis or low bone mass should have a work-up for secondary causes of bone loss. It should include a serum calcium level (corrected for albumin) to rule out hyperparathyroidism or malnutrition; a 25-hydroxyvitamin D level to assess for vitamin D deficiency or insufficiency; an alkaline phosphatase level to assess for Paget's disease, malignancy, cirrhosis, or vitamin D deficiency; liver and renal function tests to assess for abnormalities; a 24-hour urine calcium and creatinine assay to evaluate for hypercalciuria or malabsorption; a test for sprue in patients with anemia, malabsorption, or hypocalciuria; a thyrotropin level to rule out hyperthyroidism; and serum protein electrophoresis to rule out myeloma in older adults with anemia. Measurement of the parathyroid hormone (PTH) level often is needed to interpret the calcium and vitamin D levels. Total testosterone levels are recommended for men.

A more extensive work-up can be done in severe or unusual cases. A bone biopsy is rarely needed. Markers of bone turnover vary considerably in clinical practice, and these tests usually are reserved for research. However, they may be useful for assessing the rate of bone turnover after prolonged bisphosphonate use or a bisphosphonate holiday.

Radiography

Conventional radiographs and vertebral fracture assessment in adults age 50 and older can reveal a vertebral compression fracture that is diagnostic of osteoporosis (Fig. 14.4) even in the absence of a BMD. However, two thirds of vertebral compression fractures are asymptomatic. Low bone mass may not be evident on radiographs until 30% of the mass has been lost. When assessing bone mass, radiographs may be read inappropriately as a result of overpenetration or under penetration of the film. Radiographs therefore are a poor indicator of osteoporosis (with the exception of vertebral fractures), and the diagnosis is instead based on bone mineral densitometric results. A vertebral fracture assessment (VFA) can often be performed in tandem with a standard DXA and can identify vertebral compression fractures.

PREVENTION

General preventive measures for all patients include adequate calcium and vitamin D intake, exercise, and fall prevention techniques. The recommended daily allowance of calcium for adults, as reviewed by the Institute of Medicine, is 1200 mg for women 51 years or older and men 71 years or older and 1000 mg for men 50 to 70 years old. Calcium intake can be accomplished by dietary consumption, supplementation, or the combination of diet plus supplement. The supplements should be pure calcium carbonate or pure calcium citrate, taken in divided doses of approximately 500 to 600 mg twice daily. Calcium carbonate should be taken with meals for best absorption, whereas calcium citrate may be taken with or without food. Calcium supplements are available as tablets and in chewable and liquid forms. Foods such as orange juice, cereals, breads, and nutrition bars may be calcium fortified. There is no benefit to taking more than 1200 mg per day, and excess intake may increase the risk of kidney stones and cardiovascular disease (although data are controversial).

Vitamin D is important for calcium absorption and bone mineralization. Vitamin D has nonskeletal benefits and has been associated with improvement in muscle strength and prevention of falls. Vitamin D comes from two sources: diet and photosynthesis. Because dietary sources of vitamin D are limited only to certain foods (e.g., fortified milk, yogurt) and patients are often advised to avoid sun exposure for prevention of skin cancer and wrinkles, many studies have documented vitamin D deficiency and insufficiency in older adults. Older patients have a reduced ability to synthesize vitamin D in the skin. Low vitamin D levels can lead to secondary hyperparathyroidism.

Vitamin D can be taken in a multivitamin, in a calcium supplement, or in pure form and is available as cholecalciferol (D_3) or ergocalciferol (D_2). Based on data from noninstitutionalized patients without osteoporosis, the daily dose recommended by the Institute of Medicine is 600 IU per day for adults up to age 70 and 800 IU for those older than 70 years to achieve a 25-hydroxy vitamin D level of at least 20 ng/mL (50 nmol/L). However, the NOF suggests 800 to 1000 IU per day and a 25-hydroxy vitamin D level of at least 30 ng/mL for optimal calcium absorption. Elderly patients, those with malabsorption, and obese patients may need greater amounts of vitamin D. Older patients with severe vitamin D deficiency may be given 50,000 IU of vitamin D once per week for 3 months to bring serum vitamin D into the normal range to be followed by a maintenance dose of at least 1000 IU daily. The upper limit of vitamin D intake is 4000 IU/day. Activated vitamin D is rarely needed and should not be given on a regular basis for postmenopausal osteoporosis.

表 14.2　WHO 定义的骨质疏松症分类	
分类	骨密度标准
正常	骨密度≥正常年轻成人峰值骨量均值－1.0 SD
低骨量（骨量减少）	骨密度＝正常年轻成人峰值骨量均值的－1.0 SD～－2.5 SD
骨质疏松症	骨密度≤正常年轻成人峰值均值－2.5 SD

患有与低骨量或骨量丢失相关疾病或服用相关药物的成人，也应进行骨密度筛查（表 14.3）。此建议与 2018 年美国预防服务工作组（USPSTF）的指南存在差异，后者建议仅对≥ 65 岁的女性和有风险的 < 65 岁的女性进行骨密度筛查（使用筛查工具），但未推荐筛查男性骨密度。NOF 的指南与美国内分泌学会和国际临床骨密度测量学会的建议一致。参考数据库适用于白人、非裔美国人、亚裔和西班牙裔男性和女性。

FRAX 是一种骨折风险评估工具，可用于预测 40 ～ 90 岁女性和男性在未来 10 年内发生髋部或任何主要骨质疏松性骨折的风险。FRAX 综合考虑了股骨颈骨密度 T 值、年龄、性别、身高、体重及特定危险因素，包括成年后骨折史、父母髋部骨折史、当前吸烟情况、糖皮质激素使用史、类风湿关节炎、饮酒（≥ 3 杯 / 天）和继发性骨质疏松症。骨折风险预测具有种族和国家特异性，且应用于未接受治疗的患者。

使用 DXA 测定的骨密度通常可在治疗 2 年后再次评估，骨密度变化情况取决于评估部位和接受治疗的药物种类。例如，松质骨的表面积较大，代谢比皮质骨更活跃，给予强效骨吸收抑制剂治疗后可能取得更明显的改善。相比于其他部位，椎体骨量在强效骨吸收抑制剂治疗后的变化可能更为显著。虽然测量精度高，但前臂骨密度随时间的变化常不明显。足跟部位含有较高比例的松质骨，但骨密度测量的准确性欠佳，不建议监测该部位的骨密度。

所有骨质疏松症或低骨量患者均应筛查导致骨量丢失的继发性病因。筛查内容包括血清钙浓度（经白蛋白校正），以排除甲状旁腺功能亢进症或营养不良；25- 羟维生素 D 水平，以评估维生素 D 缺乏或不足；碱性磷酸酶水平，以评估骨佩吉特病、恶性肿瘤、肝硬化或维生素 D 缺乏；检测肝肾功能，以评估是否存在异常；24 h 尿钙和肌酐检测，以评估有无高钙尿症或吸收不良；贫血、吸收不良或低钙尿症患者可进行乳糜泻检测；促甲状腺激素水平，以排除甲状腺功能亢进症；老年贫血患者检测血清蛋白电泳，以排除骨髓瘤。通常需要检测甲状旁腺激素（PTH）水平，以评价钙和维生素 D 水平。男性患者建议检测总睾酮水平。

对于病情严重或疑难患者，需要完成更为广泛的检查评估。极少数患者需要进行骨活检。骨转换标志物在临床实践中变异较大，通常用于研究。然而，在长期使用双膦酸盐或其药物假期期间，骨转换标志物可用于评估骨转换率。

影像学评估

在≥ 50 岁的成人中，常规 X 线检查和椎体骨折评估可显示椎体压缩性骨折，即使在缺乏骨密度结果时也可诊断骨质疏松症（图 14.4）。然而，2/3 的椎体压缩性骨折患者无症状。只有骨量丢失＞ 30% 时，X 线检查才可能显示低骨量。在评估骨量时，透射剂量过高或过低均影响阅片结果。因此，除了椎体骨折外，X 线检查不是反映骨质疏松症的可靠指标，骨质疏松症的诊断应基于骨密度测量结果。椎体骨折评估（VFA）通常可与 DXA 同时进行，以识别椎体压缩性骨折。

预防

骨质疏松症患者的一般预防措施包括摄入充足的钙及维生素 D、运动和预防跌倒。美国医学研究所推荐的成人每日钙摄入量如下：≥ 51 岁女性和≥ 71 岁男性为 1200 mg，50 ～ 70 岁男性为 1000 mg。钙的摄入可通过饮食和（或）钙补充剂来完成。钙补充剂应选择纯碳酸钙或纯柠檬酸钙，每次 500 ～ 600 mg，2 次 / 日。为了达到最佳吸收，碳酸钙应随餐服用，而柠檬酸钙可随餐或空腹服用。钙补充剂包括片剂、咀嚼片和液体形式。食物（如橙汁、谷物、面包和营养棒）可强化添加钙。每日钙摄入量＞ 1200 mg 没有额外获益，过量摄入可能增加肾结石和心血管疾病的风险（尽管相关数据存在争议）。

维生素 D 对钙的吸收和骨骼矿化至关重要。维生素 D 不仅对骨骼有益，还与改善肌力和预防跌倒相关。维生素 D 主要有两个来源：饮食摄入和通过光合成。由于维生素 D 的饮食来源仅限于某些食物（如强化牛奶、酸奶），且患者通常因预防皮肤癌和皱纹而避免日晒，许多研究表明老年人普遍存在维生素 D 缺乏和不足。老年患者皮肤合成维生素 D 的能力降低。维生素 D 缺乏可能导致继发性甲状旁腺功能亢进症。

维生素 D 可在多种维生素、钙补充剂或纯维生素 D 中摄入。维生素 D 包括维生素 D_3 和维生素 D_2 两种形式。根据来自无骨质疏松症的非住院患者数据，美国医学研究院建议 70 岁以下成人每天摄入 600 IU 维生素 D，70 岁以上者每天摄入 800 IU 维生素 D，以使 25- 羟维生素 D ≥ 20 ng/ml（50 nmol/L）。然而，NOF 建议每天摄入 800 ～ 1000 IU 维生素 D，要求 25- 羟维生素 D ≥ 30 ng/ml，以达到适当的钙吸收。老年、吸收不良和肥胖症人群可能需要补充更多的维生素 D。对于严重缺乏维生素 D 的老年患者，可在 3 个月内每周给予 50 000 IU 维生素 D，使血清维生素 D 水平恢复到正常范围，之后的维持剂量为每天≥ 1000 IU。维生素 D 的摄入量上限为 4000 IU/d。很少需要补充活性维生素 D，且不应常规用于绝经后骨质疏松症的治疗。

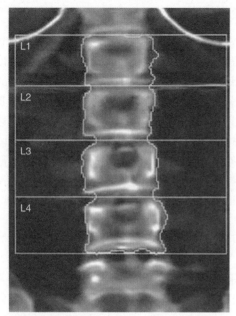
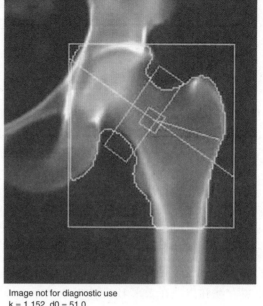

Image not for diagnostic use
k = 1.131, d0 = 47.0
116 × 117

Image not for diagnostic use
k = 1.152, d0 = 51.0
83 × 90
NECK: 49 × 15

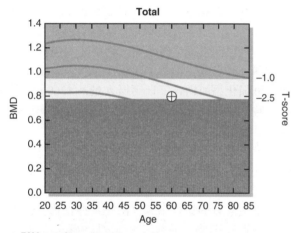

DXA results summary:

Region	Area (cm²)	BMC (g)	BMD (g/cm²)	T-score	Z-score
L1	10.29	8.63	0.839	−1.4	−0.1
L2	10.69	8.16	0.763	−2.4	−1.0
L3	11.78	9.50	0.807	−2.5	−1.1
L4	12.51	9.68	0.774	−2.6	−1.1
Total	45.27	35.97	0.794	−2.3	−0.9

Total BMD CV 1.0%, ACF = 1.039, BCF = 1.005, TH = 7.494
WHO classification: Osteopenia
Fracture risk: Increased

DXA results summary:

Region	Area (cm²)	BMC (g)	BMD (g/cm²)	T-score	Z-score
Neck	4.83	3.16	0.655	−1.7	−0.5
Total	28.61	23.10	0.807	−1.1	−0.1

Total BMD CV 1.0%, ACF = 1.039, BCF = 1.005, TH = 5.696
WHO classification: Osteopenia

Fig. 14.3 (Left) This patient has a lumbar spine (L1 through L4) bone mineral density (BMD) of 0.794 g/cm² *(white circle with cross on the graph)* as measured by dual-energy x-ray absorptiometry (DXA) and a T-score of −2.3. The reference database graph displays age- and sex-matched mean BMD levels ±2 standard deviations (SDs) derived from a normative database from the manufacturer (Hologic, Inc., Bedford, Mass.). The T-score indicates the difference in SD between the patient's BMD and that of the predicted sex-matched mean peak of a young adult; the z-value is the difference in SD between the patient's BMD and the sex-, age-, and ethnicity-matched mean BMD. (Right) This patient has a total hip BMD of 0.807 g/cm² and a femoral neck BMD of 0.655 g/cm² *(white circle with cross on the graph)* as measured by DXA, a total hip T-score of −1.1, and a femoral neck T-score of −1.7. The reference database graph displays age- and sex-matched mean BMD levels ±2 SDs derived from the third National Health and Nutrition Examination Survey. The T-score indicates the difference in SD between the patient's BMD and the predicted sex-matched mean peak young adult BMD; the z-score is the difference in SD between the patient's BMD. The 10-year fracture risk (FRAX) is 15% for a major osteoporotic fracture and 1.6% for a hip fracture (including reported risk factors: previous fracture, BMI = 24.2, using a US Caucasian database). (Bone densitometry report for the Horizon bone densitometer, Bedford, Mass., Hologic, Inc.)

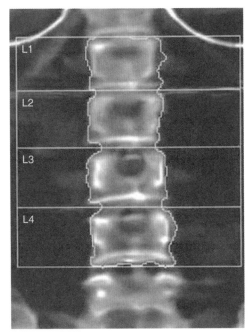

图像不用于诊断
k = 1.131, d0 = 47.0
116 × 117

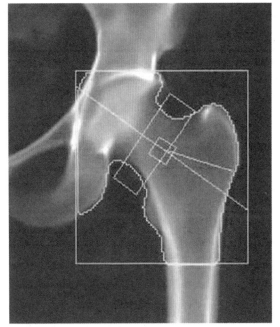

图像不用于诊断
k = 1.152, d0 = 51.0
83 × 90
股骨颈: 49 × 15

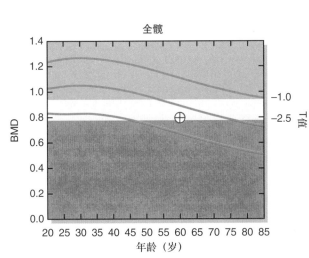

DXA结果总结:

区域	面积 (cm²)	BMC (g)	BMD (g/cm²)	T值	Z值
L1	10.29	8.63	0.839	−1.4	−0.1
L2	10.69	8.16	0.763	−2.4	−1.0
L3	11.78	9.50	0.807	−2.5	−1.1
L4	12.51	9.68	0.774	−2.6	−1.1
总体	**45.27**	**35.97**	**0.794**	**−2.3**	**−0.9**

全髋BMD CV 1.0%, ACF = 1.039, BCF = 1.005, TH = 7.494
WHO分类: 骨量减少
骨折风险: 增加

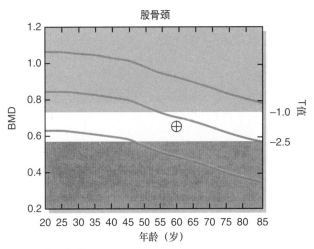

DXA结果总结:

区域	面积 (cm²)	BMC (g)	BMD (g/cm²)	T值	Z值
股骨颈	4.83	3.16	0.655	−1.7	−0.5
总体	**28.61**	**23.10**	**0.807**	**−1.1**	**−0.1**

全髋BMD CV 1.0%, ACF = 1.039, BCF = 1.005, TH = 5.696
WHO分类: 骨量减少

图 14.3 （左侧）患者通过双能 X 射线吸收法（DXA）测得腰椎（L1 ~ L4）骨密度（BMD）为 0.794 g/cm²（十字白圈），T 值为−2.3。参考数据库来自仪器厂家（Hologic，Inc.，Bedford，Mass），图中曲线代表年龄和性别匹配的 BMD 均值 ±2 个标准差（SD）。T 值表示患者 BMD 与预测的同性别正常年轻成人峰值骨密度间的标准差；Z 值是患者 BMD 与同性别、同年龄、同种族人群 BMD 均值的标准差。（右侧）患者通过 DXA 测得全髋 BMD 为 0.807 g/cm²，股骨颈 BMD 为 0.655 g/cm²（十字白圈），全髋 T 值为−1.1，股骨颈 T 值为−1.7。参考数据库来自美国第 3 次全国健康与营养调查（NHANES Ⅲ），图中曲线代表年龄和性别匹配的 BMD 均值 ±2 SD。T 值表示患者 BMD 与预测的同性别正常年轻成人峰值骨密度间的标准差；Z 值是患者 BMD 与同性别、同年龄、同种族人群 BMD 均值的标准差。FRAX 预测的未来 10 年主要骨质疏松性骨折风险为 15%，髋部骨折风险为 1.6%（报告的危险因素包括：既往骨折史、BMI = 24.2 kg/m²，使用美国白人数据库）（骨密度报告来自 Horizon 骨密度测量仪，Bedford，Mass.，Hologic，Inc.）

TABLE 14.3 National Osteoporosis Foundation Recommendations for Bone Mineral Density Testing

- Women age ≥65 yr and men ≥70 yr, regardless of clinical risk factors
- Younger postmenopausal women, women in the menopausal transition, and men age 50–69 yr with clinical risk factors for fracture
- Adults who have a fracture after age 50 yr
- Adults who have a condition (e.g., rheumatoid arthritis) or are taking a medication (e.g., glucocorticoids in a daily dose of ≥5 mg prednisone or equivalent for ≥3 mo) associated with low bone mass or bone loss

TABLE 14.4 National Osteoporosis Foundation Guidelines for Treatment

- An adult hip or vertebral fragility fracture
- Osteoporosis by DXA T-score ≤ –2.5 SD for lumbar spine, total hip, or femoral neck after appropriate evaluation
- Low bone mass by DXA T-scores between –1.0 and –2.5 SD at the lumbar spine or femoral neck and a FRAX 10-year probability of a hip fracture ≥3% or a 10-year probability of major osteoporosis-related fractures ≥20%.

DXA, Dual-energy x-ray absorptiometry; *FRAX,* fracture risk assessment tool; *SD,* standard deviation.

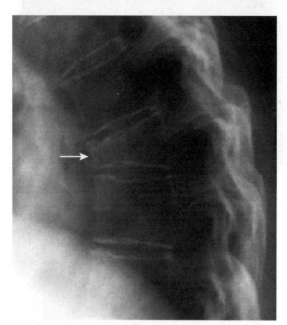

Fig. 14.4 Lateral spine radiograph demonstrates a thoracic anterior wedge compression fracture.

Weight-bearing exercise (walking, jogging, dancing, tai chi, etc.) is important for maintaining skeletal integrity. Study results are controversial concerning different types and durations of exercise by postmenopausal women and men. However, weight-bearing or resistance training exercises usually are suggested and have been shown to improve bone mass or maintain skeletal integrity. In patients with new vertebral fractures, physical therapy is important for improving posture and increasing the strength of back muscles.

Because 90% of hip fractures and a significant number of vertebral fractures occur following a fall, preventive measures are suggested for frail older patients at risk for falling. Fall-proofing the household includes installing grab bars in the bathroom and hand rails on stairways, avoiding loose throw rugs and cords, ensuring good lighting by the bedside, and moving objects within easy reach in the kitchen. Other fall prevention measures include eliminating medications that cause dizziness or postural hypotension (if possible), assessing the need for assistive devices (e.g., canes, walkers), and ensuring appropriate footwear and good vision. The benefits of hip protectors for hip fracture reduction are disappointing and controversial, and compliance with these products is often poor.

TREATMENT AND PROGNOSIS

The NOF developed treatment guidelines that incorporate a 10-year fracture risk prediction. The NOF suggests treatment for postmenopausal women and men 50 years old or older, as shown in Table 14.4. In addition, the National Bone Health Alliance (NBHA) group of experts published an expanded version that included a fourth criterion for treatment: fracture of proximal humerus, pelvis or wrist in the setting of osteopenia (T-score between –1.0 and –2.5).

Patients taking glucocorticoids can fracture despite having normal bone density. The American College of Rheumatology suggests that patients starting glucocorticoids who will be treated for 3 months or longer have a bone density test and start antiresorptive therapy if indicated according to their guidelines.

Bisphosphonates

Bisphosphonates are the mainstay of osteoporosis prevention and treatment. They inhibit the cholesterol synthesis pathway in osteoclasts, causing early apoptosis and inhibiting osteoclast migration and attachment. Unlike other agents, bisphosphonates are incorporated into bone, the half-life is long, and the agent may be recycled.

In the United States, the bisphosphonates alendronate, risedronate, ibandronate, and zoledronic acid have been approved for the prevention and treatment of osteoporosis. Alendronate can increase bone mass by about 8% at the spine and 4% at the hip over 3 years. This increase has been associated with an approximately 50% reduction in spine, hip, and forearm fractures (Table 14.5). Alendronate is prescribed at 35 mg once weekly for osteoporosis prevention and 70 mg once weekly for the treatment of osteoporosis. Alendronate has been approved for use in men and patients with glucocorticoid-induced osteoporosis.

Risedronate is approved for the prevention and treatment of osteoporosis at a dose of 35 mg per week or 150 mg per month or as a delayed dose after breakfast of 35 mg per week. Large-scale, multicenter studies have shown improvements in bone mass of about 6% to 7% at the spine and 3% at the hip over 3 years. These studies revealed approximately 50% reduction in vertebral fractures, 40% reduction in nonvertebral fractures, and 40% reduction in hip fractures (see Table 14.5). Risedronate is approved for the treatment of osteoporosis in men and for the prevention and treatment of patients with glucocorticoid-induced osteoporosis.

Oral ibandronate is approved for the prevention and treatment of postmenopausal osteoporosis. After 3 years of treatment, ibandronate increased bone density by 6.5% at the spine and 3.4% at the hip, and it reduced new vertebral fractures by approximately 60%. No reductions in nonvertebral or hip fractures occurred. Ibandronate is approved at an oral dose of 150 mg monthly and for treatment at an intravenous dose of 3 mg every 3 months.

Zoledronic acid is approved for the prevention and treatment of postmenopausal osteoporosis, osteoporosis in men, and steroid-induced bone loss. The 3-year pivotal trial demonstrated increases of 6.9% of bone density at the spine and 6.0% at the hip, and the drug reduced spinal fractures by 70%, nonvertebral fractures by 25%, and

表14.3 NOF 的骨密度检测建议
• ≥65 岁的女性和 ≥70 岁的男性，无论有无临床危险因素
• <65 岁的绝经后女性、绝经过渡期女性、具有骨折危险因素的 50～69 岁男性
• >50 岁且有骨折史的成人
• 患有某些疾病（如类风湿关节炎）的成人或正在服用某些药物（如糖皮质激素，泼尼松 ≥5 mg/d 持续 ≥3 个月）

表14.4 NOF 治疗指征
• 成人髋部或椎体脆性骨折
• DXA 测量的腰椎、全髋或股骨颈骨密度 T 值 ≤-2.5 SD，符合骨质疏松症诊断
• DXA 测量的腰椎、全髋或股骨颈骨密度 T 值为-1.0～-2.5 SD，符合低骨量诊断，且 FRAX 预测的未来 10 年髋部骨折风险 ≥3% 或主要骨质疏松性骨折风险 ≥20%

DXA，双能 X 射线吸收法；FRAX，骨折风险预测工具；SD，标准差。

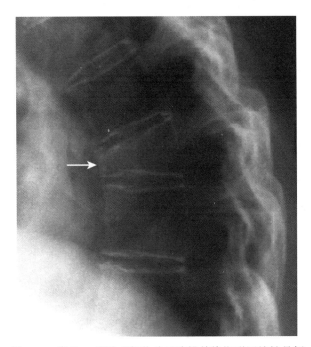

图 14.4　脊柱 X 线检查侧位片示胸椎前缘楔形压缩性骨折

负重运动（如步行、慢跑、跳舞、太极）对于维持骨骼完整性至关重要。关于不同运动类型和持续时间对绝经后女性和男性的益处尚存争议。然而，推荐进行负重或抗阻训练，其有助于改善骨量或保持骨骼完整性。对于有新发椎体骨折的患者，物理治疗可有效改善姿势和增强背部肌肉强度。

由于 90% 的髋部骨折和大多数椎体骨折发生在跌倒后，建议对存在跌倒风险的虚弱老年患者采取预防措施。家庭预防跌倒的措施包括：浴室安装抓杆、楼梯安装扶手、避免使用松散的地毯和电线、确保床旁有良好的照明、将厨房内的物品放置在容易获取的位置。其他预防跌倒的措施包括：尽可能减少使用引起头晕或体位性低血压的药物；需要时使用辅助设备（如拐杖、助行器）；确保穿着合适的鞋袜；保持良好的视力。髋部保护器减少髋部骨折的效果欠佳且存在争议，患者对这些产品的依从性通常较差。

治疗和预后

NOF 指南纳入了对未来 10 年骨折风险的预测。NOF 建议对 ≥50 岁的绝经后女性和男性骨质疏松症患者进行治疗（表 14.4）。此外，美国国家骨骼健康联盟

（NBHA）专家组发布了拓展版指南，增加了第 4 条治疗指征：骨量减少（T 值为-1.0 SD～-2.5 SD）时存在肱骨近端、骨盆或腕部骨折。

服用糖皮质激素的患者即使骨密度正常也可能发生骨折。美国风湿病学会建议，对于开始接受糖皮质激素治疗且计划疗程 ≥3 个月的患者，应评估骨密度，并根据指南开始使用抑制骨吸收的药物治疗。

双膦酸盐

双膦酸盐是预防和治疗骨质疏松症的一线药物。双膦酸盐通过抑制破骨细胞中的胆固醇合成通路，促进破骨细胞的早期凋亡，抑制破骨细胞迁移和黏附。不同于其他药物，双膦酸盐可沉积在骨骼中，半衰期较长，且可被循环利用。

在美国，阿仑膦酸钠、利塞膦酸钠、伊班膦酸钠和唑来膦酸等双膦酸盐已被批准用于预防和治疗骨质疏松症。使用阿仑膦酸钠治疗 3 年后，腰椎骨密度可增加约 8%，髋部骨密度增加约 4%。对应于骨密度的增加，椎体、髋部和前臂骨折可减少约 50%（表 14.5）。阿仑膦酸钠用于预防骨质疏松症的剂量为每周 35 mg，用于治疗骨质疏松症的剂量为每周 70 mg。阿仑膦酸钠已被批准用于治疗男性骨质疏松症和糖皮质激素性骨质疏松症。

利塞膦酸钠被批准用于预防和治疗骨质疏松症，剂量为每周 35 mg 或每月 150 mg，目前也有在早餐后服用的利塞膦酸钠缓释剂型（每周 35 mg）。大规模多中心临床研究表明，使用利塞膦酸钠治疗 3 年后，腰椎和髋部骨密度可分别增加 6%～7% 和 3%。治疗后，椎体骨折、非椎体骨折和髋部骨折可分别减少约 50%、40% 和 40%（表 14.5）。利塞膦酸钠被批准用于治疗男性骨质疏松症，以及预防和治疗糖皮质激素性骨质疏松症。

口服伊班膦酸钠被批准用于预防和治疗绝经后骨质疏松症。伊班膦酸钠治疗 3 年可使腰椎和髋部骨密度分别增加 6.5% 和 3.4%，新发椎体骨折减少约 60%，但非椎体骨折或髋部骨折发生率无显著下降。伊班膦酸钠被批准的口服剂量为每月 150 mg，静脉输注剂量为每 3 个月 3 mg。

唑来膦酸被批准用于预防和治疗绝经后骨质疏松症、男性骨质疏松症及糖皮质激素性骨质疏松症。一项为期 3 年的关键临床研究显示，唑来膦酸治疗可使腰椎和髋部骨密度分别增加 6.9% 和 6.0%，且椎体骨折和非椎体骨折可分别减少 70% 和 25%，髋部骨折可减

hip fractures by 41%. Zoledronic acid is given at a dose of 5 mg intravenously once per year for treatment and 5 mg intravenously every 24 months for prevention.

There is not a simple guide for which bisphosphonate is chosen, since the order of medication selection is often determined by the cost of the medication and insurance consideration. Generally, alendronate is the most commonly used because it is usually the least expensive.

Because oral bisphosphonates are poorly absorbed, they must be taken first thing in the morning on an empty stomach with a full glass of water. Patients must wait 30 minutes (when taking alendronate and risedronate) to 60 minutes (when taking ibandronate) before eating and must not lie down. A delayed-release form of risedronate can be taken after breakfast.

Potential side effects of bisphosphonates include epigastric distress, heartburn, and esophagitis. Intravenous bisphosphonates have been associated with an influenza-like syndrome after infusion. Bisphosphonates can also cause arthralgias and myalgias. They are contraindicated in patients with renal insufficiency (i.e., estimated glomerular filtration rate of 30 to 35 mL/minute). Osteonecrosis of the jaw (ONJ) is a rare adverse event of abnormal bone growth in the jaw, which is more often associated with high-dose intravenous bisphosphonates in patients with cancer and poor oral hygiene. Atypical femoral shaft fractures (AFF) have been reported rarely after long-term use (>5 years of oral or >3 years intravenous) of bisphosphonates. These fractures may manifest with a prodrome of unilateral or bilateral thigh pain, and fractures may occur with minimal activity. These fractures are rare after osteoporosis treatment but common in cancer patients receiving frequent high doses intravenously.

Denosumab

The receptor activator of nuclear factor-κB (RANK) and its ligand (RANKL) are mediators of osteoclast activity. Compared with placebo, denosumab, an antibody to RANKL, produced a relative increase in bone mineral density at the spine of 9.2% and hip of 6.0% over 3 years, and it reduced fractures by 68% at the spine, 40% at the hip, and 20% at nonvertebral sites. Denosumab is approved for postmenopausal women and men with osteoporosis, men with prostate cancer on androgen deprivation therapy, postmenopausal women with breast cancer on aromatase inhibitors, and men and women on glucocorticoids. It is given as a 60-mg subcutaneous injection every 6 months. Denosumab may cause hypocalcemia so calcium intake by diet or supplement is encouraged. It is rarely associated with a rash or skin infection and very rarely associated with ONJ or AFF. When therapy is stopped, bone loss and vertebral compression fractures can occur, especially in patients with a previous vertebral fracture. It is suggested patients switch to an oral or intravenous bisphosphonate. Following denosumab discontinuation, teriparatide (a recombinant version of human parathyroid hormone) treatment (see later) can lead to bone loss at some sites.

Estrogen Agonists-Antagonists

Estrogen agonists-antagonists were previously called selective estrogen receptor modulators (SERMs) because they have some estrogen-like and anti-estrogen-like benefits. Raloxifene is approved for the prevention and treatment of osteoporosis in women. The Multiple Outcomes of Raloxifene Evaluation (MORE) trial found that bone mass was increased by 4% at the spine and 2.5% at the femoral neck over 3 years. This increase was associated with an approximate 50% reduction in vertebral fractures. No reduction in nonvertebral or hip fractures was seen (see Table 14.5). Treatment was associated with improved lipid status, as shown by decreased total and low-density lipoprotein cholesterol.

Raloxifene is not associated with endometrial hyperplasia, and patients should not have bleeding or spotting. They do not have breast tenderness or swelling. Raloxifene reduces the risk for invasive breast cancer in postmenopausal women with osteoporosis and in women at high risk for invasive breast cancer. Patients have the same small risk of deep vein thrombosis or pulmonary embolus that is found with hormone therapy. Raloxifene does not relieve postmenopausal symptoms and may exacerbate hot flashes. Studies have not found a significant impact on cardiovascular disease. Raloxifene can be given with or without food in a daily oral dose of 60 mg per day.

Hormone Therapy

Investigators of the Women's Health Initiative, a large, randomized, placebo-controlled, multicenter trial evaluating estrogen therapy, reported a 34% reduction in hip and vertebral fractures after 5.2 years. In addition to improvements in bone mass, benefits include an improved lipid profile, decreased colon cancer incidence, and decreased menopausal symptoms. However, because of the potential risks of hormone therapy (i.e., cardiovascular events, breast cancer, deep vein thrombosis, pulmonary embolus, and gallbladder problems), it should be used only for prevention or management of menopausal symptoms, and other agents should be used for the treatment of osteoporosis. A combination of conjugated estrogen/bazedoxifene is also approved for prevention in postmenopausal osteoporosis and other menopausal symptoms (hot flashes).

Parathyroid Hormone

Recombinant human PTH (1-34), or teriparatide, is an osteoanabolic agent that increases spinal bone mineral density by 9.7% and hip bone mineral density by 2.6% in 18 months. It is associated with a 65% reduction in vertebral fractures and a 53% reduction in nonvertebral fractures. Teriparatide is taken for up to 2 years as a subcutaneous, 20-µg daily dose for postmenopausal women and men at high risk for fracture including patients on glucocorticoids. Side effects include nausea, headache, and dizziness and may be associated with bone loss at some sites if initiated following denosumab discontinuation. After therapy, patients benefit from antiresorptive therapy to prevent bone loss. Recombinant human PTH (1-84) is approved for use in Europe.

Parathyroid Hormone-Related Peptide

Abaloparatide analog of PTHrP (1-34) is an osteoanabolic agent that increases spine bone density by 9.8% and hip bone density by 3.4% in approximately 12 months. The pivotal trial reported a reduction of vertebral fractures by 86% and nonvertebral fractures by 43%. It can be administered as a daily subcutaneous injection of 80 mg for up to 2 years for postmenopausal women. Side effects include nausea, headache, dizziness, and palpitations. A patch form is under investigation. Following therapy, an antiresorptive agent is recommended to prevent bone loss.

Romosozumab

Romosozumab is a monoclonal antibody to sclerostin that has a dual effect mechanism of action since it increases bone formation and decreases bone resorption. In pivotal trials compared to placebo, after 12 months romosozumab increased bone density by 13.7% at the spine and 6.2% at the hip and reduced vertebral fractures by 73% and hip fractures by 38%. It is approved for postmenopausal women with osteoporosis for 12 months as a subcutaneous monthly injection of 210 mg. It should be followed by an antiresorptive therapy to prevent bone loss. It is rarely associated with ONJ and AFF. In a study where romosozumab was compared to alendronate, there was an increased risk of

少 41%。唑来膦酸的治疗剂量为 5 mg 静脉输注，每年 1 次；预防剂量为 5 mg 静脉输注，每 24 个月 1 次。

双膦酸盐的药物选择难以通过单一指南来明确，通常需要考虑药物价格和医保政策。总体来说，阿仑膦酸钠的费用最低，因此最为常用。

口服双膦酸盐吸收差，需晨起空腹用一满杯水送服。患者需在服用阿仑膦酸钠或利塞膦酸钠后 30 min、服用伊班膦酸钠后 60 min 方能进食，且其间不能平卧。缓释利塞膦酸钠可在早餐后服用。

口服双膦酸盐的潜在副作用包括上腹部不适、烧心和食管炎。双膦酸盐静脉输注后可能出现流感样症状。双膦酸盐还可能引起关节痛和肌痛。严重肾功能不全患者（即估算的肾小球滤过率为 30 ~ 35 ml/min）禁用双膦酸盐。下颌骨坏死（ONJ）是一种下颌骨生长异常的罕见不良事件，通常与恶性肿瘤和口腔卫生差的患者静脉应用大剂量双膦酸盐相关。偶有长期应用（口服 > 5 年或静脉治疗 > 3 年）双膦酸盐的患者出现非典型股骨干骨折（AFF）的报道。AFF 的前驱症状可能是单侧或双侧大腿疼痛，轻微外力下即可发生骨折。接受骨质疏松症治疗的患者中极少出现 AFF，但其常见于频繁接受大剂量静脉双膦酸盐治疗的恶性肿瘤患者。

地舒单抗

核因子 κ B 受体激活蛋白（RANK）及其配体（RANKL）参与调控破骨细胞的活性。与安慰剂相比，地舒单抗（RANKL 抗体）治疗 3 年可使腰椎和髋部骨密度分别增加 9.2% 和 6.0%，椎体骨折、髋部骨折和非椎体骨折分别减少 68%、40% 和 20%。地舒单抗已被批准用于治疗绝经后女性和男性骨质疏松症，包括接受雄激素剥夺治疗的前列腺癌患者、接受芳香化酶抑制剂治疗的绝经后乳腺癌女性患者和糖皮质激素性骨质疏松症患者。该药的治疗剂量为每次 60 mg，每 6 个月皮下注射 1 次。地舒单抗可能引起低钙血症，因此需通过饮食或补充剂摄入充足的钙。该药很少引起皮疹或皮肤感染，极少导致 ONJ 或 AFF。停止地舒单抗治疗后，可能出现骨量丢失和椎体压缩性骨折，尤其是既往有椎体骨折史的患者，建议转换为口服或静脉输注双膦酸盐治疗。停止地舒单抗治疗后，采用特立帕肽（重组人甲状旁腺激素）治疗可能会导致某些部位的骨量丢失。

雌激素激动剂-拮抗剂

雌激素受体激动剂-拮抗剂曾被称为选择性雌激素受体调节剂（SERM），因为该类药物具有类雌激素和抗雌激素的作用。雷洛昔芬被批准用于预防和治疗女性骨质疏松症。MORE（Multiple Outcomes of Raloxifene Evaluation）研究发现，雷洛昔芬治疗 3 年可使椎体骨密度增加 4%，股骨颈骨密度增加 2.5%，同时椎体骨折减少约 50%，但非椎体骨折或髋部骨折风险无明显下降（表 14.5）。雷洛昔芬治疗还可改善脂代谢，表现为总胆固醇和低密度脂蛋白胆固醇水平下降。

雷洛昔芬治疗与子宫内膜增生无关，患者不应有阴道出血或点滴出血，也不会出现乳房压痛或肿胀。对于绝经后骨质疏松症患者及具有侵袭性乳腺癌高风险的女性，雷洛昔芬可降低其罹患侵袭性乳腺癌的风险。患者出现深静脉血栓或肺栓塞的风险与绝经后激素治疗相同。雷洛昔芬不能减轻绝经症状，且可能加重潮热。研究未发现其对心血管疾病有显著影响。雷洛昔芬的治疗剂量为 60 mg/d，口服，可随餐或空腹服用。

激素治疗

女性健康倡议（Women's Health Initiative）是一项评估雌激素治疗的大型多中心随机安慰剂对照试验，研究显示，雌激素治疗 5.2 年后，髋部骨折和椎骨骨折可减少 34%。除了骨量增加，雌激素治疗还能改善脂代谢、降低结肠癌发生率、减轻绝经症状。然而，由于激素治疗的潜在不良反应（如心血管事件、乳腺癌、深静脉血栓、肺栓塞和胆囊疾病），应仅用于预防或控制绝经期症状，而选择其他药物治疗骨质疏松症。雌激素 / 巴多昔芬复方制剂也被批准用于预防绝经后骨质疏松症和其他绝经症状（如潮热）。

甲状旁腺激素

特立帕肽［重组人 PTH（1-34）］是一种骨形成促进剂，治疗 18 个月后，腰椎和髋部骨密度可分别增加 9.7% 和 2.6%，同时椎体骨折和非椎体骨折分别减少 65% 和 53%。特立帕肽的治疗剂量为 20 μg/d，皮下注射，药物最长治疗时间为 2 年，用于治疗骨折风险高的绝经后骨质疏松症、男性骨质疏松症及糖皮质激素性骨质疏松症。药物副作用包括恶心、头痛和头晕。如果地舒单抗停药后序贯特立帕肽治疗，可能导致某些部位的骨量丢失。特立帕肽治疗结束后，患者可接受骨吸收抑制剂治疗，以预防骨量丢失。重组人 PTH（1-84）在欧洲已获批用于临床。

甲状旁腺激素相关肽

阿巴洛肽是 PTHrP（1-34）的类似物，是一种骨形成促进剂，治疗约 12 个月后，腰椎和髋部骨密度可分别增加 9.8% 和 3.4%。研究显示，阿巴洛肽治疗后，椎体骨折和非椎体骨折可分别减少 86% 和 43%。用于绝经后女性的治疗剂量为 80 mg/d，皮下注射，疗程不超过 2 年。药物副作用包括恶心、头痛、头晕和心悸。目前该药的贴剂正在研究中。治疗结束后建议序贯骨吸收抑制剂，以预防骨量丢失。

罗莫佐单抗

罗莫佐单抗是硬骨抑素的单克隆抗体，具有双重作用机制，既能增加骨形成又能减少骨吸收。在关键临床研究中，与安慰剂相比，罗莫佐单抗治疗 12 个月后，椎体和髋部骨密度分别增加 13.7% 和 6.2%，椎体骨折和髋部骨折分别减少 73% 和 38%。该药已获批用

TABLE 14.5   US Food and Drug Administration–Approved Therapies for Prevention and Treatment of Osteoporosis

Agent	Prevention/ Treatment	Dosage	Vertebral Fracture Reduction	Hip Fracture Reduction	Women/ Men	Steroid-Induced OP
Antiresorptive Agents						
Alendronate[a]	Yes/yes	Prev: 35 mg/wk PO Treat: 70 mg/wk PO	Yes	Yes	Yes/yes	Yes
Ibandronate[a]	Yes[b]/yes	150 mg/mo PO, 3 mg q3mo IV	Yes	No	Yes/no	No
Risedronate[a]	Yes/yes	Prev/treat: 35 mg/wk PO, 35 mg/wk PO delayed release, 150 mg/mo PO	Yes	Yes	Yes/yes	Yes
Zoledronic acid[a]	Yes/yes	Prev: 5 mg q2yr IV Treat: 5 mg/yr IV	Yes	Yes	Yes/yes	Yes
Calcitonin	No/yes	200 IU/day Intranasal	Yes	No	Yes/no	No
Denosumab	No/yes	60 mg q6mo SC	Yes	Yes	Yes/yes	Yes
Hormone/Estrogen Therapy	Yes[c]/no	Various preparations available	Yes	Yes	Yes[d]/no	No
Raloxifene	Yes/yes	60 mg/day PO	Yes	No	Yes/no	No
Anabolic Agents						
Abaloparatide (PTHrP)	No/yes	80 µg/day SC	Yes	No	Yes/yes	No
Teriparatide (PTH [1-34])	No/yes	20 µg/day SC	Yes	No	Yes/yes	Yes
Dual-Action Agents						
Romosozumab	No/yes	210 mg/month SC	Yes	Yes	Yes/no	No

OP, Osteoporosis; *PO*, oral administration; *prev*, prevention; *PTH*, parathyroid hormone; *PTHtrP*, parathyroid hormone-related peptide; *SC*, subcutaneous administration; *Treat*, treatment.
[a]Alendronate, risedronate, ibandronate, and zoledronic acid are bisphosphonates.
[b]Oral only.
[c]Short-term prevention or management.
[d]For management.

cardiovascular events and strokes, so it should be avoided in patients who have had these events in the preceding year.

Calcitonin

Calcitonin is a 32-amino-acid peptide produced by the parafollicular cells of the thyroid gland. The pivotal clinical treatment trial did not show significant changes in bone mineral density after 3 years. However, the 200 IU dose of nasal calcitonin was associated with a 50% reduction in vertebral fractures (see Table 14.5). No reduction in nonvertebral or hip fractures was found. There is a possible association with development of cancer. Calcitonin may reduce pain following an acute vertebral compression fracture.

Choice of Therapy and Sequential Versus Combination Therapy

The initial choice of medication and sequence of therapy is important and under investigation. Currently, conventional therapy starts with a single agent. The choice of therapy is usually driven by the insurance provider, and often an oral antiresorptive bisphosphonate such as alendronate is the least expensive and provides fracture risk reduction at key vertebral, nonvertebral, and hip sites. If a patient has a contraindication to an oral bisphosphonate such as GERD, an intravenous bisphosphonate such as zoledronic acid is often initiated.

The concept of "treat-to-target" is based on the premise that starting *any* therapy may *not* be sufficient to achieve an acceptable level of risk. For high-risk patients with severe osteoporosis, the initial choice of therapy may be based on using the most potent therapy first

(anabolic), followed by a less potent therapy (antiresorptive) to maintain skeletal integrity. Recent studies have demonstrated greater vertebral fracture risk reduction with an anabolic therapy compared to an antiresorptive therapy.

Combination therapy with an anabolic and potent antiresorptive (denosumab) has been shown to increase bone mineral density more than monotherapy, but fracture reduction studies are needed. Combination of two antiresorptive therapies are not indicated.

Duration of Treatment

Osteoporosis is a chronic disease and requires lifelong management and follow-up. It is recommended that patients be reevaluated after 5 years of oral or 3 years of intravenous bisphosphate therapy. If they are osteopenic and without fracture risk they can begin a bisphosphate holiday, but reevaluation is suggested in 1 to 2 years. If they still have osteoporosis, have fractured on therapy, or are still at risk for fracture, therapy can be continued but a change to an alternative agent should be considered. After 2 years of an anabolic therapy with teriparatide or abaloparatide or 1 year of romosozumab, an antiresorptive therapy is suggested. There is no limit to the duration for denosumab, but following discontinuation of therapy an alternative antiresorptive therapy should be considered to prevent bone loss.

Vertebroplasty and Kyphoplasty

Vertebroplasty involves injection of cement (i.e., polymethylmethacrylate) into a compressed vertebra to prevent the vertebral body from

表 14.5　FDA 批准用于预防和治疗骨质疏松症的药物

药物	预防 / 治疗	剂量	减少椎体骨折	减少髋部骨折	女性 / 男性	糖皮质激素性骨质疏松症
骨吸收抑制剂						
阿仑膦酸钠 [a]	是 / 是	预防：每周 35 mg，PO 治疗：每周 70 mg，PO	是	是	是 / 是	是
伊班膦酸钠 [a]	是 [b]/ 是	每月 150 mg，PO；每 3 个月 3 mg，IV	是	否	是 / 否	否
利塞膦酸钠 [a]	是 / 是	预防 / 治疗：每周 35 mg，PO；缓释剂型每周 35 mg，PO；每月 150 mg，PO	是	是	是 / 是	是
唑来膦酸 [a]	是 / 是	预防：5 mg，每 2 年 1 次，IV 治疗：5 mg，每年 1 次，IV	是	是	是 / 是	是
降钙素	否 / 是	200 IU/d，鼻喷	是	否	是 / 否	否
地舒单抗	否 / 是	60 mg，每 6 个月 1 次，SC	是	是	是 / 是	是
激素 / 雌激素治疗	是 [c]/ 否	多种剂型可选	是	是	是 [d]/ 否	否
雷洛昔芬	是 / 是	60 mg/d，PO	是	否	是 / 否	否
骨形成促进剂						
阿巴洛肽（PTHrP）	否 / 是	80 µg/d，SC	是	否	是 / 否	否
特立帕肽［PTH（1-34）］	否 / 是	20 µg/d，SC	是	否	是 / 是	是
双重作用药物						
罗莫佐单抗	否 / 是	每月 210 mg，SC	是	是	是 / 否	否

IV，静脉注射；PO，口服；PTH，甲状旁腺激素；PTHrP，甲状旁腺素相关肽；SC，皮下注射。
[a] 阿仑膦酸钠、利塞膦酸钠、伊班膦酸钠和唑来膦酸均属于双膦酸盐类药物。
[b] 仅口服。
[c] 短期预防或治疗。
[d] 用于治疗。

于治疗绝经后女性骨质疏松症，治疗剂量为 210 mg，皮下注射，每月 1 次，疗程不超过 12 个月。治疗结束后应序贯骨吸收抑制剂，以预防骨量丢失。罕见情况下，罗莫佐单抗可引起 ONJ 和 AFF。一项罗莫佐单抗与阿仑膦酸盐的比较研究显示，罗莫佐单抗可导致心血管事件和卒中风险增加，因此在过去 1 年内曾有心脑血管事件的患者应避免使用该药。

降钙素

降钙素是甲状腺滤泡旁细胞生成的由 32 个氨基酸组成的肽。关键临床治疗研究显示，降钙素治疗 3 年后骨密度无显著变化。然而，鼻喷 200 IU 降钙素与椎体骨折减少 50% 有关（表 14.5），但未观察到非椎体骨折或髋部骨折减少。使用降钙素可能与恶性肿瘤风险增加相关。降钙素可减轻急性椎体压缩性骨折引起的疼痛。

治疗选择：序贯治疗 vs. 联合治疗

骨质疏松症的初始药物选择和治疗顺序非常重要，且仍在研究中。目前，常规治疗从单一药物开始。治疗选择通常会受医保的影响，初始药物常选择口服骨吸收抑制剂双膦酸盐，如阿仑膦酸钠，因其费用低，且能降低椎体骨折、非椎体骨折和髋部骨折的风险。如果患者存在口服双膦酸盐的禁忌证［如胃食管反流病（GERD）］，则通常选择静脉注射双膦酸盐（如唑来膦酸）。
"治疗达标"的概念基于以下前提：开始任何治疗

都不足以达到可接受的风险水平。对于骨折风险高的严重骨质疏松症患者，首选最强效的治疗方法（骨形成促进剂），然后使用次强效的治疗方法（骨吸收抑制剂）来维持骨骼的完整性。近期研究显示，骨形成促进剂比骨吸收抑制剂能够更有效地降低椎体骨折风险。

与单药治疗相比，骨形成促进剂联合强效骨吸收抑制剂（如地舒单抗）能更加显著地增加骨密度，但其减少骨折的效果仍需更多研究。不推荐联合使用两种骨吸收抑制剂。

治疗疗程

骨质疏松症是一种慢性疾病，需要终身管理和随访。建议患者在口服双膦酸盐治疗 5 年或静脉双膦酸盐治疗 3 年后重新评估骨骼状态。若骨量减少且没有骨折风险，患者可进入双膦酸盐药物假期，但停药后 1～2 年需要再次进行评估。若患者仍有骨质疏松症、在治疗中新发骨折或仍有骨折风险，可继续双膦酸盐治疗，但也应考虑更换抗骨质疏松药物。骨形成促进剂特立帕肽或阿巴洛肽治疗 2 年或罗莫佐单抗治疗 1 年后，建议序贯骨吸收抑制剂治疗。地舒单抗没有疗程限制，但在停止治疗后应考虑序贯另一种骨吸收抑制剂，以预防骨量丢失。

椎体成形术和椎体后凸成形术

椎体成形术是通过将骨水泥（如聚甲基丙烯酸甲酯）注射到压缩的椎体中，以防止椎体进一步塌陷。

further collapse. Kyphoplasty introduces a balloon into the vertebral body to expand it, followed by cement placement inside the vertebral body. This approach expands the vertebral body and may increase height. Some studies suggest a significant reduction in pain early on, but the long-term pain reduction may be similar to that of placebo. Ongoing studies are needed to determine whether differences in outcomes can be found between vertebroplasty and kyphoplasty. These procedures are recommended only for patients with significant pain from vertebral fractures and are not routinely performed in asymptomatic patients with vertebral osteoporosis.

SUGGESTED READINGS

Clinician's guide to prevention and treatment of osteoporosis, Washington, D.C., 2020, National Osteoporosis Foundation (in press).

Eastell R, Rosen CJ: Response to Letter to the Editor "Pharmalogical Management of Osteoporosis in Postmenopausal Women: An Endocrine Society Clinical Practice Guidelines," J Clin Endocrinol Metab 104(8):3537–3538, 2019.

Siu A, Allore H, Brown D, Charles ST, Lohman M: National Institutes of Health Pathways Workshop: Research Gaps for Long-Term Drug Therapies for Osteoporotic Fracture Prevention, Ann Intern Med 171(1):51–57, 2019.

U.S. Preventive Services Task Force: Screening for Osteoporosis to Prevent Fractures: US Preventative Services Task Force Recommendation Statement, JAMA 319(24):2521–2531, 2018.

Viswanathan M, Reddy S, Berkman N, Cullen K, Middleton JC, Nicholson WK, et al: Screening to Prevent Osteoporotic Fractures: Updated Evidence Report and Systematic Review for the US Preventative Services Task Force, JAMA 319(24):2532–2551, 2018.

椎体后凸成形术是通过球囊扩张椎体，然后将骨水泥注入椎体内。这些方法可以扩张椎体并可增加椎体高度。研究表明，这两种手术在骨折早期可明显减轻骨痛，但其对疼痛的长期缓解效果与安慰剂相似。未来仍需要更多研究来明确椎体成形术和后凸成形术的疗效差异。这些手术仅推荐用于椎体骨折导致明显疼痛的患者，而不常规用于无症状的椎体骨质疏松症患者。

推荐阅读

Clinician's guide to prevention and treatment of osteoporosis, Washington, D.C., 2020, National Osteoporosis Foundation (in press).

Eastell R, Rosen CJ: Response to Letter to the Editor "Pharmalogical Management of Osteoporosis in Postmenopausal Women: An Endocrine Society Clinical Practice Guidelines," J Clin Endocrinol Metab 104(8):3537–3538, 2019.

Siu A, Allore H, Brown D, Charles ST, Lohman M: National Institutes of Health Pathways Workshop: Research Gaps for Long-Term Drug Therapies for Osteoporotic Fracture Prevention, Ann Intern Med 171(1):51–57, 2019.

U.S. Preventive Services Task Force: Screening for Osteoporosis to Prevent Fractures: US Preventative Services Task Force Recommendation Statement, JAMA 319(24):2521–2531, 2018.

Viswanathan M, Reddy S, Berkman N, Cullen K, Middleton JC, Nicholson WK, et al: Screening to Prevent Osteoporotic Fractures: Updated Evidence Report and Systematic Review for the US Preventative Services Task Force, JAMA 319(24):2532–2551, 2018.

索引 Index

Page numbers followed by "f" indicate figures, "t" indicate tables, and "b" indicate boxes.

页码数字中，"f" 代表 "图"，"t" 代表 "表格"，"b" 代表 "框"。